A PRACTICAL APPROACH TO

MUSCULOSKELETAL MEDICINE

FIFTH EDITION

A PRACTICAL APPROACH TO
MUSCULOSKELETAL
MEDICINE

Assessment, Diagnosis and Treatment

Elaine **Atkins** MBE DProf MA Cert FE FCSP FSOMM

Fellow, Chartered Society of Physiotherapy
Fellow, Society of Musculoskeletal Medicine
Associate Tutor, Queen Margaret University, Edinburgh

Emily **Goodlad** MSc MCSP FSOMM

Advanced Physiotherapy Practitioner, NHS Lothian
Fellow, Society of Musculoskeletal Medicine
Visiting Lecturer, Glasgow Caledonian University

Sharon **Chan-Braddock** DProf MSc BSc MCSP FSOMM IP

Advanced Clinical Practitioner, Tier 2 MSK service and First Contact Practitioner,
Manchester University NHS Foundation Trust
Fellow, Society of Musculoskeletal Medicine
Associate Tutor, Queen Margaret University, Edinburgh
Visiting Lecturer, Salford University
HEE National Trainer for FCP Roadmap

ELSEVIER

First edition 1998
Second edition 2005
Third edition 2010
Fourth edition 2016

Notices

Practitioners and researchers must always rely on their own experience and knowledge in evaluating and using any information, methods, compounds or experiments described herein. Because of rapid advances in the medical sciences, in particular, independent verification of diagnoses and drug dosages should be made. To the fullest extent of the law, no responsibility is assumed by Elsevier, authors, editors or contributors for any injury and/or damage to persons or property as a matter of products liability, negligence or otherwise, or from any use or operation of any methods, products, instructions, or ideas contained in the material herein.

ISBN: 978-0-7020-8408-9

Content Strategist: Robert Edwards
Content Project Manager: Taranpreet Kaur
Design: Patrick Ferguson
Marketing Manager: Deborah Watkins
Illustration Manager: Akshaya Mohan

Printed in India

Last digit is the print number: 9 8 7 6 5 4 3 2 1

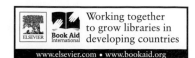

Working together to grow libraries in developing countries

www.elsevier.com • www.bookaid.org

CONTENTS

ABOUT THE AUTHORS

Elaine has collaborated with different brilliant author teams through all the editions of this textbook – Monica Kesson, Jill Kerr, Emily Goodlad and now Sharon Chan-Braddock. In keeping with the authors' tradition, each of the current team has been teaching the musculoskeletal medicine approach with the Society of Musculoskeletal Medicine for many years, both nationally and internationally, and has made an important contribution to the essential ongoing development of the Society's modules, culminating in the MSc Musculoskeletal Medicine.

Each author has developed and integrated the approach into their own clinical practice but, now retired, Elaine has drawn from the extensive knowledge and clinical experience of Emily and Sharon, in collaborating on this new edition. Both Emily and Sharon work in the NHS as Advanced Practitioners and, between them, specialise in spinal disorders, shoulder conditions, persistent pain management, injection therapy and clinical reasoning. Their contribution is evident throughout and the whole text has been streamlined and updated to reflect contemporary musculoskeletal practice, both in the NHS in multiprofessional teams and in the private sector.

The authors have continued to focus on students' learning, against the backdrop of continuing professional development and the needs of practitioners to be able to meet the requirements of evolving musculoskeletal service provision.

Elaine Atkins
Emily Goodlad
Sharon Chan-Braddock

Dr James Cyriax gained his medical qualification at St Thomas' Hospital, London in 1929. Following over two decades of innovative practice, he published his ground-breaking *'Textbook of Orthopaedic Medicine', Volume 1* in 1954. The textbook aimed to describe a method for logical, clinically reasoned, differential diagnosis of musculoskeletal conditions, based on extensive knowledge of applied anatomy, leading to effective management and treatment.

Inspired by the pragmatic clinical reasoning and ease of application into clinical practice, Monica Kesson and Dr Elaine Atkins further worked to develop the underpinning evidence base relating to the 'Cyriax approach'. Disseminating the theory and practice of orthopaedic and musculoskeletal medicine, through the first two editions of *Orthopaedic Medicine: A Practical Approach*. This insured that the concepts and philosophy of orthopaedic medicine were passed onto the next generation of musculoskeletal clinicians.

Jill Kerr and Emily Goodlad worked alongside Elaine to publish a 3rd and then a 4th edition (*A Practical Approach to Musculoskeletal Medicine*), updating the underpinning theory and evidence, and using digital technology to enhance learning and facilitate clinical excellence by enabling the readers to evaluate their learning through self-assessment tasks via the digital platform 'EVOLVE'.

The last 10 years have seen an acceleration in the evolving nature of musculoskeletal practice, with a significant surge in the musculoskeletal evidence base, and encouraging transformations in health care philosophy. Advanced practice musculoskeletal practitioners are now formally recognised across the world with a standard of practice agreed by experts in the specialty.

We were delighted to hear that a 5th edition had been proposed, with the objective of immersing the approach within contemporary evidence and practice, and further developing and evolving Musculoskeletal medicine in the context of Advanced Practice. Dr Sharon Chan-Braddock has joined forces with Elaine and Emily, to write this new edition, and they have modernised the text to support current mastery of musculoskeletal capability and clinical excellence.

Although this 5th edition may look familiar to many clinicians, keeping the Cyriax approach explicitly at its core, it conveys a current and exciting feel. The content meets the expectations of clinicians working as musculoskeletal specialists at an advanced practice level. It embodies the environmental-biopsychosocial approach, spotlighting precision rehabilitation and personalised care, whilst embracing the modern-day complexity of the assessment, diagnosis, and management.

This edition has been thoughtfully put together by the truly passionate, committed, and talented authors, reflecting the rich history of Musculoskeletal Medicine within contemporary clinical practice, to inspire the next generation of musculoskeletal practitioners.

Amanda Hensman-Crook FCSP, MSc, Dip Phys

Fellow of the Chartered Society of Physiotherapy; Health Education England National Musculoskeletal (MSK) Subject Matter Expert; Consultant MSK Physiotherapist; Visiting Lecturer University of Winchester.

Dr Tim Noblet PhD, MSc, BSc (Hons) Physiotherapy, MCSP

Consultant Physiotherapist, St George's University Hospitals NHS Foundation Trust; Hon. Associate Professor, St George's University of London, London UK and Maquarie University, Sydney, Australia; Adjunct Professor of Research, Western University, Canada.

PREFACE

Approximately one third of the UK population is living with a musculoskeletal condition (Versus Arthritis, 2021) and the healthcare world has had to adapt to provide resources to manage this significant problem.

An increasingly ageing population, the growing demands of the primary care workload and the difficulties in maintaining the General Practitioner (GP) workforce, have all led to a different model of practice, and professions allied to medicine have been identified as well-placed to support GPs as part of an integrated multidisciplinary care team.

From the latter 1980s, 'extended' roles were developed from professions' traditional scope of practice, principally in physiotherapy (Byles and Ling, 1989). Further training provided extended scope physiotherapists with additional skills such as injection therapy, requesting and interpreting investigations, independent prescribing, and an understanding of medical complexities and some non-musculoskeletal conditions, such as neurological, vascular and serious pathologies.

The development of enhanced and advanced clinical practitioner roles continued, and First Contact Physiotherapist roles were developed in 2014, followed by First Contact Practitioners (FCPs) as the roles were expanded within other allied health professions and nursing. As well as in primary care, musculoskeletal practitioners work in other sectors and specialties in the health service, where practitioners can progress to advanced and consultant levels through further education and training.

Musculoskeletal medicine (originally orthopaedic medicine) is a specialism that is dedicated to the examination, diagnosis and conservative management of disorders of the musculoskeletal system (i.e. disorders of joints, ligaments, muscles and tendons).

The specialism is founded on the life's work of Dr James Cyriax MRCP (1904-1985) who, for many years, was Honorary Consultant Physician to the Department of Physical Medicine, St Thomas' Hospital, London. The 'Cyriax' approach is still a globally understood term within musculoskeletal practice and Cyriax's key texts continue to be referred to throughout this fifth edition: Cyriax, 1982, 1984; Cyriax and Cyriax, 1993.

Since its inception in the 1920s, 'orthopaedic medicine' has been on a journey.

Initially, bidisciplinary courses in orthopaedic medicine were led by Cyriax and a teaching team of medical and physiotherapy practitioners. The bidisciplinary courses were unusual at the time, but were then lauded for providing an opportunity for medical practitioners and physiotherapists to learn together and to share their experience. This provided a strong foundation for the approach moving forwards.

The 'Society of Orthopaedic Medicine' was established as an educational charity in 1979 to continue to develop and promote the theory and practice of the approach, through its educational pathway. The Society changed its name to the Society of Musculoskeletal Medicine (SOMM) in 2013, to reflect the more widely used term to describe the clinical specialism and the conditions encountered.

A major step forward for the Society was taken to coincide with the changes in primary care early in the 2010s, and, as well as medical practitioners and physiotherapists, the Society opened its modules to all experienced, registered allied health professionals and nurses working in musculoskeletal practice.

Course modules are now attended by musculoskeletal physiotherapists, FCPs and Advanced Practitioners (APs) from a variety of levels and backgrounds; allied health professionals, such as podiatrists, nurses, musculoskeletal sonographers, osteopaths and chiropractors; and medical doctors, including Sports and Exercise Medicine (SEM) doctors, GPs with a musculoskeletal extended role, rheumatologists, radiologists and orthopaedic and pain specialists.

The Society developed the first MSc Orthopaedic Medicine (now MSc Musculoskeletal Medicine) in 2000, to inspire professionals to become research minded, and research active, and to grow and disseminate the evidence base of musculoskeletal medicine.

The Society's modules now form a flexible master's level pathway to support practitioners' continuing professional development in the specialism. The modules take place throughout the year at a variety of different venues, both nationally and internationally (https://www.sommcourses.org).

Following the introduction of FCP roles, it became clear that standards of practice would need to be developed, at master's level, to support the FCP and developing AP roles. In 2020, a 'roadmap to practice' was introduced by Health Education England (HEE), in collaboration with key stakeholders, for FCPs and APs in primary care to follow towards accreditation by the 'Centre for Advancing Practice'.

SOMM's Foundation in Musculoskeletal Medicine module has been accredited as Stage One of the HEE 'First Contact Practitioners and Advanced Practitioners in Primary Care: (Musculoskeletal) A Roadmap to Practice' (HEE, 2020) and SOMM's educational team has been closely involved in the joint project to develop standards of practice towards Advanced Practitioner and Consultant roles.

The musculoskeletal medicine approach will continue on its journey, to ensure that it remains current to the needs of the musculoskeletal practitioner while remaining based on firm principles to guide and underpin practice.

The aim of this textbook is to provide the principles of diagnosis and treatment that can be applied to any of the common soft tissue conditions encountered in musculoskeletal practice, within the context of a stepped approach to management.

The content of this textbook is structured to link to the scheme of SOMM's Foundation in Musculoskeletal Medicine module, and the book is designed as a tool to enable medical, allied health and nursing professionals to develop their skills in the management of musculoskeletal conditions.

Cyriax set high standards for innovative and reflective thinking in clinical practice and promoted the development of clinical reasoning underpinned by current evidence. Notwithstanding, the importance of expert opinion and clinical experience has always been respected and inter- and intra-disciplinary communication is encouraged throughout all SOMM's courses.

This fifth edition continues to focus on students' learning, combining those elements of best available evidence, expert opinion and clinical experience, to justify practice and to develop clinical autonomy still further. We believe that the strength of this new edition is as much in what has been removed, to focus even more on the 'need to know', as well as the extensive updating that brings the approach into line with current theory and practice.

We have reframed the text to align to the standards and competencies set out in the 'Multi-professional framework for advanced clinical practice in England' (2017), the 'Musculoskeletal core capabilities framework for first point of contact practitioners' (2018) and the knowledge, skills and attributes specified in the 'First Contact and Advanced Practitioners in Primary Care: (Musculoskeletal) A Roadmap to Practice' (2020). We have emphasised personalised care, shared decision-making and the wider public health role of musculoskeletal practitioners.

Resources have been updated on the Evolve Resources website (http://evolve.elsevier.com/Atkins/msk) and we would encourage readers to make use of these resources to challenge their understanding of the principles and practice of musculoskeletal medicine.

The musculoskeletal medicine approach puts the patient at the centre of decisions made about their care and is firmly aligned to the principle of 'making every contact count'.

Cyriax's primary aim was to develop and integrate the musculoskeletal medicine approach into musculoskeletal practice - and ultimately to benefit patients. The approach, and the Society, have come a long way but have never wavered from Cyriax's intention. Through each edition of this textbook, this has been our aim too.

Elaine Atkins, Emily Goodlad and
Sharon Chan-Braddock

REFERENCES

Byles, S.E., Ling, R.S.M., 1989. Orthopaedic out-patients – A fresh approach. Physiotherapy 75 (7), 435–437.

Cyriax, J., 1982. Textbook of Musculoskeletal Medicine, eighth ed. Baillière Tindall, London.

Cyriax, J., 1984. Textbook of Musculoskeletal Medicine, eleventh ed. Baillière Tindall, London.

Cyriax, J., Cyriax, P., 1993. Cyriax's Illustrated Manual of Musculoskeletal Medicine. Butterworth Heinemann, Oxford.

First Contact and Advanced Practitioners in Primary Care: (Musculoskeletal), 2020. A Roadmap to Practice. https://www.hee.nhs.uk/sites/default/files/documents/MSK%20July21-FILLABLE%20Final%20Aug%202021_2.pdf. Accessed 10 January 2022.

Multi-professional framework for advanced clinical practice in England, 2017. https://www.hee.nhs.uk/sites/default/files/documents/multi-professionalframeworkforadvancedclinicalpracticeinengland.pdf. Accessed 10 January 2022.

Musculoskeletal core capabilities framework for first point of contact practitioners. 2018. https://www.csp.org.uk/system/files/musculoskeletal_framework2.pdf. Accessed 10 January 2022.

Versus Arthritis. https://www.versusarthritis.org/about-arthritis/data-and-statistics/the-state-of-musculoskeletal-health/. Accessed 7 December 2021.

To Monica Kesson (1951-2012)
This book is dedicated to our dear friend and colleague Monica.
We are so grateful for her inspiration, drive and hard work
to further the musculoskeletal medicine approach, which was
tireless. She embraced the educational needs of the students
and tutors alike, always striving to nurture, improve and
develop. Monica supported us all as Fellows and encouraged our
professional development in musculoskeletal medicine at every stage.
This book is her legacy.

Tell me and I forget.
Teach me and I remember.
Involve me and I learn.

BENJAMIN FRANKLIN

ACKNOWLEDGEMENTS

We continue to acknowledge the valuable contribution of all those mentioned for the previous editions and all our current colleagues in the Society of Musculoskeletal Medicine.

We acknowledge those along the way who provided such inspiration through their enthusiasm to share their knowledge of musculoskeletal medicine. These include Stephanie Saunders, who was so instrumental in the introduction of injection therapy into physiotherapists' scope of practice; Monica Kesson, who deserves all credit for her original idea to write the 'book of the course'; and Dr James Cyriax, the founder of the specialism, who gave us all our 'light bulb moment'.

Thanks to Amanda Hensman-Crook and Dr Tim Noblet, both alumni of the Society, who are avid advocates of the approach, and of the Society of Musculoskeletal Medicine. They have worked hard to forge important collaborations, all to the good of musculoskeletal health.

Thanks to Taranpreet Kaur, our patient and hardworking Content Project Manager at Elsevier, and Robert Edwards, Executive Content Strategist, for his continuing support for the book.

And finally, we acknowledge our families who have been unwavering in their support and encouragement and so understanding of all that it has taken to see this fifth and previous editions through; our gratitude and love are extended to them. Elaine would like to thank, as always, Clive, Kate and Tess and now her sons-in-law, Oscar and Mark, and grandchildren Victor, Remy, Dudley and Georgia; Emily would like to thank John, Maggie and Finlay; and Sharon would like to give special thanks to John, Aimee and Lucas, and her mentors Paul Hattam and Dr Peter Goodwin.

Principles of Musculoskeletal Medicine

1. Clinical Reasoning in Musculoskeletal Medicine
2. Soft Tissues of the Musculoskeletal System
3. Soft Tissue Healing
4. Musculoskeletal Medicine Treatment Techniques

INTRODUCTION TO SECTION 1

Section 1 presents the theory underpinning the principles and practice of musculoskeletal medicine.

The first chapter provides an outline of pain theory relevant to the approach, followed by a presentation of the principles of assessment and clinical diagnosis.

The histology and biomechanics of the soft tissues follow, with a review of the healing process and the effects of injury and immobilisation on the soft tissues. This should enable the application of appropriate treatment to the different phases of healing, towards the restoration of full, painless function.

Building on the theory of the first chapters, the final chapter in this section explains the principles of treatment, as applied in musculoskeletal medicine, and discusses the techniques of transverse frictions, mobilisation, manipulation and injection, their use and application. An outline of the relevant pharmacology and general considerations is provided.

Clinical tips emphasise key points throughout the section.

Clinical Reasoning in Musculoskeletal Medicine

CHAPTER CONTENTS

SUMMARY

Musculoskeletal medicine (formerly orthopaedic medicine) is based on the life's work of the late Dr James Cyriax (1904 to 1985). He developed a method of assessing the soft tissues of the musculoskeletal system, using a process of diagnosis by selective tension. Selective tension applies passive movements to test the inert structures and resisted movements to test the contractile structures.

This chapter is divided into two parts. The first discusses pain and includes patterns and 'rules' of referral of pain and other symptoms from different structures. The second, clinical examination, describes the theory behind Cyriax's logical method of assessment, which, by reasoned elimination, leads to the identification of the tissue in which the lesion lies.

Screening for psychosocial factors, health comorbidities and lifestyle risk factors forms an important part of medical history, and medications and 'red flags' are considered, as well as further investigations.

PAIN AND REFERRED SYMPTOMS

Pain is most often the primary complaint for patients presenting in musculoskeletal practice, but there may be other symptoms that cause them to seek advice, such as stiffness, weakness, numbness and pins and needles. The latter can also provide clues to diagnosis, and both pain and referred symptoms will form the basis of this discussion.

At first glance, pain seems to be straightforward – hitting your thumb with a hammer hurts your thumb. Such an acute pain experience is easily understood as activation of pain receptors (nociceptors) in response to a painful stimulus, and it gives a reliable indication of where the tissue damage has occurred and where the pain is coming from. However, pain can be much more complex and there are different types of pain that frequently overlap.

The study of pain is a vast topic, most of which is outside the scope of this book. For a more detailed account, the practitioner is referred to the many other sources available.

Notwithstanding, pain and its behaviour are relevant to musculoskeletal medicine, particularly in the assessment procedures, towards the achievement of an accurate clinical diagnosis and as a guide to improve individualised care and maximise the effectiveness of the management approach.

A brief overview of pain terminology is provided here as a basis for the discussion on referred pain that follows.

Pain Terminology

The International Association for the Study of Pain (IASP) produced a revised definition of pain in 2020 describing it as 'An unpleasant sensory and emotional experience associated with, or resembling that associated with, actual or potential tissue damage' (Raja et al., 2020).

This definition can be applied to acute and persistent (chronic) pain and to all painful conditions, regardless of their biological pain mechanism.

Biological Pain Mechanisms

The term 'biological pain mechanisms' is used to describe factors that can contribute to the development, maintenance or enhancement of pain. Broadly speaking,

biological pain mechanisms can be categorised into three categories: nociceptive, nociplastic (central sensitisation) and neuropathic. These three pain mechanisms can also be influenced by psychosocial factors and movement system (motor) factors (Chimenti et al., 2018) (Fig. 1.1).

A patient may have a single pain mechanism or multiple pain mechanisms occurring at the same time. On the other hand, two individuals with the exact same diagnosis can have different underlying pain mechanisms contributing to their pain.

It can be difficult to differentiate pain mechanisms, despite the continued development of clinical methods of biological pain mechanism assessment. However, an understanding of pain mechanisms and the biopsychosocial approach to pain helps the practitioner to target specific or multiple pain mechanisms and to personalise patient management. Fig. 1.2 gives a brief description of the three biological pain mechanisms, with examples.

Nociceptive pain is caused by stimulation of *nociceptors*, sensory nerve cells (neurons) that respond to potentially damaging stimuli, sending nerve signals to the spinal cord and brain. Pain is perceived only when the signals are interpreted within the higher centres.

Pain often originates in the peripheral nervous system when nociceptors are activated due to noxious stimulation such as injury, inflammation or a mechanical

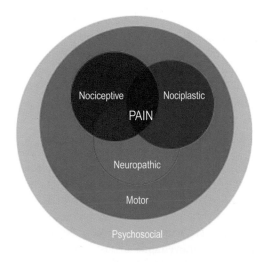

Fig. 1.1 Schematic diagram representing a mechanism-based approach to pain management. Schematic representation of three pain mechanisms occurring within the context of movement system and psychosocial factors. (From Chimenti et al., 2018.)

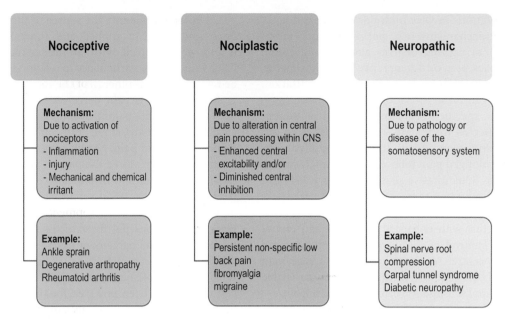

Fig. 1.2 Brief description of the three biological pain mechanisms, and examples.

irritant. Nociceptive signals are relayed to the spinal cord and then to the cortex through ascending nociceptive pathways, resulting in the perception of pain.

Peripheral sensitisation of nociceptive neurons can enhance or prolong the pain experience, even without sensitisation of central neurons (i.e. nociplastic or central sensitisation). Therefore nociceptive pain is primarily due to nociceptor activation, albeit processed through the central nervous system (CNS), typically resulting in acute localised pain, such as an ankle sprain.

Within the CNS, nociceptive signals are constantly modulated by cortical and brain stem pathways. These can be facilitatory or inhibitory and modulate both the sensory and emotional components of pain.

Nociceptive pain may also originate from 'visceral' or 'somatic' structures.

Visceral pain arises from internal organs that are highly sensitive to inflammation, stretch and ischaemia but are relatively insensitive to cutting or burning.

Somatic pain arises from the musculoskeletal tissues and can be divided into deep and superficial somatic pain. *Deep somatic pain* is initiated by stimulation of nociceptors within bones, ligaments, tendons, muscles fascia and blood vessels, and *superficial somatic pain* arises from activation of nociceptors in the skin or other superficial tissues.

Pain of visceral origin can mimic that of somatic origin (Bogduk, 2023) and vice versa. For example, pain arising from pathology in the heart may produce a spread of pain into the arm, imitating the pain of nerve root sleeve compression from a cervical lesion. Similarly, pain may be produced in the central chest region from pathology in the midthoracic spine.

Nociplastic pain, more commonly referred to as '*central sensitisation*', has been defined by the IASP as 'pain that arises from altered nociception, despite no clear evidence of actual or threatened tissue damage causing the activation of peripheral nociceptors, or evidence for disease or lesion of the somatosensory system causing the pain' (International Association for the Study of Pain [IASP], 2021). That is, tissue injury plays no role in pain associated with central sensitisation.

Nociplastic pain is due to alterations of nociceptive processing, most likely within the CNS, such as enhanced central excitability and/or diminished central inhibition. It occurs when areas in the spinal cord or brainstem become more sensitive after repeated peripheral nociceptive stimulation and weaker impulses are then needed to initiate responses. It is typically persistent and more widespread than nociceptive pain.

Nociplastic pain is thought to be a common factor contributing to many persistent pain conditions, such as fibromyalgia, persistent low back pain and migraine.

Some conditions involve both nociceptive and noci-plastic pain mechanisms (e.g. peripheral and central sensitisation) to varying degrees along a continuum, such as low back pain or degenerative knee arthropathy. Patients can have high levels of peripheral sensitisation, high levels of central sensitisation, or both.

There is no specific test for central sensitisation, but it can be suspected from signs and symptoms that can include ongoing, spontaneous and widespread pain, or severe and prolonged pain following a seemingly innocuous stimulus. 'Quantitative sensory testing' (QST) can evaluate sensitivity to a range of stimuli and can detect heightened responsiveness.

It may be that with enhanced peripheral and central sensitisation, removal of the peripheral component can eliminate the central sensitisation (e.g. total knee joint replacement) but the improvement may only be partial due to residual central sensitisation causing persistent pain.

Neuropathic pain arises from pathology within the somatosensory nervous system (transmitting sensations from the body, as opposed to sensations from specialised organs such as the ear or eye). There are many conditions which can cause damage to the somatosensory nervous system, leading to neuropathic pain. For example, this can result from a direct injury to the nerve, such as spinal nerve root compression or peripheral nerve compression (e.g. carpal tunnel syndrome), or can be due to metabolic disease, such as diabetes resulting in diabetic neuropathy.

Neuropathic pain may also be felt in areas with no tissue damage and may be experienced far from the lesion or disease (e.g. in the leg or foot associated with nerve root compression, phantom limb pain syndrome or trigeminal neuralgia). Other conditions such as shingles, excessive alcohol consumption or certain medications can also cause neuropathic pain.

Due to the variety of manifestations of neuropathic pain, it can often lead to confusion in the understanding of referred symptoms, including pain and other associated symptoms such as allodynia, hyperalgesia, itchiness, tingling sensation, numbness, prickling, burning and the sensation of electric shock.

Referred Pain

Whether right or wrong in their assessment, patients usually localise their pain as coming from a certain point and can describe the area of its spread, although sometimes only vaguely.

To be able to identify the source of the pain, a thorough knowledge of applied and functional anatomy is essential, coupled with an understanding of the behaviour of pain, particularly in relation to its ability to be referred to areas other than the causative site.

Referred pain is pain perceived at a location other than the site of the painful stimulus. The three biological pain mechanisms, alone or in combination, can contribute to referred pain. Cyriax considered that all pain is referred, and explored the pattern of referred pain to establish some rules to help to interpret its true source (Cyriax and Cyriax, 1993).

Since the end of the 19th century, there have been several suggestions put forward for the mechanism of referred pain, and agreement has yet to be reached on which, if any, is correct. The more significant suggestions are presented here.

Evidence has been provided for the mechanism that visceral and somatic primary sensory neurons converge onto common spinal neurons, causing confusion in the ascending spinal pathways and leading to misinterpretation of the origin of the pain. The message from the primary lesion could be wrongly interpreted as coming from the area of pain referral (Vecchiet and Giamberardino, 1997; Robinson, 2003; Galea, 2014). This has been dubbed the convergence–projection theory and is attributed to the original work of Sturge and Ross in 1888.

The confusion in differential diagnosis between pain arising from visceral lesions and that arising from musculoskeletal lesions is discussed further by Galea (2014), who describes how the level of the spinal cord to which visceral afferent fibres project depends on their embryonic innervation and notes that many viscera migrate well away from their embryonic derivation during development, such that visceral referred pain may be perceived at remote sites.

A sidetrack from the 'convergence–projection theory' is the 'convergence–facilitation theory', put forward by McKenzie in 1893 (cited in McMahon et al., 1995); this theory claimed that viscera are insensitive but visceral afferent activity produces an irritable focus within the spinal cord, where somatic nociceptive inputs take over to produce abnormal referred pain in the appropriate segmental distribution. This theory was not generally accepted because it denied that true visceral pain could exist.

Referred pain does not only present itself for misinterpretation between visceral and somatic structures but is also a phenomenon that may prevent accurate localisation of the primary source of symptoms within the musculoskeletal tissues.

Cyriax and Cyriax (1993) suggested that the misinterpretation of pain occurs at the cortical level, where stimuli arriving at certain cortical cells from the skin can be localised accurately to that area. When stimuli from other deeper tissues of the same segmental derivation reach those same cells, the sensory cortex makes assumptions on the basis of past experience and attributes the source of the pain to that same area of skin. This accounts for the dermatomal reference of pain, but the theory can be extended to include the referral of other symptoms from structures within the same segment.

SEGMENTAL REFERENCE

Several authors have tried to establish patterns of referred pain by examining the dermatomes. However, the dermatomes appear to vary according to the different methods for defining them and there is more overlap with some methods than with others. These methods mainly derive from embryonic development, observation of herpetic eruptions, areas of vasodilation resulting from nerve root stimulation and the areas of tactile sensation remaining after rhizotomy (surgical severance) of spinal nerve roots.

Lee et al. (2008) set out to produce a novel dermatome map based on the available evidence drawn from experiments conducted over the past century (Fig. 1.3). They proposed that the overlapping of dermatomes and their variability deserved more emphasis and that to represent dermatomes as autonomous zones of cutaneous sensory innervation is unreliable.

However, despite the experimental findings, the extent of individual dermatomes, especially in the limbs, is largely based on clinical evidence, and Standring (2015) acknowledges that this leads to a wide variation between the opinions of different disciplines.

The dermatomes given in this book are drawn mainly from the clinical experience of Cyriax and are different from those given in *Gray's Anatomy* (Standring, 2015), for example. In the authors' experience, they provide a basic guide for clinical practice and are presented as shown in Fig. 1.4.

Nerve Root Dermatomes

In general, the muscle groups lie under the dermatome which shares the same nerve supply. However, there are some apparent exceptions to this rule. This can cause confusion in the consideration of referred pain, in that a

lesion in the relevant muscle may appear to refer pain to an unrelated site and vice versa.

As mentioned earlier, the viscera may also refer pain to apparently unrelated sites, and this should be considered within the differential diagnosis. For example, Pappano and Bass (2006) present a case study describing referred shoulder pain preceding abdominal pain in a teenage girl with gastric perforation.

Pappano and Bass (2006) also highlight other conditions referring to the shoulder, including peritonitis, cholecystitis and subdiaphragmatic endometriosis. Postlaparoscopy shoulder pain is noted, where carbon dioxide used for inflation applies stretch to the diaphragm. Sloan (2008) provides further detail, listing right-sided periscapular pain in gall bladder disease and interscapular pain in aortic dissection.

The most commonly encountered discrepancies are as follows:
- Scapular muscles are supplied by C4–C7 but underlie thoracic dermatomes
- Latissimus dorsi is supplied by C6–C8 but underlies thoracic and lumbar dermatomes
- Pectoralis major is supplied by C5–T1 but underlies thoracic dermatomes
- The heart, a thoracic structure, is supplied by the vagus nerve and may refer pain into the arms, axillae, neck, jaw and chest
- The diaphragm is supplied by C3–C5, and diaphragmatic irritation may lead to pain felt in the epaulette region of the shoulder
- The gluteal muscles are supplied by L5, S1–S2 but underlie L1–L3 dermatomes
- The testicle is supplied by T11–T12 but underlies the S4 dermatome, where pain may be felt locally or can be referred to the lower thoracic or upper lumbar regions

Factors That Influence Referred Pain

Cyriax (1982) and Cyriax and Cyriax (1993) identified several factors that influence the referral of pain:
- Strength of the stimulus
- Position of the stimulus
- Depth of the structure
- Type or nature of the structure

Strength of the Stimulus

The more acutely inflamed or irritable the lesion (i.e. the greater the stimulus), the further the symptoms will be referred (Inman and Saunders, 1944). For example, an

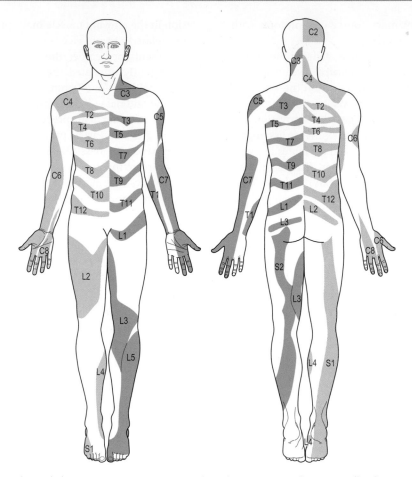

Fig. 1.3 The evidence-based dermatome map representing the most consistent tactile dermatomal areas for each spinal dorsal nerve root found in most individuals, based on the best available evidence. The dermatomal areas shown are NOT autonomous zones of cutaneous sensory innervation because, except in the midline where overlap is minimal, adjacent dermatomes overlap to a large and variable extent. Blank regions indicate areas of major variability and overlap. S3, S4 and S5 supply the perineum but are not shown for reasons of clarity. (Reproduced from Lee et al., 2008. © With permission from John Wiley & Sons, Inc.)

acutely inflamed subacromial bursitis may refer its pain to the wrist, the distal extent of the C5 dermatome, and a lumbar lesion involving compression and inflammation of the L4 nerve root may refer pain and associated symptoms to the big toe, at the distal end of the L4 dermatome.

Position of the Stimulus

Pain and tenderness tend to refer distally. Therefore a stimulus arising from a structure placed more proximally in the dermatome is capable of referring its symptoms over a greater distance.

The length or distance of dermatomal referral is particularly obvious in the limbs, where the dermatomes tend to be long. However, if the dermatome is short, even with an acutely inflamed or irritable condition, the reference will halt at the end of its dermatome, or at the most distal dermatome in the event of more than one nerve supply.

Structures within the hand and forefoot are already at the distal end of their relevant dermatome. Therefore referral of symptoms is less, or shorter, and lesions in these areas are easier to localise (Inman and Saunders, 1944).

Depth of the Structure

Skin is the only organ that provides precise localisation of pain and is, of course, the most superficial structure

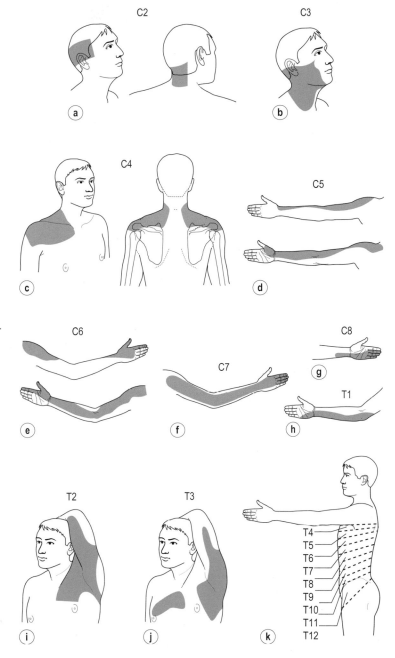

Fig. 1.4 Dermatomes. C2: side and back of the head, upper half of the ear, cheek and upper lip, nape of the neck (a). C3: entire neck, lower mandible, chin, lower half of the ear (b). C4: epaulette area of the shoulder (c). C5: anterolateral aspect of the arm and forearm as far as the base of the thumb (d). C6: anterolateral aspect of the arm and forearm, thenar eminence, thumb and index finger (e). C7: posterior aspect of the arm and forearm, index, middle and ring fingers (f). C8: medial aspect of the forearm, medial half of the hand, middle, ring and little fingers (g). T1: medial aspect of the forearm, upper boundary uncertain (h). T2: Y-shaped dermatome, medial condyle of humerus to axilla, branch to sternum and branch to scapula (i). T3: area at front of chest, patch in axilla (j). T4, T5, T6: circling trunk above, at and below the nipple area (k). T7, T8: circling trunk at lower costal margin (k). T9, T10, T11: circling the trunk, reaching the level of the umbilicus (k). T12: margins uncertain, extends into groin, covers greater trochanter and the iliac crest (k).

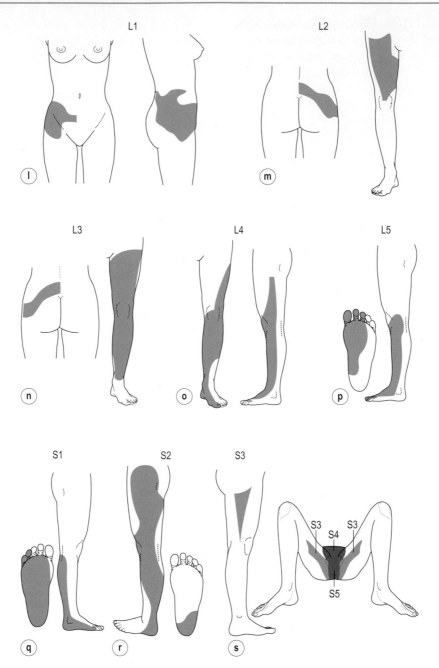

Fig. 1.4 Cont'd L1: lower abdomen and groin, lumbar region between levels L2 and L4, upper, outer aspect of the buttock (l). L2: two separate areas: lower lumbar region and upper buttock, whole of the front of the thigh (m). L3: two separate areas: upper buttock, medial aspect and front of the thigh and leg as far as the medial malleolus (n). L4: lateral aspect of the thigh, front of the leg crossing to the medial aspect of the foot, big toe only (o). L5: lateral aspect of the leg, dorsum of the whole foot, first, second and third toes, inner half of the sole of the foot (p). S1: sole of the foot, lateral two toes, lower half of the posterior aspect of the leg (q). S2: posterior aspect of the whole thigh and leg, plantar aspect of the heel (r). S3: circular area around the anus, medial aspect of the thigh (s). S4: saddle area: anus, perineum, genitals, medial upper thigh (s). S5: coccygeal area (s). (From Conesa and Argote, 1976; Cyriax, 1982; Cyriax and Cyriax, 1993).

(Gnatz, 1991). Cyriax (1982) proposed that lesions in the more deeply placed structures tend to give more vague and greater reference of pain, which was also the finding of Kellgren (1939) and Inman and Saunders (1944). The deeper structures therefore give rise to greater misunderstanding in terms of clinical diagnosis.

Joint, ligament (e.g. medial collateral and anterior cruciate ligaments) and bursa lesions tend to conform to this assumption but a notable exception is provided by lesions within bone. Pain and tenderness arising from fractures or involvement of the cortical bone tend to be well localised, even though bone itself is the most deeply placed tissue in musculoskeletal terms. Pathology involving the cancellous part of bone may give the more typical pattern of referred pain.

As mentioned later, segmental pain arising from lesions in the deeply sited viscera can also be misleading.

Nature of the Tissue

The nature of the tissue should be considered alongside the preceding depth of the structure since studies to observe the effect of lesions in tissues on patterns of referred pain are hard to dissociate.

Looking at muscle first, most practitioners are familiar with the work of Travell and Simons (1996) who identified trigger points in muscle, as a focus of hyperirritability, that give rise to local tenderness and referred pain.

Witting et al. (2000) compared local and referred pain following intramuscular capsaicin injection into the brachioradialis muscle and intradermal injection in the skin above the muscle. Intradermal injection produced more intense but localised pain, whereas referred pain was more marked after the intramuscular injection and was deeply located as well as referring to skin.

Farasyn (2007) added support to the observation that muscles refer pain, describing that a local muscle lesion can give rise to a wider area of pain, separate from the tender local injury and often described as 'burning'.

Much earlier, Kellgren (1938, 1939) observed that pain arising from the limb muscles tended to refer to the region of the joints moved by these muscles, where it could easily be confused as arising from the joint itself.

With regard to other tissues, tendon sheath and fascia gave sharply localised pain (Farasyn, 2007). Stimulation did not produce pain from articular cartilage or compact bone, but when applied to cancellous bone a deep diffuse pain was produced.

Stimulation of the interspinous ligaments gave rise to segmentally referred pain, which, as in muscle, was associated with tenderness in the deeply placed structures (Kellgren, 1938, 1939; Farasyn, 2007).

Referred Pain in the Spine
Facet Joints

Moving to the spinal joints, controversy has existed for many years as to whether the facet joints (zygapophyseal joints) or the disc are the primary source of back pain, especially when associated with pain referred to the limb.

Facet joints of the spine are well innervated by the medial branches of the dorsal rami (Bogduk, 1982a; Bogduk et al., 1982b). They have been shown to be capable of causing pain in the neck, upper and mid back and low back, with pain referred to other joints, including bilaterally (Manchikanti et al., 2004). Some evidence suggests that facet joints can be a source of pain in patients with persistent spinal pain, when using diagnostic techniques of known reliability and validity (Manchikanti et al., 2002, 2003; Boswell et al., 2003).

Conversely, the reliability of physical examination in diagnosing the specific cause of back pain has been questioned (Bogduk and McGuirk, 2002). Furthermore, it has been shown that there is a weak correlation between magnetic resonance imaging (MRI) findings and the response to lumbar facet joint intervention (Stojanovic et al., 2010).

Aprill et al. (1989) studied the reference of pain from the cervical facet joints. They found reasonably distinct and consistent segmental patterns of pain referral associated with joints between each of the levels of C2–C7, but there was no referral of pain into the arm from any of the levels tested.

In support of this pattern of referral, Cooper et al. (2007) determined the patterns of referred pain arising from cervical facet joints by using diagnostic blocks to establish pain referral patterns in symptomatic subjects. There was considerable overlap of referral areas, and patients described the symptoms in lines, spots or patches that were mostly confined to the neck and shoulder region.

Somatic Referred Pain, Radicular Pain and Radiculopathy

Somatic referred pain, radicular pain and radiculopathy are often used to describe the clinical presentation and pain mechanism in patients with spinal pathologies.

However, approximately 90% of cases of low back pain do not have a clear-cut cause. As mentioned earlier, different pain mechanisms can occur separately or together, but there may be a principal pain mechanism (e.g. neuropathic pain may be the more dominant driver of radicular pain than nociceptive pain).

There is still some confusion about the terms somatic referred pain, radicular pain and radiculopathy. To reduce unwarranted variation of communication between practitioners and to ensure an accurate explanation of diagnosis to patients, it is helpful to clarify these terms (Table 1.1).

In *somatic referred pain syndromes*, it is proposed that the source of the pain could be in any structure that receives a nerve supply, such as muscles, ligaments, facet joints, intervertebral discs, dura mater and dural nerve root sleeve. Somatic pain is not associated with neurological abnormalities, does not involve nerve root compression and is nondermatomal. The quality of somatic pain is described as dull, diffuse and difficult to localise with deeper structures but sharp, well-defined and clear to locate in superficial structures.

For *radicular pain syndromes*, a further distinction should be made between '*radicular pain' and 'radiculopathy'*.

In *radicular (root) pain*, the pain arises as a result of irritation of a spinal nerve or its roots. Disc herniation is the most common cause of radicular pain. Clinical experiments have demonstrated radicular pain to be lancinating and shooting in quality and referred into the limb in relatively narrow bands (Smyth and Wright, 1959; Bogduk, 2023). It rarely follows dermatomal patterns, and the 'line' of pain is not always clearly defined (Murphy et al., 2009; Furman and Johnson, 2019).

The common notion that radicular pain is expected to follow a specific dermatome, and that this information is useful to make a diagnosis of radicular pain, is questionable (Nitta et al., 1993; Bove et al., 2005; Murphy et al., 2009; Van Boxem et al., 2010).

In most cases, the sensitivity and specificity for the dermatomal pattern of pain are low for all nerve root levels (Murphy et al., 2009). It has been shown that radicular pain does not follow along a specific dermatome. The two possible exceptions to this are the S1 nerve root, where the pain does commonly follow the S1 dermatome (Bove et al., 2005; Murphy et al., 2009), and the C4 nerve root level (Murphy et al., 2009). If present, the dermatomal distribution of paresthesia appears to be more specific for all levels (Tarulli and Raynor, 2007).

There are several possible explanations for radicular pain not following a dermatomal pattern. Firstly, patients with radicular pain may also have other sources of pain, such as the intervertebral disc, dura mater or other tissues, which produce nociceptive, as opposed to radicular pain. Another possibility is that there can be

TABLE 1.1 Differences Between Somatic Referred Pain, Radicular Pain and Radiculopathy

Pain Terminology	Description	Mechanism
Somatic Referred Pain	Dull, aching, gnawing. Expanding pressure. Boundary difficult to localise but core of pain clear. Not dermatomal. No neurological signs.	Noxious stimulation of nerve endings within somatic structures. Nociceptive afferents from different peripheral sites converge onto common neurons that relay to higher centres, leading to confusion in localisation.
Radicular Pain	Lancinating, 'electric shock', shooting pain, in narrow bands, rarely follows dermatomal patterns and not clearly defined. May or may not be associated with radiculopathy. Typically, leg pain is worse than back pain.	Pain evoked by ectopic discharges from a dorsal nerve root or its ganglion. Disc herniation is the most common cause, provided nerve root sensitised by previous stimulation.
Radiculopathy	Objective neurological signs, including numbness, weakness and diminished or absent reflexes. Numbness can be dermatomal and weakness myotomal. May or may not be associated with pain.	Caused by the blocking of conduction along sensory (numbness) and motor axons (weakness).

From Bogduk (2009, 2023).

an overlap between dermatomes, with one dermatome encompassing one or two adjacent segments (Itomi et al., 2000). It may therefore be possible for an individual with radicular pain to have a dermatomal distribution but for this distribution to differ from the pattern in the classic dermatome maps.

From the clinical perspective, practitioners should be aware that a dermatomal distribution of pain is not always a useful factor in the diagnosis of radicular pain, and it is important to take other clinical findings into consideration towards diagnosis and onward management.

The mechanism of radicular pain is complex and is not fully understood. Current thinking is that it is a result of ectopic action potential emanating from a demyelinated or damaged axon of a nerve at the dorsal root or at the nerve root ganglion, as opposed to resulting from stimulation of the nerve's peripheral terminals (Bogduk, 2009; Baron et al., 2016).

Radicular pain is not necessarily neuropathic, because the nervi nervorum (innervating the nerve) can be a cause of nociceptive pain (Teixeira et al., 2016). In addition, 'occult' neuropathic pain can be a feature of nonneuropathic pain. For this reason, the IASP suggests simply documenting 'lower limb' pain, for example, rather than applying more specific labels (Merskey and Bogduk, 2023).

Irritation of the nerve, whether by a disc, its exudate or by foraminal stenosis, also leads to intraneural inflammation, which alone is sufficient to sensitise a nerve to movement (Dilley et al., 2005) and can spread to the spinal cord and the brain (Albrecht et al., 2018). Robinson (2003) confirmed this by stating that an inflammatory component or already damaged nerve root is necessary before a nerve root will produce pain.

The combination of compression of the dorsal root ganglion and/or intraneural inflammation, and anatomical abnormalities results in hyperexcitability and spontaneous ectopic activity in the dorsal root ganglion, which is interpreted as pain (Peng et al., 2007; Schmid, 2015). This can also contribute to central sensitisation (nociplastic pain) (Niere, 1991).

Radiculopathy is a neurological condition in which conduction is blocked in the axons of a spinal nerve or its roots. Neurological signs and symptoms associated with radiculopathy can include paraesthesia (numbness; pins and needles), muscle weakness and dull/loss of reflexes (Bogduk, 2023).

Conduction block in sensory axons results in paraesthesia, and conduction block in motor axons results in weakness and altered reflexes. Radiculopathy is a state of neurological loss. It does not necessarily result in pain in the back or in the limbs and may or may not be associated with radicular pain. The cause of both can be the same, but the mechanisms are different.

As described earlier, somatic and radicular pain syndromes can coexist (Bogduk, 1994). For example, the annulus fibrosus of the disc may be a source of somatic low back pain but may also cause secondary compression by a posterolateral displacement causing compression of the nerve root and leading to radicular pain.

O'Neill et al. (2002) demonstrated that noxious stimulation of the annulus fibrosus of the disc can give rise to low back and referred extremity pain, with the distal extent of pain produced depending on the intensity of stimulation. Nociceptors within the discal tissue may have become more sensitised in patients presenting with nonradicular leg pain, allowing provocation of peripheral symptoms at lower thresholds of stimulation (peripheral sensitisation).

O'Neill et al. (2002) and Bogduk (2023) describe referred leg pain from the somatic lumbar annulus fibrosus as being poorly localised, dull and aching, adding that it is usually less troublesome than the patient's low back pain.

They note that it is important to be able to differentiate between referred pain arising from somatic structures and radicular pain associated with nerve root compression from disc herniation, because the two types of pain have different causal mechanisms and may therefore require different treatment. They add that the traditional description 'pain radiating below the knee' as representing radicular pain rather than referred somatic pain is unreliable.

Notwithstanding, Stynes et al. (2018) include that feature within their 'cluster' of factors that suggest the cause of pain as radicular as opposed to somatic referred pain:

- Pain below the knee
- Leg pain worse than back pain
- Positive neurodynamic test
- Report of pins and needles

With consideration of the overlapping nature of somatic and radicular pain referral patterns, and the different qualities of the pain experienced, Robinson (2003) suggests that the patient's description of the pain itself may be more reliable than the location.

In this text, specific consideration of *visceral referred pain* is provided within the appropriate chapters as part of differential diagnosis. However, just as we have attempted to separate out the characteristics of somatic and radicular pain, Vecchiet and Giamberardino (1997) described general aspects of visceral pain that can be borne in mind for differential diagnosis, particularly for those conditions requiring more urgent referral, such as myocardial infarction and pancreatitis.

Initially, visceral pain is usually felt along the midline of the chest or abdomen, mainly in the lower sternal area and the epigastric region, regardless of the viscera affected. It is generally perceived as a deep, dull, vague sensation that is poorly defined and may not be able to be described.

It can vary from a sense of discomfort to one of oppression or heaviness and may be associated with autonomic signs such as pallor, sweating, nausea, vomiting and changes in heart rate, blood pressure and temperature. Strong emotional reactions are also often present and include anxiety, anguish and sometimes even feelings of impending death.

Common features of segmentally referred pain were identified by Cyriax as 'rules' of referred pain (Cyriax, 1982; Cyriax and Cyriax, 1993). As with all rules, exceptions are noted, but nonetheless they act as a general guideline in assessing pain behaviour and locating the causative lesion. Cyriax developed rules for referral of pain from unilateral structures as represented in the following box.

RULES OF REFERRED PAIN FROM UNILATERAL STRUCTURES
- It does not cross the midline
- It refers distally
- It refers segmentally
- It occupies part or all of its dermatome

A notable exception to the rules of referred pain is provided by the dura mater, which, as a centrally placed structure, produces so-called *multisegmental reference* of pain on compression or irritation.

Multisegmental Reference of Pain

Throughout his writing Cyriax referred to the phenomenon of 'extrasegmental' reference of pain (Cyriax, 1982; Cyriax and Cyriax, 1993). He used the term to explain the observation that symptoms arising from the dura mater do not obey the rules of referred pain, in terms of referring segmentally, but rather that a pattern of reference is produced that is 'outside' or 'extra' to that of the segment.

With another interpretation, the terminology may not be ideal because it implies that the pain is not experienced within the segment in which the causative lesion is housed. This is not so, and 'multisegmental' would perhaps be a more correct term.

The ventral aspect of the dura mater, the annulus fibrosus and other central spinal structures are innervated by the sinuvertebral nerve that sends branches to segments above and below its level of origin (Bogduk, 2023). This could account for the multisegmental reference of pain arising from compression of central structures.

Multisegmentally referred pain is felt diffusely across several segments, usually as a dull background ache, and is often associated with tenderness or trigger spots (Figs. 1.5–1.7). It may vary and be incomplete, and other unilateral symptoms might be superimposed upon it, as in lesions involving pressure on both the dura and the dural nerve root sleeve.

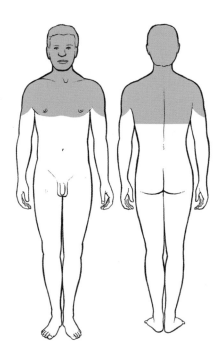

Fig. 1.5 Limits of dural multisegmental pain of cervical origin. (From A System of Orthopaedic Medicine by Ombregt, L., Reprinted by permission of Elsevier Ltd.)

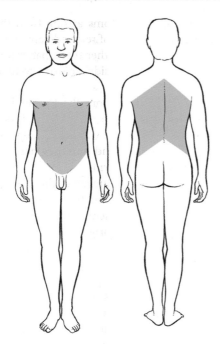

Fig. 1.6 Limits of dural multisegmental pain of thoracic origin. (From A System of Orthopaedic Medicine by Ombregt, L., Reprinted by permission of Elsevier Ltd.)

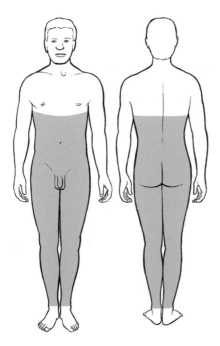

Fig. 1.7 Limits of dural multisegmental pain of lumbar origin. (From A System of Orthopaedic Medicine by Ombregt, L., Reprinted by permission of Elsevier Ltd.)

Mention of the dura mater leads to the general observation that lesions associated with compression of neural tissue produce varying patterns and nature of symptoms, according to the tissue involved. These will be listed as described in the box overleaf, beginning with the dura mater itself.

Psychosocial Factors

Having recognised the revised IASP definition of pain (i.e. pain is not just a sensory awareness of bodily harm, but is also an emotional experience that can be influenced by a number of psychosocial factors), pain is therefore considered to be a multidimensional phenomenon.

The biopsychosocial model of pain was proposed by Waddell in 1987 and continues to be the most widely accepted model to understand persistent pain and its associated disability. There is now a vast amount of literature on psychosocial factors and their relation to pain and disability.

Nociceptive, nociplastic and neuropathic pain mechanisms can be influenced by psychosocial factors directly or indirectly. In persistent pain, pain is more likely to be contributed to by psychosocial factors (e.g. depression), behavioural (e.g. fear-avoidance behaviour) and cognitive factors (e.g. pain belief and negative attitudes), than physical factors (Moseley, 2003, 2007).

Misinterpretation of pain as a sign of physical harm results in fear and avoidance behaviour, which consequently leads to a vicious cycle of anxiety, avoidance, disability and worsening pain (Vlaeyen and Linton, 2012).

A large meta-analysis on 15,623 patients with chronic musculoskeletal pain found that higher levels of fear-of-pain, fear-avoidance behaviour and anxiety were statistically significant when associated with pain and disability (Martinez-Calderon et al., 2019). Therefore addressing maladaptive psychosocial factors and adopting a multimodal management approach can optimise treatment outcomes for acute and persistent pain conditions.

Nevertheless, an initial organic basis should not be ignored. Shaw et al. (2007) looked at shared and independent associations of psychological factors among men with low back pain and suggested that early intervention will do much to avoid chronicity with its attendant psychosocial factors and persistent work disability.

Early identification and assessment of significant psychosocial influence will allow an early and appropriate management approach for individual patients

Dura Mater
- Multisegmental reference of pain and tenderness (see Figs. 1.5–1.7).

Spinal Cord
- No pain, multisegmental reference of paraesthesia (i.e. in both feet or all extremities if associated with cervical lesions).
- May produce upper motor neuron lesion with increased muscle tone, overactive reflexes, muscle weakness and possible muscle wasting.
- May produce a spastic gait.
- May produce an extensor plantar response.

Dural Nerve Root Sleeve
- Pain produced on compression of the tissue (i.e. the pressure or 'compression phenomenon') (Cyriax, 1982).
- Segmental reference of pain may be in all or part of the dermatome, but is mostly nondermatomal.
- Difficult to ascribe an aspect to the pain (e.g. anterior or lateral).
- Difficult to define an edge to the pain.

Nerve Root
- Neurological signs and symptoms are produced on compression through the dural sleeve:
  - segmental reference of paraesthesia is usually felt at the distal end of the dermatome
  - lower motor neuron lesion with muscle weakness and wasting

- absent or reduced reflexes
- may become pain sensitive

Nerve Trunk
- Symptoms produced on release of pressure (i.e., the 'release phenomenon') (Cyriax, 1982): for example, after sitting on a hard gate with pressure placed on the sciatic nerve trunk for a period of time, a shower of 'painful pins and needles' will be experienced in the leg until the nerve recovers.
- Sensation of deep painful paraesthesia in the cutaneous distribution of the nerve trunk.
- Some aspect; no edge to the symptoms.
- The longer the compression, the greater the length of time before the onset of pins and needles: for example, the thoracic outlet syndrome produces diffuse pins and needles in all five digits of one or both hands after going to bed at night, several hours after the compression has been released from the brachial plexus.

Peripheral Nerve
- Compression produces paraesthesia and possible wasting.
- Clear edge and aspect to the symptoms: for example, carpal tunnel syndrome producing paraesthesia in the cutaneous distribution of the lateral three and a half digits on the palmar aspect of the hand, or meralgia paraesthetica involving compression of the lateral cutaneous nerve of the thigh, which is associated with a clearly demarcated area of paraesthesia in the anterolateral aspect of the thigh.

(see page 22). It also provides a contraindication for some of the techniques used in musculoskeletal medicine, most notably the manipulative treatments used for spinal pain.

Cyriax (1982) presented characteristics which, if recognised in patients, give an indication that affective influences are a predominant feature of the complaint and should be taken into account in arriving at a diagnosis, as well as in subsequent treatment selection or appropriate referral.

He suggested that any or all of the following features might be present:
- No recognisable pattern of symptoms or signs in the history or examination
- Poor cooperation throughout the assessment
- Overenthusiastic assistance from the patient, often accompanied by an element of 'triumph' if the clinical diagnosis remains obscure
- Patients may seek the answer expected of them

- Mutually contradictory signs through the patient's incomplete knowledge of the condition
- 'Juddering' (quick, jerking movements), which is a response occasionally noted on resisted testing, but there is no evidence for any neurological condition that allows muscles to work in spasms of effort to produce such a juddering pattern.

Severe pain usually produces an 'all-or-nothing' effort where resistance is lost completely as a result of pain, for example, in resisted wrist extension as a test for tennis elbow where the wrist 'breaks' due to the sharp pain elicited. This is also not the cogwheel phenomenon encountered in Parkinson's disease.

Active movements are cited later in this chapter as a useful means of establishing the patient's willingness to perform the movement. This can relate to the psychosocial influence as well as allowing consideration of any unwillingness caused by actual pain or fear of producing it.

Waddell (1992, 2004), after extensive study in the field of problematic back pain, described behavioural symptoms and signs that provide information and raise awareness of illness behaviour. In contrast, Adams et al. (2012) warned that the balance of back pain research has swung too far towards psychosocial issues to the neglect of the physical.

To balance the focus on psychosocial issues, Waddell emphasised the need for careful assessment, warning that a 'galaxy of signs does not exclude a remediable condition'. Furthermore, students on musculoskeletal medicine courses are cautioned against the misinterpretation of unusual signs and symptoms by the statement: '*beware of the bizarre but consistent patient*', whose behaviour could be indicative of underlying serious pathology.

The central aim for management should be to avoid acute back pain becoming persistent and to avoid the emergence of a dominant psychosocial component (Shaw et al., 2007).

Several effective approaches have been devised in the treatment of persistent pain (Chartered Society of Physiotherapy, 2006a, 2006b). These are generally based on the concept of increasing activity and fitness levels and promoting the maxim that 'hurt does not equate to harm'. Skilled counselling such as cognitive behavioural therapy may also be required.

Tools have been devised to match patients to the most appropriate treatment package for them, to be able to decrease disability and the development of persistent pain, for example the STarT Back approach devised by Keele University (STarT Back, 2021).

This text has set out to acknowledge the possible influence of psychosocial factors but does not intend to expand further on its management. The interested practitioner is referred to texts relating to this important field.

Movement (Motor) System Factors

Assessment and treatment of the movement system are key in the management of patients with musculoskeletal pain. Pain can produce increased muscle contraction, tone or trigger points, which can result in physical deconditioning, muscle inhibition or fear-avoidance behaviours, leading to disuse or disability or both (Vlaeyen et al., 1995).

The relationship between pain and the movement system is complex and often highly variable between individuals (Hodges et al., 2013). Pain can also result in both a physical and psychological vicious cycle (Fig. 1.8), which is often a contributing factor to persistent pain for many patients.

A lower level of physical activity leads to physical changes such as muscle atrophy, changes in metabolism,

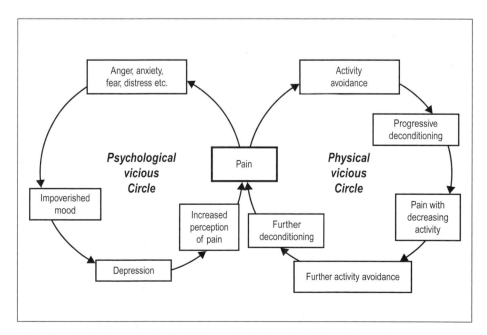

Fig. 1.8 Psychological and physical vicious circle of pain. (Adapted from Vlaeyen and Linton, 2012.)

decreased muscle strength and obesity, as well as psychosocial and behavioural changes such as distress, depression, anxiety and avoidance behaviour (Verbunt et al., 2003).

From a motor control perspective, maladaptive movement and motor control impairment, in response to pathophysiological pain and psychosocial factors, lead to abnormal tissue loading and ongoing peripheral nociceptive sensitisation (O'Sullivan, 2005).

From a neurophysiological perspective, poor motor function is likely to increase sensitivity of the CNS (Woolf, 2011), activate the pain neuromatrix (Moseley, 2007) and influence pain modulation (Zusman, 2002; O'Sullivan, 2005). This in turn reduces the pain threshold, lowers tissue nociceptive tolerance and further fuels pain and disability.

Therefore targeted intervention may help to reduce motor responses that exacerbate pain, and improve function. The integration of the practitioner's expertise in the movement system with the other biological pain mechanisms has the potential to optimise the level of care and to support planning in the management of pain conditions.

CLINICAL EXAMINATION

In the course of a consultation, not only do we need to establish a clinical diagnosis, we need to rule out red flags, establish rapport and trust, and explore ideas, concerns, worries and expectations. We also need to decide on a management plan, via shared decision making with the patient, sometimes all in 10 to 20 minutes.

We can have complex interactions with patients, and there are many ways we communicate: verbal, nonverbal, paraverbal and active listening. It is important to be aware that there are many tools and models available, especially based in medicine, to help us with this vital skill. For example, the biopsychosocial, 'Neighbour' and 'Calgary-Cambridge' models all have advantages and disadvantages.

Over more recent years, motivational interviewing has been implemented into our assessments to help patients change their behaviour, especially regarding lifestyle changes to improve health. Motivational interviewing is a person-centred, goal-orientated, communication style which aims to elicit and strengthen a person's intrinsic motivation and commitment to change (Miller and Rollnick 2009).

Patients should receive personalised care, which builds on the relationship between people, professionals and the health and social care system. Personalised care derives from making the most of the expertise, capacity and potential of people, families and communities.

It is accessed through six key components: patient choice, shared decision making, patient activation and supported self-management, social prescribing and community-based support, personalised care and support planning, and personal health budgets (National Health Service [NHS], 2021).

To support *shared decision making*, patients' wishes, goals, attitudes, beliefs and circumstances should be taken into consideration. They should be given details of their diagnosis and be fully informed of the risks, benefits and expected outcomes of the proposed treatment regime, to enable them to give their informed consent (National Institute for Health and Care Excellence [NICE], 2021a).

It is important to highlight that both assessment and treatment are absolutely contraindicated in the absence of informed patient consent. Consent is the patient's agreement, written or oral, for a health professional to provide care. It may range from an active request by the patient for a particular treatment regime to the passive acceptance of the health professional's advice.

The process of consent, within the context of the musculoskeletal medicine approach, is 'fluid', rather than one instance in time when the patient gives consent, and it underpins the elements of clinical examination and management throughout each of the chapters presented in Section 2.

For further information on consent, the practitioner is referred to the 'Reference guide to consent for examination or treatment (second edition)' (Department of Health, 2009) (current at the time of writing).

Cyriax's starting point in the development of musculoskeletal medicine was the premise that all pain has a source. It was a simple extension of that logic that, to be effective, all treatment must reach the source and all treatment must benefit the lesion.

Cyriax was intrigued by the number of patients passing through orthopaedic clinics who presented with normal X-ray findings and acknowledged the soft tissues as the source of the complaints. He devised a logical and methodical mechanism of clinical examination that was deliberately pared to the minimum needed to establish the source of the pain. This resonated with the claim of Sir Robert Hutchison in 1897 that 'every good method of case taking should be both comprehensive and concise' (Hunter and Bomford, 1963).

An important emphasis of this examination procedure is that negative findings are as significant as the positive, eliminating from the enquiry those structures which are *not* at fault. The systematic approach devised by Cyriax produces a set of findings that can be interpreted through logical reasoning, integrating the assessment with existing knowledge towards clinical diagnosis.

The term 'diagnosis' at this stage implies the hypothesis against which we all work, which becomes proven or disproven in light of the patient's subsequent response.

In recent years, much work has been devoted to developing areas of specialist assessment. However, the musculoskeletal medicine examination procedure gives practitioners a sound framework from which to start and any special examination techniques can be added to it.

For example, once a basic spinal assessment has been carried out, additional neural tissue sensitising tests can be included to search for aspects of neural tension; repeated or combined movements can be included; or localised joint palpation and mobility tests can be applied.

A further aim of the examination is to establish whether the condition is suitable for the treatments offered in musculoskeletal medicine or other allied treatment modalities or whether the patient would be more suitably referred onwards to the multiprofessional team.

More detailed tests such as blood tests, X-rays, ultrasound and MRI scans and arthrograms can be used as necessary but do not form part of the basic examination procedure.

The musculoskeletal medicine assessment procedure follows a set model for the collection of clinical information. It contains the following elements, which will be discussed in turn:

- **Observation**, noting face, gait and posture
- A detailed history
- **Inspection** for bony deformity, colour changes, muscle wasting and swelling
- **Palpation** for heat, swelling and synovial thickening
- **State at rest**
- **Examination** by selective tension, assessing active, passive and resisted movements
- **Palpation** for the site of the lesion, once the causative structure has been identified

OBSERVATION

OBSERVATION
- Face
- Posture
- Gait

Note the patient's *face*, *posture* and *gait*.

A general observation is made as the patient is met. Observe the patient's face for any signs of sleeplessness and pain. Serious disease accompanied by unrelenting pain is usually indicated in the patient's overall demeanour. It can be useful to note whether the patient's appearance matches the history, because important clues can be provided, particularly relating to the psychosocial component of the condition.

Certain postures indicate specific conditions. An antalgic posture (one assumed by the patient to avoid pain) is often adopted in neck pain, such as a torticollis (wry neck), or as a lateral shift when associated with a lumbar lesion.

In the upper limb, note any apparent guarding, perhaps with an altered arm swing associated with a painful shoulder, elbow or even wrist.

The patient's gait pattern may be altered, with a limp indicating symptoms on weight-bearing. An altered stride may be due to limitation of movement at a joint, or protection from weight bearing. The use of an aid such as a stick or crutches provides an obvious clue to the need for extra support to avoid or to assist with weight bearing. As part of the overall observation, a check may also be made on whether such aids are being used correctly.

HISTORY

HISTORY
- Age, occupation, sports, hobbies and activities
- Site and spread
- Onset and duration
- Symptoms and behaviour
- Medical history
- Other joint involvement
- Medications

A complete history is taken from the patient to discover as much information as possible about the condition. With respect to diagnosis, the history is more relevant at some joints than at others. For instance, the history of the knee joint may give many clues to diagnosis, whereas at the hip and shoulder, with commonly encountered conditions such as capsulitis, the history gives far fewer clues.

The term 'history' implies a chronological account of how the condition has progressed, but it has a much broader scope to include other features, such as aggravating and alleviating factors and past medical history, and is the subjective part of the examination procedure. It is traditional in clinical practice to use a model for the collection of clinical data from the patient (Beckman and Frankel, 1984).

Most models, including the model used in musculoskeletal medicine, involve the categorisation of the history under different headings to ensure that all information is collected. However, if this pattern is adhered to too rigidly, it can be restricting for the patient.

The use of closed questions to steer patients' responses results in interviews being practitioner-led. Constant interruptions may restrict the fluency of patients' accounts such that they are prevented from presenting the true nature of the problem (Beckman and Frankel, 1984; Blau, 1989).

Studies on the process of history taking revealed that physicians interrupted and took control of the interview on average 18 seconds into the consultation and that by asking specific closed questions they halted the spontaneous flow of information (Beckman and Frankel, 1984).

However, if allowed to continue uninterrupted, and with no specific guidance, patients talked on average for less than 2 minutes, during which time most of the information required by the physician was disclosed (Blau, 1989). This study was repeated by Wilkinson (1989), who found the time taken to be even shorter, with 89 of 100 patients surveyed speaking for less than 1½ minutes and 41 of those for less than 30 seconds.

Bearing the previous points in mind, although it is necessary to consider the categories of the history adopted in musculoskeletal medicine, in clinical practice it is better to begin the patient interview with an open question such as 'What brings you here today?' and then to allow the history to be expressed in the patient's own words. Anything not mentioned can be searched for after the patient has finished speaking.

Of course, not all patients will reveal a succinct history, and some guidance will be required to keep to the relevant. Nonetheless, a balance should still be sought between allowing the patient time to speak and controlling the interview to prevent irrelevant deviation (Blau, 1989).

The model for history taking in musculoskeletal medicine will now be described. The practitioner should note the relevant details from the history on the patient's record and clinical reasoning will continue throughout the interview.

Age, Occupation, Sports, Hobbies and Activities

The *age* of the patient may be relevant because certain conditions predominantly affect certain age groups. For example, children may suffer from Perthes disease or slipped epiphysis in the hip, pulled elbow, or loose bodies associated with osteochondritis dissecans in the knee.

Adolescents may suffer from Osgood–Schlatter disease, altered biomechanics and maltracking problems in the knee, or juvenile idiopathic arthritis. Mechanical lumbar lesions, ligament or tendon injuries are common in the working-aged, and degenerative arthropathy is usually a problem in the older age group.

Occupation can be relevant in terms of the postures adopted while at work and the activities involved in the patient's job. In this respect, it is important to explore the job's requirements rather than just to note the job title.

Sports, hobbies and activities, including level of activity, can provide clues to the cause and nature of the condition, as well as indicating the requirements for rehabilitation back to full activity. For example, tendon or muscle belly lesions frequently occur in sports requiring explosive activity, as in tennis and squash, and the specific requirements of the sport will need to be considered to be able to devise an appropriate rehabilitation programme.

Change in use can lead to tendinopathy, and appropriate advice will need to be given.

Those engaged in a more sedentary occupation or lifestyle might be prone to back pain and will need to be encouraged to increase their general activity as part of management and to prevent recurrence.

Site and Spread

Patients usually complain of pain, but there may be other symptoms that lead them to seek advice, such as numbness and pins and needles (paraesthesia), for example. Much information can be gained towards diagnosis by establishing where the symptoms began, where they are currently and their overall spread.

For instance, low back pain often travels into the leg but normally becomes less apparent in the back as it does so, which is a typical presentation of radicular pain. Low back pain moving into the leg without remission in the back implies central sensitisation, or a spreading lesion, and could require different interpretation and management.

Several factors can influence the site and spread of pain, and these were described in the first part of this chapter. The site and spread of pain can be an indication of the overall irritability of the lesion, as well as providing a clue to the structure at fault by considering the 'rules' (mentioned earlier) for the referral of symptoms that can arise from different somatic and neurological structures.

Onset and Duration

The mode of onset of the lesion can provide information that leads to a clinical diagnosis and can also contribute to the treatment selection and overall prognosis of the condition. Was the onset sudden or gradual? Acute muscle belly lesions come on suddenly, whereas tendon and bursa problems associated with change of use, usually have a gradual onset.

Fractures usually have a sudden onset associated with trauma, but systemic conditions, benign tumours or serious pathology such as malignancy have an insidious onset. None of these latter conditions is suitable for treatment within the specialism of musculoskeletal medicine, and they require urgent referral.

In the lumbar spine, the mode of onset can provide a guideline for treatment selection. For example, a sudden onset may respond to manipulation whereas a gradual onset may respond more effectively to treatment with traction, in the absence of contraindications.

The duration of the symptoms is important as an indicator of the acute or chronic stage in healing, which gives guidance for the treatment approach to be adopted and indicates the likely effectiveness and progress of treatment.

For example, an acutely sprained ligament requires a gentle approach to treatment aiming to reduce swelling, to promote healing and to prevent adverse scar tissue formation. In contrast, a chronic ligamentous lesion requires a firmer approach, aiming to restore range and function, with stretching and manipulative techniques as appropriate.

Symptoms and Behaviour

Symptoms can include pain, stiffness, weakness, numbness and pins and needles (paraesthesia), all of which are important within clinical reasoning.

The way the symptoms behave will help diagnosis. With pain, musculoskeletal lesions usually have aggravating and easing factors rather than constant pain and they are normally better with rest and worse on activity. In addition, changing posture can alter the pain. Ligamentous lesions are eased by movement and are usually worse after a period of resting. If pain does not alter with activities or positioning, the practitioner should be alerted that the pathology could be a nonmusculoskeletal-related condition.

Pain rating scales can be used to provide patients with a means of communicating levels of pain and to provide a basis for assessment of treatment outcomes.

What is the daily pattern of the symptoms? Joint stiffness more marked in the morning, and lasting more than one hour, indicates the presence of inflammatory arthropathy, as in rheumatoid arthritis, for example. If the lesion was associated with sudden trauma, asking whether the patient could continue with the activity can provide information on the severity of the lesion and/or instability.

Serious pathology may present with unrelenting pain, and night pain is likely to be a feature, along with other 'red flag' features (see page 25).

In distinguishing between serious pathology and an irritable musculoskeletal lesion, it can be helpful to distinguish whether the pain prevents sleep or disturbs sleep, with possible serious pathology being implicated in the former. With musculoskeletal lesions it may be that specific postures have to be adopted to allow sleep, such as sitting up for neck pain.

There will be special questions at each joint that are relevant to the patient's symptoms. For example, how do stairs affect knee pain? How does a cough or sneeze affect back pain? Does the patient with neck pain experience any visual disturbances? Pertinent questions asked at each joint region will help clinical reasoning and, importantly, will also rule out any contraindications to treatment.

Medical History and Screening
Medical History

Establish general health, and ask about past and present existence of serious illness, any ongoing conditions and treatment, or any planned surgery. Unexplained weight loss, operations, past or recent trauma or recent infection can be important indicators towards diagnosis. For example, an old fracture of the tibia may lead to degenerative changes in the ankle joint, or a mastectomy for breast malignancy may be followed by the formation of bony secondaries in the spine. Recent infection may trigger reactive arthritis.

The mnemonic **THREADSSFC** can be a helpful prompt for past and current medical history:

- **T** – Thyroid
- **H** – Heart
- **R** – Rheumatoid arthritis
- **E** – Epilepsy
- **A** – Asthma
- **D** – Diabetes
- **S** – Surgery
- **S** – Steroid intake
- **F** – Fracture
- **C** – Cancer

Consider family history, which might be relevant for inflammatory or other nonmusculoskeletal conditions and can aid differential diagnosis.

Explore any previous episodes of the current complaint, other previous or current musculoskeletal problems, any treatment given and the outcome of treatment. Spinal pain may be a progression of the same condition, and a lesion may characteristically present as increasing episodes of worsening pain.

Screening

A biopsychosocial model of pain has been widely adopted by the health community to reflect certain aspects of persistent pain and disability more accurately (Waddell and Aylward, 2010). Biopsychosocial assessment evaluates the integrated 'whole person' and recognises biological, psychological and social components of pain and illness.

To adopt a person-centred active approach to treating musculoskeletal pain and disability, practitioners should screen for *psychological, socioeconomical* and *occupational risk factors* (Fig. 1.9), as well as considering *health comorbidities* and *lifestyle risk factors.*

Psychosocial Factors

Emerging evidence demonstrates that musculoskeletal pain disorders, such as knee, hip, neck, shoulder and back pain, frequently coexist and share common psychosocial

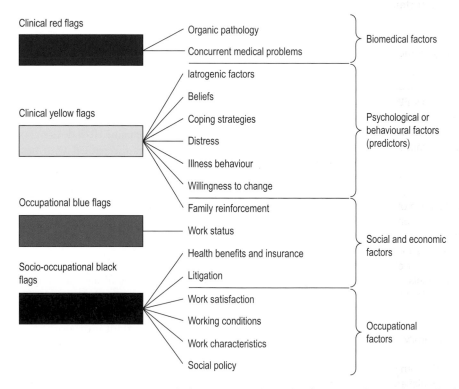

Fig. 1.9 Biological, psychological, socioeconomical and occupational risk factors which may contributing to persistent pain and disability.

risk profiles for pain and disability (Hannibal and Bishop, 2014; Kittelson et al., 2014; Hartvigsen et al., 2018; Lewis and O'Sullivan, 2018; Lin et al., 2020).

Irrespective of body region, there is broad consensus across clinical guidelines and recommendations for best practice, that a shift is needed to focus on the person's context and modifiable psychosocial factors ('yellow flags'), which can influence their pain and disability (Lin et al., 2020; Caneiro et al., 2020).

Evidence also suggests that psychosocial factors can have a greater influence than biomedical or biomechanical factors in the transition from acute to persistent pain (Gatchel et al., 1995; Picavet et al., 2002; Waddell, 2004; Carragee et al., 2005; Chou et al., 2009) and are associated with poor outcomes (Pincus et al., 2013).

Therefore routine assessment of psychosocial factors (i.e. to assess whether these factors may act as a main driver, form a barrier to recovery or a return to usual activity or work) should be embedded into musculoskeletal practice. Such information guides clinical decision making and helps to develop therapeutic targets for patient care.

Context is an important factor to consider in persistent pain and disability. Context is influenced by our attitude, beliefs, knowledge and understanding, emotions and past experience. For example, the context of persistent pain and disability can be influenced by pain belief, coping strategies, misunderstanding of the explanation of diagnosis/scan result by health professionals, or fearing to move, which can lead to avoidance behaviour.

Health Comorbidities

'Comorbidity is associated with worse health outcomes, more complex clinical management, and increased healthcare costs' (Valderas et al., 2009). Several definitions have been suggested for 'comorbidity', but it is essentially the presence of more than one distinct condition in an individual (Valderas et al., 2009). Conditions described as comorbidities are often long-term conditions. They can be present at the same time or successively (one condition occurs after the other).

Patients with multiple long-term conditions are becoming the norm rather than the exception, and the number of people with comorbidities has continued to increase in England from 1.9 million in 2008 to approximately 3 million at the time of writing (Department of Health, 2012).

There are many different possibilities of comorbidities. For example, obesity is known to predispose to other comorbid conditions such as diabetes, cardiovascular diseases, osteoarthritis and depression (Alexander, 2018).

Depression and anxiety disorder are common examples of comorbidity in the mental health field; nearly 60% of those with anxiety also have symptoms of depression and vice versa (Salcedo, 2019). Both are strongly associated with persistent musculoskeletal pain and disability (Bair et al., 2008).

As part of the musculoskeletal assessment, practitioners should explore comorbidities and consider how this may impact on their musculoskeletal health. It is also important to consider each patient's individual needs, preferences for treatment, health priorities, lifestyle and goals. The NICE guideline 'Multimorbidity: clinical assessment and management' provides additional recommendations (National Institute for Health and Care Excellence [NICE], 2016).

Lifestyle Risk Factors

Lifestyle factors such as smoking, obesity, alcohol, poor diet and physical inactivity increase the risk of morbidity and mortality (Department of Health, 2014). They also have a significant impact on musculoskeletal health.

The mnemonic **ABCDEFW** can be a helpful prompt for psychosocial assessment (Hague and Shenker, 2014):

A – Attitude – pain is indicative of severe damage. Passive attitude linked to poor outcome.

B – Belief and behaviour – unhelpful beliefs about pain such as pain means harm; pain behaviour such as passive coping strategies; avoidance of activities due to expectations of pain and possible reinjury.

C – Compensation – ongoing litigation/insurance or compensation issue

D – Diagnosis – misunderstanding about diagnosis (e.g. slipped disc) or different diagnosis by different health professionals

E – Emotion – e.g. fear-avoidance, stress, depression, anxiety, feeling worry

F – Family and friends – social and family context (e.g. overprotective family or family shows no support/ sympathy)

W – Work – delayed return to work is major factor in staying off sick; unsatisfied with their job, poor support from line manager, occupational risk factors such as excessive postural strain

A multicohort study (Virtanen et al., 2018) showed that the most common cause of sickness absence associated with lifestyle factors is musculoskeletal conditions. Therefore practitioners should take account of the potential for musculoskeletal symptoms (e.g. degenerative arthropathy of the knee, persistent low back pain) or potential for nonmusculoskeletal conditions (e.g. vitamin D deficiency, vascular claudication) to be affected by lifestyle factors.

Smoking affects bone mass and increases the risk of osteoporosis and fracture (Yoon et al., 2012). It also increases the risk of developing degenerative disc disease and low back pain (Shiri et al., 2010).

Excessive alcohol reduces normal absorption of vitamin D and calcium, which increases the risk of osteoporosis and affects bone healing and bone health (Mikosch, 2014). Excessive alcohol consumption may also contribute to the development and exacerbation of persistent pain (Zale et al., 2015) via dysregulation of the endogenous opioid system (Egli et al., 2012) and via an increased risk of traumatic injury and deleterious effects on the musculoskeletal system (Brennan et al., 2011; Brennan and Soohoo, 2013).

Physical inactivity has a number of harmful effects on health and well-being. It causes 6% to 10% of the major noncommunicable diseases of coronary heart disease, type 2 diabetes and breast and colon malignancy (Lee and Kean, 2012). It is also associated with musculoskeletal conditions (Holth et al., 2008), symptoms of depression and anxiety (Ströhle, 2009) and is a risk factor for low back pain and disability (Teichtahl et al., 2015).

According to The Lancet Global Burden of Disease reports, *poor diet* now generates more disease than physical inactivity, alcohol and smoking combined (Malhotra et al., 2015). Poor diet has been associated with obesity (Macfarlane et al., 2007; Livingstone and McNaughton, 2016), hypertension (Livingstone and McNaughton, 2016), cardiovascular disease (Vandenkerkhof et al., 2011), type 2 diabetes (Hu et al., 2001), stroke (Strong et al., 2007), gout (Mead et al., 2014), malignancy (Zhang et al., 2019), mental health (e.g. low mood, depression and anxiety) (Scott and Happell, 2011), vitamin D deficiency (Pearce and Cheetham, 2010), vitamin B12 deficiency and folate deficiency anaemia (Allen, 2008).

The association between *obesity* and degenerative knee arthropathy is well documented (Blagojevic et al., 2010; Lee and Kean, 2012). Obesity is also associated with increased risk of diabetes (Hu et al., 2001), malignancy (Lauby-Secretan et al., 2016), persistent low-back

pain, pain-related disability and reduced quality of life (Marcus, 2004; Heuch et al., 2013). It can also be associated with fatty tendons and tendinopathy.

Vitamin D deficiency constitutes a largely unrecognised epidemic worldwide (Holick and Chen, 2008). It has been associated with cardiovascular disease (Ginde et al., 2009; Dobnig et al., 2012), type 2 diabetes (Pittas et al., 2007), bowel and breast cancer (Yin et al., 2009; Chen et al., 2010), multiple sclerosis (Munger et al., 2006) and type 1 diabetes (Zipitis and Akobeng, 2008). It also has been associated with diffuse skeletal pain, low back pain, noninflammatory arthritis and rheumatoid arthritis (Heidari et al., 2010). It can exacerbate bone loss and increase fracture risk (Laird et al., 2010).

> **KEY LIFESTYLE RISK FACTORS FOR MUSCULOSKELETAL CONDITIONS**
> - Smoking
> - Excessive alcohol
> - Physical inactivity
> - Obesity
> - Poor diet

Other Joint Involvement

Other joint involvement gives clues to the patient's pain being associated with systemic joint disease. It will alert the examiner to the presence of inflammatory arthritis, such as rheumatoid arthritis and polymyalgia rheumatica, and also to degenerative arthropathy, all of which have a distinctive pattern of onset and joints affected.

Consider the signs and symptoms of the different forms of inflammatory arthritis. For instance, rheumatoid arthritis often presents with significant early morning stiffness (i.e. more than one hour) and persistent synovitis of unknown cause (which often involves more than one joint), and it affects the small joints of the hands or feet (NICE, 2020).

Axial spondyloarthritis usually occurs before the age of 45, with low back pain of more than 3 months, and it may display four or more features such as buttock pain, waking during the second half of the night due to symptoms, a first-degree relative with spondyloarthritis, and current or past arthritis, enthesitis or psoriasis (NICE, 2017a; NICE, 2021c).

Psoriatic arthritis is likely to be asymmetrical and may present with skin-related symptoms such as a chronic itch, bleeding, scaling and nail involvement (NICE, 2017b).

Polymyalgia rheumatica often has a rapid onset of symmetrical muscle pain in the proximal girdle regions (i.e. shoulder and pelvic girdle), with stiffness lasting for at least 45 minutes after waking or a period of rest, and often accompanied by raised inflammatory markers (erythrocyte sedimentation rate [ESR] and/or C-reactive protein [CRP]) (NICE, 2021b).

Inflammatory joint disease, most notably rheumatoid arthritis, provides a contraindication to manipulative treatment, especially in the cervical spine.

Medications

Medications give a clue to past or underlying disease. For example, the use of tamoxifen or Herceptin may indicate a history of breast cancer, the use of hormone therapy may indicate a history of prostate cancer, the use of anticoagulant and antiplatelet medications may indicate a history of cardiac disease or stroke, and long-term steroids may indicate inflammatory joint disease.

Anticoagulants are a contraindication for spinal manipulation and a caution for the application of the technique for some peripheral joints, because manipulation may cause disruption of capillaries, and the prolonged bleeding time induced by anticoagulant therapy may lead to haematoma formation.

Steroids may not be a contraindication in themselves, but consideration needs to be given to the underlying pathology that requires their prescription.

Antidepressants can give an indication of the emotional state of patients, which may provide a contraindication to some treatments. However, it should also be noted that anticonvulsants and low-dose antidepressants may be used as an adjunct to analgesics in the management of persistent pain.

The quantity and regularity of the dose of analgesic and nonsteroidal antiinflammatory drugs (NSAIDs) provide an indication of the level of pain being experienced by the patient. They can be used as objective markers to monitor the progress of treatment in terms of noting whether higher or lower doses are needed to control the pain.

It is important to consider drug interaction and the side effects of medications. For example, the use of both oral NSAIDs and anticoagulant medication increases the risk of bleeding. If the patient has asthma and is aspirin sensitive, the use of oral NSAIDs may cause severe bronchospasm. The common side effects of co-codamol are constipation, dizziness and drowsiness, which can be unpleasant and unsafe for elderly patients (risk of falls).

Patients can access some common musculoskeletal medications over the counter, without knowing the potential risk of using medications concurrently.

When reviewing a patient's medication, it is important to consider all the medications in relation to each other (polypharmacy) and in relation to the patient's age and general health, particularly liver, heart and kidney health. Due to the increased concurrence of multiple chronic and acute diseases, older people are the main users of healthcare resources, and it has been estimated that more than 10% of the older population receives 10 or more concomitant medicines (Strampelli et al., 2019).

Red Flags

'Red flags' have been used in medicine since 1949, and they became more widely known after the publication of the work of the Clinical Standards Advisory Group in 1994. The profile of red flags has evolved, and they are now recognised as a key component towards patient safety in clinical practice.

Red Flags are possible indicators of serious pathology, including:
- **Malignancy**
- **Infection**
- **Fracture**
- **Cauda equina syndrome (CES)**

They are not diagnostic tests or certain predictors of diagnosis or prognosis. The use of red flags should not replace clinical judgement and reasoning, and they are used as an adjunct to the process (Ferguson et al., 2010). The main role of red flags is that, when combined, they help to raise the practitioner's index of suspicion.

A single red flag would not necessarily provide a strong indication of serious pathology. It should be considered in the context of a person's history (e.g. history of trauma, history of cancer, immunosuppression), symptoms (e.g. onset and progress of pain and neurological deficit) and clinical findings on examination (Mercer et al., 2006; Finucane et al., 2020a).

Prognostic factors, such as age and gender, and risk factors, such as lifestyle factors (e.g. smoking, alcohol), should also be considered.

Individually, each red flag can be significant, but greater emphasis is placed on the presence of concurrent red flags (Greenhalgh and Selfe, 2010). For example, weight loss, history of malignancy or age greater than 55 years would cause some concern individually, but the presence of all

UPDATED HIERARCHICAL LIST OF RED FLAGS

- Age >50 years + history of cancer + unexplained weight loss + failure to improve after 1 month of evidence-based conservative therapy

- Age <10 and >51 years
- Medical history (current or past) of:
  - Cancer
  - Tuberculosis
  - Human immunodeficiency virus (HIV)/acquired immune deficiency syndrome (AIDS) or intravenous drug use
  - Osteoporosis
- Weight loss >10% body weight (3–6 months)
- Severe night pain precluding sleep
- Loss of sphincter tone and altered S4 sensation
- Bladder retention or bowel incontinence
- Positive extensor plantar response

- Age 11–19
- Weight loss 5%–10% body weight (3–6 months)
- Constant progressive pain
- Band-like pain
- Abdominal pain and changed bowel habits, but with no change of medication
- Inability to lie supine
- Bizarre neurological deficit
- Spasm
- Disturbed gait

- Loss of mobility, difficulty with stairs, falls, trips
- Legs misbehave, odd feelings in legs, legs feeling heavy
- Weight loss <5% body weight (3–6 months)
- Smoking
- Systemically unwell
- Trauma
- Bilateral pins and needles in hands and/or feet
- Previous failed treatment
- Thoracic pain
- Headache
- Physical appearance
- Marked partial articular restriction of movement

From Greenhalgh and Selfe (2010). Reprinted by permission of Elsevier Ltd.

three has a sensitivity of nearly 100% for identifying an underlying malignancy (Jarvick and Deyo, 2002).

Red flags indicative of cauda equina syndrome (CES) (i.e. urinary incontinence, saddle anaesthesia or paraesthesia and retention) are a potential surgical emergency and require urgent specialist review (New Zealand Guidelines Group [NZGG], 2004; van Tulder et al., 2006; Royal College of General Practitioners [RCGP], 2009).

Serious pathology as a cause of musculoskeletal conditions is considered rare. For example, serious spinal pathology accounts for approximately 1% in patients with low back pain (Ferguson et al., 2010). However, if suspected, it needs to be managed either as an emergency or as requiring urgent onward referral, as directed by local pathways.

Finucane et al. (2020b) produced a summary to help towards the recognition of serious pathology and suggest that it should be considered as a differential diagnosis if a person presents:

- With escalating pain and progressively worsening symptoms (e.g. gait disturbance, worsening neurological symptoms) that do not respond to conservative management or medication as expected
- As systemically unwell (fever, night sweats, unexplained weight loss, recent infection, rash, respiratory problem)
- With night pain that prevents sleep due to escalating pain and/or difficulty in lying flat.

They further categorise potential serious pathologies into those conditions requiring emergency or urgent referral. Local pathways should always be consulted.

Emergency referral – these serious pathologies must be dealt with on the day as an emergency (Finucane et al., 2020b):

- CES
- Metastatic spinal cord compression (MSCC)
- Spinal Infection
- Septic arthritis

Urgent referral – these pathologies must be managed as onward urgent referral (Finucane et al., 2020b):

- Primary or secondary cancers – if patient becomes systemically unwell, this needs to be escalated to local emergency pathway
- Insufficiency fracture
- Major spinal-related neurological deficit
- Cervical spondylotic myelopathy (CSM)
- Acute inflammatory arthritis and suspected rheumatological conditions

'Safety netting' describes the technique of communicating uncertainty in diagnosis. Patients are provided with

clear information, and a plan is put into place to ensure timely reassessment. Safety netting advice may include information on the natural history of the condition, worrying symptoms to look out for that could lead to the diagnosis being reconsidered and specific information on how and when to seek help (Jones et al., 2019). Written information and patient leaflets can be given to reinforce verbal advice (Jarvis, 2021).

Safety netting is usually conducted alongside the principle of 'watchful wait', where the patient's condition is watched closely but treatment is not given or altered unless symptoms appear or change.

Full documentation is essential throughout the process. That is, the specific advice given should be documented rather than just 'advice given' (Jarvis, 2021).

CLINICAL CONTEXT
- Serious pathology diagnosis in primary care is complex
- Patients rarely present with classic red flags
- Red flags need to be assessed in combination
- Patients often present their symptoms in the context of other illness
- Do not underestimate your clinical judgment and trust if it 'doesn't feel right'
- Should level of suspicion be high, consider onward referral as directed by local pathways. Also 'safety net', apply watchful wait and ensure full documentation.

INSPECTION

After the history is completed, the patient is inspected, suitably undressed and in a good light, paying particular attention to any *bony deformity*, *colour changes*, *muscle wasting* or *swelling*.

INSPECTION
- Bony deformity
- Colour changes
- Muscle wasting
- Swelling

Bony Deformity

This can broadly apply to the posture adopted, but it may also include spinal asymmetry, leg length discrepancy, excessive valgus or varus deformity at joints, bony lumps or exostoses. Obvious distortion of bony or joint contours following trauma could indicate fracture or dislocation.

Colour Changes

Redness may indicate the presence of joint activity, which can be acute inflammation or infection. It is one of the four cardinal signs of inflammation or infection: redness, heat, swelling and pain. There may be signs of bruising following trauma, which may be distal to the site of the lesion, or pallor, mottling or reddening associated with circulatory or sympathetic involvement. The presence of scars and rashes may also be indicative of relevant pathology.

Muscle Wasting

Any obvious muscle wasting is noted. This may have its origin in a neurological condition, which is usually nerve root compression at the relevant spinal level or a neuritis, or as a consequence of disuse, possibly due to pain. The cause of the wasting will usually become apparent as the examination proceeds.

Swelling

Swelling is indicative of the activity within the tissue or joint, resulting from trauma or overuse, as in tenosynovitis, bursitis, arthritis or infection. Swelling that presents immediately indicates bleeding in the area. Other swellings may include haematomas, ganglia, lipomas and soft tissue nodules.

PALPATION

PALPATE A PERIPHERAL JOINT
- Heat
- Swelling
- Synovial thickening

At this stage of the examination, peripheral joints are palpated for signs of activity, associated with inflammatory conditions or infection, in the form of heat, swelling and synovial thickening. It may also be necessary to palpate for peripheral pulses at this stage if circulatory disturbance is suspected.

The area is not palpated for tenderness – this must wait until the end of the examination when the structure at fault has been identified through the rest of the examination procedure.

Heat

The joint is palpated for heat using the back of the hand and comparing the same aspect on each side. The same hand is used throughout because the dominant hand may be a few degrees warmer than the nondominant hand, and may lead to a discrepancy. Any bandaging or support that the patient has been wearing, which could have warmed the area, should be considered.

Swelling

Swelling is often apparent on inspection alone, but it may be palpated for, particularly to detect minor swelling (e.g. in the knee).

Synovial Thickening

Synovial thickening has a 'boggy' feel to it and indicates the presence and level of inflammation in a joint. It is particularly evident in rheumatoid arthritis at the wrist, ankle and knee.

STATE AT REST

The state at rest must be established before any examination requiring joint movement or muscle activity takes place, to provide a baseline against which the effect of the movements applied can be noted. There may or may not be any symptoms at rest but comparison can still be made with subsequent movements, which may produce the symptoms or make them better or worse.

An open question such as 'How do you feel as you are standing/sitting there?' usually draws out the status quo and avoids the leading use of the word 'pain'.

Based on the observation that normal tissue functions painlessly whereas abnormal tissue does not, Cyriax devised a method of applying appropriate stress to the structures surrounding each joint to test their function.

Passive movements are applied to test the so-called inert structures such as joint capsules and ligaments, whereas resisted tests are used to test the contractile structures, incorporating muscle, tendon and attachments to bone. This is the method of applying *selective tension* to tissues (Cyriax, 1982; Cyriax and Cyriax, 1993), and the movements will now be described.

EXAMINATION BY SELECTIVE TENSION

Throughout this discussion of examination by selective tension and within the examination in the following

regional chapters, comparison should be made with the other side, where appropriate.

Active Movements

> **ACTIVE MOVEMENTS**
> - Range
> - Pain
> - Power
> - Willingness
> - Painful arc

Active movements give an idea of the *range* of movement available in the joint, the *pain* experienced by the patient and the *power* in the muscle groups. They are not carried out routinely at all joints because they are nonselective and use both inert and contractile tissues.

However, they are useful in establishing the *willingness* of the patient to perform the movements, as an indicator of the level of pain being experienced within each range. In this role they can act as a guide to the range of movement available before applying passive stresses to the joint and can be used at any joint to gain that information if necessary.

Active movements can also be used to eliminate neighbouring joints as a potential source of pain. For example, as part of the shoulder examination, six active neck movements are performed. If the patient's pain is not reproduced, then the cervical spine is eliminated at that initial stage.

Active movements are also most important in illustrating how willing the patient is to move, with respect to the pain experienced as well as psychosocial factors, and particularly noting any unusual or bizarre responses. The patient's response can be significant in the subsequent selection of treatment techniques.

A particular sign known as the *painful arc* is demonstrated by active movement. By definition, a painful arc is an arc of pain with pain-free movement on either side. It implies that a structure is being compromised at that point of the movement and is a useful finding towards diagnosis.

For example, if the pathology is within the subacromial bursa or at the teno-osseous attachments of supraspinatus, infraspinatus or subscapularis, a painful arc may be found on active abduction at the shoulder, where pain may be provoked within structures as they pass under the coracoacromial arch, before passing beyond it and into the pain-free range. The painful arc is not usually found in isolation, and positive findings on other tests will further incriminate the causative structure.

Passive Movements

> **PASSIVE MOVEMENTS**
> - Pain
> - Range
> - End-feel

Passive movements test the *inert structures* that include the joint capsule, joint menisci, ligaments, fascia, bursae, dura mater and the dural nerve root sleeve. Relaxed muscle and tendon can act as inert structures when they are stretched by their opposite passive movement. Passive movements principally give information on *pain*, *range* and *end-feel*.

The observation of pain and range of movement will be familiar to all practitioners working with soft tissue lesions. However, the notion of end-feel may be a new concept that is particularly valuable in the assessment of the soft tissues and is inherent in the musculoskeletal medicine approach.

End-feel is the specific sensation imparted through the practitioner's hands at the end of passive movement (Cyriax, 1982; Cyriax and Cyriax, 1993).

Normal End-feel

> **NORMAL END-FEEL**
> - Hard
> - Soft
> - Elastic

Normal end-feel is divided into three categories: hard, soft and elastic. Normal bone-to-bone approximation, as in extension of the elbow, gives a characteristic *hard end-feel* to passive movement.

A *soft end-feel* is characteristic of a stop to the movement brought about by approximation of tissue, as in passive knee or elbow flexion.

An *elastic end-feel* is felt when the tissues are placed on a passive stretch and is the elastic resistance produced in the inert tissues at the end of range in normal joints. Examples are provided in stretching the end of range of lateral rotation at the shoulder or hip.

There may be a range of end-feels within the 'elastic' group, but all are indicative of normal tissue tension, such as the 'leathery' end-feel of passive pronation and supination of the forearm, or the even tighter 'rubbery'

end-feel of ankle plantarflexion and wrist flexion where the resistance to the movement is in part provided by the tendons spanning the joint.

Pain is a component at the end of range of normal movements, acting as a protection and to prevent continuation of movement to the point of producing tissue damage.

Abnormal End-feel

> **ABNORMAL END-FEEL**
> - 'Hard'
> - Springy
> - Empty

The sensation imparted in an abnormal end-feel falls into three categories: 'hard', springy and empty.

The cause of an abnormal *'hard' end-feel* is different from that of the normal hard bone-to-bone end-feel, and it is a particular feature of the movements limited in arthritis.

In mild arthropathy (e.g. degenerative arthropathy of the hip or 'frozen shoulder'), joint movement is initially limited by pain, and involuntary muscle spasm halts the movement (Cyriax, 1982). This involuntary muscle spasm provides a brake to the movement and feels 'hard' to the examiner. The end-feel feels harder than expected, but in the early stages some elasticity is preserved.

Mild degenerative arthropathy of the hip, for example, may produce a 'hard' end-feel on either passive flexion or medial rotation, but it should be emphasised that this is not caused by bony degenerative change blocking the joint movement. This difference is important because it aids the practitioner in the selection of treatment techniques.

In moderate degenerative arthropathy, the 'hard' end-feel is also due to capsular or ligamentous contracture (Cyriax, 1982). The capsular resistance together with the involuntary muscle spasm may still allow some 'give' at the end of range, but it will not feel as elastic as the earlier stage.

In severe degenerative arthropathy, bony changes may occur, leading to a genuine hard end-feel and the crepitus associated with advanced degeneration, as well as that arising from involuntary muscle spasm and capsular contracture.

An abnormal *springy end-feel* is associated with mechanical joint displacement, usually a loose body. The sensation imparted to the practitioner is one of not quite getting to the end of range, with the joint springing or bouncing back. It is similar to the sensation of trying to close a door with a small piece of rubber or grit caught in the hinge that causes the door to spring open again.

An *empty end-feel* occurs when the practitioner does not have the opportunity to appreciate the true end-feel because the patient calls a halt to the movement prematurely and urgently because of pain, often raising a hand to prevent further movement. The sensation imparted to the practitioner is 'empty', as described, in that the complaint of serious pain comes on before any spasm or tissue resistance.

The empty end-feel can be associated with serious pathology such as fracture, neoplasm or septic arthritis. A further cause may be a highly irritable lesion such as acute subacromial bursitis where the empty end-feel is instantly apparent on passive abduction of the shoulder.

The abnormal 'hard' end-feel associated with involuntary muscle spasm is different from that produced by voluntary muscle spasm. Voluntary muscle spasm halts the movement abruptly and indicates acute pain or serious pathology. If the pain is very severe, it may also be associated with an empty end-feel.

The assessment of end-feel together with the restriction of movement at each joint produces a particular pattern that is either 'capsular' or 'noncapsular'.

Capsular Pattern

> **CAPSULAR PATTERN**
> - Indicates an arthropathy
> - Varies from joint to joint
> - Limits movement in a fixed proportion

The *capsular pattern* is a limitation of movement in a defined pattern that is specific to each joint and indicates the presence of an arthropathy. The pattern varies from joint to joint and is characterised by limitation of movement in a fixed proportion. It is the same whatever the cause of the arthropathy (Cyriax, 1982; Cyriax and Cyriax, 1993), and the history will suggest whether it is degenerative, inflammatory or traumatic.

Characteristically, the movements restricted in the capsular pattern take on the 'hard' end-feel of arthropathy, which is different from the expected normal elastic capsular resistance.

The reason for the development of the capsular pattern is not really understood but could be the presence of joint effusion, causing the joint to assume the position of ease and/or protective muscle spasm (Eyring and Murray, 1964). An effusion is often present in arthritis, and the acuteness of the condition determines the quantity of the effusion. Joints with symptomatic effusions are held in the aforementioned position of ease, and movements out of this position produce pain.

In addition, the involuntary muscle spasm, in protecting the painful, inflamed joint, prevents use, and if the range of movement is underused, it will become limited. In arthropathy, the individual joints resent some movements more than others; hence the capsule contracts disproportionately, making some movements more limited than others and giving rise to the characteristic pattern of limitation.

For example, the position of minimum pressure for the elbow was found to be between 30 and 70 degrees of flexion. The pressure was not influenced by either pronation or supination. This aligns with the capsular pattern of the elbow joint which is proportionally more limitation of flexion than extension but without involvement of pronation or supination (Eyring and Murray, 1964).

The capsular patterns described in Table 1.2 provide a useful guide to the diagnosis of arthropathy but research support is mixed.

Noncapsular Pattern

> **NONCAPSULAR PATTERN**
> - Intra-articular displacement
> - Ligamentous lesion
> - Extra-articular lesion

The *noncapsular pattern* of a joint is, quite simply, anything other than the capsular pattern. That is, it is a limitation of movement that does not conform to the capsular pattern and occurs as a result of a component or part of the joint being affected rather than the whole joint.

A lesion such as an intra-articular displacement produces the noncapsular pattern, which may be evident at the spinal joints, in a loose body at the elbow joint or a meniscal tear at the knee. A meniscal lesion in a degenerative joint may produce a noncapsular pattern superimposed on the capsular pattern.

A ligamentous lesion will give pain and possible limitation of the movement that stretches the structure. However, injury to ligaments that form an integral part of the capsule itself, such as the anterior talofibular ligament of the ankle and the medial collateral ligament of the knee, cause a secondary capsulitis, and hence a

TABLE 1.2   Capsular Patterns

Joint	Capsular Pattern
Shoulder joint	Most limitation of lateral rotation Less limitation of abduction Least limitation of medial rotation
Elbow joint	More limitation of flexion than extension
Radioulnar joints	Pain at end of range of pronation and supination
Wrist joint	Equal limitation of flexion and extension Eventual fixation in the midposition
First carpometacarpal joint	Most limitation of extension
Metacarpophalangeal joints	Limitation of radial deviation and extension Joints fix in flexion and drift into ulnar deviation
Interphalangeal joints	Slightly more limitation of flexion than extension
Cervical spine	*Demonstrated by the cervical spine as a whole*: Equal limitation of rotations Equal limitation of side flexions Some limitation of extension Usually full flexion
Thoracic spine	*Demonstrated by the thoracic spine as a whole*: Equal limitation of rotations Equal limitation of side flexions Some limitation of extension Usually full flexion
Hip joint	Most limitation of medial rotation Less limitation of flexion and abduction Least limitation of extension
Knee joint	More limitation of flexion than extension
Ankle joint	More limitation of plantarflexion than dorsiflexion
Subtalar joint	Increasing limitation of supination Eventual fixation in pronation
Midtarsal joint	Limitation of adduction and inversion. Forefoot fixes in abduction and eversion
First metatarsophalangeal joint	Marked limitation of extension Some limitation of flexion
Other metatarsophalangeal joints	*May vary*: Tend to fix in extension
Interphalangeal joints	Fix in flexion
Lumbar spine	*Demonstrated by the lumbar spine as a whole*: Most limitation of extension Equal limitation of side flexions Usually full flexion

noncapsular pattern is superimposed on the capsular pattern.

Because a contractile unit can be stretched by passive movement, the unit may respond as an inert structure when relaxed, producing pain when it is stretched by the passive movement opposite to its functional active movement.

For example, the subscapularis muscle and tendon, which produce medial rotation at the shoulder, will be stretched by passive lateral rotation. This is also particularly evident in acute tenosynovitis when the tendon involved is pulled through its inflamed synovial sheath. For example, in acute tenosynovitis at the wrist, pain will be produced on the appropriate resisted test and the opposite passive movement, for example, passive thumb flexion and wrist ulnar deviation in de Quervain's tenosynovitis.

An extra-articular lesion, such as bursitis, produces a noncapsular pattern and commonly presents as a 'muddle' or mixture of signs involving passive and resisted tests. Any movement that squeezes or stretches the inflamed bursa will produce positive signs.

Resisted Tests

RESISTED TESTS
- Pain
- Power

Resisted isometric muscle tests assess the *contractile unit* – comprising the muscle, musculotendinous junction, tendon and the teno-osseous attachment to bone – for *pain* and *power*. Tendon is not strictly a contractile structure but is tested as part of the functional contractile unit.

When assessing the resisted tests, it is important to look for reproduction of the patient's presenting pain. There are specific points to bear in mind, which ensure that only the contractile unit is being tested rather than the inert structures, as far as possible. It is accepted that, although joint movement may be inhibited, isometric muscle contraction will cause compression and joint shearing and a rise in intradiscal pressure in the spinal joints (Lamb, 1994).

The joint should be placed in the midposition with the inert structures relaxed so that minimal stress falls upon them. The muscle group is tested isometrically, as strongly as possible, encouraging maximal voluntary contraction without allowing movement to occur at the joint. This also ensures that minor lesions will be detected.

The patient's and practitioner's body positioning should be such that all muscles that are not being tested are eliminated from the testing procedure. Appropriate positioning will be demonstrated within each of the chapters in Section 2.

In addition to the active, passive and resisted tests, a neurological examination is included as part of the routine examination for a spinal joint, testing for root signs (see Chapters 8, 9, 13 and 14).

After the history and examination sequence are completed, the causative structure will, in almost all cases, have been identified (Cyriax, 1982; Cyriax and Cyriax, 1993).

RESISTED TESTS MAY PRODUCE ANY OF SEVERAL FINDINGS, EACH OF WHICH HAS A DIFFERENT IMPLICATION. THE TEST MAY BE:
- Strong and painless – normal
- Strong and painful – contractile lesion
- Weak and painless – neurological weakness; complete rupture
- Weak and painful – partial rupture or serious pathology such as fracture or bone tumour
- Painful on repetition – claudication or provocation of overuse injury or less irritable lesion
- All resisted tests about the joint painful or juddering – serious pathology, or marked psychosocial component
---

PALPATION

At this stage, palpation of the structure determined to be at fault may be made to identify the site of the lesion to which appropriate treatment can be applied.

If the diagnosis is still unclear, further tests and imaging may be required.

CONSIDERATIONS FOR CLINICAL DIAGNOSIS AND MANAGEMENT ON COMPLETION OF THE ASSESSMENT
- Is this a musculoskeletal or nonmusculoskeletal condition?
- What else could be the cause of presentation?
- Consider red flags, neurological, internal/visceral, cardiovascular, inflammatory conditions, psychosocial involvement
- What, if any, diagnostic investigations are required?
- Are there any psychosocial factors, comorbidities and lifestyle factors that may contribute to or exacerbate symptoms?
- What are the patient's goals and expectations?

Further Investigations

At the end of the examination, the practitioner may consider further investigations such as blood tests, radiological imaging and other diagnostic procedures. Investigations should be guided by the suspected cause, and as an extension to the clinical examination process within clinical reasoning.

Practitioners should understand the indications and limitations of different investigations to inform decision making. Additional training is often required to be able to refer for further investigations and to ensure appropriate referral and a good level of understanding for the interpretation of results, to correlate clinical findings.

> **CONSIDER FURTHER INVESTIGATION IF IT HELPS:**
> - to make or confirm diagnosis
> - differential diagnosis
> - to add value to the patient's management plan
> - to direct appropriate onward referral, including emergency/urgent referral for red flags, such as primary malignancy or metastatic tumours, infection or septic arthritis, inflammatory arthropathy and fracture/dislocation, surgery, rheumatology, pain team or other medical specialities (e.g. a vascular or neurological team)

It is also important to be familiar with local referral guidelines, referral pathways and the expertise of all members of the multidisciplinary team, to optimise the integration of patient care.

Indications for Blood Tests

Blood tests can be considered if the practitioner suspects: serious pathology (e.g. myeloma screening), infection, inflammation, inflammatory arthritis (e.g. rheumatoid arthritis, axial spondyloarthritis), systemic conditions such as type II diabetes, thyroid disease and vitamin deficiency.

Should the symptoms be associated with a nonmusculoskeletal condition, appropriate onward referral should be made according to local referral guidelines and pathways. For example, for suspected rheumatoid arthritis, a blood test for rheumatoid factor and anti-cyclic citrullinated peptide (CCP) antibodies (if they are negative for rheumatoid factor) can be considered (NICE, 2020). For patients presenting with symptoms of polymyalgia rheumatica and older than the age of 50, blood tests requesting an erythrocyte sedimentation rate (ESR)/plasma viscosity and/or C-reactive protein (CRP), in addition to other blood tests, help to rule in/out polymyalgia rheumatica (NICE, 2021c).

Radiological Imaging

Imaging in musculoskeletal medicine is most effective when used as an extension to the clinical examination process.

Table 1.3 considers the indications and pros and cons of the different imaging, nerve conduction and electromyographic investigations.

> **DECISION CONSIDERATIONS FOR RADIOLOGICAL INVESTIGATION**
> - Does it help to answer a clinical question or add value to the patient's management plan and/or onward referral following clinical examination?
> - Local policies and referral guidelines – cost, availability, indications and contraindications
> - Clinical guidelines and evidence
> - Patient's choice and consent
> - Patient's expectations
> - Radiation exposure (Table 1.4)

TABLE 1.3   To Show Different Types of Imaging and Investigations

Investigation	Indication	Pros and *cons*
X-ray	**Indication:** Bones and joints pathology **Example:** Arthritis, fracture, dislocation, calcification/ossification, prosthesis loosening, tumour, infection, deformities.	• Cheap, quick and available • Plain film X-ray prior to injection may be best practice to avoid possible incidental findings • Can be used as baseline • Can be imprecise • *Radiation*
Ultrasound scan (USS)	**Indication:** Superficial soft tissues; extra-articular pathology **Example:** Tendon, tendon sheath, bursa, calcification, plantar fascia, ganglion/cyst, ligament	• Portability • Quick and dynamic assessment • Particularly useful in shoulder – subacromial pain syndrome (SAPS), rotator cuff tendon pathology, acromioclavicular joint (ACJ) arthropathy • Noninvasive as no ionising radiation • Patient friendly and good level of patient satisfaction due to immediate feedback • *Poor quality for deep or intra-articular pathology* • *Poor quality if limited movements and obese patient* • *Operator dependent and machine dependent* • *Need expert interpretation*

Continued

TABLE 1.3   To Show Different Types of Imaging and Investigations—Cont'd

Investigation	Indication	Pros and *cons*
Magnetic resonance imaging (MRI)	**Indication-** Intra-articular pathology, deeper soft tissues or joints **Example:** Intervertebral disc, spinal canal and nerve root, spinal cord, bone marrow, most ligaments, articular cartilage, meniscus, some labrum tear (with contrast)	• Detailed and good quality image- all around best imaging • More comprehensive image of bones and deeper soft tissues compared with ultrasound scan (USS) • Absence of ionising radiation • *Costly* • *Metallic objects to consider (e.g. pace maker or cardiac defibrillator device)* • *Claustrophobic* • *Takes 20–30 min each area. Some patients unable to tolerate*
Contrast agents	**Indication:** Deep soft tissues pathology, specific organs, blood vessels or tissues, when images not clearly evident on conventional radiology **Example:** Labral tear, capsular damage, instability, ligament injuries	• Can be used in X-ray and MRI to improve the visibility of pathologies • Low level of adverse reaction (0.004%) • Pros and cons as per MRI • *Magnetic resonance angiograms (MRAs) have high false positives, some studies show 37% accuracy in imaging shoulder labral tears*
Computed tomography (CT) scan	**Indication:** Great for bone loss and instability; often considered prior to surgery if bone loss is of major concern. CT scan and computer software used in planning for hip, shoulder replacements and correcting fractures in order to customise **Example:** Fracture and arthritis, reviewing osseous union	• Quick • Offer three-dimensional (3D) imaging • Has the best 3D bone anatomy, if metal work in situ (e.g. for those who are not eligible for MRI) • *More ionising radiation than X-ray*
Isotope bone scan	**Indication:** Localised bone pathologies; used as a complementary study to further investigate abnormalities found on other diagnostic images (x-ray, CT or MRI) **Example:** Primary bony malignancies or metastatic disease, Paget disease, fractures from osteoporosis, avascular necrosis, infection	• To evaluate and localise bony pathologies • *Radiation, some patients may not be able to tolerate (e.g. patients may have to stay still for prolonged period of time; and it can take up to 4 h)*
Nerve conduction study and electromyography (EMG)	**Indication:** peripheral nerve and muscle disorders **Example:** peripheral nerve entrapment such as carpal tunnel syndrome and tarsal tunnel syndrome, polyneuropathy such as diabetics neuropathy	• Generally safe with no long-term side effects and few contraindications • *Can be uncomfortable for patients* • *Be cautious with patients with some pacemakers* • *Be cautious with patients on anticoagulant medication*

TABLE 1.4 Radiation Doses From Common Diagnostic Imaging Tests

Imaging Modality	Specific Test	Effective Radiation Dose (Approximate)	Comparison With Natural Background Radiation in Years	Estimated Lifetime Risk of Fatal Cancer*
X-ray	X-ray spine	1.5 millisievert (mSv)	6 months	Very low
	X-ray chest	0.1 mSv	10 days	Minimal
	X-ray extremity	0.001 mSv	3 h	Negligible
	X-ray upper gastrointestinal (GI)	6 mSv	2 years	Low
	X-ray lower GI	8 mSv	3 years	Low
	X-ray intraoral (dental)	0.005 mSv	1 day	Negligible
	Intravenous pyelogram (IVP)	3 mSv	1 year	Low
Computed tomography (CT) scan	CT head	2 mSv	8 months	Very low
	CT head (with contrast)	4 mSv	16 months	Low
	CT spine	6 mSv	2 years	Low
	CT chest	7 mSv	2 years	Low
	CT chest (lung cancer screening, low-dose CT scan)	1.5 mSv	6 months	Very low
	CT abdomen and pelvis	10 mSv	3 years	Low
	CT abdomen and pelvis (with contrast)	20 mSv	7 years	Moderate
	Coronary CT angiography (CTA)	12 mSv	4 years	Low
	Cardiac CT for calcium scoring	3 mSv	1 year	Low
Nuclear Medicine	Positron emission tomography (PET)/CT scan	25 mSv	8 years	Moderate
	Bone densitometry (DXA) scan	0.001 mSv	3 h	Negligible

Kolla et al. (2017) and RadiologyInfo.org. (2022).

REVIEW QUESTIONS

1. Can you explain the differences between the terms somatic referred pain, radicular pain and radiculopathy?
2. What is the significance of the referral patterns of paraesthesia, and edge and aspect?
3. Explain the term multisegmental pain; which structures can give rise to this pain distribution?
4. Consider the three types of the onset of pathology: sudden, gradual and insidious; which one is more likely to be a red flag?
5. Explain the terms 'capsular pattern' and 'empty end-feel'.

REFERENCES

Adams, M., Bogduk, N., Burton, K., et al., 2012. The Biomechanics of Back Pain, third ed. Churchill Livingstone, Edinburgh.

Albrecht, D., Ahmed, S., Kettner, N., et al., 2018. Neuroinflammation of the spinal cord and nerve roots in chronic radicular pain patients. Pain 159 (5), 968.

Alexander, L., 2018. Diseases Related to Obesity. Obesity Medicine Association, Centennial.

Allen, L.H., 2008. Causes of vitamin B12 and folate deficiency. Food Nutr. Bull. 29 (Suppl. 2), S20–S34.

Aprill, C., Dwyer, A., Bogduk, N., 1989. Cervical apophyseal joint pain patterns. II: a clinical evaluation. Spine 15, 458–461.

Bair, M.J., Wu, J., Damush, T.M., et al., 2008. Association of depression and anxiety alone and in combination with chronic musculoskeletal pain in primary care patients. Psychosom. Med. 70 (8), 890–897.

Baron, R., Binder, A., Attal, N., et al., 2016. Neuropathic low back pain in clinical practice. Eur. J. Pain 20 (6), 861–873.

Beckman, H.B., Frankel, R.M., 1984. The effect of physician behaviour on the collection of data. Ann. Intern. Med. 101, 692–696.

Blagojevic, M., Jinks, C., Jeffery, A., et al., 2010. Risk factors for onset of osteoarthritis of the knee in older adults: a systematic review and meta-analysis. Osteoarthritis Cartilage 18 (1), 24–33.

Blau, J.N., 1989. Time to let the patient speak. Br. Med. J. 298, 39.

Bogduk, N., 1982a. The clinical anatomy of the cervical dorsal rami. Spine 7, 35–45.

Bogduk, N., Wilson, A.S., Tynan, W., 1982b. The human lumbar dorsal rami. J. Anat. 134, 383–397.

Bogduk, N., 1994. Innervation, pain patterns and mechanisms of pain production. In: Twomey, L.T. (Ed.), Clinics in Physical Therapy, Physical Therapy of the Low Back, second ed. Churchill Livingstone, Edinburgh, pp. 93–109.

Bogduk, N., McGuirk, B., 2002. Assessment. In: Bogduk, N. McGuirk, B. (Eds.) Medical Management of Acute and Chronic Low Back Pain. An Evidence-Based Approach: Pain Research and Clinical Management, vol. 13. Elsevier Science, Amsterdam, pp. 127–138.

Bogduk, N., 2009. On the definitions and physiology of back pain, referred pain, and radicular pain. Pain 147 (1), 17–19.

Bogduk, N., 2023. Clinical and Radiological Anatomy of the Lumbar Spine, sixth ed. Churchill Livingstone, Edinburgh.

Boswell, M.V., Singh, V., Staats, P.S., et al., 2003. Accuracy of precision diagnostic blocks in the diagnosis of chronic spinal pain of facet or zygapophysial joint origin. Pain Phys. 6, 449–456.

Bove, G.M., Saheen, A., Bajwa, Z., 2005. Subjective nature of lower limb radicular pain. J. Manipulative. Physiol. Ther. 28 (1), 12–14.

Brennan, P.L., Schutte, K.K., SooHoo, S., et al., 2011. Painful medical conditions and alcohol use: a prospective study among older adults. Pain Med. 12, 1049–1059.

Brennan, P.L., Soohoo, S., 2013. Pain and use of alcohol in later life: prospective evidence from the health and retirement study. J. Aging Health 25, 656–677.

Caneiro, J.P., Roos, E.M., Barton, C.J., et al., 2020. It is time to move beyond 'body region silos' to manage musculoskeletal pain: five actions to change clinical practice. Br. J. Sports Med. 54, 438–439.

Carragee, E.J., Alamin, T.F., Miller, J.L., et al., 2005. Discographic, MRI and psychosocial determinants of low back pain disability and remission: a prospective study in subjects with benign persistent back pain. Spine J. 5, 24–35.

Chartered Society of Physiotherapy, 2006a. Clinical Guidelines for the Physiotherapy Management of Persistent Low Back Pain (LBP): Part 1 Exercise. CSP, London.

Chartered Society of Physiotherapy, 2006b. Clinical Guidelines for the Physiotherapy Management of Persistent Low Back Pain (LBP): Part 2 Manual Therapy. CSP, London.

Chen, P., Hu, P., Xie, D., et al., 2010. Meta-analysis of vitamin D, calcium and the prevention of breast cancer. Breast Cancer Res. Treat. 121 (2), 469–477.

Chimenti, R.L., Frey-Law, L.A., Sluka, K.A., 2018. A mechanism based approach to physical therapist management of pain. Phys. Ther. 98 (5), 302–314.

Chou, R., Fu, R., Carrino, J.A., et al., 2009. Imaging strategies for low-back pain: systematic review and meta-analysis. Lancet 373, 463–472.

Conesa, S.H., Argote, M.L., 1976. A Visual Aid to the Examination of Nerve Roots. Baillière Tindall, London.

Cooper, G., Bailey, B., Bogduk, N., 2007. Cervical zygapophyseal joint pain maps. Am. Acad. Pain Med. 8, 344–352.

Cyriax, J., 1982. Textbook of Orthopaedic Medicine, eighth ed. Baillière Tindall, London.

Cyriax, J., Cyriax, P., 1993. Cyriax's Illustrated Manual of Orthopaedic Medicine. Butterworth Heinemann, Oxford.

Department of Health (DoH), 2009. Reference guide to consent for examination or treatment, second ed. Department of Health., https://www.gov.uk/government/publications/reference-guide-to-consent-for-examination-or-treatment-second-edition. Accessed 3 September 2021.

Department of Health (DoH), 2012. Long Term Conditions Compendium of Information, third ed. Department of Health., https://www.gov.uk/government/publications/long-term-conditions-compendium-of-information-third-edition. Accessed 3 September 2021.

Department of Health (DoH), 2014. Comorbidities: A framework of principles for system-wide action. Department of Health., https://assets.publishing.service.gov.uk/government/uploads/system/uploads/attachment_data/file/307143/Comorbidities_framework.pdf. Accessed 3 September 2021.

Dilley, A., Lynn, B., Pang, S.J., 2005. Pressure and stretch mechanosensitivity of peripheral nerve fibres following local inflammation of the nerve trunk. Pain 117 (3), 462–472.

Dobnig, H., Pilz, S., Scharnagl, H., et al., 2012. Independent association of low serum 25-hydroxyvitamin D and 1,25-dihydroxyvitamin D levels with all-cause and cardiovascular mortality. Arch. Intern. Med. 168, 1340–1349.

Egli, M., Koob, G.F., Edwards, S., 2012. Alcohol dependence as a chronic pain disorder. Neurosci. Biobehav. Rev. 36, 2179–2192.

Eyring, E.J., Murray, W.R., 1964. The effect of joint position on the pressure of intraarticular effusion. J. Bone Joint Surg. 46A, 1235–1241.

Farasyn, A., 2007. Referred muscle pain is primarily peripheral in origin: the barrier-dam theory. Med. Hypotheses 68, 144–150.

Ferguson, F., Holdsworth, L., Rafferty, D., 2010. Low back pain and physiotherapy use of red flags: the evidence from Scotland. Physiotherapy. 96, 282–328.

Finucane, L.M., Downie, A., Mercer, C., et al., 2020. International framework for red flags for potential serious spinal pathologies. J. Orthop. Sports Phys. Ther. 50 (7), 350–372.

Finucane, L., Cumming, D., Griffiths, B., et al., 2020b. Guidance to recognise serious pathology as a cause of musculoskeletal symptoms requiring urgent or emergency referral to secondary care. Positioning Paper. NHS England.

Furman, M.B., Johnson, S.C., 2019. Induced lumbosacral radicular symptom referral patterns: a descriptive study. Spine J. 19 (1), 163–170.

Galea, M., 2014. Neuroanatomy of the nociceptive system. In: van Griensven, H., Strong, J., Unruh, A.M. (Eds.), Pain: A Textbook for Health Professionals, second ed. Churchill Livingstone, Edinburgh.

Gatchel, R.J., Polatin, P.B., Mayer, T.G., 1995. The dominant role of psychosocial risk factors in the development of chronic low back pain disability. Spine 20 (24), 2702–2709.

Ginde, A.A., Scragg, R., Schwartz, R.S., et al., 2009. Prospective study of serum 25-hydroxyvitamin D level, cardiovascular disease mortality and all-cause mortality in older U.S. adults. J. Am. Geriatr. Soc. 57 (9), 1595–1603.

Gnatz, S.M., 1991. Referred pain syndromes of the head and neck. Phys. Med. Rehabil. 5 (3), 585–596.

Greenhalgh, S., Selfe, J., 2010. Red Flags II – A Guide to Solving Serious Pathology of the Spine. Churchill Livingstone, Edinburgh.

Hague, M., Shenker, N., 2014. How to investigate: chronic pain. Best Pract. Res. Clin. Rheumatol. 28 (6), 860–874.

Hannibal, K.E., Bishop, M.D., 2014. Chronic stress, cortisol dysfunction, and pain: a psychoneuroendocrine rationale for stress management in pain rehabilitation. Phys. Ther. 4 (94), 1816–1825.

Hartvigsen, J., Hancock, M.J., Kongsted, A., et al., 2018. What low back pain is and why we need to pay attention. Lancet 391, 2356–2367.

Heidari, B., Shirvani, J.S., Firouzjahi, A., et al., 2010. Association between nonspecific skeletal pain and vitamin D deficiency. Int. J. Rheum. Dis. 13 (4), 340–346.

Heuch, I., Heuch, I., Hagen, K., et al., 2013. Body mass index as a risk factor for developing chronic low back pain: a follow-up in the Nord-Trøndelag Health Study. Spine 38 (2), 133–139.

Hodges, P.W., Coppieters, M.W., MacDonald, D., et al., 2013. New insight into motor adaptation to pain revealed by a combination of modelling and empirical approaches. Eur. J. Pain 17 (8), 1138–1146.

Holick, M.F., Chen, T.C., 2008. Vitamin D deficiency: a world wide problem health consequences. Am. J. Clin. Nutr. 87 (Suppl) 1080S1086S

Holth, H.S., Werpen, H.K.B., Zwart, J.A., et al., 2008. Physical inactivity is associated with chronic musculoskeletal complaints 11 years later: results from the Nord-Trøndelag Health Study. BMC Musculoskelet. Disord. 9 (1), 1–7.

Hu, F.B., Manson, J.E., Stampfer, M.J., et al., 2001. Diet, lifestyle, and the risk of type 2 diabetes mellitus in women. N. Engl. J. Med. 345 (11), 790–797.

Hunter, D., Bomford, R.R., 1963. Hutchison's Clinical Methods, fourteenth ed. Saunders, Elsevier.

Inman, V.T., Saunders, J.B., 1944. Referred pain from skeletal structures. J. Nerv. Ment. Dis. 99, 660–667.

International Association for the Study of Pain (IASP), 2021. IASP Taxonomy. http://www.iasp-pain.org/Education/Content.aspx?ItemNumber=1698&navItemNumber=576. Accessed 3 September 2021.

Itomi, K., Kakigi, R., Maeda, K., et al., 2000. Dermatome versus homunculus; detailed topography of the primary somatosensory cortex following trunk stimulation. Clin. Neurophysiol. 111 (3), 405–412.

Jarvick, J.G., Deyo, R.A., 2002. Diagnostic evaluation of low back pain with emphasis on imaging. Ann. Intern. Med. 137, 586–597.

Jarvis, S., 2021. Playing it safe – safety netting advice. https://mdujournal.themdu.com/issue-archive/issue-4/playing-it-safe—safety-netting-advice. Accessed 3 September 2021.

Jones, D., Dunn, L., Watt, I., et al., 2019. Safety netting for primary care. Br. J. Gen. Pract. 69 (678), e70–e79.

Kellgren, J.H., 1938. Observations on referred pain from muscle. Clin. Sci. 3, 175–190.

Kellgren, J.H., 1939. On the distribution of pain arising from deep somatic structures with charts of segmental pain areas. Clin. Sci. 4, 35–46.

Kittelson, A.J., George, S.Z., Maluf, K.S., et al., 2014. Future directions in painful knee osteoarthritis: harnessing complexity in a heterogeneous population. Phys. Ther. 94, 422–432.

Kolla, B.C., Roy, S.S., Duval, S., et al., 2017. Cardiac imaging methods for chemotherapy-related cardiotoxicity screening and related radiation exposure: Current practice and trends. Anticancer Res. 37 (5), 2445–2449.

Laird, E., Ward, M., McSorley, E., et al., 2010. Vitamin D and bone health: Potential mechanisms. Nutrients 2 (7), 693–724.

Lamb, D.W., 1994. A review of manual therapy for spinal pain. In: Boyling, J.D., Palastanga, N. (Eds.), Grieve's Modern Manual Therapy, second ed. Churchill Livingstone, Edinburgh.

Lauby-Secretan, B., Scoccianti, C., Loomis, D., et al., 2016. Body fatness and cancer–viewpoint of the IARC working group. N. Engl. J. Med 375 (8), 794–798.

Lee, M.W.L., McPhee, R.W., Stringer, M.D., 2008. An evidence-based approach to human dermatomes. Clin. Anat. 21, 363–373.

Lee, R., Kean, W.F., 2012. Obesity and knee osteoarthritis. Inflammopharmacology 20, 53–58.

Lewis, J., O'Sullivan, P., 2018. Is it time to reframe how we care for people with non-traumatic musculoskeletal pain? Br. J. Sports. Med. 52 1543–154

Lin, I., Wiles, L., Waller, R., et al., 2020. What does best practice care for musculoskeletal pain look like? Eleven consistent recommendations from high-quality clinical practice guidelines: systematic review. Br. J. Sports Med. 54, 79–86.

Livingstone, K.M., McNaughton, S.A., 2016. Diet quality is associated with obesity and hypertension in Australian adults: a cross sectional study. BMC Public Health 16 (1), 1–10.

Macfarlane, G.J., Jones, G.T., Knekt, P., et al., 2007. Is the report of widespread body pain associated with long-term increased mortality? Data from the mini-Finland health survey. Rheumatology 46, 805–807.

McMahon, S.B., Dmitrieva, N., Koltzenburg, M., 1995. Visceral pain. Br. J. Anaesth. 75, 132–144.

Malhotra, A., Noakes, T., Phinney, S., 2015. It is time to bust the myth of physical inactivity and obesity: you cannot outrun a bad diet. Br. J. Sports Med. 49, 967–968.

Manchikanti, L., Singh, V., Pampati, V., et al., 2002. Is there correlation of facet joint pain in lumbar and cervical spine? Pain Phys. 5 (4), 365–371.

Manchikanti, L., Staats, P.S., Singh, V., et al., 2003. Evidence-based practice guidelines for interventional techniques in the management of chronic spinal pain. Pain Phys. 6 (1), 3–80.

Manchikanti, L., Boswell, M.V., Singh, V., et al., 2004. Prevalence of facet joint pain in chronic spinal pain of cervical, thoracic, and lumbar regions. BMC Musculoskelet. Disord. 5, 15.

Marcus, D.A., 2004. Obesity and the impact of chronic pain. Clin. J. Pain 20 (3), 186–191.

Martinez-Calderon, J., Jenson, M.P., Morales-Asencio, J.M. et al., 2019. Pain catastrophizing and function in individuals with chroninc musculoskeletal pain: A systematic review and meta-analysis. Clin. J. Pain 35(3), 279–293.

Mead, T., Arabindoo, K., Smith, B., 2014. Managing gout: there's more we can do. J. Fam. Pract. 63 (12), 707–714.

Mercer, C., Jackson, A., Hettinga, D., et al., 2006. Clinical guidelines for the physiotherapy management of persistent low back pain, part 1: exercise. Chartered Society of Physiotherapy, London.

Merskey, H., Bogduk, N., 2012. Classification of Chronic Pain. IASP Pain Terminology. International Association for the Study of Pain., https://www.iasp-pain.org/resources/terminology/. Accessed 3 September 2021.

Mikosch, P., 2014. Alcohol and bone. Wien. Med. Wochenschr. 164 (1), 15–24.

Miller, W.R., Rollnick, S., 2009. Ten things that motivational interviewing is not. Behav. Cogn. Psychother. 37 (2), 129–140.

Moseley, G.L., 2003. A pain neuromatrix approach to patients with chronic pain. Man. Ther. 8 (3), 130–140.

Moseley, G.L., 2007. Reconceptualising pain according to modern pain science. Phys. Ther. Rev. 12 (3), 169–178.

Munger, K.L., Levin, L.I., Hollis, B.W., et al., 2006. Serum 25-hydroxyvitamin D levels and risk of multiple sclerosis. JAMA. 296, 2832–2838.

Murphy, D.R., Hurwitz, E.L., Gerrard, J.K., et al., 2009. Pain patterns and descriptions in patients with radicular pain: Does the pain necessarily follow a specific dermatome? Chiropr. Osteopat. 17, 9.

National Health Service, 2021. Personalised care. https://www.england.nhs.uk/personalisedcare/. Accessed 3 September 2021.

National Institute for Health and Care Excellence (NICE), 2016. Multimorbidity: clinical assessment and management. NICE., https://www.nice.org.uk/guidance/ng56. Accessed 3 September 2021.

National Institute for Health and Care Excellence (NICE), 2017a. Spondyloarthritis in over 16s: diagnosis and management. NICE., https://www.nice.org.uk/guidance/ng65. Accessed 3 September 2021.

National Institute for Health and Care Excellence (NICE), 2017b. Psoriasis: assessment and management. NICE., https://www.nice.org.uk/guidance/cg153. Accessed 3 September 2021.

National Institute for Health and Care Excellence (NICE), 2020. Rheumatoid arthritis in adults: management. NICE., https://www.nice.org.uk/guidance/ng100. Accessed 3 September 2021.

National Institute for Health and Care Excellence (NICE), 2021a. Shared decision making. NICE., http://www.nice.org.uk/guidance/ng197. Assessed 1 August 2021.

National Institute for Health and Care Excellence (NICE), 2021b. Management of polymyalgia rheumatica?. NICE, CKS., https://cks.nice.org.uk/topics/polymyalgia-rheumatica/management/management/. Accessed 3 September 2021.

National Institute for Health and Care Excellence (NICE), 2021c. Polymyalgia rheumatica. https://cks.nice.org.uk/topics/polymyalgia-rheumatica/. Accessed 3 September 2021.

New Zealand Guidelines Group. 2004. New Zealand acute low back pain guide, incorporating the guide to assessing psychosocial yellow flags in acute low back pain. https://www.healthnavigator.org.nz/media/1006/nz-acute-low-back-pain-guide-acc.pdf. Accessed 3 September 2021.

Niere, K., 1991. Understanding referred pain. Sports Train. Med. Rehabil. 2, 247–256.

Nitta, H., Tajima, T., Sugiyama, H., et al., 1993. Study on dermatomes by means of selective spinal nerve block. Spine 18 (13), 1782–1786.

Ombregt, L., 2013. A System of Orthopaedic Medicine, third ed. Churchill Livingstone, Edinburgh.

O'Neill, C.W., Kurganky, M.E., Derby, R., et al., 2002. Disc stimulation and patterns of referred pain. Spine. 27 (24), 2776–2781.

O'Sullivan, P., 2005. Diagnosis and classification of chronic low back pain disorders: maladaptive movement and motor control impairments as underlying mechanism. Man. Ther. 10 (4), 242–255.

Pappano, D.A., Bass, S., 2006. Referred shoulder pain preceding abdominal pain in a teenage girl with gastric perforation. Pediatr. Emerg. Care 22, 807–809.

Pearce, S.H., Cheetham, T.D., 2010. Diagnosis and management of vitamin D deficiency. Br. Med. J. 340, b5664.

Peng, B., Wenwen, W., Zhenzhou, L., et al., 2007. Chemical radiculitis. Pain 127, 11–16.

Picavet, H.S., Vlaeyen, J.W., Schouten, J.S., 2002. Pain catastrophizing and kinesiophobia: predictors of chronic low back pain. Am. J. Epidemiol. 156, 1028–1034.

Pincus, T., Kent, P., Bronfort, G., et al., 2013. Twenty-five years with the biopsychosocial model of low back pain - is it time to celebrate? A report from the Twelfth International Forum for Primary Care Research on Low Back Pain. Spine 38 (24), 2118–2123.

Pittas, A.G., Lau, J., Hu, F.B., et al., 2007. The role of vitamin D and calcium in type 2 diabetes: a systematic review and meta-analysis. J. Clin. Endocrinol. Metab. 92, 2017–2029.

RadiologyInfo.org, 2022. Radiation dose. https://www.radiologyinfo.org/en/info/safety-xray. Accessed 10 June 2022.

Raja, S.N., Carr, D.B., Cohen, M., et al., 2020. The revised International Association for the Study of Pain definition of pain: concepts, challenges, and compromises. Pain 161 (9), 1976–1982.

Robinson, J., 2003. Lower extremity pain of lumbar spine origin: differentiating somatic referred and radicular pain. J. Man. Manip. Ther. 11 (4), 223–224.

Royal College of General Practitioners, 2009. Low back pain: Early management of persistent non-specific low back pain. https://www.ncbi.nlm.nih.gov/books/NBK11702/. Accessed 3 September 2021.

Salcedo, B., 2019. The comorbidity of anxiety and depression. National Association of Mental Illness (NAMI)., https://www.nami.org/Blogs/NAMI-Blog/January-2018/The-Comorbidity-of-Anxiety-and-Depression. Accessed 3 September 2021.

Schmid, A., 2015. The peripheral nervous system and its compromise in entrapment neuropathies. Grieve's Modern Musculoskeletal Physiotherapy, fourth ed. Elsevier, Edinburgh.78–89.

Scott, D., Happell, B., 2011. The high prevalence of poor physical health and unhealthy lifestyle behaviours in individuals with severe mental illness. Issues Ment. Health Nurs. 32 (9), 589–597.

Shaw, W.S., Means-Christensen, A., Slater, M.A., et al., 2007. Shared and independent associations of psychosocial factors on work status among men with subacute low back pain. Clin. J. Pain 23 (5), 409–416.

Shiri, R., Karppinen, J., Leino-Arjas, P., et al., 2010. The association between smoking and low back pain: a meta-analysis. Am. J. Med. 123 (1), e7–e35. 87

Sloan, J., 2008. Soft tissue injuries: introduction and basic principles. Emerg. Med. J. 25 (1), 33–37.

Smyth, M.J., Wright, V., 1959. Sciatica and the intervertebral disc: an experimental study. J. Bone Joint Surg. 40A, 1401–1408.

Standring, S., 2015. Gray's Anatomy: The Anatomical Basis of Clinical Practice, forty-first ed. Churchill Livingstone, Edinburgh.

STarT Back, 2021. Health Faculty, Keele University. https://startback.hfac.keele.ac.uk/. Accessed 26 June 2021.

Stojanovic, M.P., Sethee, J., Mohiuddin, M., et al., 2010. MRI analysis of the lumbar spine: Can it predict response to diagnostic and therapeutic facet procedures. Clin. J. Pain 26, 110–115.

Stynes, S., Konstantinou, K., Ogollah, R., et al., 2018. Clinical diagnostic model for sciatica developed in primary care patients with low back-related leg pain. PloS One 13 (4), e0191852.

Strampelli, A., Cerreta, F., Vucic, K., 2019. Medication use among older people in Europe: Implications for regulatory assessment and co-prescription of new medicines. Br. J. Clin. Pharmacol. 86 (10), 1912–1920.

Ströhle, A., 2009. Physical activity, exercise, depression and anxiety disorders. J. Neural Transm. 116 (6), 777–784.

Strong, K., Mathers, C., Bonita, R., 2007. Preventing stroke: saving lives around the world. Lancet Neurol. 6 (2), 182–187.

Tarulli, A.W., Raynor, E.M., 2007. Lumbosacral radiculopathy. Neurol. Clin. 25 (2), 387–405.

Teichtahl, A.J., Urquhart, D.M., Wang, Y., et al., 2015. Physical inactivity is associated with narrower lumbar intervertebral discs, high fat content of paraspinal muscles and low back pain and disability. Arthritis Res. Ther. 17 (1), 1–7.

Teixeira, M.J., Almeida, D.B., Yeng, L.T., 2016. Concept of acute neuropathic pain. The role of nervi nervorum in the distinction between acute nociceptive and neuropathic pain. Rev. Dor. 17, 5–10.

Travell, J.G., Simons, D.G., 1996. Trigger Point Flipcharts. Lippincott Williams & Wilkins, Philadelphia.

Valderas, J.M., Starfield, B., Sibbald, B., et al., 2009. Defining comorbidity: implications for understanding health and health services. Ann. Fam. Med. 7 (4), 357–363.

Van Boxem, K., Cheng, J., Patijn, J., et al., 2010. 11. Lumbosacral radicular pain. Pain Pract. 10 (4), 339–358.

Vandenkerkhof, E.G., Macdonald, H.M., Jones, G.T., et al., 2011. Diet, lifestyle and chronic widespread pain: results from the 1958 British Birth Cohort Study. Pain Res. Manag. 16 (2), 87–92.

van Tulder, M., Becker, A., Bekkering, T., 2006. European guidelines for the management of acute non-specific low back pain in primary care. Eur. Spine J. (Suppl. 2), S169–S191. (Chapter 3)

Vecchiet, L., Giamberardino, M.A., 1997. Referred pain: clinical significance, pathophysiology, and treatment. Phys. Med. Rehabil. Clin. N. Am. 8 (1), 119–136.

Verbunt, J.A., Seelen, H.A., Vlaeyen, J.W., et al., 2003. Disuse and deconditioning in chronic low back pain: concepts and hypotheses on contributing mechanisms. Eur. J. Pain 7 (1), 9–21.

Virtanen, M., Ervasti, J., Head, J., et al., 2018. Lifestyle factors and risk of sickness absence from work: a multicohort study. Lancet Public Health 3 (11), e545–e554.

Vlaeyen, J.W., Kole-Snijders, A.M., Boeren, R.G., et al., 1995. Fear of movement/(re) injury in chronic low back pain and its relation to behavioral performance. Pain 62 (3), 363–372.

Vlaeyen, J.W., Linton, S.J., 2012. Fear-avoidance model of chronic musculoskeletal pain: 12 years on. Pain 153 (6), 1144–1147.

Waddell, G., 1992. Understanding the patient with back pain. In: Jayson, M. (Ed.), The Lumbar Spine and Back Pain, fourth ed. Churchill Livingstone, Edinburgh, pp. 469–485.

Waddell, G., 2004. The Back Pain Revolution, second ed. Churchill Livingstone, Edinburgh.

Waddell, G., Aylward, M., 2010. Models of Sickness and Disability Applied to Common Health Problems. The Royal Society of Medicine Press, London.

Wilkinson, C., 1989. Time to let the patient speak [letter]. Br. Med. J. 298, 389.

Witting, N., Svensson, P., Gottrup, H., et al., 2000. Intramuscular and intradermal injection of capsaicin: a comparison of local and referred pain. Pain 84, 407–412.

Woolf, C.J., 2011. Central sensitization: implications for the diagnosis and treatment of pain. Pain 152 (3), S2–S15.

Yin, L., Grandi, N., Raum, E., et al., 2009. Meta-analysis: longitudinal studies of serum vitamin D and colorectal cancer risk. Aliment. Pharmacol. Ther. 30, 113–125.

Yoon, V., Maalouf, N.M., Sakhaee, K., 2012. The effects of smoking on bone metabolism. Osteoporosis Int. 23 (8), 2081–2092.

Zale, E.L., Maisto, S.A., Ditre, J.W., 2015. Interrelations between pain and alcohol: an integrative review. Clin. Psychol. Rev. 37, 57–71.

Zhang, F.F., Cudhea, F., Shan, Z., et al., 2019. Preventable cancer burden associated with poor diet in the United States. JNCI Cancer Spectr. 3 (2), pkz034.

Zipitis, C.S., Akobeng, A.K., 2008. Vitamin D supplementation in early childhood and risk of type 1 diabetes: a systematic review and meta-analysis. Arch. Dis. Child. 93, 512–517.

Zusman, M., 2002. Forebrain-mediated sensitization of central pain pathways: 'non-specific' pain and a new image for MT. Man. Ther. 7 (2), 80–88.

Soft Tissues of the Musculoskeletal System

CHAPTER CONTENTS

SUMMARY

Musculoskeletal medicine involves the examination, diagnosis and treatment of soft tissue lesions. To understand the relevant mechanisms of injury and repair and the rationale for treatment of soft tissue lesions, the soft tissues themselves need to be defined and examined.

The principal soft tissues of concern in musculoskeletal medicine comprise the connective tissues, muscle tissue and nervous tissue. Within this chapter, the basic histology and biomechanics of the soft tissues relevant to musculoskeletal medicine will be explored, to provide background knowledge for clinical practice.

CONNECTIVE TISSUE

Connective tissue is one of four classes of biological tissues, the others being epithelial, muscular and nervous tissue. It is responsible for providing tensile strength, substance, elasticity and density to the body, as well as facilitating nourishment and defence. It also has a major role in repair following trauma, a mechanical role in providing connection and leverage for movement and prevents friction, pressure and shock between mobile structures.

Connective tissue consists primarily of cells embedded in an extracellular matrix, which is composed of fibres and an interfibrillar ground substance (Fig. 2.1). The synthesis, degradation and maintenance of the matrix depend on the cells within it (September et al., 2007).

Not all types of connective tissue cells are found in each tissue, and the cell content can alter, with some cells being resident in the tissue and others brought to specific areas at times of need. Generally, the cells make up approximately 20% of the tissue volume and consist mainly of fibroblasts, macrophages and mast cells.

Connective Tissue Cells
Fibroblasts

Fibroblasts, usually the most abundant of the connective tissue cells, are responsible for producing the contents of the extracellular matrix – namely, fibres and ground substance.

They are found lying close to the bundles of fibres they produce and are closely related to chondroblasts and osteoblasts, the cells responsible for producing

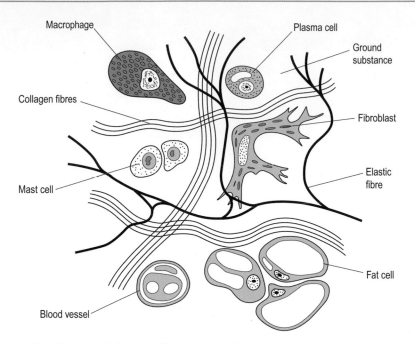

Fig. 2.1 Irregular connective tissue, cellular and fibre content. (Adapted from Cormack, 1987 with permission.)

cartilage and bone matrix. The inactive mature fibroblasts are known as fibrocytes.

Since fibroblasts produce the contents of the extracellular matrix, they play a key role in the repair process after injury. Stearns (1940) observed that once fibre formation was initiated, the fibroblast was able to produce an extensive network of fibrils in a remarkably short time.

Myofibroblasts are specialised cells that contain contractile filaments producing similar properties to smooth muscle cells. They assist wound closure after injury.

Macrophages (Histiocytes or Mononuclear Cells)

Macrophages may be resident in the connective tissues or circulating as monocytes that migrate to an area of injury and modulate into tissue macrophages (Fowler, 1989). They are large cells that have two important roles. The first is phagocytosis, and the second is to act as director cells, in which role they have a considerable influence on scar formation (Hardy, 1989).

As a phagocyte, the macrophage acts as a housekeeper to the wound, ingesting cellular debris and subjecting it to lysosomal hydrolysis, thus debriding the wound in preparation for the fibroblasts to begin the repair process. Matter such as bacteria and cellular debris is engulfed by the phagocyte on contact.

As a director cell, the macrophage chemically activates the number of fibroblasts required for the repair process.

Macrophages also play an important role in muscle regeneration, leading to increased satellite cell differentiation and muscle fibre proliferation (Grefte et al., 2007; Liu et al., 2017). A reduced number of macrophages in muscle tissue has been shown to lead to reduced muscle regeneration (Shen et al., 2008; Chazaud, 2020).

Corticosteroids can inhibit the function of the macrophage in the early inflammatory stage, resulting in a delay in fibre production (Dingman, 1973; Leibovich and Ross, 1974; Fowler, 1989), which is caused by the inhibition of vascular permeability and matrix synthesis by corticosteroid (Hashimoto et al., 2002). This should be taken into consideration when exploring treatment options in the early stage of healing.

CLINICAL TIP

Gentle mobilisation techniques that agitate tissue fluid increase the chance contact of the macrophage with debris and can be applied during the early stages of inflammation to promote phagocytosis (Evans, 1980).

Mast Cells

Mast cells are large, round cells containing secretory granules that store several inflammatory mediators, including heparin, histamine and possibly serotonin. The contents of the mast cell granules are released in response to mechanical or chemical trauma and they play a role in the early stages of inflammation.

Heparin temporarily prevents coagulation of the excess tissue fluid and blood components in the injured area while histamine causes a brief vasodilatation in the neighbouring non-injured area (Wilkerson, 1985; Hardy, 1989). Serotonins are internal nociceptive substances released during platelet aggregation in response to tissue damage. They cause contraction of blood vessels and activate pain signals (Kapit et al., 1987).

Extracellular Matrix

The extracellular matrix accounts for about 80% of the total tissue volume, with approximately 30% of its substance being solids and the remaining 70% being water. It consists of fibres and an interfibrillar ground substance, which is responsible for supporting and nourishing the cells. The ground substance also determines the compliance, mobility and integrity of the connective tissue.

The fibrous portion of connective tissue is responsible for determining the tissue's biomechanical properties. Two major groups of fibres exist within connective tissue: collagen fibres and elastic fibres.

Collagen Fibres

Collagen is a protein in the form of fibre and is the body's 'glue'. It possesses two major properties – great tensile strength and relative inextensibility – and forms the major fibrous component of connective tissue structures (i.e. tendons, ligaments, fascia, sheaths, bursae, bone and cartilage).

Individual collagen fibres are normally mobile within the ground substance, producing discrete shear and gliding movement as well as responding to compression and tension. Collagen is also the main constituent of scar tissue, in which it demonstrates its versatility by adapting to the structure it replaces.

Collagen fibres are large in diameter and appear to be white in colour. They are arranged in bundles and do not branch or anastomose. They are flexible but are inelastic individually.

The bundles of fibres are laid down parallel to the lines of the main mechanical stress, often in a wavy,

sinusoidal or undulating configuration. This gives the tissue an element of crimp (small folds) when not under tension.

Collagen fibre bundles elongate under tension to their physiological length and recoil when the tension is released. Crimp provides a buffer so that longitudinal elongation can occur without damage and it also acts as a shock absorber along the length of the tissue to control tension (Amiel et al., 1990).

Collagen fibres are strong under tensile loading but weak under compressive forces when they tend to buckle. The orientation of the collagen fibres determines the properties of structures. Crimp patterns are dependent upon function and therefore differ in different tissues. For example, the arrangement of collagen fibres perpendicular to the surface in articular cartilage provides a cushioning force for weight-bearing, while the parallel arrangement in tendons provides great tensile strength for transmitting loads and resisting pull. Crimp patterns may also vary between different ligaments and different tendons.

Production and Structure of Collagen Fibres and Collagen Cross-Linking

Procollagen, the first step in collagen fibre formation, is produced intracellularly by the fibroblast. Amino acids are assembled to form polypeptide chains that are twisted into triple helices and held together by weak intramolecular hydrogen bonds known as *cross-links* (Fig. 2.2).

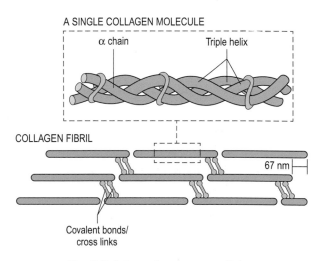

Fig. 2.2 Intramolecular cross-links.

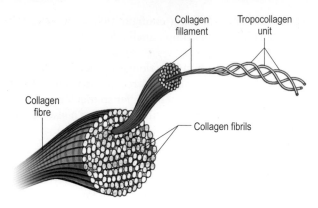

Fig. 2.3 Collagen aggregation.

The procollagen molecules are exocytosed from fibroblasts into the extracellular space. Once outside the fibroblast, the polypeptide chains are known as tropocollagen molecules, and several tropocollagen molecules become bonded by intermolecular cross-links to form a filament or microfibril (Fig. 2.3).

With the maturation into tropocollagen, the cross-links are stronger covalent bonds and occur at specific nodal intercept points, making the structure more stable (Nimni, 1980; Donatelli and Owens-Burkhart, 1981; Hardy, 1989).

Many microfibrils make up a collagen fibril, and many collagen fibrils make up a collagen fibre. Collagen fibrils gain their strength from intermolecular cross-links as they mature (Stauber et al., 2020). Cross-links exist at every level of the organisation of collagen, acting to weld the units together into a rope-like structure. The greater the intermolecular cross-linking, the stronger the collagen structure, with bone being the most highly cross-linked tissue (Hardy, 1989).

Collagen turnover, the dynamic state of the tissue, may be related to the number of cross-links, with fibres being continuously and simultaneously produced and broken down. When collagen production exceeds breakdown, more cross-links develop and the structure resists stretching. If collagen breakdown exceeds production there is a reduction in the number of cross-links and the structure stretches more easily (Alter, 2014).

Excessive cross-link formation can be prevented in immature scar tissue by early mobilisation. Treatment aims to mobilise established cross-links in adhesive scar tissue and then to encourage the longitudinal orientation of the fibres through the application of graded mobilisation. In some instances, manipulative rupture of adhesive scar tissue is indicated (see Chapter 4).

> **CLINICAL TIP**
> Transverse frictions used in musculoskeletal medicine aim to mobilise the tissues.

Collagen fibres continue to aggregate together into larger and larger bundles, and the production, aggregation and orientation of collagen are strongly influenced by mechanical tension and stress.

Bundles of collagen are arranged in a specific pattern to accommodate the function of each individual connective tissue structure (Chamberlain, 1982).

It has been demonstrated that when fibroblasts grown in tissue culture are subjected to regional tension, the cells exposed to the tensile forces multiply more rapidly and orientate themselves in parallel lines in the direction of the tension (Le Gros Clark, 1975).

> **CLINICAL TIP**
> The influence of mechanical stress and tension on collagen alignment can be used to advantage in musculoskeletal medicine during the repair process, when collagen fibres are initially laid down in the early repair phase and in the later remodelling phase of healing. In order to promote tissue gliding and to regain tissue length, the use of graded mobilisation techniques is advocated.

Immobilisation produces rapid changes of collagen tissue as it adapts to its new resting length. Collagen that develops in the absence of mechanical stress (i.e. in the absence of movement) has a random orientation, a change in the numbers and thickness of the fibres and loss of ground substance. This reduction in the lubricating interfibrillar gel allows greater adherence at the fibre–fibre interface (Hardy and Woodall, 1998).

Collagen takes on many forms and functions. In tendons it is tough and inelastic, in cartilage it is resilient, while in bone it is hard. This difference in structure is related to the diameter, orientation and concentration of the fibres. Collagen fibres have been classified into groups (Nimni, 1980):

- **Type I** – The most common form, consisting of large-diameter fibres and found abundantly in structures subjected to tensile forces, e.g. tendon, ligament and the annulus fibrosus of the intervertebral disc.

- **Type II** – Consists of a mixture of large- and narrow-diameter fibres and is abundant in structures subjected to pressure or compressive forces, e.g. articular cartilage and the nucleus pulposus of the intervertebral disc.
- **Type III** – Known as reticulin, is a delicate supporting network of fragile fibres thought to be present in the earliest stages of soft tissue repair. It tends to be replaced by type I collagen as the tissue matures, particularly in regular connective tissue structures (Nassari et al., 2017).

Elastic Fibres

Elastic fibres, consisting of the protein elastin, are yellow in colour and are much thinner and less wavy than collagen fibres. They run singly and freely branch and anastomose.

Elastic fibres provide the tissue with extensibility so that it can be extended in all directions, but if tension is constantly exerted in one direction the elastic fibres may be laid down in sheets known as lamellae, e.g., the ligamentum flavum (the 'yellow ligament').

Elastic fibres are found in ligaments, joint capsules, fascia and connective tissue sheaths, and to a small extent in tendons.

Ground Substance

The connective tissue extracellular matrix comprises interfibrillar ground substance and its fibrous content.

As well as maintaining the mobility and integrity of the tissue structure at a macrostructural level, the ground substance is responsible for nourishing the living cells by facilitating the diffusion of gases, nutrients and waste products between the cells and capillaries.

It contains carbohydrates bound to protein (Standring, 2015). The carbohydrate is in the form of polysaccharides, hexuronic acid and amino sugars, alternately linked to form long-chain molecules called glycosaminoglycans (GAGs). The predominant GAGs in the connective tissue matrix are hyaluronic acid, chondroitin-4-sulphate, chondroitin-6-sulphate and dermatan sulphate (Donatelli and Owens-Burkhart, 1981).

When GAGs are covalently bonded to proteins, the molecules are called proteoglycans (Cormack, 1987). These proteoglycan molecules form a supporting substance for the fibre and cellular components and have the property of attracting and retaining water (Bogduk, 2023). The hydration of structures depends on the proportion of proteoglycans and the flow of water into the extracellular matrix.

Increased hydration creates rigidity in the extracellular matrix, allowing it to exist as a semisolid gel, which improves the tissue's ability to resist compressive forces. Therefore, tissues that are subjected to high compressive forces, such as bone and articular cartilage, have a high proteoglycan content.

Decreased hydration allows the substance to exist as a viscous semisolution, which improves the tissue's ability to resist tensile forces. Therefore, tissues that are subjected to high tensile forces, such as tendons and ligaments, have a low proteoglycan concentration (Levangie et al., 2019).

The ground substance forms a lubricant, filler and spacing buffer system between collagen fibres, fibrils, microfibrils and the intercellular spaces (Akeson et al., 1980). It reduces friction, maintains distance between fibres and facilitates the discrete shear and gliding movement of individual collagen fibres and fibrils.

It is the lubrication and spacing at the fibre–fibre interface that are crucial to the gliding function at nodal intercept points where the fibres cross in the tissue matrix (Amiel et al., 1982). If the tissues are allowed to become immobile, anomalous cross-links form at the nodal intercept points, decreasing the ability to glide.

A balance between the cross-link formation relative to the tissue's tensile strength and mobility is important for normal connective tissue function. Excessive cross-linking and loss of proteoglycans and water volume result in loss of the critical distance between the fibres. The fibres come into contact with each other and stick together, leading to altered tissue function and pain and resulting in loss of extensibility and increased stiffness.

The elasticity of connective tissue fibres together with the viscosity of the ground substance give connective tissue structures viscoelastic properties, which ensure that normal connective tissues are mobile.

CLINICAL TIP

The aim in musculoskeletal medicine is to maintain normal connective tissue mobility through the phases of acute inflammation, proliferation and remodelling and to regain mobility in the chronic situation. This mobility is essential to function, and musculoskeletal medicine treatment techniques aim to preserve the mobility of connective tissue structures.

The biomechanical properties of connective tissue depend on the number and orientation of collagen fibres and the proportion of ground substance present. Each connective tissue structure is specifically designed for function, but the tissues can be grouped simply into regular and irregular connective tissue.

REGULAR CONNECTIVE TISSUE

Regular connective tissue has a highly organised structure, with fibres running in the same linear direction in a precise arrangement that is related to function (Fig. 2.4)

The main collagen fibre bundles are aligned parallel to the line of major mechanical stress, which functionally suits structures such as tendons and ligaments that are mainly subjected to unidirectional stress (Donatelli and Owens-Burkhart, 1981).

The following examples of regular connective tissue are important in musculoskeletal medicine.

Tendons

Muscles and tendons are distinct tissues, although they act functionally as one structure, the contractile unit.

Tendon cells are derived from the embryonic mesenchyme, the tissue occupying the areas between the embryonic layers, classifying tendon as a connective tissue (Standring, 2015).

Muscle cells are derived from mesoderm, the intermediate embryonic layer, such that muscle itself belongs to a separate tissue group.

Tendon tissue does not renew after the age of approximately 17, making it a relatively stable inert structure (Rudavsky and Cook, 2014). The tendon does not contract, but as part of the contractile unit, it is directly involved in muscle action and is assessed by resisted testing via the muscle belly.

A tendon provides tensile force transmission, and storage and release of elastic energy during locomotion, which is important for many sports and activities (Witvrouw et al., 2007).

FUNCTION OF TENDONS
- To attach a muscle to bone
- To transmit the force of muscle contraction to the bone to produce functional movement
- To set the muscle belly in the optimal position for functional movement and to affect the direction of muscle pull
- To be able to glide within the surrounding tissues, accepting stress and tensile forces with minimal drag

---

Tendons are exposed to strong, unidirectional forces. To function, they require great tensile strength and inelastic properties. They can withstand much greater tensile forces than ligaments and are composed of closely packed parallel bundles of collagen microfibrils, fibrils and fibres, bound together by irregular connective tissue sheaths into larger bundles (Fig. 2.5). Most fibres are oriented in one direction, parallel to the long axis, which is the direction of normal physiological stress (Alter, 2014; Nassari et al., 2017).

The tendon extracellular matrix is rich in type I collagen (Nassari et al., 2017), but tendons contain only a small proportion of elastic fibres (1% to 2% of the dry mass of the tendon) (Kannus, 2000), as their muscle belly acts as an energy damper (Akeson, 1990). They do have the ability to store and release elastic energy;

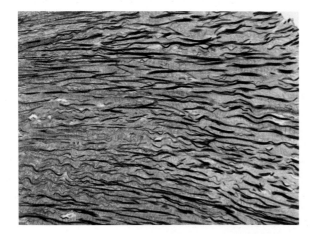

Fig. 2.4 Regular connective tissue. (Tendon; elastic-Van Gieson stain.) (Provided by Dr T Brenn.)

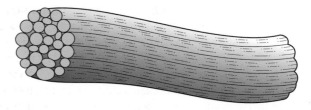

Fig. 2.5 Structure of a tendon.

however, and rehabilitation programmes should aim to increase tendon elasticity. Tendon elasticity has been shown to increase significantly with ballistic stretching (Witvrouw et al., 2007).

Tendon fibres are mainly large-diameter type I collagen and are suited to accept tensile forces. The proteoglycans are packed in between the fibres, and because the tendon is so compact, there is little room for the tendon cells or blood supply. The vascularisation of tendons is relatively sparse compared with that of muscles (Alfredson et al., 2002), and the tendon's blood vessels lie in the epitenon and the endotenon (Gelberman et al., 1983).

Calcification may occur within the tendon structure, which is generated by extracellular organelles known as matrix vesicles. Proteoglycans in the tendon usually suppress the mineralisation, but ageing and diabetes may alter proteoglycan levels, thus allowing calcification of the normally unmineralised extracellular matrix (Gohr et al., 2007).

Tendons are surrounded by a fibroelastic paratenon functioning as an elastic sleeve to facilitate their gliding properties and permit free movement in the surrounding tissues. Under the paratenon, the entire tendon is surrounded by the thin connective tissue sheath of the epitenon; the two together are sometimes referred to as the peritendon. On its inner surface, the epitenon is continuous with the endotenon, which invests each tendon fibre (Józsa and Kannus, 1997).

The *musculotendinous junction* is the area where tension generated in the muscle fibres is transmitted from intracellular contractile proteins to extracellular connective tissue proteins. It is a relatively weak area, making it susceptible to injury (Józsa and Kannus, 1997).

The *teno-osseous* junction is the point of insertion of the tendon into the bone where the viscoelastic tendon transmits force to the rigid bone. At this point, the tendon goes through a transition from tendon to fibrocartilage, mineralised fibrocartilage and finally bone. The mechanism of overuse injuries involving the teno-osseous junction, or enthesis, is not well understood.

An *aponeurosis* is a flat sheet of fibrous tissue that increases the muscle or tendinous attachment to bone, but the term is also applied to the fascial thickenings of the palmar and plantar aponeuroses.

Aponeuroses are usually arranged in layers with the bundles of collagen fibres arranged at different angles in adjacent layers, distributing the muscle or tendon forces,

and increasing the tendon's mechanical advantage, e.g. biceps aponeurosis.

Within each layer, the fibres have a regular arrangement, but the varying angles throughout the whole structure occasionally lead to the classification of aponeurosis as irregular connective tissue by some authors. Mobility needs to be retained throughout the aponeurotic structure to enable it to perform its function.

Ligaments and Joint Capsules

> **PROPERTIES OF LIGAMENTS AND JOINT CAPSULES**
> - Flexibility, requiring elastic properties, to allow normal movement to occur at a joint
> - Resilience, requiring tensile strength, to be tough and unyielding to excessive movement at a joint

The joint capsule and its supporting ligaments are similar in function, both allowing and restraining joint movement.

Ligaments are compact bands of fibrous regular connective tissue that join two or more bones and reinforce the joint capsule in areas of special stress. They vary in size, shape and orientation of fibres, and their prime function is to stabilise joints both at rest and during their normal range of movement.

Ligaments, together with the fibrous capsule, guide and stabilise the articular surfaces. When excessive stresses are applied to a joint, proprioceptive impulses recruit a muscle response so that the passive stabilising effect of the ligament is reinforced by dynamic muscle stabilisation (Akeson et al., 1987; Hauser and Dolan, 2011).

To meet its functional requirements of resisting shear, as well as tensile and compressive forces, the structure of a ligament is different from that of a tendon. The main ligamentous fibres are 70% to 80% collagen laid down in bundles, which assume a wavy, 'crimp' configuration providing an element of elongation and recoil to facilitate movement (Fig. 2.6).

Interwoven with these main fibre bundles are 3% to 5% elastic fibres to enhance extensibility and elasticity (Akeson et al., 1987), as well as proteoglycans and other proteins and glycoproteins (Hauser and Dolan, 2011). When ligaments are put under longitudinal tensile stress, the parallel wavy bundles of collagen straighten out to prevent excessive movement and to elongate without sustaining structural damage (Hauser and Dolan, 2011) (Fig. 2.6).

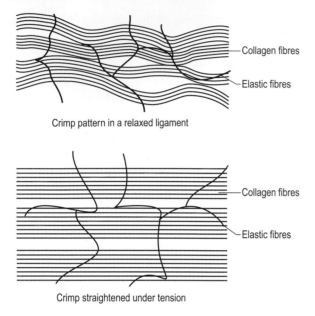

Fig. 2.6 Structure of a ligament.

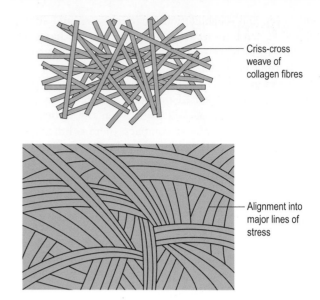

Fig. 2.7 Structure of the joint capsule.

As inert tissue structures, ligaments are assessed by passive movements, which should be applied at the end of available range to test function.

Although the *joint capsule* is similar in function to ligaments, its structure is different. The capsule consists of sheets of collagen fibres that form a fibrous cuff joining opposing bony surfaces.

The fibrous structure is predominantly collagen, but rather than a parallel array of fibres, its pattern is more a criss-cross weave, with the fibres becoming more parallel as the capsule is loaded (Fig. 2.7) (Amiel et al., 1990; Woo et al., 1990).

The ability of the fibres to change and straighten depends on them being mobile and able to slide independently of one another. Capsular contractures, in the form of disorganised collagen, will prevent independent fibre gliding, considerably reducing function and causing pain.

The joint capsule has two layers: an outer fibrous capsule and an internal synovial membrane.

The outer *fibrous capsule* is strong and flexible but relatively inelastic. It is supported functionally by its ligaments, which may be intrinsic, forming an integral part of the joint capsule (e.g. coronary and medial collateral ligaments of the knee), or accessory, being either intracapsular (e.g. the cruciate ligaments) or extracapsular (e.g. lateral collateral ligaments of the knee).

The fibrous capsule is perforated by vessels and nerves and contains afferent sensory nerve endings, including mechanoreceptors and nociceptors.

The *synovial membrane* (synovium) is mainly a loose connective tissue membrane with a degree of elasticity to prevent its folds and villi becoming nipped during movement. It covers all surfaces within the joint except the articular surfaces themselves and menisci.

The synovial membrane is a highly cellular membrane containing synoviocytes (i.e. the synovium-producing cells) and collagen fibres. It has a rich nerve, blood and lymphatic supply. A capillary network is situated on the inner surface of the synovium to produce synovial fluid (Ballard et al., 2012).

Synovial fluid is pale yellow and viscous. It lubricates the ligamentous structures of the joint and nourishes cartilage and menisci through a mechanism of trans-synovial flow aided by movement (Akeson et al., 1987).

In joint arthropathy, pain initially prevents full range of movement. The relative immobility causes changes to occur in the connective tissue that lead to capsular contracture, further loss of function and pain. This is seen clinically as the capsular pattern (see Chapter 1).

Cartilage

Cartilage is a weight-bearing connective tissue displaying a combination of rigidity, which is resistant to compression, resilience and some elasticity. It is relatively avascular and relies on tissue fluid for nourishment.

There are three main types:
- Elastic cartilage
- Fibrocartilage
- Hyaline cartilage

Elastic cartilage consists of a matrix of yellow elastic fibres and is very resilient. It is found in the external ear, the epiglottis and the larynx.

Fibrocartilage has a large proportion of type I collagen fibres in its matrix, providing it with great tensile strength. It is found in the annulus fibrosus of the intervertebral discs, the menisci of the knee joint, the acetabular and glenoid labra, the articular disc of the acromioclavicular and wrist joints, the lining of the grooves that house tendons, and as a transitional cartilage at the teno-osseous junction of tendons (Cormack, 1987; Standring, 2015; Soames and Palastanga, 2018).

Hyaline cartilage is *articular cartilage*. Its relatively solid gel-like matrix provides a weight-bearing surface that is elastic and resistant to compression. It moulds to the shape of the bones, presenting a smooth articular surface for movement.

Hyaline cartilage is composed of scantily deposited chondroblasts and chondrocytes that produce the gel extracellular matrix consisting of type II collagen fibres and ground substance. The extracellular matrix contains distinctive large super-molecular proteoglycan aggregates that provide a network for trapping and retaining water, which contributes significantly to the resilience of cartilage (Cormack, 1987).

The collagen fibres themselves are relatively weak under compression. Therefore, the water-enhanced matrix compensates for this by providing a resilient weight-bearing surface.

Four separate structural zones exist in hyaline articular cartilage that contribute to its biomechanical functions (Nordin and Frankel, 2020):
- A superficial zone helps to prevent friction between the joint surfaces and to distribute the compressive

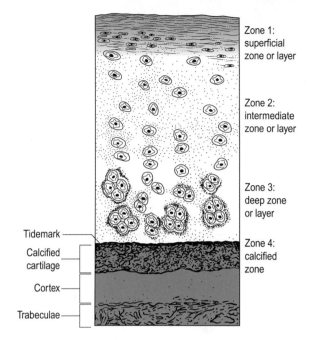

Fig. 2.8 Zonal arrangement of articular cartilage. (From Orthopaedic and Sports Physical Therapy by Gould JA and Davies GJ. Reprinted by permission of Elsevier Ltd.)

forces. It consists of fine, tangential, densely packed fibres lying in a plane parallel to the articular surface (Fig. 2.8).
- In the middle zone, the cells are arranged in vertical columns, perpendicular to the surface, with scattered collagen fibres. The middle layer allows deformation of the collagen fibres and absorbs some of the compressive forces.
- The deep zone forms a transition between the articular cartilage and the underlying calcified cartilage layer (calcified zone); the fibres are arranged in radial bundles.

The zonal arrangement of articular cartilage provides a 'well-sprung mattress' arrangement to cope with compressive forces. The variation in collagen fibre orientation in each zone enables the articular cartilage to vary its material property with direction of the load.

Hyaline cartilage has no blood vessels and depends on fluid flow through compressive forces for nutrition. This fluid flow depends on the magnitude and duration of the compressive force, and a balance of weight-bearing and non-weight-bearing is important to its health (Levangie et al., 2019).

The fluid content of articular cartilage is responsible for its nutrition as well as its mechanical properties, allowing diffusion of nutrients and products between the cells and the synovial fluid. When cartilage is loaded, the fluid in the 'sponge' moves, which is important for the mechanical properties of the cartilage as well as for joint lubrication. Intermittent loading creates a pumping effect, but prolonged loading will eventually press fluid out of the cartilage and prevent uptake of new fluid, leading to degeneration.

> **CLINICAL TIP**
> Articular cartilage requires movement for nutrition and to maintain fluid levels within its matrix to withstand compressive forces. Prolonged loading reduces fluid levels in the matrix through the action of tissue creep, which may lead to degenerative changes. It is essential, therefore, to maintain the mobility of inflamed or degenerate joints.

IRREGULAR CONNECTIVE TISSUE

In contrast to regular connective tissue, irregular connective tissue does not display a highly organised structure. It consists of a mixture of collagen and elastic fibres interwoven to form a loose meshwork that can withstand stress in any direction (Fig. 2.9). Its main function is to support and protect regular connective tissue structures.

The following examples of irregular connective tissue are important in musculoskeletal medicine.

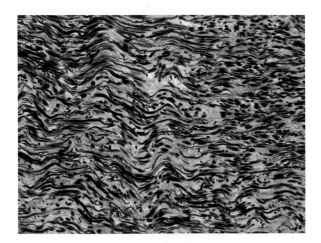

Fig. 2.9 Irregular connective tissue. (Paratenon; elastic-Van Gieson stain.) (Provided by Dr T Brenn.)

The *dura mater* is the outermost of three irregular connective tissue sleeves that enclose the brain and the spinal cord. It is extended to form the dural nerve root sleeve that invests the nerve roots within the intervertebral foramen. Within or just beyond the intervertebral foramen, the dural nerve root sleeve fuses with the epineurium of the nerve root.

The dura mater and dural nerve root sleeve extensions are formed of sheets of collagen and elastic fibres providing a tough but loose fibrous tube. The dura mater is separated from the bony margins of the vertebral canal by the epidural space that contains fat, loose connective tissue and a venous plexus.

The dura mater and dural nerve root sleeve are mobile in a non-pathological state and can accommodate normal movement (Iannotti and Parker, 2012; Standring, 2015; Soames and Palastanga, 2018). Adhesions may develop within the dura mater and the dural nerve root sleeve, compromising their mobility and giving rise to clinical symptoms.

Layers of irregular tissue are found within *muscle*. The *epimysium* is a layer of irregular connective tissue surrounding the whole muscle. The *perimysium* surrounds the fascicles within the muscle, and the *endomysium* surrounds each individual muscle fibre.

In a similar arrangement, a fibrous sheath, the *epineurium*, surrounds each nerve. The *perineurium* surrounds each fascicle, and each individual nerve fibre is invested in a delicate sheath of vascular loose connective tissue, the *endoneurium*.

Since connective tissue mobility is important to the function of muscle, its arrangement in nerve structure implies that it is also important to the function of nervous tissue. For example, tight hamstrings can increase the mechanosensitivity and tension of the sciatic nerve (Boyd et al., 2009).

Returning to tendon, the *paratenon* is an irregular connective tissue fibroelastic sheath, adherent to the outer surface of all tendons. It is composed of relatively large amounts of proteoglycans to provide a gliding surface around the tendon, allowing it to move freely among other tissues with a minimum of drag (Merrilees and Flint, 1980).

True *tendon synovial sheaths* are found most commonly in the hand and foot where they act to reduce friction between the tendon and surrounding tissues. The synovial sheath consists of two layers: an outer fibrotic sheath and an inner synovial sheath that has parietal and visceral layers.

Between these two layers is an enclosed space containing a thin film of synovial fluid. The synovial sheath may also assist in tendon nutrition (Józsa and Kannus, 1997).

Like the synovial tendon sheaths, *bursae*, flat synovial sacs, also prevent friction and pressure and facilitate movement between adjacent connective tissue structures. Bursae can be subcutaneous (e.g. the olecranon bursa), subtendinous (e.g. psoas bursa), sub- or intermuscular (e.g. gluteal bursa), or adventitious—developing in response to trauma or pressure (e.g. subcutaneous Achilles bursa).

Fascia lies in sheets to facilitate movement between the various tissue planes. *Deep fascia* has a more regular formation as it forms a tight sleeve to retain structures, adds to the contours of the limbs and is extended to form the intermuscular septa. It provides a compressive force that facilitates venous return and may act as a mechanical barrier preventing the spread of infection.

Fascia may develop *retinacula* (bands of thickened fascia), which hold tendons in place, preventing a bowstring effect on movement, such as the retinacula at the ankle. It may produce thickenings, forming protective layers such as the *palmar* and *plantar aponeuroses*, or it may form envelopes to enclose and protect major neurovascular bundles, such as the femoral sheath in the femoral triangle.

> **CLINICAL TIP**
> Tissue injury involves the surrounding and supporting irregular connective tissue as well as the regular connective tissue structure itself. It is therefore important to recognise the extensive nature of irregular connective tissue and its close relationship with the regular connective tissue structures encountered in musculoskeletal medicine.

MUSCLE

Muscle tissue is a separate tissue responsible for contraction and functional movement. Skeletal muscle consists of cells known as muscle fibres due to their long, narrow shape. Muscle has a large connective tissue component that supplies its nutrients for metabolism and facilitates contraction by providing a continuous connective tissue harness.

As mentioned, this continuous harness comprises the epimysium, perimysium and endomysium (Fig. 2.10). Each end of the harness is continuous with strong connective tissue structures that anchor it to its attachments.

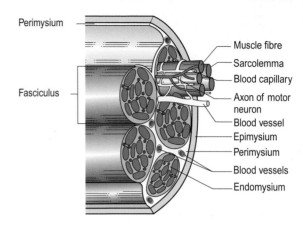

Fig. 2.10 Connective tissue component of skeletal muscle. (From Soames and Palastanga, 2018. Reprinted by permission of Elsevier Ltd.)

With muscle lesions, mobility is maintained through transverse frictions, to preserve the muscle's ability to broaden as it contracts, and graded mobilisation.

NERVOUS TISSUE

Nervous tissue is designed for the conduction of nerve impulses and initiation of function. The central nervous system is largely devoid of connective tissue, being made up of specialised tissue held together by neuroglia, the supporting cells of the central nervous system.

Three connective tissue meninges (pia mater, arachnoid mater and dura mater) and the cerebrospinal fluid protect the system inside its bony framework.

The peripheral nervous system is not as delicate, with connective tissue constituting part of the nerves, providing strength and resilience. As mentioned, the epineurium is an outer connective tissue sheath enclosing large nerves; the perineurium surrounds each fascicle or bundle of nerve fibres and the endoneurium invests each individual nerve fibre.

The maintenance of mobility within and around nervous tissue is important for restoring the dynamic balance between the neural tissues and surrounding mechanical interfaces, thereby allowing reduced intrinsic pressures on the neural tissues and promoting optimum physiological function of both neural and non-neural structures (Ellis and Hing, 2008; López et al., 2019).

CONNECTIVE TISSUE RESPONSE TO MECHANICAL STRESS

Excessive mechanical stress is responsible for connective tissue injury, but manual techniques utilise mechanical stresses to mobilise scar tissue.

Understanding the mechanical response of connective tissue structures to stress is helpful in interpreting mechanisms of injury and rationalising treatment programmes. However, it should be appreciated that most experimental evidence has been derived from animal and cadaveric specimens in the laboratory setting, and physical principles have been adapted to explain the mechanical properties demonstrated.

Connective tissue can change its structure and function in response to applied forces by altering the composition of the extracellular matrix, demonstrating its dynamic nature and the relationship between form and function (Levangie et al., 2019).

The *stress*, or *load*, is the mechanical force applied to the tissue. The *strain* is the resultant deformation produced by the applied stress.

The *stress–strain curve* is a way of illustrating the reaction of connective tissue structures to loading (Fig. 2.11). Experimentally, a tensile stress is applied to collagen until it ruptures. The applied stress or elongating force is plotted on the *y* axis, and the strain, the extent to which collagen elongates, measured as a percentage of its original length, is plotted along the *x*-axis.

Collagen at rest is crimped. As stress is applied, the fibres straighten initially, responding with an elastic form of elongation and the crimp pattern is lost (Akeson et al., 1987; Hardy and Woodall, 1998; Bogduk, 2023).

The straightening out of the fibres is represented by the first part of the curve, known as the *toe region*. Crimp straightens easily and there is little or no resistance to the applied stress.

At the end of the toe region, some of the elongation may be due to recoverable sliding of the collagen fibres in the interfibrillar gel (Nordin and Frankel, 2020; Stauber et al., 2020). The capacity of the tissues to lengthen is

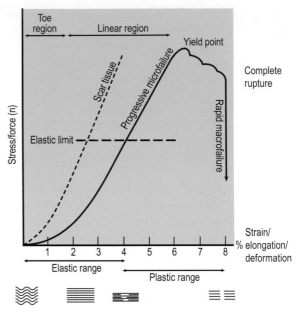

Fig. 2.11 Stress–strain curve.

initially determined by their structural weave, that is, the more regularly oriented the collagen fibres, the shorter the toe region. For example, a ligament displays a shorter toe region than the more loosely woven joint capsule, but a longer toe region than the more regularly arranged tendon (Threlkeld, 1992; Hardy and Woodall, 1998).

The second part of the curve is known as the *linear region*. The straightened fibres realign in the linear direction of the applied stress, and the structure becomes longer and thinner.

In the first half of the linear region, water and proteoglycans are displaced and the chemical cross-links between fibres and fibrils are strained, producing a resistance or stiffness in the tissue so that a progressively greater stress is required to produce equivalent amounts of elongation.

The steeper the stress–strain curve, the stiffer the tissue. If the deforming stress is removed at this point, the elastic properties of the collagen tissue allow the structure to return to its original resting length.

In the early part of the linear region, a point is reached at which slack is taken up in connective tissue, and this represents the end of the passive range. As strain increases past this point, fibre and fibril sliding becomes increasingly non-recoverable (Stauber et al., 2020).

> **CLINICAL TIP**
> Passive movements applied during clinical examination represent the stress applied to take up the slack. The strain is represented by the range of movement observed and the end-feel of the movement.

In the second half of the linear region, stress causes some of the strained cross-links to break and *microfailure* begins to occur in a few overstretched fibres. Microfailure is said to occur somewhere after 4% of elongation has been achieved (Bogduk, 2023), at which point the collagen is said to have reached its *elastic limit*.

A traumatic stress applied at this stage produces minor pain and swelling but no clinical laxity (equivalent to a Grade I injury. See Chapter 11 for definitions of the grades of injury as applied to the medial collateral ligament of the knee).

Once the elastic limit of collagen has been exceeded, collagen exhibits *plastic properties* (i.e. the property of the tissue to deform permanently when loaded beyond its elastic limit).

Progressive microfailure produces permanent elongation once the deforming stress is removed. A traumatic stress applied within the plastic range produces more pain and swelling together with some clinical laxity (equivalent to a Grade II injury. See Chapter 11 for definitions of the grades of injury as applied to the medial collateral ligament of the knee).

A further increase in stress causes major collagen fibre failure and the *yield point* is reached, represented by the peak of the stress–strain curve, where a large number of cross-links are irreversibly broken.

The stress–strain curve drops rapidly, indicating *macrofailure*, or complete rupture, where the structure is unable to sustain further stress even though it may remain physically intact (equivalent to a Grade III injury. See Chapter 11 for definitions of the grades of injury as applied to the medial collateral ligament of the knee)

Threlkeld (1992), reporting Noyes et al., stated that the estimated macrofailure of connective tissue occurs at approximately 8% of elongation. Wang et al. (2006) propose that this is a conservative figure and state 12% as the percentage value for complete rupture. They suggest that even this value could be an underestimation and that it might be as much as 14% of elongation.

A traumatic stress that produces complete rupture causes severe pain initially, which is followed by less pain and gross clinical laxity.

The stress applied to tissues can be divided into several categories (Norris, 2004; Bogduk, 2023):
- *Tensile stress* – a pulling or elongating force applied longitudinally, parallel to the long axis of the structure
- *Compressive stress* – a pushing or squashing force applied perpendicular to the long axis of the structure
- *Shear stress* – a sliding force applied across the long axis of the structure
- *Torsional stress* – a twisting force or torque applied in opposite directions about an axis of rotation.

Collagen does not have pure elastic properties, and the presence of the ground substance provides a viscous fluid factor. Therefore, the viscoelastic properties of collagen may be affected by the type of stress applied and the speed of application, influencing the outcome of the different mobilisation techniques used in musculoskeletal medicine, as discussed in Chapter 4.

The *stiffness* of a structure is its resistance to deformation under the applied stress. A stiff structure displays reduced elastic properties and a shorter toe phase.

Scar tissue, which forms within a connective tissue structure, is not as elastic as the surrounding normal tissue (see Fig. 2.11). Therefore, slack will be taken up sooner in the adherent scar tissue, and mobilisation techniques can be applied to produce elongation or rupture.

Tough scar tissue requires considerable force or stress to deform it, and it does not easily resume its original shape. Once the failure point of scar tissue is reached, it ruptures relatively quickly (Norris, 2004).

The *viscoelastic properties* of connective tissue structures cause them to behave differently under different loading rates. If the structure is loaded quickly, it behaves more stiffly than the same tissue loaded at a slower rate (Threlkeld, 1992).

Tendons, for example, are more easily deformed at low strain rates where they absorb more energy but are less effective at transmitting loads. At high strain rates, they become stiffer and are less easily deformed but are more effective at moving large loads (Wang et al., 2006).

Higher-force, short-duration stretching at normal or lower temperatures favours recoverable elastic tissue deformation, whereas low-force, long-duration stretching at higher temperatures favours permanent plastic deformation (Warren et al., 1971; Leban, cited in Alter, 2014).

This behaviour of the tissue is utilised in tissue mobilisation techniques. Adhesions may be ruptured by a quickly applied shear stress or stretched by a slow

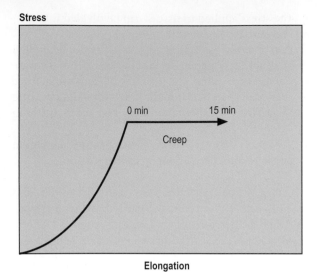

Fig. 2.12 Stress–strain curve illustrating creep. Despite maintenance of a constant load, elongation occurs within the passage of time. (From Bogduk, 2023. Reprinted by permission of Elsevier.)

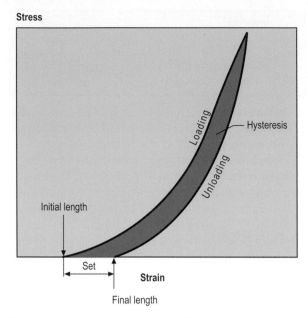

Fig. 2.13 Stress–strain curve illustrating hysteresis. When unloaded, a structure regains shape at a rate different to that at which it deformed. Any difference between the initial and final shape is the 'set'. (From Bogduk, 2023. Reprinted by permission of Elsevier.)

sustained tensile stress. Increasing the temperature of a structure allows lower sustained loads to achieve greater elongation (Warren et al., 1971; Usuba et al., 2007).

Creep is a property of viscous structures that occurs when a prolonged stress is applied in the linear phase. Creep, or elongation of the tissue, is inversely proportional to the velocity of the stress and the slower the applied stress, the greater the lengthening (Hardy and Woodall, 1998) (Fig. 2.12).

Deformation occurs through a gradual rearrangement of the collagen fibres, proteoglycan gel and water and/or through straining and perhaps breaking some of the collagen fibre cross-links (Bogduk, 2023).

When the stress is released, resumption of the original length of the structure occurs at a slower rate than its deformation. This mechanical behaviour is known as *hysteresis*. The loading and unloading stress–strain curves are not identical, as would be demonstrated in a purely elastic structure, and the original length may not be achieved. The difference between the two lengths is known as *set* (Fig. 2.13).

Repeated or cyclical loading may achieve an increment of elongation with each loading cycle. This may lead to eventual failure of the structure through accumulated fatigue. A larger load requires fewer repetitions

to produce failure, but a certain minimum load must be applied to achieve this effect (Norris, 2004).

> **CLINICAL TIP**
> The aim of mobilisation is to maintain or regain the gliding function and length of the tissues, allowing or restoring full painless function.

Mobilisation to maintain tissue function is conducted within the elastic range, while mobilisation aimed at elongating or rupturing established scar tissue adhesions occurs by applying appropriate stress at the end of the linear region and within the plastic range of the tissue.

Timing of the application of the mobilisation stress is important and is determined by the grade of the injury, the resultant irritability of the tissues and the stage in the healing process. Young scar tissue is 'ripe' for mobilisation and can be altered by stress parameters that do not affect older scar tissue.

The tensile strength limitations of the healing tissues should be respected and uncontrolled or overaggressive mobilisation avoided (Madden cited in Hardy and Woodall, 1998).

REVIEW QUESTIONS

1. What are the main functions of the macrophage?
2. What are the key differences in structure of regular and irregular connective tissue and how does this relate to the function of different structures?
3. Why do anomalous cross-links form during collagen synthesis? What is the relevance of movement during the healing process?
4. What is the key function of the fibroblast?
5. With reference to the stress–strain curve, how does scar tissue behave in response to loading?

REFERENCES

Akeson, W., 1990. The response of ligaments to stress modulation and overview of the ligament healing response. In: Daniel, D., Akeson, W.H., O'Connor, J.J. (Eds.), Knee Ligaments: Structure, Function, Injury and Repair. Lippincott Williams & Wilkins, Philadelphia, pp. 315–327.

Akeson, W., Amiel, D., Woo, S.L.-Y., 1980. Immobility effects on synovial joints, the pathomechanics of joint contracture. Biorheology 17, 95–110.

Akeson, W., Amiel, D., Abel, M.F., et al., 1987. Effects of immobilisation on joints. Clin. Orthop. Relat. Res. 219, 28–37.

Alfredson, H., Bjur, D., Thorsen, K., et al., 2002. High intratendinous lactate levels in painful chronic Achilles tendinosis. An investigation using microdialysis technique. J. Orthop. Res. 20 (5), 934–938.

Alter, M.J., 2014. Science of Flexibility, third ed. Human Kinetics, Champaign, IL.

Amiel, D., Woo, S.L.-Y., Harwood, L., Akeson, W.H., 1982. The effect of immobilization on collagen turnover in connective tissue: a biochemical–biomechanical correlation. Acta Orthop. Scand. 53, 325–332.

Amiel, D., Billings, E., Akeson, W., 1990. Ligament structure, chemistry and physiology. In: Daniel, D., Akeson, W.H.O., Connor, J.J. (Eds.), Knee Ligaments: Structure, Function, Injury and Repair. Lippincott Williams & Wilkins, Philadelphia, pp. 77–90.

Ballard, B.L., Antonacci, J.M., Temple-Wong, M.M., et al., 2012. Effect of tibial plateau fracture on lubrication function and composition of synovial fluid. J. Bone Joint Surg. Am 94 (10), e64.

Bogduk, N., 2023. Clinical and Radiological Anatomy of the Lumbar Spine, sixth ed. Churchill Livingstone, Edinburgh.

Boyd, B.S., Wanek, L., Gray, A.T., Topp, K.S., 2009. Mechanosensitivity of the lower extremity nervous system during straight-leg raise neurodynamic testing in healthy individuals. J. Orthop. Sports Phys. Ther. 39 (11), 780–790.

Chamberlain, G.J., 1982. Cyriax's friction massage: a review. J. Orthop. Sports Phys. Ther. 4, 16–22.

Chazaud, B., 2020. Inflammation and skeletal muscle degeneration: Leave it to the macrophages! Trends in Immunology 41 (6), 481–492.

Cormack, D.H., 1987. Ham's Histology, ninth ed. Lippincott Williams & Wilkins, Philadelphia.

Dingman, R.O., 1973. Factors of clinical significance affecting wound healing. Laryngoscope 83 (9), 1540–1555.

Donatelli, R., Owens-Burkhart, H., 1981. Effects of immobilisation on the extensibility of periarticular connective tissue. J. Orthop. Sports Phys. Ther 3, 67–72.

Ellis, R.F., Hing, W.A., 2008. Neural mobilization: a systematic review of randomized controlled trials with an analysis of therapeutic efficacy. J. Man. Manip. Ther. 6 (1), 8–22.

Evans, P., 1980. The healing process at cellular level: A review. Physiotherapy 66, 256–259.

Fowler, J.D., 1989. Wound healing: An overview. Semin. Vet. Med. Surg. 4, 256–262.

Gelberman, R.H., Vande Berg, J.S., Lundberg, G.N., Akeson, W.H., 1983. Flexor tendon healing and restoration of the gliding surface. J. Bone Joint Surg. 65A, 70–83.

Gohr, C., Fahey, M., Rosenthal, A., 2007. Calcific tendonitis: A model. Connect. Tissue Res. 48, 286–291.

Gould, J.A., Davies, G.J., 1985. Orthopaedic and Sports Physical Therapy. Elsevier Health Sciences (Mosby), London.

Grefte, S., Kuijpers-Jagtman, A.M., Torensma, R., et al., 2007. Skeletal muscle development and regeneration. Stem Cells Dev. 16, 857–868.

Hardy, M.A., 1989. The biology of scar formation. Phys. Ther. 69, 1014–1023.

Hardy, M., Woodall, W., 1998. Therapeutic effects of heat, cold and stretch on connective tissue. J. Hand Ther. 11 (2), 148–152.

Hashimoto, I., Nakanishi, H., Shono, Y., et al., 2002. Angiostatic effects of corticosteroid on wound healing of the rabbit ear. J. Med. Invest. 49 (1/2), 61–66.

Hauser, R.A., Dolan, E., 2011. Ligament injury and healing: An overview of current concepts. J. Prolother. 836–846.

Iannotti, J.P., Parker, R., 2012. The Netter Collection of Medical Illustrations: Musculoskeletal System, Volume 6, Part 1. Saunders, Philadelphia.

Józsa, L., Kannus, P., 1997. Human Tendons: Anatomy, Physiology and Pathology. Human Kinetics, Champaign, IL.

Kannus, P., 2000. Structure of the tendon connective tissue. Scand. J. Med. Sci. Sports 10, 312–320.

Kapit, W., Macey, R., Meisami, E., 1987. The Physiology Coloring Book. HarperCollins, New York.

Le Gros Clark, W.E., 1975. The Tissues of the Body, sixth ed. Oxford University Press, Oxford.

Leibovich, S.J., Ross, R., 1974. The role of the macrophage in wound repair. Am. J. Pathol. 78, 71–91.

Levangie, P., Norkin, C., Lewek, M.D., 2019. Joint Structure and Function: A Comprehensive Analysis, sixth ed. F.A. Davis, Philadelphia.

Liu, X., Liu, Y., Zhao, L., Zeng, Z., et al., 2017. Macrophage depletion impairs skeletal muscle regeneration: The roles of regulatory factors for muscle regeneration. Cell. Biol. Int. 41, 228–238.

López, L.L., Torres, J.R., Rubio, A.O., et al., 2019. Effects of neurodynamic treatment on hamstrings flexibility: A systematic review and meta-analysis. Phys. Ther. Sport 40, 244–250.

Merrilees, M.J., Flint, M.H., 1980. Ultrastructural study of tension and pressure zones in a rabbit flexor tendon. Am. J. Anat. 157, 87–106.

Nassari, S., Duprez, D., Fourier-Thibault, C., 2017. Non-myogenic contribution to muscle development and homeostasis: The role of the connective tissues. Front. Cell Dev. Biol. 5, 22.

Nimni, M.E., 1980. The molecular organisation of collagen and its role in determining the biophysical properties of the connective tissues. Biorheology 17, 51–82.

Nordin, M., Frankel, V.H., 2020. Basic Biomechanics of the Musculoskeletal System, fifth ed. Lippincott Williams & Wilkins, Philadelphia.

Norris, C.M., 2004. Sports Injuries: Diagnosis and Management for Physiotherapists, third ed. Butterworth-Heinemann, Oxford.

Rudavsky, A., Cook, J., 2014. Physiotherapy management of patellar tendinopathy (jumper's knee). J. Physiother. 60, 122–129.

September, A.V., Schwellnus, M.P., Collins, M., 2007. Tendon and ligament injuries: the genetic component (review). Br. J. Sports Med. 41 (4), 241–246.

Shen, W., Li, Y., Zhu, J., Schwendener, R., Huard, J., 2008. Interaction between macrophages. TGF-beta1, and the COX-2 pathway during the inflammatory phase of skeletal muscle healing after injury. J. Cell. Physiol. 214, 405–412.

Soames, R., Palastanga, N.R., 2018. Anatomy and Human Movement, seventh ed. Elsevier, Oxford.

Standring, S., 2015. Gray's Anatomy: The Anatomical Basis of Clinical Practice, forty-first ed. Churchill Livingstone, Edinburgh.

Stauber, T., Blache, U., Snedeker, J.G., 2020. Tendon tissue microdamage and the limits of intrinsic repair. Matrix Biol. 85–86, 68–79.

Stearns, M.L., 1940. Studies on the development of connective tissue in transparent chambers in the rabbit's ear, II. Am. J. Anat. 67, 55–97.

Threlkeld, A.J., 1992. The effects of manual therapy on connective tissue. Phys. Ther. 72, 893–902.

Usuba, M., Akai, M., Shirasaki, Y., Miyakawa, S., 2007. Experimental joint contracture correction with low torque–long duration repeated stretching. Clin. Orthop. Relat. Res. 456, 70–78.

Wang, J., Losifidus, M., Fu, F., 2006. Biomechanical basis for tendinopathy. Clin. Orthop. Relat. Res. 443, 320–332.

Warren, C.G., Lehmann, J.F., Koblanski, J.N., 1971. Elongation of the rat tail tendon: Effect of load and temperature. Arch. Phys. Med. Rehabil. 52, 465–474.

Wilkerson, G.B., 1985. Inflammation in connective tissue: Etiology and management. Athl. Train. 20, 298–301.

Witvrouw, E., Mahieu, N., Roosen, P., McNair, P., 2007. The role of stretching in tendon injuries. Br. J. Sports Med. 41 (4), 224–226.

Woo, S.L.-Y., Wang, C.W., Newton, P.O., et al., 1990. The response of ligaments to stress deprivation and stress enhancement. In: Daniel, D., Akeson, W.H., O'Connor, J.J. (Eds.), Knee Ligaments: Structure, Function, Injury and Repair. Lippincott Williams & Wilkins, Philadelphia, pp. 337–349.

Soft Tissue Healing

CHAPTER CONTENTS

SUMMARY

The previous chapter explored the histology and biomechanics of the soft tissues relevant to musculoskeletal medicine. This chapter examines the different phases of healing in soft tissue lesions and briefly outlines relevant pathology.

The process of scar tissue formation is explored and its implication in restoring or preventing pain-free function. A general overview of lesions is provided and factors that promote or impede healing are considered.

SOFT TISSUE LESIONS

Lesions encountered in musculoskeletal medicine include joint and ligamentous lesions, muscle belly lesions, tendinopathy, tenosynovitis, bursitis and mechanical joint displacements.

An injury causes disruption of connective tissue unity. The body's response to this is generally one of inflammation, proliferation and remodelling, to restore anatomical structure and normal function to the damaged tissue. However, studies have questioned the presence of inflammatory changes in chronic overuse tendon lesions, and the inflammatory model has been challenged.

We shall begin by outlining the different phases of healing and will expand the discussion from there to address the lesions referred to previously.

After an initial, relatively short bleeding phase, the inflammatory phase prepares the area for healing, the proliferation phase rebuilds the structure and the remodelling phase provides the final form of the tissue (Hardy, 1989; Broughton et al., 2006; Watson, 2009). The different phases of connective tissue healing are not separate and each is overlapped by the other, with one response signalling another until the wound is bridged by scar tissue (Fig. 3.1).

INFLAMMATORY PHASE

The degree of inflammation in response to injury depends on the degree of trauma. A minor injury causes a minimal response, whereas a major injury will produce a significant inflammatory response that will usually pass through acute, subacute and chronic phases.

Acute inflammation is significant, and the patient can usually recall the precise time and mode of onset. Following injury, the inflammatory response is rapid with noticeable pain and swelling, which can last for hours or days.

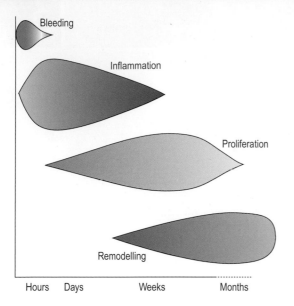

Fig. 3.1 Tissue repair phases and timescale. (Available from: http://www.electrotherapy.org. Reprinted by permission of Professor Tim Watson.)

With chronic inflammation, the patient cannot usually recollect the onset, and the reaction is low-grade with less noticeable pain and swelling. Chronic inflammation can occur as a progression from acute inflammation, or it can result from change in use and can last for weeks, months or even years.

The initial inflammatory reaction involves vascular and cellular changes. Injury is rapidly followed by transient vasoconstriction, lasting for 5 to 10 minutes, and is succeeded by vasodilatation, which may result in haemorrhage. If the lesion is still bleeding at the time of treatment, this will need careful management.

Fig. 3.2 illustrates the components of acute and chronic inflammatory responses and their principle functions, which will be referred to below. As described in Chapter 2, connective tissue comprises cells embedded in an extracellular matrix of fibres with an interfibrillar ground substance, occupying the background spaces in the figure.

In the early stage of inflammation, the blood vessel walls become more permeable and plasma and leukocytes leak into the surrounding tissues as inflammatory exudate or oedema.

Swelling may take a few hours to develop and the amount of swelling is determined by the type of tissue involved in the injury. For example, muscle bellies may produce considerable swelling and bleeding, but the structure of tendons prevents the collection of fluid. They do not swell as easily, but they do thicken, which can give the appearance of swelling.

Similarly, ligaments themselves do not usually show dramatic swelling but capsular ligaments (e.g. the medial collateral ligament of the knee) may provoke traumatic arthritis of the joint, causing considerable pain and swelling. Swelling may also be restricted physically by fascial bands and intermuscular septa.

The vascular response is directly due to damage of blood vessel walls and indirectly due to the influence of chemical mediators. These chemical mediators include heparin and histamine, released by the mast cells (see Fig. 3.2); bradykinin, originating from plasma and plasma proteins; serotonin, from platelets; and prostaglandins, hormone-like compounds produced by all cells in the body.

- Heparin temporarily prevents coagulation of the excess tissue fluid and blood in the area.
- Bradykinins have multiple effects. They are potent mediators of the inflammatory response, can directly cause pain and vasodilatation, can activate the production of substance P and can enhance prostaglandin release.
- Prostaglandins may provoke or inhibit the inflammatory response.
- Histamine and serotonin produce a short-lived vascular effect.
- Both bradykinins and prostaglandins promote more long-term vasodilatation (Broughton et al., 2006).

Substance P is also a key early responder to injury. It is a potent peptide found in most tissues where it amplifies or stimulates cellular processes. It promotes vasodilatation, increases vascular permeability and promotes phagocytosis and mast cell degranulation with the subsequent release of histamine and serotonin.

The overall vascular activity is responsible for the gross signs of inflammation: heat (calor), redness (rubor), swelling (tumor), pain and tenderness (dolor) and disturbed function (functio laesa) (Peery and Miller, 1971).

Inflammation causes pain and tenderness. Mechanical pain is due to mechanical stress, tissue damage, muscle spasm and the accumulated oedema, causing excess pressure on surrounding tissues. Chemical pain arises as a result of the release of inflammatory chemical mediators that go on to sensitise or activate surrounding nociceptors (Woller et al., 2017; Armstrong and Herr, 2019).

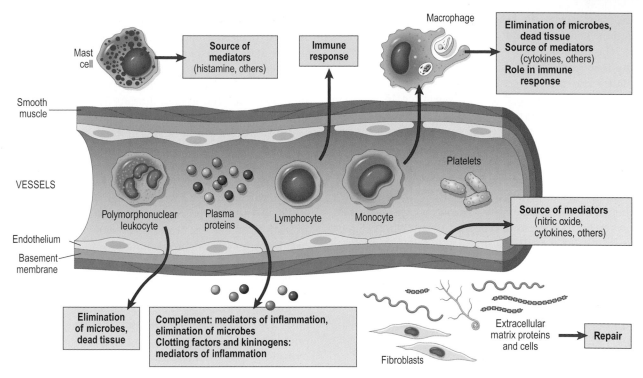

Fig. 3.2 The components of acute and chronic inflammatory processes: circulating cells and proteins, cells of blood vessels, and cells and proteins of the extracellular matrix. (From Kumar et al., 2020. Reprinted by permission of Elsevier Ltd.)

Chemical pain is also induced by certain inflammatory chemical mediators such as histamine, serotonin, bradykinins and prostaglandins, all released into the tissues during this inflammatory phase. The inflammatory substances may cause extreme irritation of nerve fibres without necessarily causing them damage.

The nociceptors become progressively more sensitive the longer the pain stimulus is maintained. Proinflammatory prostaglandins are believed to sensitise nociceptors, leading to a state of hyperalgesia—an increased response to a painful stimulus (Wilkerson, 1985; Kloth and Miller, 1990).

Attempts must be made to stop any continued bleeding, as blood is a strong irritant and will cause chemical and mechanical pain, as well as prolong the inflammatory process (Dingman, 1973; Evans, 1980).

Early Inflammatory Phase

In the first few hours of the early inflammatory phase, fibronectin, a structural glycoprotein that acts as a tissue 'glue', appears in the wound, deposited along strands of fibrin in the clot (Broughton et al., 2006; Standring, 2015).

This fibrin–fibronectin meshwork is associated with immature fibroblasts, which deposit type III collagen fibres to provide a scaffold for platelet adhesion and anchorage for further invading fibroblasts (Nimni, 1980; Lehto et al., 1985).

In minor injury, the inflammatory process is short and the scar tissue produced is minimal. The red blood cells break down into cellular debris and haemoglobin pigment, and the platelets (see Fig. 3.2) release thrombin, an enzyme that changes fibrinogen into fibrin. The fibrin forms a meshwork of fibres, which traps the blood clot, and an early scar is formed.

Phagocytic Phase

If the injury is significant, the next stage of the inflammatory phase is phagocytic. Circulating monocytes modulate into macrophages (Fowler, 1989) (see Fig. 3.2) and join the resident macrophage population to clear the debris from the site of injury through phagocytic action (Leibovich and Ross, 1974).

The macrophages increase in great numbers during the first 3 or 4 days (Dingman, 1973). They engulf any matter with which they come into contact, clearing the wound and preparing it for subsequent repair.

As well as performing a phagocytic role, the macrophage acts as a director cell, directing the repair process by chemically influencing an appropriate number of fibroblast cells activated in the area.

Macrophages also have a role in muscle regeneration, stimulating the production of satellite cells that align themselves to muscle fibres, where they can form new muscle fibres or restore damaged muscle fibres (Grefte et al., 2007; Liu et al., 2017).

Neovascularisation Phase

A stage of neovascularisation is reached, with capillaries starting to develop after about 12 hours and continuing to develop for a further 2 or 3 days (Daly, 1990). The new vessels supply oxygen and nourishment to the injured tissues; they are delicate and easily disrupted.

Inflammation is a normal response to either trauma or infection and to have no inflammatory response would mean that healing would not occur. Too little inflammation will delay healing, and too much inflammation will lead to excessive scarring.

Fig. 3.3 summarises the possible outcomes of acute inflammation and the features of complete resolution, healing by fibrosis or chronic inflammation.

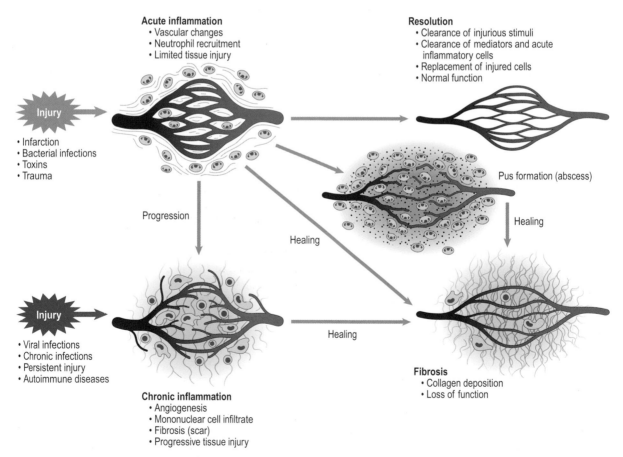

Fig. 3.3 Outcomes of acute inflammation: resolution, healing by fibrosis or chronic inflammation. The components of the various reactions and their functional outcomes are listed. (From Kumar et al. (2020). Reprinted by permission of Elsevier Ltd.)

PROLIFERATIVE PHASE

The proliferative, or repair, phase happens at the same time as the inflammatory phase and overlaps the remodelling phase.

Some tissues, for example, the synovial lining of the joints, bone and skeletal muscle, are capable of direct regeneration. All other connective tissues are incapable of regeneration, and repair of these structures involves a reconstruction process of the damaged tissue by collagen fibre or scar tissue formation.

Scar tissue does not have exactly the same properties or tensile strength as the tissue it is rebuilding, but its structure comes to resemble that tissue closely to ensure that normal function is regained (Douglas et al., 1969; Hardy, 1989; Watson, 2009).

Once the wound has been prepared by phagocytosis, the macrophage becomes the director of repair and signals an appropriate number of fibroblasts to the area. As the inflammatory phase subsides, the fibroblast becomes the dominant cell in the repair phase and synthesises the connective tissue matrix, comprising the ground substance and collagen (see Fig. 3.2).

Fibroblasts may appear in the wound during the first 24 hours after injury, but maximum numbers are not achieved until days 5 to 10 (Bryant, 1977; Chamberlain, 1982; Fowler, 1989). They do not decrease in number until 3 weeks after the injury (Chamberlain, 1982).

Fibroblasts secrete the ground substance, which provides the cross-linking mechanism for the collagen fibres it also synthesises. This arrangement 'glues' the wound together, with cross-links forming at appropriate nodal intersect points (see Chapter 2).

Once the fibroblasts are stimulated to produce collagen, there is rapid closure of the healing breach. Collagen fibres are laid down approximately 5 to 10 days after injury, and the repair process continues as they arrange themselves into larger units or bundles (Stearns, 1940b; Chamberlain, 1982).

Macrophages continue to stimulate the production of satellite cells, important for the regeneration and repair of muscle tissue. At the proliferation stage, the satellite cells become myoblasts that may either fuse to each other to create new myofibres or may fuse to existing damaged myofibres for repair (Grefte et al., 2007; Liu et al., 2017).

Fig. 3.3 summarises the components of acute and chronic inflammatory process and their principal functions.

The rate of repair is directly related to the size of the wound (Stearns, 1940a, 1940b). A small wound with approximated edges will heal quickly with a minimal inflammatory response, and collagen fibres will be laid down early to bind the edges together, provided that the edges remain in apposition. Consider a clean, stitched skin wound when the stitches are usually safely removed after 7 days and the wound has sufficient tensile strength to withstand movement.

Large, unapproximated wounds are deep as well as wide, and healing initially requires the formation of granulation tissue. It may be several days after injury before the fibroblasts initiate fibre formation and several weeks before there is sufficient collagen to provide enough tensile strength for the wound to withstand normal movement.

It is important to highlight that all timings mentioned throughout the healing process are approximate, and the practitioner needs to conduct a thorough assessment to establish the level of irritability of the tissues as a guide for the application of the appropriate graded mobilisation (see Chapter 4).

> **CLINICAL TIP**
> The level of irritability and stage in the healing process provide a guide to the application of the appropriate graded mobilisation.

Initial collagen fibre formation is random. The number of collagen fibres and the tensile strength of the wound increase substantially during the first 3 weeks after injury to become approximately 15% to 20% of the normal strength of the tissue (Hardy, 1989; Daly, 1990; Hardy and Woodall, 1998). However, the tensile strength does not depend entirely on the number of fibres, since after this time the number of collagen fibres stabilises but the tensile strength of the wound continues to increase.

Tensile strength is related to a balance between the synthesis and degradation of collagen (the production and breakdown of collagen; a continuous, dynamic process), the development of collagen cross-links and the orientation of collagen fibres into the existing weave.

This process of maturation is known as the remodelling phase (van der Meulen, 1982; Standring, 2015).

REMODELLING PHASE

The final stage of healing is the remodelling, or maturation phase, during which the new collagen or scar tissue attempts to take on the physical characteristics of the tissue it is replacing.

It begins in earnest approximately 21 days after injury and continues for 6 months or more, possibly even for years. Broughton et al. (2006) suggest that the process can begin much earlier than the peak of 21 days, from approximately 8 days, and support that the remodelling stage continues for 1 year.

Remodelling is responsible for the final structural orientation and arrangement of the fibres as well as the tensile strength. Initial, immature scar tissue is weak, and the fibres are oriented in all directions through several planes. Remodelling allows these randomly arranged fibres to become rearranged in both a linear and a lateral orientation into a 'well-mannered network' (Broughton et al., 2006). The orientation of collagen fibres occurs through induction and through tension.

Normal tissue adjacent to the wound induces structure in the replacement scar tissue. Thus, dense tissue induces dense, highly cross-linked scar tissue, while pliable tissue induces loose, less cross-linked scar tissue (Hardy, 1989). The final physical weave of the collagen formed is responsible for the functional behaviour of the wound within the connective tissue it is replacing.

Internal and external stresses (e.g. muscle tension, joint movement, passive gliding of fascial planes, connective tissue loading and unloading, temperature changes and mobilisation) apply tension to the wound during the remodelling phase (Hardy, 1989). Both mobilisation and immobilisation can strongly influence the structural orientation of collagen fibres (Stearns, 1940a, 1940b; Akeson et al., 1987).

During the maturation phase of scar formation, immature scar tissue is converted to mature scar tissue and the cross-linking system changes from weak hydrogen bonding to strong covalent bonding (Price, 1990).

While the scar tissue is relatively immature, the weak electrostatic bonding forms reducible cross-links that allow scar tissue to be mobilised with a gentle, steady stress. During this stage, transverse frictions and mobilisation are appropriate, within the limits of pain, to maintain the mobility of immature scar tissue. The graded mobilisation promotes the alignment of fibres.

Remodelling involves the reorganisation of a scar while it matures, with fibres being absorbed, replaced and reorientated. When stresses arising from mobilisation are applied to collagen fibres, the resultant piezo-electric effect (generation of small voltages called streaming potentials) is believed to be responsible for the production, maintenance, alignment and absorption of collagen fibrils (Price, 1990; Standring, 2015).

Cross-linking is responsible for the tensile strength of new, desirable scar tissue, but if the cross-linking becomes excessive, it will be responsible for the toughness and lack of resilience of unwanted fibrous adhesions (Kloth and Miller, 1990). Immobilisation causes loss of the ground substance, which reduces the interfibrillar distance, causes friction between the collagen subunits and facilitates the formation of excessive cross-links (Akeson et al., 1967; Donatelli and Owens-Burkhart, 1981; Akeson, 1990).

Collagen fibre formation and orientation conform to lines of stress within connective tissue and are similar in this respect to osseous alignment (Le Gros Clark, 1975; Price, 1990; Standring, 2015).

As mentioned, collagen synthesis and remodelling continue following injury with the tissue usually returning to its normal state of activity 6 to 12 months after injury (Daly, 1990). However, the increase in tensile strength in tendons, ligaments, fascia and other dense connective tissues is thought to take much longer (Dingman, 1973).

As the scar matures, it becomes tough and less pliable than immature scar tissue. The developing stable cross-links become more prolific and the stronger covalent bonds that form do not yield as readily to applied stresses (Price, 1990).

Synthesis and degradation, together with orientation of the collagen fibres (i.e. remodelling), ensure the final form of scar tissue. A balance is needed between collagen synthesis and degradation for an appropriate turnover of collagen, and sufficient stress should be applied to the tissue to stimulate fibre orientation but without disrupting the healing breach. This has implications for the grade of mobilisation applied and is discussed in Chapter 4.

Excessive scar tissue, adhesions or contracture within any soft tissue structure will impede function and cause pain. In the connective tissue structures important to musculoskeletal medicine, excessive production of scar tissue may be apparent as adhesion formation and contracture, either within the healing structure or within the surrounding tissues.

Abnormal excessive production of scar tissue may result in hypertrophic or keloid scars (Daly, 1990; Price, 1990). Hypertrophic scars develop when excessive collagen is deposited within the original wound site while keloid scarring involves excessive collagen deposits in the tissues surrounding the scar.

Pain itself, as a characteristic of inflammation, acts as an inhibitor to normal function and, if a state of chronic inflammation is maintained, the function of the tissue will continue to deteriorate. This self-perpetuating inflammation presents an ongoing chronic functional problem that may be difficult to treat.

Ligament Healing

Ligament injuries disrupt the balance between joint mobility and stability, which can lead to abnormal transmission of forces throughout the joint and possible damage to intra- and extra-articular structures (Hauser and Dolan, 2011).

Ligaments heal through the phases described earlier in this chapter. They need strong scar tissue fibres within their parallel wavy weave to be capable of resisting excessive joint stresses, as well as being able to relax and fold when the tension is removed. The scar tissue formed between the ligament and bone must mimic the normal weave to allow normal movement of the joint (Hardy, 1989).

The whole process of tissue healing can take many months to years and can be unpredictable, with some ligaments healing better than others. Many ligaments do not regain their normal tensile strength.

Despite the return of the properties listed, the structure within ligament scars remains different from normal ligament tissue. The collagen is relatively disorganised compared with normal ligament tissue with smaller collagen fibrils and flaws between fibres. Immature cross-links and more type III collagen are found dispersed throughout the tissue matrix with a higher density of cells. The turnover of cells and matrix is higher (Frank et al., 1999) (Fig. 3.4).

Incomplete healing can result in ligament laxity and joint instability which can lead to further injury as well as chronic pain, diminished function and eventual degenerative osteoarthropathy of the affected joint (Hauser and Dolan, 2011).

Muscle Healing

Skeletal muscle injury is a common problem in musculoskeletal practice and is often associated with contusion following direct trauma.

Figs 3.5 and 3.6 compare ultrasound scans of normal muscle fibre orientation in the semitendinosus muscle belly and a tear within the semitendinosus muscle belly.

The healing process of skeletal muscle is complex but consists of three phases, as described at the beginning of this chapter (Liu et al., 2017). Following trauma, muscle does demonstrate some regenerating properties.

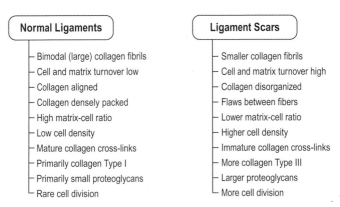

Normal Ligaments	Ligament Scars
– Bimodal (large) collagen fibrils	– Smaller collagen fibrils
– Cell and matrix turnover low	– Cell and matrix turnover high
– Collagen aligned	– Collagen disorganized
– Collagen densely packed	– Flaws between fibers
– High matrix-cell ratio	– Lower matrix-cell ratio
– Low cell density	– Higher cell density
– Mature collagen cross-links	– Immature collagen cross-links
– Primarily collagen Type I	– More collagen Type III
– Primarily small proteoglycans	– Larger proteoglycans
– Rare cell division	– More cell division

Fig. 3.4 Differences between normal ligaments and ligament scars. (From Hauser and Dolan, 2011.)

Normal muscle fibre orientation
in semitendinosus muscle belly

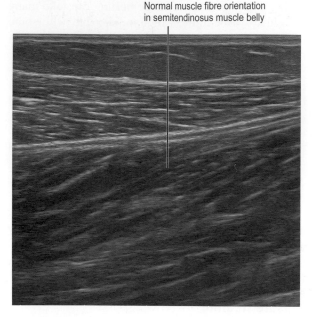

Fig. 3.5 Ultrasound scan of normal semitendinosus muscle. (Provided by Kjetil Nord-Varhaug.)

Tear within semitendinosus
muscle belly

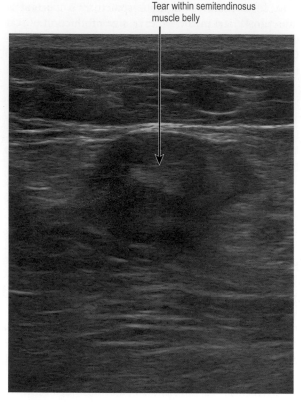

Fig. 3.6 Ultrasound scan demonstrating a tear within the semitendinosus muscle belly. (Provided by Kjetil Nord-Varhaug.)

- The first phase is *degeneration and inflammation* and is marked by local swelling at the injury site, haematoma formation, necrosis of muscle tissue, degeneration and the inflammatory response. Macrophages are important in muscle regeneration since their infiltration leads to increased satellite cell proliferation and differentiation.
- The second phase of *myofibre regeneration* occurs 5 to 10 days after injury and includes phagocytosis of the injured muscle tissue and regeneration of muscle fibres. Satellite cells, located next to the muscle fibres, can form completely new muscle fibres or restore damaged muscle fibres (Grefte et al., 2007; Nassari et al., 2017). The satellite cells become myoblasts that may either fuse to each other to create new myofibres or may fuse to existing damaged myofibres for repair.
- As healing moves into the third phase, the *muscle fibres mature and scar tissue is formed*. Most muscle injuries heal without dysfunctional scar tissue, but large muscle belly lesions resulting from major trauma will be filled with a mixture of disorganised scar tissue and new muscle fibres, which can inhibit regeneration and lead to incomplete functional recovery.

Chazaud (2020) highlights how important inflammation and the role of macrophages is to muscle healing and emphasises that the natural response of the pro-inflammatory stage of tissue injury should not be 'blunted' or 'fought' by applying an anti-inflammatory treatment too early, as it can be detrimental to healing. He advises against the use of ice or non-steroidal anti-inflammatory drugs (NSAIDs) for a few days after severe skeletal muscle injury, although it may not be as important with milder muscle injuries.

Shen et al. (2008) and Liu et al. (2017) stress the crucial role of macrophages in skeletal muscle regeneration, and a reduced number of macrophages in muscle tissue is associated with reduced muscle regeneration.

Scar tissue formed within a muscle belly needs to be flexible to allow the muscle fibres to broaden as the muscle contracts and extensible enough to allow the muscle to lengthen when stretched.

Muscle tissue is highly responsive to changes in functional demands and after a brief period to allow the scar tissue to stabilise progressive loading should be started to minimise atrophy and to encourage faster and more complete regeneration (Khan and Scott, 2009).

Tendinopathy

The term *tendinopathy* describes a clinical condition affecting tendons and is normally used to describe a symptomatic tendon. 'Tendinitis' used to be the common term, but the inflammatory model of tendon pain has been challenged (Cook et al., 2000; Khan and Cook, 2000); and 'tendinopathy' has been adopted as more appropriate since it does not commit to pathology.

The terms 'tendinosis', 'paratendinitis' and 'tendinitis' are reserved as histopathological labels and *tendinopathy* will be used throughout this text to indicate a painful tendon lesion.

Characteristics of tendinopathy include a combination of pain, thickening and impaired performance. The aetiology of tendinopathy appears to be multifactorial and the pathogenesis is unclear. It is found in those who participate in recreational and elite sport but is also found in those with a more sedentary lifestyle.

A sudden increase or decrease in activity may be a cause of tendinopathy, and tendons can respond adversely to both overuse and underuse Rees et al. (2006). 'They don't like rest, and they don't like change' (J.L. Cook, Tendinopathy Masterclass, Nov 2012).

Tendons have evolved primarily to transmit tensile load and their fibrous, inelastic structure reflects their function. As well as increased or repetitive tensile stresses, compression has been proposed as a contributory factor to tendinopathy, particularly in those tendons that have a close relationship with a bony prominence (Cook and Purdam, 2012).

Other factors such as vascular supply, adiposity, age and genetics can also play a part in the pathogenesis of tendinopathy (Wang et al., 2006; Scott et al., 2013, Cook et al., 2016, Ahmad et al., 2020), as well as local hypoxia, repetitive microtrauma or impaired wound healing (Richards et al., 2005). Heat generated during prolonged locomotion may be another factor that could contribute to tendon injury (Ahmad et al., 2020).

Ahmad et al. (2020) classify factors contributing to tendon pathology as 'intrinsic' or 'extrinsic' (Table 3.1).

TABLE 3.1 Factors Implicated in Chronic Tendinopathy

Intrinsic Factors	Extrinsic Factors
Age	Occupation
Vascular	Sport
Nutrition	Physical load
Anatomical variants	Training errors
Laxity of joint	Shoes and equipment
Muscle weakness	Environmental condition
Gender	

From Ahmad et al., 2020.

Contributing factors for specific tendon lesions and their management are discussed in the chapters that follow in Section 2.

If a tendon and its blood supply are ruptured or torn, a classic inflammatory response is seen, passing through the three overlapping phases of inflammation, proliferation and remodelling (Cook et al., 2016; Ahmad et al., 2020).

In tendinopathy, the tendon's response is complex and the inflammatory response is not traditional (Cook et al., 2016). Inflammatory cells or signs of chemical inflammation are absent in chronically painful tendons, and the pathological process in tendinopathy may involve degenerative rather than inflammatory changes (Cook et al., 2000; Khan and Cook, 2000; Wang et al., 2006).

Degenerative changes are observed in chronic tendon lesions, which include collagen fibre breakdown, irregular fibre arrangement, a high concentration of glycosaminoglycans, increased ground substance, neovascularisation, increased number of nerve filaments and increased immunoreactivity of substance P and calcitonin (Alfredson et al., 2002; Tasto et al., 2003; Richards et al., 2005; Wang et al., 2006, Kragsnaes et al., 2014).

Where the pain comes from in tendon lesions is still unclear (Cook et al., 2016). Alfredson et al. (2002) suggested that neovascularisation might be involved, and some treatments, such as prolotherapy and aprotinin injections, aim to reduce vascularity in the tendon and thus reduce tendon thickening and pain.

Rees et al. (2006) also put forward mechanical, neural and vascular theories, suggesting that the pain arises from a combination of factors. Rudavsky and Cook (2014) refer to more recent evidence that appears to support that central sensitisation or abnormal up-regulation of the central nervous system could have a role in the pain experienced in tendinopathies.

There is evidence for both tendon-based nociceptive contributions and extensive mechanisms within the peripheral and central nervous systems. Tendon pain remains complex and requires thorough assessment of musculoskeletal and neural contributing factors, including potential central mechanisms (Rio et al., 2014).

The most marked change in tendon degeneration is decreased tensile strength. Collagen cross-linking increases and alters the mechanical properties of the tendon. The ability to withstand load, viscoelasticity and tensile strength all decrease, and there is an increase in mechanical stiffness (Kannus et al., 2005; Eliasson et al. 2007).

Repetitive strain can reduce the ability of the tendon to endure further tension, disrupting its microscopic and macroscopic structure. The structural damage noted in tendinopathy can include partial tearing of the collagen fibres, possibly leading to partial and complete tendon tears (Józsa and Kannus, 1997).

Whilst acknowledging the degenerative features in chronic tendinopathy, Cook and Purdam (2009) have suggested that the degenerative model does not fully explain how the signs and symptoms and the histological changes can improve or reverse, as observed in the clinical situation. They propose that there is a continuum of tendon pathology that transitions through three stages: reactive tendinopathy, tendon disrepair and degenerative tendinopathy (Fig. 3.7).

Reactive tendinopathy usually results from acute overload associated with a burst of unaccustomed activity, often after a period of rest or relative immobilisation, or a direct blow to the tendon. A short-term reaction occurs with tendon thickening and changes in the tissue structure.

In *tendon disrepair*, attempts at tendon healing are apparent alongside a greater breakdown of the matrix

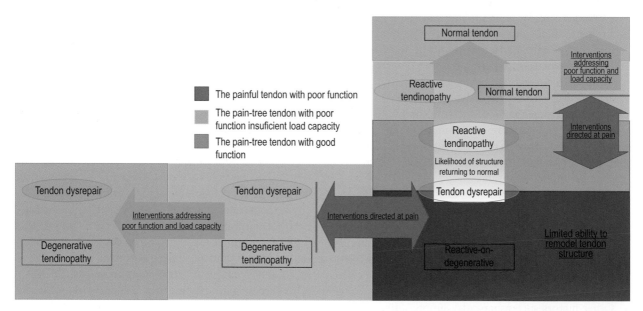

Fig. 3.7 Schematic representation of how we may phenotype patients with tendinopathy in relation to the continuum and target treatments. The aim of treatment is to push the tendon into the green section with relatively little pain and good function. Tendon structure can be normalised in the early stages of the continuum where rehabilitation can push the tendon 'up the continuum'. In the latter stages of the continuum, 'moving up the continuum' may not be possible, so interventions should be focused in 'moving the tendon sideways'. It is important to note that interventions directed solely at pain will not drive the tendon to a positive outcome as they do not address dysfunction, such as motor inhibition, strength and power deficits, or tendon load capacity. Interventions that target structure may improve tendon structure and direct the tendon 'upwards along the continuum'; however, it will not address functional deficits (effect on pain is inconclusive) or load capacity and may leave the tendon vulnerable to reinjury. (Reproduced from Cook et al., 2016. With permission from BMJ Publishing Group.)

and an overall increase in the number of cells, predominantly chondrocytes and myofibroblasts, that leads to a marked increase in proteoglycans and collagen production. Increased vascularity and neural in-growth may be apparent at this stage.

At the third stage of the continuum, *degenerative tendinopathy*, the histopathological changes described previously have progressed, with further degradation of the matrix and acellularity as a sign of cell death (apoptosis).

In revisiting the continuum model, Cook et al. (2016) emphasise that some tendons may have discrete regions that are in different stages at the same time, producing an important clinical presentation of 'reactive-on-degenerative tendinopathy'.

Tendon is a dynamic, mechanoresponsive tissue that is sensitive to changes in physical load and can respond favourably to controlled loading after injury (Khan and Scott, 2009). In the earlier stages, the condition can be influenced by initially removing and then progressively adding load to allow the tendon to adapt and return to full function (optimal or progressive loading) (Cook and Purdam, 2009).

Khan and Scott (2009) explain the beneficial effects of loading through 'mechanotransduction', the process whereby cells convert physiological mechanical stimuli into biomechanical responses. They describe the process in three steps: mechanocoupling, where the physical loading acts as a trigger or catalyst for cell-to-cell communication; cell-to-cell communication, which leads to a wide array of responses in cells that are distant from the site of the stimulus; and the effector cell response, which promotes cell proliferation, tissue repair and remodelling within the tendon.

Several factors affect the mechanical forces that act on tendons and influence their adaptation in response. The different types of activity, location of the tendon in the body and joint position induce different levels of force on tendons, such that different tendons are subject to different levels of mechanical loading.

Once in the degenerative phase of the continuum, there is little capacity for the reversal of pathological changes. Transverse frictions, extracorporeal shock wave therapy, ultrasound and other physical treatments that stimulate cell activity, increase protein production and restructure the matrix are appropriate for the degenerative stage (Cook and Purdam, 2009; Ahmad et al., 2020). Progressive loading is also appropriate.

Cook and Purdam (2009) note that pain may, or may not, be associated with any stage along their proposed continuum, regardless of pathology, and may possibly be complicated by associated bursitis. In addition to providing a subjective marker for improvement, pain can also be used to guide the application of progressive loading in tendon rehabilitation.

Heavy load eccentric exercise programmes may be highly provocative in the reactive stage (Cook et al., 2016). Over the long term, however, they can reduce swelling, affect type I collagen production and increase tendon volume, which is an important consideration in the rehabilitation of tendinopathies (Alfredson and Cook, 2007), especially in the latter stages of the continuum proposed by Cook and Purdam (2009).

Cook and Purdam (2012) suggest that stretching increases compression where tendons pass over a bony prominence, especially where there is some tension in the muscle as well. They advise that in this situation, it is probably better to address muscle length and compliance in the muscle–tendon unit by using massage techniques rather than stretching.

Other treatment options for tendinopathy include prolotherapy (sclerosant injections) and autologous blood injections (Brukner et al., 2017). Surgery may be appropriate in some cases and for some tendons but only once the more conservative stages of a stepped approach have been exhausted.

Transverse frictions and injections are described in Chapter 4, and management for specific tendon lesions is discussed for specific lesions within the relevant chapters in Section 2.

In summary, tendinopathy is a long-standing condition that takes many months to resolve and requires ongoing monitoring and management towards full rehabilitation. The development of treatment and rehabilitation programmes for patients presenting with symptomatic tendinopathy requires complex clinical reasoning. Rehabilitation varies considerably depending on the site and stage of tendinopathy, functional assessment and activity status, contributing biomechanical issues, comorbidities and concurrent presentations (Scott et al., 2013).

Tenosynovitis is distinct from tendinopathy and occurs in ensheathed tendons, involving the synovial sheath of a tendon rather than the tendon itself (Vuillemin et al., 2012); for example, De Quervain's stenosing tenosynovitis of the sheath containing the abductor pollicis longus and extensor pollicis brevis tendons. Tendon sheaths are filled with a lubricating fluid, allowing the tendons to move smoothly and freely through them. Inflammation of the synovium produces pain on movement and adhesions can form, which may produce palpable crepitus (Cyriax, 1982).

Treatment includes mobilising the sheath around the tendon, through the application of transverse frictions, or injection of corticosteroid within the synovial space.

Arthropathy

Arthropathy is a generic term used to describe pain, swelling and stiffness in a joint. There are many different types of arthropathy with the most common being degenerative and inflammatory, for example, rheumatoid arthritis.

Despite the underlying histopathology, 'arthritis' appears to be used commonly for all forms of arthropathy. The term 'arthritis' may be more widely understood when communicating with patients but this text will use 'arthropathy' throughout unless referring to inflammatory joint conditions.

Degenerative arthropathy is the most common form. Prevalence ranges between 15% and 20% in Western populations and it becomes more common with age. It is estimated that around 8.75 million people in the UK have consulted a medical practitioner about 'osteoarthritis' (Versus Arthritis, 2021).

Degenerative arthropathy is a condition affecting synovial joints. There is progressive deterioration and loss of articular cartilage, which is associated with structural and functional changes in the whole joint, including the synovium, periarticular ligaments and subchondral bone (Mobasheri and Batt, 2016).

Despite the distinction between 'degenerative' and 'inflammatory' arthritis, inflammation is an accepted feature of degenerative arthropathy, marked by the presence of synovitis and with a direct association between joint inflammation and disease progression (Mobasheri and Batt, 2016). Notwithstanding, much of the focus of attention has been on the articular component of the disease and specifically articular cartilage in the context of injury, ageing and degeneration.

Inflammatory mediators with mechanical and oxidative stress compromise the function of chondrocytes and they undergo hypertrophic differentiation and early senescence, or ageing. This increases their sensitivity to the effects of pro-inflammatory and pro-catabolic mediators and leads to further cartilage degeneration.

Degenerative arthropathy is complex and multifactorial, and there are many different types. The knowledge base on the pathophysiology of degenerative arthropathy is expanding and multiple mediators are appearing as regulators of the disease process.

NICE guidelines (2020) recommended a stepped approach to the management of degenerative arthropathy. Patients diagnosed with degenerative arthropathy, irrespective of age, comorbidity, pain severity or disability should all be offered a core treatment plan and individualised self-management plan. This includes exercise, education, pacing, ice/heat application, activity and work modification, orthotics, and weight reduction for overweight or obese patients.

Should symptoms persist, less invasive treatments can be considered in addition to core treatment, including simple analgesics and NSAIDs, and physiotherapy (e.g. exercise, manual therapy, gait re-education). When symptoms remain irritable, e.g. night pain and impaired function, more invasive treatments, such as corticosteroid injection, can be considered in addition to core treatment. These measures may delay the need for surgical intervention (Mobasheri and Batt, 2016).

General indications for surgery are persistent severe symptoms (e.g. pain and significant impact on function), and when good quality non-surgical interventions have failed (NICE, 2020).

Bursitis

A bursa is a fluid filled sac lined with synovial membrane which secretes viscous synovial fluid into the bursal cavity. Bursae are associated with most of the peripheral joints in the body where they help to reduce friction between structures and provide lubrication for free movement.

Subcutaneous bursae are flat sacs of synovial membrane, supported by irregular connective tissue within the loose areolar tissue between skin and bone. They contain a thin film of synovial fluid, and examples of bursae may be found at the elbow and knee.

Most synovial bursae lie between tendons and bones or ligaments (subtendinous), and others are found between muscle and a bone, tendon or ligament (submuscular). Many communicate with the nearby joint, for example, the psoas bursa and subscapularis bursa.

Adventitious bursae arise in adulthood at sites where subcutaneous tissue becomes subject to high pressure and friction, for example, the subcutaneous calcaneal bursa.

An inflamed bursa is associated with swelling and pain. It tends to produce a 'muddle' of signs with some passive movements and some resisted tests being painful when the bursa is compressed or stretched.

Bursitis may be associated with biomechanical factors that need to be addressed. It can respond to treatment with NSAIDs, can be aspirated or injected with corticosteroid. Care must be taken with infected bursitis. Aspiration can be considered and antibiotic medication is normally required. Corticosteroid injection is not appropriate for infected bursitis.

Management of specific bursal lesions is discussed within the relevant chapters in Section 2.

Mechanical Joint Displacements

The term 'mechanical joint displacement' can be applied to a range of lesions that can include loose bodies (e.g. knee and elbow) and meniscal lesions (e.g. knee and wrist).

They are 'mechanical' as opposed to inflammatory and indicate that something is blocking normal movement and may be the cause of pain. The lesions important in musculoskeletal medicine will be covered individually in the relevant chapters.

Factors That May Affect Wound Healing

> **CLINICAL TIP**
> In considering various factors that can promote, delay or lead to poor repair, assessment of connective tissue lesions should take into account the following factors:
> - Time of onset and the time lapse since injury
> - Extent of the lesion
> - Grade of injury
> - Inappropriate or overaggressive mobilisation relating to irritability of the lesion
> - First aid and initial management of the injury
> - Stage reached in the inflammation, repair and remodelling phases
> - Anatomical structures involved directly and indirectly in the lesion
> - General health such as poor nutrition, obesity and inactivity
> - Medical conditions that may affect wound healing, such as cardiovascular disorders, blood clotting disorders, diabetes and immunosuppressive conditions
> - Age
> - Medications that might affect management and healing, such as anticoagulants, analgesics, anti-inflammatory drugs, and immunosuppressant drugs

Chronic trauma can cause excessive movement or tension on devitalised tissues, promoting unwanted scarring. This may be the mechanism of chronic overuse syndromes in which repeated movement disrupts tissue unity.

Haematoma formation slows the healing process by acting as an irritant, producing a mechanical blockage that separates the torn edges and provides a medium for infection (Dingman, 1973). Infection of the injured tissue presents a serious complication that delays the healing process.

Ageing can delay cell migration and proliferation, wound contracture and collagen remodelling and decrease the tensile strength of the wound, increasing the chance of wound splitting (Mulder, 1990).

Chemical changes in the gel–fibre ratio have been noted in such tissues as the skin and the nucleus pulposus of older individuals (Akeson et al., 1968). Changes occurring with age are consistent with the changes occurring with immobilisation. Contractures tend to occur more frequently, after less trauma and after shorter periods of time in the relatively immobile joints of the elderly.

Some medications, therapies and conditions may also affect healing. While anti-inflammatory medication may not be the most appropriate treatment for acute inflammation, its use in chronic lesions is appropriate for suppressing inflammation and relieving pain. NSAIDs do not cause a significant change in collagen synthesis but they inhibit the production of histamine, serotonin and prostaglandins (Wilkerson, 1985). In addition to its anti-inflammatory function, aspirin inhibits platelet aggregation and may prolong bleeding (Ritter et al., 2020).

The oral intake of corticosteroids inhibits collagen synthesis, reduces tensile strength and delays wound healing (Dingman, 1973; Ahonen et al., 1980; Mulder, 1990). Corticosteroids administered in the acute inflammatory phase interfere with macrophage migration but if delivered after the macrophage invasion, i.e. after 3 days, their effect on wound healing is much less severe (Fowler, 1989).

Anticoagulants, such as heparin and warfarin, prolong bleeding and delay healing.

The effect of chemotherapy depends on the drugs used and their dosage, but fibroblast proliferation may be affected and collagen synthesis delayed (Carrico et al., 1984).

Radiotherapy radiation can damage fibroblasts, cause vascular damage and decrease collagen production, but it depends on the dose, frequency and location of the irradiated area in relation to the injury site (Mulder, 1990).

Acquired immune deficiency syndrome patients are in a state of immunosuppression and this will delay the healing process.

Diabetes appears to affect the inflammatory stage rather than collagen synthesis, implying that insulin is important in the early phase of healing (Carrico et al., 1984).

Other factors that could affect healing include vitamin A and C deficiency, protein deprivation, low temperature (Watson, 2009), systemic vascular disorders and systemic connective tissue disorders.

REVIEW QUESTIONS

1. Describe the role of the macrophage in soft tissue healing.
2. What process happens during the remodelling phase?
3. What pathological changes take place during the healing process if the tissue is immobilised?
4. What is your understanding of the different stages of the pathophysiology of tendinopathy?
5. What is meant by the term 'progressive loading' when referring to the rehabilitation of tendinopathy?

REFERENCES

Ahmad, Z., Parkar, A., Shepherd, J., et al., 2020. Revolving door of tendinopathy: definition, pathogenesis and treatment. Postgrad. Med. J. 96, 94–101.

Ahonen, J., Jiborn, H., Zederfeldt, B., 1980. Hormone influence on wound healing. In: Hunt, T.K. (Ed.), Wound Healing and Wound Infection: Theory and Surgical Practice. Appleton Century Croft, New York, pp. 95–105.

Akeson, W., 1990. The response of ligaments to stress modulation and overview of the ligament healing response. In: Daniel, D., Akeson, W.H., O'Connor, J.J. (Eds.), Knee Ligaments: Structure, Function, Injury and Repair. Lippincott, Williams & Wilkins, Philadelphia, pp. 315–327.

Akeson, W., Amiel, D., La Violette, D., 1967. The connective tissue response to immobility: a study of chondroitin-4 and 6-sulfate and dermatan sulfate changes in periarticular connective tissue of control and immobilised knees of dogs. Clin. Orthop. Relat. Res. 51, 183–197.

Akeson, W., Amiel, D., LaViolette, D., 1968. The connective tissue response to immobility: an accelerated ageing response? Exp. Gerontol. 3, 289–301.

Akeson, W., Amiel, D., Abel, M.F., 1987. Effects of immobilisation on joints. Clin. Orthop. Relat. Res. 219, 28–37.

Alfredson, H., Cook, J., 2007. A treatment algorithm for managing Achilles tendinopathy: new treatment options. Br. J. Sports Med. 41 (4), 211–216.

Alfredson, H., Bjur, D., Thorsen, K., et al., 2002. High intra-tendinous lactate levels in painful chronic Achilles tendinosis. An investigation using microdialysis technique. J. Orthop. Res. 20 (5), 934–938.

Armstrong, S.A., Herr, M.J., 2019. Physiology, Nociception. StatPearls Publishing. https://www.ncbi.nlm.nih.gov/books/NBK551562/. Accessed 3 September 2021.

Broughton, G., Janis, J., Attinger, C., 2006. The basic science of wound healing. Plast. Reconstr. Surg. 117 (7S), 12S–34S.

Brukner, P., Clarson, B., Cook, J., et al., 2017. Clinical Sports Medicine, fifth ed. Injuries, Volume 1, McGraw-Hill, Sydney.

Bryant, W., 1977. Wound healing. Clin. Symp. 29, 2–28.

Carrico, T.J., Mehrhof, A.I., Cohen, I.K., 1984. Biology of wound healing. Surg. Clin. N. Am. 64, 721–731.

Chamberlain, G.J., 1982. Cyriax's friction massage: a review. J. Orthop. Sports Phys. Ther. 4, 16–22.

Chazaud, B., 2020. Inflammation and skeletal muscle degeneration: Leave it to the macrophages! Trends Immunol. 41 (6), 481–492.

Cook, J.L., Purdam, C.R., 2009. Is tendon pathology a continuum? A pathology model to explain the clinical presentation of load-induced tendinopathy. Br. J. Sports Med. 43, 409–416.

Cook, J.L., Purdam, C.R., 2012. Is compressive load a factor in the development of tendinopathy? Br. J. Sports Med. 46, 163–168.

Cook, J.L., Khan, K.M., Maffulli, N., et al., 2000. Overuse tendinosis, not tendinopathy, part 2: applying the new approach to patellar tendinopathy. Phys. Sports Med. 28 (6), 31–41.

Cook, J.L., Rio, E., Purdam, C.R., et al., 2016. Revisiting the continuum model of tendon pathology: what is its merit in clinical practice and research? Br. J. Sports Med. 50, 1187–1191.

Cyriax, J., 1982. Textbook of Orthopaedic Medicine, eighth ed., vol. 1, Baillière Tindall, London.

Daly, T.J., 1990. The repair phase of wound healing – re-epithelialization and contraction. In: Kloth, L.C., McCullock, J.M., Feedar, J.A. (Eds.), Wound Healing: Alternatives in Management. F.A. Davis, Philadelphia, pp. 14–29.

Dingman, R.O., 1973. Factors of clinical significance affecting wound healing. Laryngoscope 83, 1540–1554.

Donatelli, R., Owens-Burkhart, H., 1981. Effects of immobility on the extensibility of periarticular connective tissue. J. Orthop. Sports Phys.Ther. 3 (2), 67–72.

Douglas, D.M., Forrester, J.C., Ogilvie, R.R., 1969. Physical characteristics of collagen in the later stages of wound healing. Br. J. Surg. 56, 219–222.

Eliasson, P., Fahlgren, A., Pasternak, B., et al., 2007. Unloaded rat Achilles tendons continue to grow, but lose viscoelasticity. J. Appl. Physiol. 103, 459–463.

Evans, P., 1980. The healing process at cellular level: a review. Physiotherapy 66, 256–259.

Frank, C., Shrive, N., Hiraoka, N., et al., 1999. Optimization of the biology of soft tissue repair. J. Sci. Med. Sport. 2, 190–210.

Fowler, J.D., 1989. Wound healing: an overview. Semin. Vet. Med. Surg. 4, 256–262.

Grefte, S., Kuijpers-Jagtman, A.M., Torensma, R., et al., 2007. Skeletal muscle development and regeneration. Stem Cells Dev. 16 857–168

Hardy, M.A., 1989. The biology of scar formation. Phys. Ther. 69, 1014–1023.

Hardy, M., Woodall, W., 1998. Therapeutic effects of heat, cold and stretch on connective tissue. J. Hand Ther. 11 (2), 148–152.

Hauser, R., Dolan, E., 2011. Ligament injury and healing: An overview of current clinical concepts. J. Prolotherap. 3 (4), 836–846.

Józsa, L., Kannus, P., 1997. Human Tendons: Anatomy, Physiology and Pathology. Human Kinetics, Champaign, IL.

Kannus, P., Paavola, M., Józsa, L., 2005. Aging and degeneration of tendons. In: Maffulli, N., Renström, P., Leadbetter, W.B. (Eds.), Tendon Injuries: Basic Science and Clinical Medicine. Springer-Verlag, London, pp. 25–31.

Khan, K.M., Cook, J.L., 2000. Overuse tendon injuries: where does the pain come from? Sports Med. Arthrosc. Rev. 8, 17–31.

Khan, K.M., Scott, A., 2009. Mechanotherapy: how physical therapists' prescription of exercise promotes tissue repair. Br. J. Sports Med. 43, 247–251.

Kloth, L.C., Miller, K.H., 1990. The inflammatory response to wounding. In: Kloth, L.C., McCullock, J.M., Feedar, J.A. (Eds.), Wound Healing: Alternatives in Management. F.A. Davis, Philadelphia, pp. 14–29.

Kragsnaes, M.S., Fredberg, U., Stribolt, K., Kjaer, S.G., Bendix, K., Ellingsen, T., 2014. Stereological quantification of immune-competent cells in baseline biopsy specimens from achilles tendons: results from patients with chronic tendinopathy followed for more than 4 years. Am. J. Sports Med. 42 (10), 2435–2445.

Kumar, V., Abbas, A., Aster, J., 2020. Robbins & Cotran Pathologic Basis of Disease, tenth ed. Elsevier, Amsterdam.

Le Gros Clark, W.E., 1975. The Tissues of the Body, sixth ed. Oxford University Press, Oxford.

Lehto, M., Duance, V.C., Restall, D., 1985. Collagen and fibronectin in a healing skeletal muscle injury. J. Bone Joint Surg. 67B, 820–827.

Leibovich, S.J., Ross, R., 1974. The role of the macrophage in wound repair. Am. J. Pathol. 78, 71–91.

Liu, X., Liu, Y., Zhao, L., Zeng, Z., et al., 2017. Macrophage depletion impairs skeletal muscle regeneration: The roles of regulatory factors for muscle regeneration. Cell. Biol. Int. 41, 228–238.

Mobasheri, A., Batt, M., 2016. An update on the pathophysiology of osteoarthritis. Ann. Phys. Rehabil. Med. 59 (5–6), 333–339.

Mulder, G.D., 1990. Factors complicating wound repair. In: Kloth, L.C., McCullock, J.M., Feedar, J. (Eds.), Wound Healing: Alternatives in Management. F.A. Davis, Philadelphia, pp. 43–51.

Nassari, S., Duprez, D., Fourier-Thibault, C., 2017. Non-myogenic contribution to muscle development and homeostasis: the role of the connective tissues. Front. Cell Dev. Biol. 5, 22.

National Institute for Health and Care Excellence (NICE), 2020. Osteoarthritis: care and management. NICE. https://www.nice.org.uk/guidance/cg177 Accessed 3 September 2021.

Nimni, M.E., 1980. The molecular organisation of collagen and its role in determining the biophysical properties of the connective tissues. Biorheology 17, 51–82.

Peery, T.M., Miller, F.N., 1971. Pathology: A Dynamic Introduction to Medicine and Surgery, second ed. Little, Brown, Boston.

Price, H., 1990. Connective tissue in wound healing. In: Kloth, L.C., McCullock, J.M., Feedar, J. (Eds.), Wound Healing: Alternatives in Management. F.A. Davis, Philadelphia, pp. 31–41.

Rees, J., Wilson, A., Wolman, R., 2006. Current concepts in the management of tendon disorders. Rheumatology 45, 508–521.

Richards, P., Win, T., Jones, P., 2005. The distribution of microvascular response in Achilles tendinopathy assessed by colour and power Doppler. Skeletal Radiol. 34 (6), 336–342.

Rio, E., Moseley, L., Purdam, C., et al., 2014. The pain of tendinopathy: Physiological or pathophysiological. Sports Med. 44, 9–23.

Ritter, J.M., Flower, R., Henderson, G., et al., 2020. Rang and Dale's Pharmacology, ninth ed. Elsevier, Edinburgh.

Rudavsky, A., Cook, J., 2014. Physiotherapy management of patellar tendinopathy (jumper's knee). J. Physiother. 60, 122–129.

Scott, A., Docking, S., Vicenzino, B., et al., 2013. Sports and exercise-related tendinopathies: a review of selected topical issues by participants of the second International Scientific Tendinopathy Symposium (ISTS) Vancouver 2012. Br. J. Sports Med. 47, 536–544.

Shen, W., Li, Y., Zhu, J., 2008. Interaction between macrophages. TGF-beta1, and the COX-2 pathway during the inflammatory phase of skeletal muscle healing after injury. J. Cell Physiol. 214, 405–412.

Standring, S., 2015. Gray's Anatomy: The Anatomical Basis of Clinical Practice, forty-first ed. Churchill Livingstone, Edinburgh.

Stearns, M.L., 1940a. Studies on the development of connective tissue in transparent chambers in the rabbit's ear, I. Am. J. Anat. 66, 133–176.

Stearns, M.L., 1940b. Studies on the development of connective tissue in transparent chambers in the rabbit's ear, II. Am. J. Anat. 67, 55–97.

Tasto, J.P., Cummings, J., Medlock, V., et al., 2003. The tendon treatment center: new horizons in the treatment of tendinosis. Arthroscopy 19 (Suppl. 1), 213–223.

van der Meulen, J.H.C., 1982. Present state of knowledge on processes of healing in collagen structures. Int. J. Sports Med. 3, 4–8.

Versus Arthritis. https://www.versusarthritis.org. Accessed 21 August 2021.

Vuillemin, V., Guerini, H., Bard, H., et al., 2012. Stenosing tenosynovitis. J. Ultrasound 15 (1), 20–28.

Wang, J., Losifidus, M., Fu, F., 2006. Biomechanical basis for tendinopathy. Clin. Orthop. Relat. Res. 443, 320–332.

Watson, T., 2009. Tissue repair phases and timescale. Available from: http://www.electrotherapy.org.

Wilkerson, G.B., 1985. Inflammation in connective tissue: etiology and management. Athl. Train. 20, 298–301.

Woller, S.A., Eddinger, K.A., Corr, M., Yaksh, T.L., 2017. An overview of pathways encoding nociception. Clin. Exp. Rheumatol. 107 (5), 40–46.

4

Musculoskeletal Medicine Treatment Techniques

CHAPTER CONTENTS

SUMMARY

Over the years, the emphasis of treatment for musculoskeletal lesions has moved from total immobilisation to early mobilisation. The benefits of early mobilisation have become clear, and, while a short period of immobilisation may still be necessary, the overall aim of musculoskeletal medicine treatment techniques is to restore full painless function to the connective tissues through appropriate, progressive mobilisation.

The selection of techniques depends on several factors that include the stage the lesion has reached in the healing cycle, with particular attention to the overall irritability. An accurate assessment and clinical diagnosis allow the effective application of the selected treatment techniques and the development of an agreed management programme.

Treatment techniques used in musculoskeletal medicine fall into two broad categories of mobilisation and injection and are listed in Table 4.1.

After a review of the general principles of management, this chapter is divided into two parts. The first part will discuss mobilisation and the techniques used

TABLE 4.1   Treatment Techniques in Musculoskeletal Medicine

Mobilisation	Injection
Transverse frictions	Corticosteroid
Grade A mobilisation	Local anaesthetic
Grade B mobilisation	Hyaluronic acid
Grade C manipulation	Epidural
	Platelet-rich plasma
Traction	Prolotherapy

in musculoskeletal medicine, on the basis of the theory presented in the preceding chapters. The second part will discuss and describe injection techniques.

GENERAL PRINCIPLES OF MUSCULOSKELETAL MEDICINE MANAGEMENT

The management approach for the soft tissue lesions discussed in the previous chapter is guided by the stage of healing of the condition, severity of symptoms, clinical findings and shared decision making.

A stepped approach is normally taken to management, starting with non-surgical options, such as pharmacological management, physiotherapy, education, ice/heat application, exercise rehabilitation, pacing and activity modification. Depending on the site of lesion, myofascial release, deep tissue massage, orthotics, acupuncture and electrotherapy may be indicated. Injection may also be an option and aims to provide a window of opportunity for exercise and ongoing rehabilitation.

In persistent cases or where patients fail to improve despite good-quality conservative management, surgical management can be considered.

The overall management and rehabilitation of soft tissue injuries requires careful judgement as well as knowledge of the stages of healing, as described in Chapter 3. The progression through the earlier stages of healing is described here. The principles of ongoing rehabilitation will be discussed at the appropriate points within the relevant chapters in Section 2.

At the earliest stage, the aim is to protect the tissues and then to apply progressive loading to stimulate, but not to disrupt, the healing tissues.

Various acronyms have been developed over the years to guide the management of acute injuries, and a new one seems to have become in vogue as we have prepared each edition of this text. We have moved from 'ICE' to 'RICE' to 'PRICE' and to 'POLICE'. There was a 'NICE' as well, which advocated the since-disputed early use of non-steroidal anti-inflammatory drugs (NSAIDs).

The more recent POLICE principle of employing protection, optimal (progressive) loading, ice, compression and elevation in the early stages provides a guide to control heat, swelling and pain, reduce inflammation and promote tissue repair (Bleakley et al., 2012). The inclusion of the optimal loading ('OL') highlights the importance of mobilisation at the appropriate stage of healing.

Dubois and Esculier (2020) observe that within each of the acronyms above, the focus has been on acute management of soft tissue injuries, without reference to rehabilitation. They advocate the novel acronym 'PEACE' for the early stages, leading onto 'LOVE' to guide ongoing rehabilitation (Fig. 4.1).

Summarising the key points of all the acronyms above, in the acute phase following injury, the recommendation continues to be to unload the tissues, avoiding movements in the plane of injury as a minimum. After the acute phase, prolonged immobilisation of the tissues should be avoided and progressive loading should be applied, appropriate for the level of severity and irritability and avoiding an increase in pain.

As described in Chapter 3, the process of healing is divided into four phases: bleeding, inflammation, proliferation and remodelling, and the latter three overlap (Velnar et al., 2009). In general, inflammatory exudate production is highest during the inflammatory phase and decreases as healing progresses (Schultz et al., 2011).

From the treatment perspective, the tissues should be protected in the early inflammatory stage to avoid aggravating the injury and to allow bleeding to stop. The control of swelling is important towards regaining function, since the greater the amount of inflammatory exudate, the greater the amount of fibrin in the area, which becomes organised into scar tissue (Evans, 1980). Elevation and compression are appropriate, but high levels of compression should be prevented and care taken in lowering the body part after a period of elevation.

The use of heat is contraindicated as it will increase bleeding from the fragile vessels (Hardy, 1989).

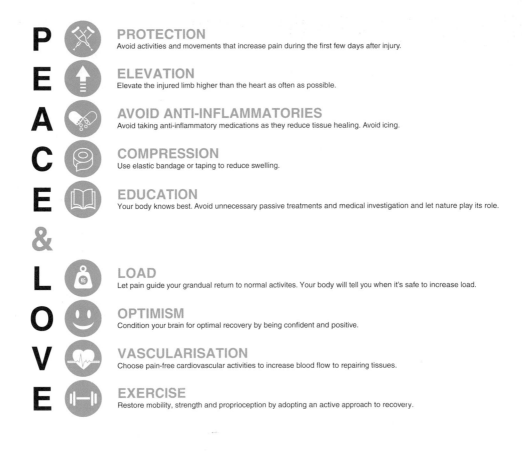

P PROTECTION
Avoid activities and movements that increase pain during the first few days after injury.

E ELEVATION
Elevate the injured limb higher than the heart as often as possible.

A AVOID ANTI-INFLAMMATORIES
Avoid taking anti-inflammatory medications as they reduce tissue healing. Avoid icing.

C COMPRESSION
Use elastic bandage or taping to reduce swelling.

E EDUCATION
Your body knows best. Avoid unnecessary passive treatments and medical investigation and let nature play its role.

&

L LOAD
Let pain guide your grandual return to normal activites. Your body will tell you when it's safe to increase load.

O OPTIMISM
Condition your brain for optimal recovery by being confident and positive.

V VASCULARISATION
Choose pain-free cardiovascular activities to increase blood flow to repairing tissues.

E EXERCISE
Restore mobility, strength and proprioception by adopting an active approach to recovery.

Fig. 4.1 PEACE and LOVE Acronyms. (From Dubois and Esculier, 2020.)

Conversely, ice has traditionally been advocated to reduce bleeding and swelling (Bleakley et al., 2012). However, its use has been questioned by Dubois and Esculier (2020).

They acknowledge the analgesic effects of ice but claim that there is no high-quality evidence on the efficacy of ice in the treatment of soft tissue injuries. They propose that it could potentially disrupt the inflammatory phase, delay neutrophil and macrophage infiltration and lead to impaired tissue repair.

The current advice is that if ice is used to reduce pain after an injury, it should be applied for short periods only (up to 10 minutes) and removed for an appropriate amount of time to allow the circulation to recover (approximately 20 minutes). The process can then be repeated once or twice more in the initial few hours following injury, and applied for 3 to 7 days to reduce pain and swelling and improve recovery time (Timestra, 2012).

Evidence from a large-scale systematic review suggested that intermittent ice applications of 10 minutes are the most effective at reducing tissue temperature in both injured animal and healthy human models (MacAuley, 2001). Such ice applications have been shown to reduce skin temperature by 5°C immediately after treatment (Ebrall et al., 1992).

Cooling the skin surface temperature to below approximately 15°C is also thought to exert a localised analgesic effect by inhibiting nerve conduction velocity (Chesterton et al., 2002; Algafly and George, 2007). Another study also found that intermittent ice applications are more effective than continuous ice at reducing pain on activity after ankle ligament injury (Bleakley et al., 2006).

Each stage of the inflammatory phase is essential to the repair process, and suppression in the early stages can delay healing (Leibovich and Ross, 1975; Hardy, 1989). It is wise to avoid NSAIDs for at least the first 2 or 3 days after injury since they will tend to delay healing (Boruta et al., 1990; Watson, 2009; Chazaud, 2020; Dubois and Esculier, 2020). Instead, it is appropriate to allow the body's natural inflammatory response to proceed with simple analgesics, such as paracetamol, and/or physical measures, such as mobilisation or massage, as more suitable methods of pain control.

The use of corticosteroid injections for soft tissue lesions is contraindicated in the acute inflammatory phase as they inhibit macrophage activity, which delays debridement of the wound and scar tissue production by delaying the onset and proliferation of the fibroblasts (Leibovich and Ross, 1975; Campagnolo et al., 2010)

There are a limited number of studies on the effect of corticosteroid in acute soft tissue lesions, and the majority of these are animal studies. Wiggins et al. (1994) found that corticosteroid impaired the healing process in rabbit ligament at 10 days and 3 weeks after injury, compared to the control group. Lee et al. (2015) concluded that early steroid injection (<7 days) may alter the collagen composition within the extracellular matrix and may interfere with the early stage of the healing process in injured rabbit tendon. However, the changes appeared to normalise after the early inflammatory healing phase.

The main weakness of both studies is that both used animals, but the evidence could imply that the early use of corticosteroid injection of soft tissues may reduce the ability to withstand the mechanical loads of early mobilisation and rehabilitation.

Graded mobilisation should be encouraged as early as possible to promote healing, to stimulate the alignment of fibres and to prevent adverse scar tissue formation (see below). Mobilisation should be introduced carefully, with pain and irritability as the guide, to avoid disrupting the early fragile scar and setting up a secondary inflammatory response, which could lead to excessive scar tissue formation and persistent pain.

Careful consideration should be given to the application of other treatment modalities along with the application of appropriate mobilisation, either simultaneously or consecutively. An approach based on clinical reasoning is appropriate and this underpins current musculoskeletal medicine practice.

Musculoskeletal medicine mobilisation techniques (transverse frictions and the specific mobilisation techniques, Grades A, B and C) are graded on the basis of patient feedback and observation, against the underpinning knowledge of the different phases of healing and the experience of the practitioner.

The appropriate grade and depth of the mobilisation technique is applied according to the severity of the lesion, and this is determined in part by assessment of irritability, rather than in terms of length of time from the onset. In approaching management in this way, the practitioner can judge the treatment needed and the appropriate time to apply it.

In summary, the aim of mobilisation treatment techniques applied in musculoskeletal medicine, including transverse frictions, is to prevent or to reverse the connective tissue changes associated with a period of immobilisation and to stimulate healing. It is important to recognise that stress deprivation causes rapid structural changes (see below), and recovery is much slower. This should be taken into account when preparing treatment programmes.

MOBILISATION

Connective tissue structures are more responsive to a decrease in mechanical demand than they are to progressive increases (Tipton et al., 1986). Therefore, depriving the healing soft tissues of motion and stress can lead to a number of structural changes within the articular and periarticular connective tissues. These are similar to the changes seen in the degenerative ageing process and may be difficult to reverse.

The length of connective tissue structures tends to adapt to the shortest distance between origin and insertion, which produces the consequences of immobilisation that can lead to pain and long-term loss of function.

The changes can include all or some of the following:

- Random deposition of new collagen fibres within the existing collagen weave and disorganised fibre orientation.
- Development of anomalous cross-linking of existing and new collagen fibres, i.e. adhesion formation at the fibre–fibre interface (Fig. 4.2)

- Alteration of the dynamics of collagen turnover (synthesis/degradation)
- Adhesion formation between ligaments, tendons and their surrounding connective tissue; loss of gliding capacity
- Reduced tensile strength of ligaments, tendons and muscles; weakening of ligament and tendon insertion points
- Loss of sarcomeres and inhibition of muscle fibre regeneration by scar tissue
- Proliferation of fibrofatty tissue into muscle tissue and the joint space with adherence to cartilage surfaces
- Decrease in the volume of synovial fluid with adhesion formation between synovial folds
- Cartilage erosion with ulcerations at points of contact and osteophyte formation (Burke-Evans et al., 1960; Akeson et al., 1967, 1973, 1980, 1986; Enneking and Horowitz, 1972; Woo et al., 1975, 1990; Arem and Madden, 1976; Woo, 1982; Videman, 1986; Hardy, 1989; Akeson, 1990; Järvinen and Lehto, 1993; Gracies, 2005).

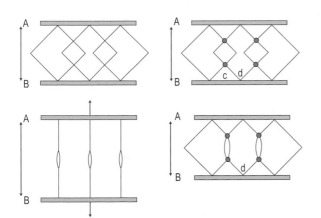

Fig. 4.2 Schematic diagram of the weave pattern of collagen fibres. (A and B) represent individual collagen fibres with cross-linkage in place to stabilise the structure. In normal tissue, represented by the left-hand diagrams, some separation is allowed between the fibres and the fibres can move apart. Adhesion formation at nodal intercept points at the fibre–fibre interface is represented in the right-hand diagrams at c and d; this adhesion formation will interfere with the free gliding of fibres and inhibit normal tissue function. (Reproduced from Woo et al. (1975), with permission of John Wiley and Sons.)

As a result of the reduced quantity and quality of ground substance, the critical distance and separating effects between adjacent collagen fibres is decreased, and the interfibrillar lubrication is reduced.

Collagen turnover (synthesis/degradation) is a dynamic process that is influenced by stress and motion. When deprived of these physical forces through immobilisation, the balance of collagen turnover is affected, and a greater ratio of immature collagen fibres is present with a potential for the formation of increased anomalous, reducible cross-links.

It is important to note that the formation of cross-links is a normal part of the repair process, and it cannot be prevented entirely. However, it is possible to prevent excessive or unwanted adhesions, or to mobilise them, and pliable young scar tissue is ready for early mobilisation techniques that will prevent or reduce the formation of anomalous cross-links.

The careful, controlled application of normal stress and motion will also stimulate new collagen to be laid down in parallel with the existing weave, and the collagen tissue will maintain its elasticity, plasticity and tensile strength.

The following section will discuss the application of Transverse Frictions and will be followed by a description of the Graded Mobilisation Techniques used in musculoskeletal medicine.

TRANSVERSE FRICTIONS

Massage is the manipulation of the soft tissues of the body with the hands, using varying degrees of force (Carreck, 1994), and it is used widely for its therapeutic effects.

In the early 1900s, Mennell (cited in Chamberlain, 1982) first introduced specific massage movements called 'friction'. Cyriax further developed and popularised this technique, adding movement for the treatment of pain caused by trauma. He described 'deep' friction massage, which reaches deep structures of the body, such as ligaments, muscles and tendons, to distinguish it from the general massage described earlier (Cyriax, 1984).

In reviewing the history of the management of tendinopathy, Joseph et al. (2012) credit Cyriax with proposing frictions as one of the first manual treatments for tendon disorders. Transverse frictions have been refined to encourage the technique to be adapted, according to the irritability of the lesion and patient feedback.

Transverse frictions are applied precisely to move the target tissues – tendons, muscles and ligaments. They are applied prior to and in conjunction with graded mobilisation techniques to produce their effects.

The term 'deep' transverse frictions has been deliberately avoided in this text, to prevent misuse of the technique. Unfortunately, deep transverse frictions have been taught to many practitioners as just that, and the technique has not been adapted or graded to suit the lesion.

Consequently, it has developed a reputation for being very painful for the patient and tiring for the practitioner, often being abandoned for these reasons (Ingham, 1981; Woodman and Pare, 1982; de Bruijn, 1984; Cyriax and Cyriax, 1993). It is an underrated modality at our fingertips (pun intended) and, when applied correctly, it is an extremely useful technique.

Transverse frictions can be graded in depth and duration and can be adapted for acute irritable lesions and for chronic non-irritable lesions in response to patient feedback and through clinical reasoning. If applied correctly, an analgesic effect is achieved, and it should not be a painful experience for the patient.

There is limited evidence supporting the effectiveness of transverse frictions. Specifically addressing their use in tendinopathy, Joseph et al. (2012) performed a systematic review to establish the level of evidence for transverse frictions. They concluded that the variety of locations, study designs, causes and outcome measures made it difficult to come to a firm conclusion. They did find some evidence for the use of frictions in tennis elbow and supraspinatus tendinopathy but acknowledged that it was mostly anecdotal.

With the studies on tennis elbow, findings generally show that the addition of transverse friction massage to standard care improves patient outcomes in the short term (Baltaci et al., 2001; Smidt et al., 2002; Nagrale et al., 2009; Dasm, 2012; Viswas et al., 2012). Most studies are at high risk of bias, however, including lack of randomisation, poor reporting, heterogeneity in study population, study treatment, and lack of long-term follow-up.

Traditional models of research tend not to take into account the multimodal approach to therapeutic management, and studies often use terms such as 'traditional' and 'standard therapy' to indicate the use of combined modalities. This tends to 'muddy the waters' for being able to assess the effect of individual techniques.

A number of studies do exist that suggest plausible reasons for the physiological effects of the technique.

Cyriax observed at an early stage that a mechanical signal is vital to tissue healing, and this was supported by Davidson et al. (1997) and Gehlsen et al. (1998).

Gregory et al. (2003) used an animal model to demonstrate the ultrastructural changes occurring in previously normal muscle tissue following 10-minute deep transverse frictions. Obvious reddening of the skin was present immediately after deep transverse frictions (which is the observation in clinical practice) with inflammation and changes in myofibre morphology still apparent 24 hours later.

The application of deep transverse frictions to chronic lesions clinically produces tenderness in the region, which can take time to settle. Gregory et al. (2003) also noted that the observed ultrastructural changes following transverse frictions could take up to 6 days to resolve, and both of these findings may have implications for considering the frequency of the application of the technique.

Further discussion on evidence associated with specific lesions is included in the relevant chapters.

Despite the paucity of evidence, transverse frictions remain in common use in clinical practice. J. Kerr (unpublished work, 2006) conducted a survey in Scotland and analysed 86 questionnaires to establish musculoskeletal physiotherapists' current practice in the use of frictions for treating soft tissue lesions. Transverse frictions were used by 83.7% of those surveyed at that time.

A consensus on a standardised method of application amongst practitioners is hard to reach, but Kerr's survey revealed that treatment times ranged from 3 to 5 minutes for acute lesions and at just below 10 minutes for chronic lesions.

The survey also provided a useful snapshot of practice, and Table 4.2 lists the 'top 10' lesions treated with frictions in the trust studied in Scotland. The table indicates the breadth of soft tissues for which transverse frictions were judged to be an appropriate treatment.

Albeit based on anecdotal evidence, good clinical results have been observed with the inclusion of transverse frictions in the management of soft tissue lesions, and the principles underpinning the technique are discussed in the following section.

TABLE 4.2 'Top 10' Lesions Treated With Transverse Frictions (86 Respondents)

Position	Lesion
1	Lateral collateral ligament of the ankle
2	Rotator cuff tendons
3	Tennis elbow
4	Medial collateral ligament of the knee
5	Achilles tendinopathy
6	Muscle strain
7	Patella tendinopathy
8	Tendinopathy
9	Golfer's elbow
10	De Quervain's tenosynovitis

Use of Transverse Frictions

USE OF TRANSVERSE FRICTIONS
- To induce pain relief
- To produce therapeutic movement
- To produce a traumatic hyperaemia in chronic lesions
- To improve function

To Induce Pain Relief

Pain relief following the application of transverse frictions has been observed clinically, and a number of working hypotheses are proposed to substantiate this. The reduction in pain is experienced as a numbing or analgesic effect and a decrease in pain perceived by the patient, who will often acknowledge this by saying that you have 'moved off the spot'.

Following treatment, the comparable signs can be reassessed and a reduction in pain and an apparent increase in strength is usually noted. This induced analgesia is used to allow the application of graded mobilisation techniques in acute lesions.

If a Grade C manipulation is the appropriate treatment, the transverse frictions are applied just to gain some analgesia before the manipulation is performed.

In chronic lesions, analgesia may be produced through changes in the local microenvironment of the tissues via an increased blood flow, which is associated with the hyperaemia induced by the application of deeper graded transverse frictions over a longer period of time. These changes may include removal of the chemical irritants that sensitise or excite local nociceptors, as well as a decrease in local oedema and pressure.

The technique is started gently to achieve an initial analgesic effect and is then continued with increasing depth, appropriate to the stage of healing, irritability and site of the lesion, after which the graded mobilisation is applied.

An in-depth discussion of the pain-relieving effects of manual therapy techniques is outside the scope of this book, but a brief outline of possible mechanisms is provided here.

Pain modulation is induced through several complex phenomena, including spinal and central nervous system mechanisms acting individually or in combination, to produce desired effects.

Theories of pain modulation include the gate control theory proposed by Melzack and Wall in 1965, that the passage of sensory information is mediated at spinal cord level, especially nociceptive impulses. Pressure stimulates low-threshold mechanoreceptors, the A-beta fibres, that reduce the excitability of the nociceptor terminals by presynaptic inhibition, effectively 'closing the gate' on the pain. The greater the mechanoreceptor stimulation, the greater the level of pain suppression (Bowsher, 1994; Wells, 1994).

Transverse frictions, like rubbing or scratching the skin, are a form of noxious counterirritation that leads to a desired analgesic effect (de Bruijn, 1984). Inhibition, which produces lasting pain relief, is believed to be through the descending inhibitory control systems via the periaqueductal grey (PAG) area – the key centre for endogenous opioid analgesic mechanisms. Endogenous opioids are inhibitory neurotransmitters that diminish the intensity of the pain transmitted to higher centres (de Bruijn, 1984; Melzack and Wall, 1988; Goats, 1994).

Put simply, the initial 'rubbing' of the painful spot reduces pain, enabling the transverse frictions to be graded in depth specific to individual lesions, thus producing their beneficial effects. The reduction in pain is then fairly long-lasting, possibly longer than either the patient or the practitioner expects.

De Bruijn (1984) observed that the time required to produce analgesia during the application of transverse frictions to a variety of soft tissue lesions was 0.4 to 5.1 minutes (mean 2.1 minutes) while the post-massage analgesic effect lasted 0.3 minutes to 48 hours (mean 26 hours).

Transverse frictions as a form of massage may also have a placebo effect, being especially reassuring if the patient perceives that 'you've hit the spot'.

To Produce Therapeutic Movement

Transverse frictions aim to mobilise the target tissues – muscles, tendons and ligaments – to prevent or to mobilise adhesions (Wieting and Cugalj, 2004).

It is important that the depth of application of transverse frictions should reach the target tissue if possible, albeit via the skin and superficial tissues. The transverse movement, together with graded mobilisation, discourages anomalous cross-link formation.

By combining transverse frictions and mobilisation in this way, the technique aims to reduce abnormal fibrous adhesions and to improve scar tissue mobility by encouraging normal alignment of soft tissue fibres and enhanced tensile strength (Brosseau et al., 2002; Wieting and Cugalj, 2004).

The therapeutic movement of the transverse frictions, followed by graded mobilisation, aims to restore the function of the target soft tissue. The nature of the tissue needs to be considered for positioning and application of the technique to be able to achieve this. For example, muscle bellies are placed into a shortened position, to facilitate broadening of the muscle, and tendons in a sheath are put on a stretch to allow mobilisation of the sheath against the tendon (see page 82).

In chronic lesions, transverse frictions produce therapeutic movement and prepare the structure for graded mobilisations that aim to apply longitudinal stress.

To Produce a Traumatic Hyperaemia in Chronic Lesions

Increasing the depth of transverse frictions, together with an increase in time of the application of the technique, produces a controlled traumatic hyperaemia and is used exclusively for chronic lesions. The hyperaemia is caused by the mechanical action of the technique (Brosseau et al., 2002).

A superficial erythema (redness) develops in the skin through dilatation of the arterioles (Gregory et al., 2003) and it is assumed that a similar reaction occurs in the deeper tissues where the effect is required (Winter, 1968). The area of redness that develops under the finger may also be slightly raised and warm, indicating increased permeability of the capillary walls that allows tissue fluid to flow into the surrounding area (Norris, 2004).

Gregory et al. (2003) observed the local redness of the skin following the application of 10-minute transverse frictions to rabbit muscle and suggested this may be sufficient to stimulate a controlled inflammatory reaction and to boost the repair process in chronic lesions. Although no clinical evidence exists to support an exact timing after achieving an analgesic effect, 5 to

10 minutes is the approximate time taken to induce and observe the skin changes in clinical practice.

Pain and function may improve after the technique, however, and as mentioned earlier, some tenderness may persist in the target and overlying tissues. Therefore, at least 48 hours is recommended between the treatment sessions in chronic lesions to allow the tenderness to subside.

Although the traumatic hyperaemia may be desirable in chronic lesions (except prior to a Grade C manipulation), this is not the case in acute lesions where the response is already excessive. Transverse frictions are applied gently to acute lesions and are performed with reduced depth and time to avoid stimulating this traumatic hyperaemia.

> **CLINICAL TIP**
> The depth and duration of the application of transverse frictions is determined by the irritability of the lesion and feedback from the patient, but the aim should be to reach the target tissue.

To Improve Function

The therapeutic movement achieved and pain relief induced by transverse frictions normally produce an immediate clinical improvement in function of the structure treated. This can be demonstrated by reassessment of the comparable signs immediately after treatment and provides an optimum situation for the application of other graded mobilising techniques.

Kelly (1997) and Iwatsuki et al. (2001) conducted studies which demonstrated that transverse frictions improved strength of contraction and increased range of movement (extensibility) in normal gastrocnemius muscle.

Principles of Application of Transverse Frictions

Transverse frictions should be applied to the exact site of the lesion. This relies on clinical diagnosis and palpation of the lesion, based on anatomical knowledge. Tenderness alone is not necessarily an accurate localising sign. It is important that a clinical diagnosis has been reached through assessment and the use of selective tension before palpation. Palpation must reproduce the patient's pain and be different in comparison with the other limb.

Transverse frictions are always applied transversely across the longitudinal fibre orientation of the structure

(Fig. 4.3). Application of the technique in this way aims to mobilise the tissue.

Transverse frictions are applied with sufficient sweep to cover the full width of the structure, aiming to affect the connective tissue fibres across the whole site of the lesion. The practitioner must be positioned to ensure that this sweep is maintained through the application of body weight.

> **READER TIP**
> With the transverse friction techniques demonstrated in the photographs within this book, the direction of friction usually follows the direction in which the fingers or thumbs are pointing. Arrows have been included where the direction of movement differs from that 'rule' or to emphasise the direction where it may not be clear.

Transverse frictions are applied with sufficient depth, aiming to reach and benefit the target tissue. Knowledge of anatomy is paramount.

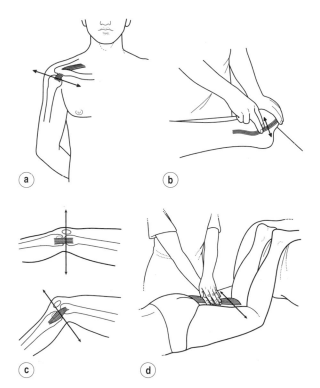

Fig. 4.3 Transverse frictions to: (a) a tendon (supraspinatus); (b) a tendon in sheath (peronei); (c) a ligament (medial collateral) in flexion and extension; (d) muscle belly (hamstring).

The grading, duration of application and depth of the technique are dependent upon the irritability of the lesion and feedback from the patient. In acute lesions, it may be necessary to work through soft tissue swelling associated with the injury to be able to reach the target site. The initial sweeps should always start gently to gain an analgesic effect before proceeding with the effective frictions.

The depth is maintained by applying the technique slowly and steadily, and care must be taken to maintain the depth, as increasing the speed of the technique tends to lift the effect towards the more superficial tissues.

> **CLINICAL TIP**
> When applying transverse frictions, progress steadily through the superficial tissues to achieve an analgesic effect by the time you reach the target tissue.
> Transverse frictions should take irritability into account and should be applied:
> • to the exact site of the lesion
> • transversely across the tissue fibres
> • with sufficient sweep to cover the full extent of the lesion
> • with sufficient depth to reach the lesion

The patient is positioned with regard to the accessibility of the structure and the degree of stretch or relaxation appropriate (Table 4.3):
• Tendons in a sheath are placed on the stretch to allow the transverse frictions to roll the sheath around the firm base of the tendon, facilitating functional movement between the tendon and its sheath.
• Tendons are placed into a position of accessibility, with the lesion commonly lying at the teno-osseous junction. Consideration is given to anatomy.

TABLE 4.3 Principles of Applying Transverse Frictions to Soft Tissue Lesions	
Structure	**Position**
Tendon in sheath	Place on stretch
Body of tendon; teno-osseous junction	Place in accessible position
Musculotendinous junction	Place in accessible position
Muscle belly	Place in shortened position
Ligament	Place in accessible position

- Musculotendinous junctions usually respond well to transverse frictions and need to be placed in a position of accessibility.
- Muscle bellies are placed in a shortened, relaxed position to facilitate broadening of the muscle fibres, imitating function.
- Ligaments are put under a small degree of tension to tighten the overlying soft tissues, allowing the target tissue to be reached.

Specific advice for how to achieve these positions is included for the treatment of lesions described within the relevant chapters in Section 2.

Transverse frictions can place considerable strain on the hands (Sevier and Wilson, 1999) and the practitioner should adopt a position that uses body weight optimally to support the application of the technique and to ensure sufficient sweep and depth.

Snodgrass et al. (2003) looked at factors relating to thumb pain in physiotherapists, and manual techniques in general were highlighted as the cause of pain for all symptomatic subjects studied.

Handheld devices have been developed to apply mobilisations and transverse frictions to help to prevent occupational injury, but strain on the digits can be greatly reduced by using body weight and sway to perform the technique.

Care should be taken to adopt a position that places the practitioner at a mechanical advantage. Sitting is possible, but the most effective position to apply body weight is with the patient placed on a lower plane than the practitioner.

Consideration should also be given to the variety of ways the hands can be used to avoid fatigue and overuse (Fig. 4.4). The therapist's finger and the patient's skin and superficial tissues should move 'as one' to avoid raising a blister on the patient's skin and to ensure that the superficial tissues are moving over the underlying target tissue.

The most efficient way of achieving this is to apply the technique in both directions. Pressure is first directed

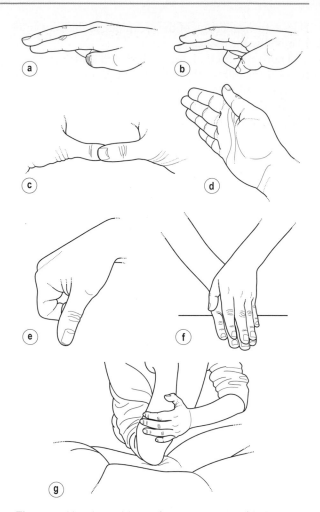

Fig. 4.4 Hand positions for transverse frictions. (a) Index finger reinforced by middle finger; (b) middle finger reinforced by index finger; (c) thumbs; (d) ring finger; (e) pinch grip; (f) hands; (g) hand guiding the flat of the elbow.

CLINICAL TIP

Keep a steady pressure and rhythm in both directions and ensure that you cover the width, depth and entire extent of the lesion.

---

downwards onto or against the structure and this is maintained while the transverse sweep is applied.

Contraindications to transverse frictions are few (see box below). The technique is never applied to active conditions: for example, areas of active infection, or active inflammatory arthritis in which the connective tissue structures are too irritable. Care is required if there is fragile skin or if the patient is currently undergoing anticoagulant therapy. Bursitis may be aggravated.

> **CONTRAINDICATIONS TO TRANSVERSE FRICTIONS**
>
> **Contraindications**
> - Local infection
> - Inflammatory arthritis
> - Cutaneous malignancy
> - Active skin disease
> - Deep vein thrombosis
>
> **Cautions**
> - Fragile skin
> - Anticoagulant therapy and blood clotting disorders
> - Bursitis

GRADED MOBILISATION TECHNIQUES

Grade A, B and C mobilisations (Saunders, 2000) are specific mobilisation techniques applied to achieve a particular purpose. Each mobilisation described is an individual technique aiming to achieve specific effects and one is not intended to be a progression of the other.

> **CLINICAL TIP**
> The application of appropriate stress by graded mobilisation will mimic normal tissue function and help to guide collagen fibre orientation throughout the tissue.

The terms are used in different ways when referring to peripheral and spinal joints, and the similarities and differences will be highlighted throughout this section. *Peripheral graded mobilisation* techniques will be explained first, followed by a description of the *spinal graded mobilisation* techniques.

PERIPHERAL GRADED MOBILISATION TECHNIQUES

Peripheral Grade A Mobilisation

Peripheral Grade A mobilisation is a passive, active or assisted/active mobilisation performed within the patient's pain-free range of movement, aiming to provide or maintain mobility. It is applied within the *elastic range* (see Chapter 2).

It is applied to irritable, acutely inflamed or painful lesions where it may be facilitated by the previous application of transverse frictions. The movements are initially of small amplitude, slow, pain-free, without force and repeated often.

The range and vigour of Grade A mobilisation are progressed as the signs and symptoms improve to achieve full, pain-free function.

Use of Peripheral Grade A Mobilisation
To Promote Tissue Fluid Agitation

Peripheral Grade A mobilisation, either active or passive, produces a gentle soft tissue movement agitating tissue fluid in the acute inflammatory phase and facilitating the phagocytic action of the macrophages (Evans, 1980).

> **CLINICAL TIP**
> Gentle mobilisation will agitate tissue fluid and increase the chance contact of the macrophage with cellular debris, promoting healing (Evans, 1980).

To Apply a Longitudinal Stress to Connective Tissue Structures

Peripheral Grade A mobilisation aims to impart sufficient longitudinal stress to promote orientation of collagen fibres within the existing parallel collagen weave.

As acute lesions subside, and once it is judged that there is sufficient tensile strength in the wound, the patient may begin to 'nudge' pain to provide longitudinal stress without disrupting the healing breach.

Grade A mobilisations performed in this way are of short duration, are not forceful and are repeated often. This form of mobilisation is appropriate for the proliferation phase of connective tissue injuries, and, as progress is made, an increasing range of movement is encouraged.

In this way, the developing scar tissue is stressed, not stretched (to avoid over-stressing the healing tissues), aiming to restore full functional range. Tissues that heal within the presence of movement in this way should not need 'traditional' stretching into the painful range.

To Promote Normal Function

Peripheral Grade A mobilisation is applied early in the inflammatory phase to ensure that function is regained rapidly. Healing within the presence of movement promotes a return to function; that is, form follows function.

The range of movement is gradually increased, applying sufficient stress to the wound to promote the orientation of fibres. As mentioned earlier, controlled mobilisation of acute lesions should prevent the need for stretching tissue.

The function of a muscle belly is maintained by performing active inner-range, isometric, pain-free contractions aiming to broaden muscle fibres. The function of a ligament is promoted by performing active pain-free movement, maintaining the ligament's ability to glide over the underlying bone.

In lesions, such as tendinopathy, the patient maintains normal function by performing movement within the pain-free range, beginning with isometric contractions and gently increasing the load and range as the pain reduces, avoiding the painful extremes of movements.

In chronic injuries, once the lesion is rendered pain-free, which may be by the use of transverse frictions or corticosteroid injection, normal movement will promote remodelling, alignment of fibres and restoration of function.

To Prevent Anomalous Adhesion Formation

Peripheral Grade A mobilisation promotes movement within connective tissue structures to prevent anomalous adhesion formation. In the acute phase of inflammation, the movement should occur without stress or disruption of the healing breach.

The patient is instructed to exercise up to the point of discomfort, but not into or through pain, and must understand the importance of this controlled, precise movement. In this way, an optimal amount of movement is applied to prevent adhesions but not to delay healing.

> **CLINICAL TIP**
>
> To avoid adverse scar tissue formation, transverse frictions and a progressively increasing range of mobilisation should be continued until a full pain-free range of movement is restored. This aims to prevent excessive cross-links occurring between individual fibres and encourages fibre alignment. Applying appropriate stress to restore length should avoid the necessity to stretch.

To Reduce a Loose Body or Bony Subluxation in a Peripheral Joint

To reduce a peripheral joint loose body (e.g. in the hip, knee or elbow) or a bony subluxation (e.g. carpal bone), a Grade A mobilisation is performed in mid-range under strong traction, which is the principal component of the technique, giving the fragment space to move.

Peripheral Grade B Mobilisation

A peripheral Grade B mobilisation is a mobilisation performed at the end of available range into the *plastic range* (see Chapter 2). It is a specific, sustained stretching technique that aims to facilitate permanent elongation of connective tissue.

Use of Peripheral Grade B Mobilisation
To Stretch Capsular Adhesions

In the early stages of arthropathy, pain causes the joint to be held in a position of ease, restricting movement of some parts of the joint capsule. Characteristically, the joint is limited in the capsular pattern with the restricted movements demonstrating a 'hard' end-feel (see Chapter 1). Peripheral Grade B mobilisation aims to restore the movements limited in the capsular pattern.

The shoulder (frozen shoulder) and hip joints commonly demonstrate this loss of movement and respond well to peripheral Grade B mobilisation, provided the joints are in a non-irritable state. However, the technique could be applied to any non-irritable capsulitis in which pain and loss of movement are clinical features.

Peripheral Grade B mobilisation is applied at the end of available range, guided by the end-feel and the patient's pain tolerance. To be successful, the end-feel should still have some elastic quality, but the sensation of muscle spasm may also be apparent, since the technique is applied into the painful range.

The technique is a slow, sustained and repeated stretch. As soon as the end range position is released, an immediate relief of pain should be felt. If pain lingers at this stage, the joint may be too irritable and the technique inappropriate.

Theoretically, the stretch is applied towards the end of the elastic limit and into the plastic range to achieve permanent lengthening (Chapter 2). Since the capsular tissue possesses viscoelastic properties, the stretch applied uses the viscous flow phenomenon, which enables contracted scar tissue to creep or lengthen gradually (Amis, 1985; Hardy and Woodall, 1998; Usuba et al., 2007). This also contributes to an increased range of movement.

Lengthening, under these circumstances, is inversely proportional to the velocity of the applied stretch, with a slowly applied force meeting with less resistance or stiffness (it is easier to move slowly through a viscous medium). *Hysteresis* (the slower rate at which the structure recovers from the elongating force) may also play a role and can be linked to cyclical loading where repeated applications of peripheral Grade B mobilisation achieve a modest increment of increased length with each mobilisation applied.

Successful treatment is dependent upon patient compliance, as the subsequent management of the condition is long term. The structural changes occurring in the mobilised tissue may produce a low-grade tissue response, and the patient should be warned about post-treatment soreness. The importance of continued movement to maintain the range achieved cannot be stressed enough, and the patient must be given an appropriate exercise programme to ensure this.

The optimum duration and frequency of the static stretch has yet to be determined, but the work of Brandy and Irion (1994) and Brandy et al. (1997) suggests that, in order to achieve an increase in range of knee extension, a static stretch of 30 seconds applied to the hamstring muscles is sufficient. In the musculoskeletal medicine approach, each stretch is maintained for 'as long as can be tolerated', and constant observation of the patient with feedback is required as the technique is applied.

The application of heat relieves pain and lowers the viscosity of collagen tissue, allowing a greater elongation of collagen tissues for less force (Warren et al., 1971). The mechanism of combined application of temperature and load affects the viscous flow properties of collagen, and, by increasing the temperature of a structure, lower sustained loads achieve greater elongation (Warren et al., 1971; Usuba et al., 2007).

Raising local temperature to between 40°C and 45°C (40°C is the temperature of a very hot bath) achieves this useful therapeutic effect. Usuba et al. (2007) found from their previous studies that heat combined with stretching was more effective than stretching alone, and this was also the conclusion of a meta-analysis conducted by Bleakley and Costello (2013).

To achieve its best effects, heat should be applied concurrently with the peripheral Grade B mobilisation. However, for practical purposes, it is usually applied beforehand. For home exercises, the advice can be to apply the stretches after a hot bath or shower, or after the application of a heat pad or hot water bottle.

'Heat, hold, repeat' is a neat mantra to describe the application of the Peripheral Grade B mobilisation.

To Reduce Pain

In degenerative arthropathy, the inflammatory changes involve both the synovial lining of the joint and the fibrous capsule. The capsule develops small lesions that undergo scar tissue formation, producing adhesions or capsular thickenings. The adhesions are affected by joint movement, which, through abnormal tension, stimulates the free nerve endings lying in the capsule, producing mechanical pain.

Malfait and Schnitzer (2013) describe the pain in degenerative arthropathy as being generated and maintained through nociceptive input from the arthritic joint, which is modulated at different levels of the peripheral and central nervous system as the pain becomes more chronic. The pain and associated involuntary muscle spasm reduce movement.

The nerve endings also respond to the chemical products of inflammation – histamine, kinins and prostaglandins. Impulses are transported in the non-myelinated C fibres and a 'slow', aching, throbbing pain is produced that is poorly defined (i.e. chemical pain) (Norris, 2004).

Central sensitisation or complex somatosensory changes may also contribute to the pain of chronic arthropathy (Malfait and Schnitzer, 2013).

Sustained or repetitive passive joint movement may modify the firing responses in large-diameter mechanoreceptor joint afferents, particularly when the capsular stretch is maintained at or near the end of range. This suggests an explanation to account for the pain-relieving effects of end-range mobilisation, including manipulation as well as passive peripheral Grade B stretching techniques.

> **CLINICAL TIP**
> Peripheral Grade B mobilisation produces some treatment soreness. The amount of after-treatment soreness is an indicator of the irritability of the lesion and guides the progression of treatment.

The permanent lengthening achieved by peripheral Grade B mobilisation increases the pain-free range, and normal movement patterns are restored.

To Improve Function

The increase in joint range and pain relief achieved by peripheral Grade B mobilisation improves overall function. However, the gradual onset of loss of movement through capsular contraction can considerably alter movement patterns.

Exercise has been demonstrated to be crucial in the management of arthropathy (Davis and MacKay, 2013; Larmer et al., 2014). In addition to applying capsular stretches, careful assessment of the patient is necessary to agree on and plan a self-managed treatment programme that considers all components of the dysfunction, including altered biomechanics, muscle weakness and neural tension.

In chronic muscle, tendon and ligament lesions, adaptive shortening may be part of an overall dysfunction. The shortened tissues can be stretched by applying the principles of peripheral Grade B mobilisation, both by the practitioner and as a home treatment regime.

Grade B mobilisation is applied once the structure has been rendered functionally pain-free by transverse frictions, and contractile structures need to be pain-free on resisted testing.

Peripheral Grade C Manipulation

Peripheral Grade C manipulation is a passive movement performed at the end of available range and is a minimal amplitude, high-velocity thrust. For clarity, it is not sustained and should be applied with a small, quick overpressure once all the slack has been taken up.

Manipulation applied to shortened scar tissue may be appropriate in peripheral lesions. The aim of the technique is to mobilise unwanted adhesions, producing permanent elongation and restoring full painless function.

Threlkeld (1992) expands on the viscous properties of connective tissue and describes that when the tissue is loaded more quickly it behaves more stiffly than the same tissues loaded more slowly. Thus, adhesions may be mobilised more readily by stress applied quickly, as in manipulation.

The short toe-phase of the adhesions ensures that the slack is taken up more rapidly in the adhesions than in the surrounding normal tissue, and that the minimal amplitude, high-velocity thrust causes macrofailure of the adhesions while the normal tissue remains intact.

It is important that the elongation achieved should be maintained by the patient. In musculoskeletal medicine, peripheral Grade C manipulation is applied in two situations, as described below.

Use of Peripheral Grade C Manipulation
To Mobilise Unwanted Adhesions Between a Ligament and Bone

Peripheral Grade C manipulation is applied to a chronic ligamentous sprain of two ligaments in the lower limb – the medial collateral ligament at the knee and the lateral collateral ligament at the ankle.

Unwanted adhesions may have developed between the ligament and the underlying bone that disrupt the normal functional movement of the joint. On examination, a non-capsular pattern of pain and limitation of movement will be found. Provided that tests for instability have been performed and are negative, the ligament is prepared by transverse frictions to achieve an analgesic effect and the manipulation follows immediately.

Effective manipulation should achieve instant results and vigorous exercise is required to maintain the lengthening and movement achieved. Rehabilitation must address all components contributing to the dysfunction.

To Mobilise Adherent Scar Tissue at the Teno-Osseous Junction of the Common Extensor Tendon ('Tennis Elbow')

A special manipulation (Mills' manipulation) is applied at the teno-osseous junction of the common extensor tendon as a treatment for tennis elbow (see Chapter 6).

The manipulation aims to mobilise adhesions interfering with the mobility of the tendon at its insertion and within the adjacent tissues. The tendon is first prepared by transverse frictions to gain some pain relief, followed by the manipulation. The elongation gained must be maintained through exercise.

> **CLINICAL TIP**
> When performing a Grade C peripheral manipulation for appropriate chronic lesions, the transverse frictions are ONLY applied to gain some analgesia and should not be continued post numbing, as when used in isolation.

As mentioned above, the Mills' manipulation has traditionally been a 'special' manipulation, and this is the only example of a teno-osseous junction being manipulated in current musculoskeletal medicine practice.

This is challenged by Stasinopoulos and Johnson (2007), however, and other sites suitable for manipulation may emerge through continuing reflection on practice; possibly spurred on by the emergence of evidence to support the use of the technique.

SPINAL GRADED MOBILISATION TECHNIQUES

Spinal Grade A Mobilisation

At the spinal joints, and specifically at the cervical spine, the term 'Grade A' is used to indicate that the mobilisation technique is applied to mid-range (i.e. the middle of the available range).

A pain-free mobilisation should be used to reduce the patient's pain and to facilitate movement. This is particularly indicated in the treatment of an acute, irritable spinal lesion.

Spinal Grade B Mobilisation

At the spinal joints, the term 'Grade B mobilisation' is used to indicate that the mobilisation technique is performed to the end of the available range. It aims to reduce pain and facilitate movement.

Grade B mobilisation at the spinal joints is not sustained and should never be applied into pain or muscle spasm. The technique should be stopped immediately if either is provoked.

Spinal Grade C Manipulation

The definition of a Grade C manipulation is shared by both peripheral and spinal joints: Grade C manipulation is a passive movement performed at the end of available range and is a minimal amplitude, high-velocity thrust.

It is worth repeating that, as for peripheral joints, spinal Grade C manipulation is not sustained and should be applied with a small, quick overpressure, only when all the slack has been taken up and provided there is no reproduction of pain at the end of range.

Within the musculoskeletal medicine approach, spinal Grade C manipulation can be applied to the cervical, thoracic and lumbar spine and to the sacroiliac joint.

Despite the positive findings of clinical trials, the mechanisms through which spinal manipulation acts are not fully established. Hypoalgesia has been associated with spinal manipulation and there is growing evidence to support its clinical effectiveness (see below).

Evidence is particularly strong when patients are classified into sub-groups by patterns suggesting the likelihood of a favourable response (Flynn et al., 2002; Childs et al., 2004; Cleland et al., 2006).

Contraindications to spinal mobilisation and manipulation are discussed in the relevant chapters in Section 2.

Table 4.4 summarises the differences between peripheral and spinal joints in the application of graded mobilisation techniques.

Use of Spinal and Sacroiliac Joint Manipulation
To Restore Movement

In the spinal or sacroiliac joints in which a non-capsular pattern exists, manipulation aims to restore full, painless function. As suggested earlier, the effects of mobilisation

TABLE 4.4 Differences in the Application of Grade A, B and C Mobilisation Techniques in Peripheral and Spinal Joints

	Peripheral Joints	Spinal Joints
Grade A	Passive, active or active-assisted mobilisation performed within patients' pain-free range of movement within elastic range	Mobilisation technique applied to mid available range
Grade B	Sustained passive mobilisation performed at the end of available range into the plastic range	Mobilisation technique applied to the end of available range (not sustained)
Grade C	Passive minimal amplitude, high-velocity thrust manipulation applied at the end of available range	Passive minimal amplitude, high-velocity thrust manipulation applied at the end of available range.

and manipulation are not simple and are probably multifactorial, involving all adjacent tissues and pain mechanisms.

To Relieve Pain

Manipulation-induced hypoalgesia (pain relief) is well documented (Wright, 1995; Vicenzino et al., 1998; Goodsell et al., 2000; Vernon, 2000; Sterling et al., 2001; Vicenzino et al., 2001; Paungmali et al., 2003a; Paungmali et al., 2003b; Mohammadian et al., 2004; Paungmali et al., 2004; George et al., 2006; Bialosky et al., 2008). Restoration of functional movement may in itself lead to reduction in pain, but relief of pain may also be required first to achieve this.

The exact underlying mechanisms of spinal manipulation hypoalgesia are not fully established. Spinal manipulation may have a direct neurophysiological effect on pain perception through dorsal horn inhibition (Hanai, 1998; Cuellar et al., 2005; George et al., 2006; Guan et al., 2006; Bialosky et al., 2008, 2009). Other factors such as placebo and patients' expectations (Bialosky et al., 2008), and reduction or prevention of neuroplastic changes associated with central sensitisation (George et al., 2006), may also be contributing factors in pain relief.

Pain relief may occur through stimulation of the mechanoreceptors within the joint capsule and spinal ligaments to effect the 'pain-gate mechanism', or through stimulation of the descending inhibitory controls. Spinal manipulation provides an appropriate stimulus to activate the descending pain inhibitory systems from the periaqueductal grey (PAG) area to the spinal cord (Wright, 1995).

Two different forms of analgesia may be produced: an opioid form that appears to be associated with sympathetic inhibition and takes a period of time to develop, and a non-opioid form that is associated with sympathetic excitation and has a more rapid onset.

Spinal manipulation can have an immediate effect, producing pain relief within seconds or minutes due to the non-opioid form. Over a period of about 20 to 45 minutes the analgesia changes to the opioid form associated with sympathetic inhibition.

The relief of pain achieved reduces the reflex muscle spasm, and an increase in the range of movement can occur.

Principles of Application of Spinal and Sacroiliac Joint Manipulation

Certain principles need to be considered in order to apply the technique effectively.

A short- or long-lever arm is used and a torque or twisting force is usually applied, taking up the slack in the surrounding connective tissue to induce a passive movement at one or more spinal joints (Hadler et al., 1987).

The minimal amplitude, high-velocity thrust is of great importance, since tissues loaded quickly behave more stiffly and have a higher ultimate strength (see Chapter 2).

Manipulative reduction is more likely to succeed if the joint space is increased. Therefore, an element of distraction is usually included. Spinal manipulation, in particular, requires skilful handling that takes time and practice to acquire. The practitioner's hands must be sensitive to the end-feel of the joints constantly, and any abnormal end-feel, such as bony resistance or muscle spasm, should alert the practitioner to stop the procedure.

Successful manipulation requires sound clinical reasoning and the choice of the right patient with knowledge of the effects, contraindications and limits of the technique. Thought, care and expert skill are essentials,

together with an explanation to the patient of the diagnosis, treatment and possible complications, in order to gain informed consent. Safety is essential and the precautions necessary will be discussed in the appropriate chapters.

TRACTION

The terms *traction* and *distraction* have the same meaning in describing a force applied to produce separation of joint surfaces and widening of the joint space. There is a convention that traction is applied to spinal joints and distraction to peripheral joints, but this is not a hard and fast rule, and the term traction is used here to apply to both.

This section briefly considers the effects of traction techniques used in musculoskeletal medicine for both peripheral and spinal joints. The general indications for traction and distraction will be mentioned, but these, together with the contraindications for treatment, will be discussed in greater detail in the following chapters.

Use of Traction
To Relieve Pain

Pain relief through the use of traction is gained by relieving pressure. Traction reduces the compression force, muscles relax and the pressure on the joint and pain-sensitive structures is reduced. Stimulation of mechanoreceptors may also have a role (Brumagne et al., 2000; Gay et al., 2005).

To Create Space

The application of distraction creates a degree of space within the joint, allowing a 'loose body' or a displaced carpal bone room to move.

To Produce a Negative Pressure Within a Joint

Creating space within the joint creates a suction effect that helps to move a displaced intra-articular fragment.

To Tighten Ligaments Around a Joint

Tightening the ligaments around the joint produces a centripetal force. A disc displacement will tend to be pushed towards the centre as the traction is applied.

To Reduce a Loose Body in a Peripheral Joint

Distraction is the main element of the manoeuvre. Grade A mobilisation is applied under strong traction and the aim is to move the displaced fragment to another area of the joint, where it does not block joint movement.

Indications for Traction at Peripheral Joints

Stiff, degenerative, arthropathic joints respond well to distraction, as do joints demonstrating the capsular pattern following adaptive changes in response to traumatic arthritis. The distraction is applied to increase mobility, using longitudinal or lateral distraction techniques, which produces separation of joint surfaces and assist mobilisation by stretching the joint capsule and capsular ligaments.

Distraction may be applied manually as a treatment in itself or in conjunction with mobilisation and manipulation techniques.

Where signs and symptoms indicate the presence of a loose body in a joint, or a carpal bone needs to be relocated, distraction before Grade A mobilisation is applied. The distraction of joint surfaces allows space for movement of the fragment, assisted by the accompanying suction effect that distraction tends to produce.

Indications for Spinal Traction

In the cervical spine most of the mobilisation and manipulation techniques are performed under manual traction.

Despite the lack of evidence to support the effectiveness of mechanical traction, many practitioners continue to use it, primarily as an additional modality (Madson and Hollman, 2015). Expert opinion, theoretical models, and some research evidence suggest that certain patients with spinal conditions may respond positively to traction. Therefore, careful patient selection, consideration of the patient's clinical presentation and a previous response to treatment with traction should be considered to integrate it into the management plan.

Cyriax (1982) identified factors from the patient's history, together with certain symptoms and signs, that he believed were characteristic of a disc herniation. Treatment with sustained traction was therefore indicated to reduce the herniation.

He stated that, with a disc herniation, the pain is usually of gradual onset, often with no recollection of the mode or time of onset. There is little central pain, but referred pain is usually present in the arm or leg. The pattern of spinal movement is non-capsular and the movements provoke the limb pain.

Mathews and Hickling (1975) suggested that traction should be applied to a defined syndrome rather than a specific condition. This would appear to be a more satisfactory premise against which practitioners from the myriad of musculoskeletal backgrounds can apply the basic principles, while the debate on pathology continues as fresh evidence emerges.

Models guiding treatment selection will be proposed in the appropriate chapters within Section 2.

> **CLINICAL TIP**
> When applying the techniques of traction to the cervical spine or peripheral joints, the following principles should be employed:
> - Appropriate body weight should be used
> - The application of body weight should be achieved by leaning out with straight arms
> - The distraction/traction should be sustained for a few seconds before proceeding with the technique

MUSCULOSKELETAL MEDICINE INJECTION TECHNIQUES

This part of the chapter provides an outline of the principles and application of injection therapy. In musculoskeletal medicine, injection techniques are often used as an alternative, or in addition to, transverse frictions, mobilisation techniques, and other treatment modalities as part of an agreed management plan.

Transverse frictions and mobilisation appear to be most efficacious when used together and with other measures, including education, activity modification and exercise. This also applies to the use of injection techniques, which benefit from attention to biomechanical and causative factors to prevent recurrence. In the majority of musculoskeletal conditions, they should not be used in isolation.

The main indication for injection therapy is that pain and function impairment have become a barrier to patients' rehabilitation and have resulted in a significant impact on their day-to-day activities. Injection techniques aim to provide a window of opportunity to allow progressive movement or loading, after a period of relative rest and protection, to gain the maximum benefit from the injection. The drugs administered often have beneficial effects for some time after they have been administered, and they must be given time to achieve these.

There is a large volume of published literature on injection therapy, and a high proportion of studies are at a high/medium risk of bias, mainly due to small sample size, poor methodological quality and heterogeneity of the study population or treatment protocols. The general theme drawn from studies supports injection therapy's short-term effectiveness, and it is a safe treatment option for a wide variety of musculoskeletal conditions. However, its long-term effectiveness is generally poor.

Therefore, injection therapy is normally used in conjunction with other treatments such as exercise rehabilitation, manual therapy, education and self-management. Patients should also be fully informed of the risks, benefits and expected outcomes of injection therapy, and regard it as an integral part of their management plan. The need for collaboration between the patient and practitioner, and shared decision making, is emphasised to decide on the best management plan for the patient.

The main injections used in musculoskeletal medicine are corticosteroid and local anaesthetic. These will form the main focus of the following text, with notes on their use, side effects and contraindications. The appropriate sizes of needles and syringes to use will also be described.

Hyaluronic acid (HA) (viscosupplementation) injections have become much more widely used in musculoskeletal practice and these will also be discussed, along with short sections on epidural injections, platelet-rich plasma (PRP) injections and prolotherapy.

Since the publication of the previous edition of this textbook, significant changes have been introduced with regard to independent prescribing, and the following update is provided as context for the subsequent sections.

An independent prescriber is a practitioner who is responsible and accountable for the assessment of patients with undiagnosed or diagnosed conditions, and who can make prescribing decisions to manage the clinical condition of the patient. Medical practitioners and dentists are already independent prescribers on completion of their training.

Post-registration pharmacists, nurses, optometrists, physiotherapists and podiatrists can all train to become independent prescribers. This allows suitably qualified practitioners to prescribe any licenced medicine relevant to their scope of practice and to mix medicines prior to administration.

With regard to mixing the drugs, at the time of writing the mixing of corticosteroid and local anaesthetic in the same syringe as part of a patient group directive (PGD), is still inhibited under the Medicines for Human

Use Regulations (1994), since that would be considered to create a new product that is unlicenced for use (CSP, 2008).

Practitioners working under a PGD, regardless of whether they are an independent prescriber or not, will need to modify their injection practice and not mix medicines, such as lidocaine and Kenalog. This will involve choosing to use a pre-mixed commercially available preparation, giving two separate injections, or not using local anaesthetic. Administration techniques can also be adjusted so that products do not mix in the syringe, for example, using separate syringes for each drug.

A patient specific direction (PSD) is a written prescription from a medical practitioner, dentist or other independent prescriber in which the patient is identified by name. Non-independent prescriber practitioners can mix the drugs under a PSD, in accordance with the medical or non-medical prescriber's directions, and in these situations the mixing of drugs is the prescriber's direct responsibility.

Corticosteroid Injections

There are two ways of influencing the inflammatory process:
- Phospholipase A_2 (PLA$_2$) inhibition (using corticosteroids)
- Cyclooxygenase (COX) inhibition (using NSAIDs)

Corticosteroid inhibits PLA$_2$ action which prevents the production of arachidonic acid, thereby halting the inflammatory process higher in the inflammatory cascade. As a consequence, this inhibits the inflammatory mediators prostaglandins, and other inflammatory proteins and inflammatory genes, which are responsible for provoking, accelerating, or prolonging the inflammatory response.

NSAIDs inhibit COX activity and are involved in reducing inflammation further down the inflammatory cascade. Because corticosteroids inhibit the inflammatory cascade higher or earlier than NSAIDs, corticosteroids are much more effective. With corticosteroids having a potent anti-inflammatory effect, they can be used therapeutically in musculoskeletal medicine to achieve this effect.

Corticosteroids are applied intra-articularly or intralesionally for chronic inflammatory lesions, including inflammatory arthritis. The intense anti-inflammatory effect is also beneficial in some acute lesions (e.g. acute flare in osteoarthritis, acute calcific tendinopathy or acute tenosynovitis) but is unwanted in other acute conditions (e.g. acute muscle belly lesions, acute teno-osseous lesions or acute ligamentous lesions) because of its detrimental effects during the early healing process.

USES OF CORTICOSTEROID INJECTIONS IN MUSCULOSKELETAL MEDICINE
- Inflammatory arthritis and acute episodes of degenerative arthropathy
- Acute and chronic bursitis
- Acute and chronic tenosynovitis
- Some tendinopathies
- Nerve entrapment syndromes
- Epidural, via sacral hiatus

As well as their anti-inflammatory effect, corticosteroids have other potent effects, including immunosuppression and a delay in the normal physiological process of healing. These effects cannot be separated from the beneficial effects of corticosteroids. However, much of the reported unwanted effects of corticosteroids involve systemic, high-dose applications of the drugs for long periods of time.

A locally applied injection of corticosteroid in musculoskeletal medicine aims to achieve a rapid and intense local anti-inflammatory effect. The local effect will depend on the dose applied, the relative potency of the corticosteroid and its solubility, which determines the length of time it stays in the tissues.

The aim is to give the lowest possible effective dose that will achieve the desired effect, although there is some expert opinion that larger doses may give better results in some conditions. For instance, degenerative arthropathy of the knee and hip and capsulitis at the shoulder.

Intra-articular injections are most appropriate if there is an inflammatory component; therefore, they are indicated whenever a joint capsule is inflamed, such as in rheumatoid arthritis, traumatic arthritis and acute episodes of degenerative arthropathy.

Intralesional injections can be considered for bursitis, tenosynovitis, nerve entrapment syndromes and some tendinopathies.

The use of corticosteroids would seem to affect all phases of the inflammatory process: the initial acute inflammatory phase, the proliferative phase and throughout remodelling.

Corticosteroids also produce a potent immunosuppressive effect, which is why it is so important to adhere to a 'no touch' technique, in order to prevent risk of local infection, to lower the risk of worsening viral infections and/or prolonging viral illness, such as influenza or Covid-19.

In this text, the corticosteroid referred to is *triamcinolone acetonide*. Two different concentrations of triamcinolone acetonide, Adcortyl (10 mg/mL) and Kenalog (40 mg/mL), provide versatility for different applications.

Adcortyl can be used for larger volume injections, while Kenalog can be used in both small and large volume injections and is therefore in wider use.

Recommended dosages of triamcinolone acetonide are usually obtained by drawing up the appropriate volume of Kenalog boosted to the total volume required by local anaesthetic or saline. Adcortyl is still currently used by some practitioners, but Kenalog only will be referred to from here on.

Corticosteroid Injection Technique

The appropriate dose or volume of injection (corticosteroid alone, or mixed with local anaesthetic or saline) will be determined by the size of the joint or lesion to be injected and the previous response to injection, if any. For many of the injections in this book, a range is provided for the dose of corticosteroid, and clinical judgement will be needed to guide selection.

CLINICAL TIP
mg – dose of steroid
mL – volume
5 mL – volume of a teaspoon

Table 4.5 provides a broad outline of dosages for different lesions and more specific details are provided within the relevant chapters.

Given the potential deleterious effect of corticosteroid on joints, bones and soft tissues, and that the biological half-life of triamcinolone acetonide is approximately 12 to 36 hours after injection (Pekarek et al., 2011), it is important that sudden increases in load on the structure(s) are avoided for the first few days.

Depending on which corticosteroid is being used, some steroid injections have a shorter duration of action and some have a longer duration (e.g. methylprednisolone acetate has a duration of approximately 3 weeks). The effectiveness also depends on patient factors (such as age, medical history, drug history, social history and treatment compliance), and the condition (such as severity of degenerative changes and severity of inflammation).

TABLE 4.5   Guideline Summary for Injections

Structure	Area/Size	Guide to Steroid (mg)	Guide to Total Volume (mL)	Technique
Joints	Hip	40–80	5	Bolus
	Knee	30–60	4	Bolus
	Ankle	20–40	3	Bolus
	Smaller joints of foot	10–20	1	Bolus
	Shoulder	20–40	4	Bolus
	Elbow	20–40	3	Bolus
	Wrist	20–30	3	Bolus
	1st Trapezio-metacarpal joint	10–20	1	Bolus
	Smaller joints of hand	5–10	1	Bolus
Bursa	Large acute	20–40	3–4	Bolus
	Large chronic	20–40	8–10	Bolus
	Small acute/chronic	10	1	Bolus
Teno-osseous junctions	Large tendons	20	2	Peppering
	Small tendons	10	1	Peppering
Tendons in a sheath	All	10	1	Bathe tendon within sheath

RELATIVE REST AND AFTER CARE FOLLOWING CORTICOSTEROID INJECTION

- Patients should be fully informed of the risks, benefits and expected outcomes of injection therapy
- After injection it is important that sudden increases in load on the structure(s) are avoided for the first few days
- Patients should minimise or modify normal activities for 2 weeks following injection. Corticosteroid tends to weaken the tissues injected and they need to be protected from excessive stress
- Movement and exercise are encouraged (including weight-bearing exercise) as soon as pain allows, in order to return to normal function
- Patients should be encouraged to recommence their progressive exercise rehabilitation based on their individual needs and treatment goals, and regard it as an integral part of their management plan

Triamcinolone acetonide has a duration of effect for 2 to 3 weeks (Drugs.com). As a general rule, it is reasonable to minimise or modify normal activities for 2 weeks following injection to avoid the possible deleterious effect of corticosteroid at the injected site. However, movements and exercise are permitted (including weight-bearing exercise) as soon as pain and symptoms allow, in order to harness the benefits of normal function. Patients should be encouraged to re-commence their exercise rehabilitation (e.g. progressive loading) based on the individual's needs and treatment goals.

Kenalog 40mg/mL is a suspension usually contained in 1 mL vials (Fig. 4.5).

Accurate needle placement is essential. This depends on clinical diagnosis. Knowledge of anatomy will allow accurate location of the lesion and avoid unnecessary complications. Points to consider are:

- The tissue in which the lesion lies
- How deep the lesion lies
- The extent of the lesion
- Adjacent structures to avoid
- The position of the patient to make the site of the lesion accessible
- The direction in which the needle should be inserted
- The length of needle and the size of syringe required.

Unwanted Side Effects and Possible Complications of Corticosteroid Therapy

Most of the unpleasant side effects of corticosteroid therapy relate to large, long-term doses of the drugs taken systemically. Systemic effects do not ordinarily occur with intra-articular or intralesional injections

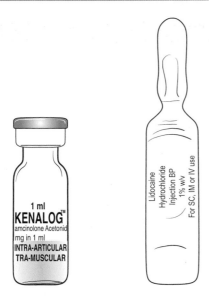

Fig. 4.5 Containers of drugs in common use for musculoskeletal injections.

when the recommended techniques of administration and the dosage regimes are observed.

Triamcinolone acetonide can gradually disseminate into the systemic circulation from the local site of the injection over a period of a few weeks. However, clinically significant systemic levels after a single intra-articular or a single intralesional injection are unlikely to occur, except perhaps following treatment of large joints with high doses (Wittkowski et al., 2007).

Post-injection flare is the most common local side effect of intra-articular corticosteroid. It is characterised by a localised inflammatory response that can last 2 to 3 days (Young and Homlar, 2016) and a flare occurs in 2% to 25% of corticosteroid injection cases (Brown et al., 1953; Hollander et al., 1961; Friedman and Moore, 1980; Young and Homlar, 2016).

Symptoms usually resolve within 48 to 72 hours and should improve with simple analgesics and/or NSAIDs and the application of an ice pack. Although it is very rare to have a severe post-injection flare to a corticosteroid injection, it is important for practitioners to inform patients of this potential local side effect, and safety netting should be applied for symptoms of infection, particularly if symptoms do not settle in the expected time.

Subcutaneous atrophy and skin depigmentation may occur with inaccurate needle placement and/or leakage of fluid into the superficial tissues. They are more

likely to occur at a superficial site (e.g. tennis elbow), and when using the relatively insoluble and more potent steroids, such as methylprednisolone and triamcinolone. Corticosteroid injections have been documented to promote fat necrosis, dermal atrophy, senile purpura, depigmentation and subcutaneous atrophy (Ponec et al., 1977; Marks et al., 1983; Grillet and Dequeker, 1990; Park et al., 2013; Durmuş et al., 2016).

These subcutaneous changes may be reversible, or the patient may be left with long-lasting evidence of injection. The best way to minimise the risk of this side effect is to use accurate needle placement and good needle proprioception. Some practitioners also advise using hydrocortisone for superficial injections as, being more soluble, it is less likely to cause these problems.

Connective tissue weakening may occur because of the effect of corticosteroid on the mechanical properties of tendon, which could result in tendon necrosis and loss in tensile strength. The detrimental effects on the tendon ranges from tendinopathy to potential tendon rupture (Knobloch, 2016), with repeated corticosteroid injections appearing to increase the risk (Boussakri and Bouali, 2014). The Achilles tendon is affected most often in terms of tendinopathy and/or subsequent tendon rupture.

However, ascribing cause and effect is often difficult. For example, poor practice such as excessive repeated injection, and poor patients' compliance to continue overloading the tendon may also be contributing factors causing drug induced tendon disorder.

> **CLINICAL TIP**
>
> Injection should NOT be first-line management at any stage of tendinopathy. Manual therapy and rehabilitation should be considered as first-line management to increase the strength of the tendon.

Corticosteroid will affect the normal tissue as well as the affected tissue. During its time of action, corticosteroid potentially causes a weakening of collagen fibres – normal and degraded – and this should be recognised as a potential hazard.

For this reason, it is especially important that corticosteroid should not be injected into the body of a tendon, only into its sheath, the teno-osseous junction or peritendinously.

In all cases, the patient is instructed to rest from aggravating activities while normal, pain-free function

> **CLINICAL TIP**
> It is advisable to perform an ultrasound scan prior to injections for tendinopathy to avoid injecting severely degenerative tendons. Check with local policy.

is encouraged to provide mechanical stimulus for the new fibres. A description of 'relative rest' is provided in the box on page 92.

Steroid arthropathy describes the deterioration of the joint surface as a result of corticosteroid injection. Both animal and human research have shown consistently that corticosteroid injections into normal and degenerate knees accelerate the arthritic process (Hauser, 2009).

From animal studies, corticosteroids have been shown to produce severe deleterious effects on the joint and articular cartilage, both mechanical and physiological, which is corticosteroid dose-related. Corticosteroids have an inhibitory effect on cartilage metabolism which is manifested by damage to, and death of, chondrocytes. Because chondrocytes decrease in number and function, collagen and proteoglycan synthesis decline. The net result of these effects is articular cartilage degeneration, such as articular cartilage necrosis, thinning of articular cartilage and a decrease of cartilage growth and repair (Shaw and Lacey, 1973; Rusanen, 1986; Chunekamrai, 1989; El-Hakim et al., 2005; Shapiro et al., 2007).

Therefore, the administration of corticosteroid injections, particularly in weight-bearing joints, must be considered with caution, and restricted to no more than three per year (NICE, 2020).

Iatrogenic (clinician induced) septic arthritis is a rare but potentially serious side-effect of intra-articular joint injection. Delayed or suboptimal treatment for septic arthritis can lead to irreversible joint damage and permanent disability (Mohamed et al., 2019).

Other conditions can mimic the condition and should be considered within differential diagnosis. These include reactive or rheumatoid arthritis, transient synovitis, osteomyelitis and avascular necrosis (Long et al., 2018).

It is difficult to establish the exact incidence after corticosteroid injection, but Tuqan and Koretz (2014) refer to studies that estimate the incidence as between 2 and 4.6 cases per 100,000 injections. Risk factors include diabetes and antibiotic-resistant organisms (Tan et al., 2021); immunosuppression; and inflammatory or degenerative arthropathy.

The cause of septic arthritis after injection is presumed to be the introduction of bacteria from the skin's surface via the intra-articular or peri-articular needle insertion (Tuqan and Koretz, 2014). The 'no-touch' technique (described on page 97) is important to avoid this complication.

Systemic effects include the possibility of transient hyperglycaemia in a diabetic patient and should be considered. In clinical practice, some patients report high levels of blood glucose following corticosteroid injections, while some do not. Evidence for the risk of developing transient hyperglycaemia in diabetic patients is also mixed. This is likely to be due to a number of variables that may also contribute to its development such as age, medical history, drug history, diabetic control, dose of steroid to be used, and area to be injected (Donihi et al., 2006).

As a general theme, evidence shows that a single intra-articular or intralesional injection can elevate blood sugar for 3 to 6 days (Wang and Hutchinson, 2006; Baumgarten, 2008; Catalano et al., 2012; Stepan et al., 2014; Blonna et al., 2018). A significant increase in blood glucose level has been reported particularly on day 1 and day 2 after injection (Stepan et al., 2014; Blonna et al., 2018). Therefore, it is sensible to inform the patient of the possibility of transient hyperglycaemia. Advice should be given to monitor blood sugar levels regularly for at least 3 days; and particularly on days 1 and 2 after the injection (Stepan et al., 2014; Blonna et al., 2018).

In addition, checking patients' Hb1Ac level and their normal diabetic control before injection is important to minimise risk of significant transient hyperglycaemia. Local policy should be adhered to.

Other systemic effects are facial flushing appearing in the first 2 to 3 days (possibly lasting a day or 2) and menstrual disturbance, including postmenopausal bleeding.

> **UNWANTED SIDE EFFECTS AND POSSIBLE COMPLICATIONS OF CORTICOSTEROID INJECTION**
> - Post-injection flare
> - Local soft tissue atrophy and pigment changes
> - Connective tissue weakening
> - Steroid arthropathy
> - Iatrogenic (clinician induced) septic arthritis
> - Systemic effects – hyperglycaemia, facial flushing, post-menopausal bleeding

Local Anaesthetic

Local anaesthetics work by penetrating the nerve sheath and axon membrane. They produce a reversible blockade to impulse conduction and do this more readily in small-diameter, myelinated and unmyelinated nerve fibres. Nociceptive and sympathetic impulses are therefore blocked more readily (Ritter et al., 2019).

The pain-relieving effect of local anaesthetic is utilised in musculoskeletal medicine for its therapeutic and diagnostic effects. Given together with corticosteroid, local anaesthetic allows immediate reassessment of the patient to confirm diagnosis.

It gives the patient initial pain relief and may reduce the effects of post-injection flare from corticosteroid injection. It is also useful to distribute the corticosteroid throughout

---

USES OF LOCAL ANAESTHETIC IN MUSCULOSKELETAL MEDICINE
- Used together with corticosteroids for diagnostic purposes and therapeutic pain relief during and after injection
- To increase volume of injection to distribute steroid and to produce possible distention effect
- As part of an epidural injection via the sacral hiatus

---

the extent of the lesion and can provide an element of distention that may be useful in joints and bursae.

In this text, lidocaine hydrochloride is used. It has a rapid rate of onset and moderate duration. It may be used as 0.5%, 1% or 2% solution and the maximum dose is 200 mg (equal to 20 mL of a 1% solution, for example). It is provided in an ampoule (see Fig. 4.5).

This dose is within safe limits to give by infiltration to a fit adult of average weight, but it would be unsafe to give this dose intravenously.

Unwanted Side Effects and Possible Complications of Local Anaesthetic

It is important to recognise the maximum dose of local anaesthetic in order to avoid unwanted side effects and complications (Ritter et al., 2019), and patients should always be questioned about sensitivity to previous injections.

Steps should be taken to ensure that the needle does not lie in a blood vessel by performing a safety aspiration before injection to avoid giving the dose intravenously.

Allergic reactions range from a mild rash to rare anaphylaxis, which can be life threatening. It is therefore a prerequisite that any practitioner using local anaesthetic must be trained to recognise and manage these complications.

Central nervous system effects may be due to stimulation and may initially include feelings of inebriation and light-headedness, restlessness, tremor and confusion progressing to extreme agitation. Further increase in drug levels leads to depression of the central nervous system that may present as sedation, twitching, convulsion or respiratory depression, which is potentially life-threatening.

Cardiovascular effects may present as a combination of myocardial depression and vasodilatation producing sudden hypotension, which may be life-threatening. Myocardial depression occurs as a result of inhibition of sodium current in cardiac muscle. Vasodilatation is due to the local anaesthetic effect on the smooth muscle of the arterioles and sympathetic inhibition.

Effects on articular cartilage have been considered more recently. There is increasing evidence suggesting that the use of local anaesthetics, such as lidocaine 1% or 2% and bupivacaine, may be chondrotoxic in intra-articular injections, but long-term effects on articular cartilage and the risk of developing degenerative arthropathy are unclear.

A number of studies have demonstrated local anaesthetic chondrotoxicity in vivo and in vitro in both human and animal cartilage (Piper et al., 2011; Syed et al., 2011; Braun et al., 2012; Jayaram et al., 2019).

Evidence suggested that commonly used local anaesthetics, such as lidocaine, reduce cell viability (Grishko et al., 2010; Dragoo et al., 2012; Sherman et al., 2015), lead to a substantial chrondrotoxic effect (Piper et al., 2011; Sherman et al., 2015) and significantly increase chondrocyte death (Karpie and Chu, 2007; Lo et al., 2009).

Local anaesthetics have also been reported to have dose- and time- dependent deleterious effects on chondrocytes, which appear to be made worse by the co-administration of corticosteroid on human knee articular cartilage (Jayaram et al., 2019).

In summary, a single-dose intra-articular administration of local anaesthetic may impede chondrocyte metabolism and may lead to a deleterious effect on chondrocytes and articular cartilage. Therefore, practitioners should apply clinical reasoning when using local anaesthetic injections, and they should be performed only with low concentrations for selected diagnostic purposes and painful joints.

UNWANTED SIDE EFFECTS AND COMPLICATIONS OF LOCAL ANAESTHETIC
- Allergic reactions
- Central nervous system effects
- Cardiovascular effects
- Cartilage effects (chondrotoxicity)

Contraindications to Corticosteroid or Local Anaesthetic Injection

Contraindications
- Absence or withdrawal of patient consent
- Allergy to corticosteroid or local anaesthetic
- Sepsis
  - Systemic – significant/febrile (e.g. active tuberculosis)
  - Local
  - Suspected

Cautions
- Poorly controlled diabetes. Some services have policies to check recent blood glucose levels to ensure that a patient is a stable diabetic before injecting. As always, local policy should be established before proceeding.
- Anticoagulants or blood clotting disorders. Policies vary with regard to this. Some services provide limits for clotting time, as indicated by the International Normalisation Rate (INR) (usually less than 2.5–3.0), while some services prohibit the use of any corticosteroid injections for patients on some anticoagulants.
- Recent joint surgery or planned within the next 3–6 months. This appears to be standard policy as there is evidence that recent injection can increase the risk of postoperative infection.
- Regular doses or a recent course of systemic steroids
- Immunosuppressed patient
- Tuberculosis (non-active)
- Pregnancy
- Young adults and children under 16 years of age. Please refer to local policies, as local care pathways vary for the provision of corticosteroid injection to those under 16.
- Unstable hypertension
- Has had, or due to have, live vaccination

Needle Sizes

Fig. 4.6.

Syringes

Fig. 4.7.

> **CLINICAL TIP**
> The syringe selected must be suitable for the total injection volume (mL). Aim to use the finest needle to be able to reach the lesion.

Two techniques are generally used to deliver the injection (see Table 4.5):

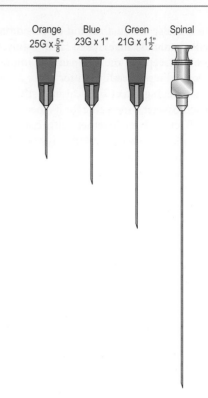

Fig. 4.6 Needles in common use for musculoskeletal injections.

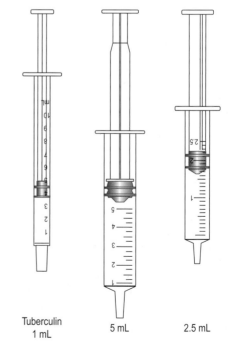

Fig. 4.7 Syringes in common use for musculoskeletal injections.

- A *bolus technique* is used for joint and bursae injections where no resistance is felt on pressing the plunger.
- A *peppering technique* is used for tendon insertions and ligaments where a series of small droplets is delivered throughout the substance of the structure to cover the extent and depth of the lesion.

'No-touch' Technique

A 'no-touch' technique is essential to minimise the risk of infection. It is essential to avoid injecting in the presence of infection because the corticosteroid also has an immunosuppressive effect.

The full injection procedure will now be described, incorporating the 'no-touch' technique:

- Having jointly decided that injection is appropriate for your patient and after screening for *contraindications*, discuss the treatment options, ensure that the patient understands the proposed treatment, including all risks and benefits and the need for relative rest after the injection, and *gain informed consent*.
- *Position the patient* making sure that the lesion and injection site are accessible.
- *Assemble equipment* – needles, syringes, alcohol swabs, cotton wool, sharps bin, plaster; check and record drugs.
- *Wash hands* – soap and water/surgical scrub.
- *Draw up* the corticosteroid and local anaesthetic – *change needle* for delivery.
- *Mark skin*.
- *Apply gloves or wash hands*.
- *Clean the skin* – alcohol swabs, etc.
- *Insert the needle* – without touching the needle or the injection site:
- Perform a *safety aspiration* prior to infiltration, to confirm that the needle is not in a blood vessel, by drawing on the syringe slightly to see if any blood is taken up through the needle
- Use appropriate peppering or bolus technique to *deliver the injection*
- *Withdraw* and dispose of all equipment appropriately
- *Apply plaster/dressing*, ensuring there are no allergies to these.
- *Reassess* after 5 minutes, keep the patient in the department for up to 30 minutes to check that there is no reaction.
- *Advise relative rest* for approximately 2 weeks.
- *Reassess the outcome* in 2–3 weeks time.

Lack of response to corticosteroid injection will require a review of the diagnosis and the technique. Patients may be provided with a follow-up appointment after 2 to 3 weeks or encouraged to initiate follow-up, depending on the treatment outcome.

If the condition is very painful, other analgesics, such as paracetamol, may be administered along with other measures, such as short applications of ice and/ or elevation.

Hyaluronic Acid Injections

Hyaluronic acid (viscosupplementation) (HA) injections can be an alternative to corticosteroid injections to reduce pain and improve function in degenerative arthropathic joints, due to its lubrication, viscoelastic and anti-inflammatory properties (Necas et al., 2008). It can be considered as a prophylactic or therapeutic treatment, or an option for patients when surgery is not advisable due to comorbidities or when the patient declines surgery.

After more than 20 years of use, HA is generally recognised as a safe and well-tolerated treatment of knee degenerative arthropathy and other joints, both in current literature and from expert opinion (Henrotin et al., 2015). In recent years, HA has also been used in tendon pathologies (Kaux et al., 2015).

Despite its positive evaluation by practitioners, and extensive research, international guidelines on the therapeutic use of HA injections are not consistent (Jevsevar et al., 2013; Bannuru et al., 2019; Kolasinski et al., 2019; NICE, 2020; Sellam et al., 2020). The UK NICE guideline for the care and management of osteoarthritis (NICE, 2020) does not currently recommend the use of HA for degenerative arthropathy. This may be based on economic impact, methodological heterogeneity and meta-analysis of randomised trials, which showed the treatment effect size to be too small to be considered clinically relevant.

Notwithstanding, HA injection is used mainly in degenerative arthropathy, particularly in the knee joint, where its effectiveness is well-documented (Bannuru et al., 2011; Bannuru et al., 2014; Bannuru et al., 2016; Maheu et al., 2016; Smith et al., 2019). Since it is a naturally occurring glycosaminoglycan, it negates many of the possible deleterious effects associated with intralesional/ intra-articular corticosteroid injections and the patient is not limited with regard to ongoing injection therapy, or the number of injections they can have.

While the precise mechanism of action responsible for the clinical benefit of HA in degenerative arthropathy is not entirely understood, several biological mechanisms have been proposed.

Maheu et al. (2019) explain that HA is a glycosaminoglycan molecule found within the knee joint where it provides viscoelastic properties similar to synovial fluid. During the course of degenerative arthropathy, the synovial fluid undergoes degradation in a similar way to other tissues in the joint. This manifests as a decrease in the amount and the average molecular weight of HA, which correlates with joint pain and functional impairment.

Injection of HA into the joint acts to restore intra-articular lubrication, consequently improving joint movement. The residence time of intra-articular HA is only 2 to 3 days, however, and more prolonged effects lasting for several weeks post-injection suggest that other mechanisms of action must be at work.

Intra-articular HA has been found to: stimulate the synthesis of HA and the components of the extracellular matrix by fibroblasts; promote chondroprotection by mitigating proteoglycan loss and death of chondrocytes; reduce HA degradation by decreasing the production of pro-inflammatory cytokines; and reduce the induction of pain mediators (Maheu et al., 2019).

Evidence of the numerous mechanisms by which HA acts on joint structure and function provides support that intra-articular HA may be clinically beneficial in knee osteoarthritis, not only by providing pain relief but also by delivering potential disease-modifying effects. The evidence is promising but further investigation is needed to confirm the disease-modifying effects.

Both corticosteroids and HA have been shown to improve pain and function in arthropathy. Evidence from randomised controlled trials (RCTs) and meta-analysis indicate that intra-articular HA offers the best benefit/risk balance amongst the various pharmacological treatments for symptomatic degenerative knee arthropathy (Bannuru et al., 2015; Henrotin et al., 2015; Maheu et al., 2016; Trojian et al., 2016).

A systemic review and meta-analysis by Trellu et al. (2015) showed that corticosteroids are superior for providing pain relief, but HA provides improved functional outcomes when compared against placebo, or each other, in patients with degenerative thumb arthropathy.

A recent review (Latourte and Lellouche, 2021) concluded that corticosteroids have a short-term effect (4 to 6 weeks) while HA has a longer-term effect (8 to 24 weeks) in the treatment of degenerative arthropathy. An extensive literature review and experts' opinion provided a consensus statement that HA is an effective treatment for mild to moderate knee degenerative arthropathy, but it is not an alternative to surgery in advanced hip degenerative arthropathy (Henrotin et al., 2015).

To summarise, in general, HA injections appear to provide short- and longer-term effectiveness in degenerative arthropathy, and it is a safe treatment option with very few side effects (e.g. small risk of infection, and temporary pain and swelling after the injection).

Practitioners should apply clinical reasoning and consider patients' individual factors, such as the stage of degenerative arthropathy, severity of symptoms, previous treatment history, and comorbidities during the shared decision-making process.

If available, hyaluronic acid injections can be considered as an alternative to corticosteroid injections.

> **CLINICAL TIP**
> Consider hyaluronic acid injections as an alternative to corticosteroid injections, or as an option when surgery is not advisable due to comorbidities, or when the patient declines surgery.

Epidural Injections

The use of epidural injections may be appropriate in the management of low back pain, particularly if radicular pain is also present (see Chapter 13). The musculoskeletal medicine approach is injection via the caudal route with the aim of bathing the dura mater and sensitised nerve roots with an anti-inflammatory solution, with or without local anaesthetic, to relieve pain.

Practitioners considering performing epidural injections should check with their professional body to ensure that appropriate insurance is in place.

Bush and Hillier (1991) discuss three possible mechanisms of pain relief, citing Bhatia and Parikh and Gupta

> **USES OF EPIDURAL INJECTIONS IN MUSCULOSKELETAL MEDICINE**
> - Chronic back or leg pain
> - Radicular pain, with or without neurological deficit
> - Trial treatment for pain relief prior to consideration for surgery

et al., who join Cyriax (1984) in the suggestion that the introduction of the fluid local anaesthetic into the epidural space is enough in itself to influence the relationship between the disc and nerve root.

Bush and Hillier (1991) also cite Melzack and Wall in describing how, in spite of its short action, the local anaesthetic may nonetheless break the pain cycle.

Corticosteroid is usually added to the solution, however, with the logic of reducing both the swelling and inflammation at the disc–nerve root interface as an additional benefit of the large-volume injection (Bush and Hillier, 1991).

Studies have shown that although local anaesthetic in the epidural mixture gives short-term pain relief (a few hours), it makes no difference to the outcome in the medium to long term. Accuracy of needle placement is improved considerably if the injection is given with the aid of imaging and this, combined with prior magnetic resonance imaging (MRI), is likely to increase accuracy and reduce the number of epidural injections needed overall (Bush, 2012).

It should be stressed that, although epidural injection via the caudal route can be performed as an outpatient procedure, the injection should only be carried out by an experienced medical practitioner who has undergone appropriate training.

The injection typically involves the introduction of 80 mg triamcinolone acetonide in 20 to 25 mL procaine, lidocaine or bupivacaine via the sacral hiatus, using a no-touch technique. Mixing the steroid with saline is an alternative that is safer and has the same efficacy, but it does not give the initial short-term pain relief that may be helpful diagnostically.

With regard to the effects on blood glucose levels in patients with diabetes (see page 94), Even et al. (2012) noted that with just 40 mg of steroid there was a systemic elevation of blood glucose in 85% of patients for 1 to 2 days after an epidural steroid injection. As well as conforming with local policy, it is important to warn patients of this as the possible side effects can include fatigue, glycosuria and infection.

Most studies of epidural reveal an overall efficacy rate (removal of pain or worthwhile reduction) of approximately 70%.

Platelet-Rich Plasma Injection

Platelet-rich plasma (PRP) injection is another injection option for musculoskeletal sports injuries and soft tissue lesions, including lesions in tendons, muscles and ligaments (Middleton et al., 2012). PRP therapy has grown in popularity since the 2010s. Not only has there been an increasing number of clinical studies, but there has also been a rising level of public awareness following the increasing use of PRP by team physicians in elite athletes.

In musculoskeletal practice, PRP injections are most commonly used to treat chronic tendinopathies including tennis elbow, plantar fasciopathy, Achilles tendinopathy and patellar tendinopathy (Lee, 2013; NICE, 2013a, 2013b).

PRP injections can also be used in degenerative arthropathy of the knee (Latourte and Lellouche, 2021), avascular necrosis of the femoral head (Guadilla et al., 2012), and some acute injuries, such as acute muscle tears, medial collateral ligament tears, and ankle sprains (Lee, 2013).

PRP is concentrated platelet plasma obtained by centrifuging the patient's venous blood, which is believed to be rich in anti-inflammatory or pro-anabolic growth factors (Bennell et al., 2017). The platelet concentration from PRP injection is typically five times more concentrated than the physiological concentration found in healthy whole blood (Marx et al., 1998).

The strong growth factors may help in the healing process of chronic injuries (Middleton et al., 2012). Injection aims to deliver growth factors in blood directly to the site of lesion, stimulating the healing process and leading to partial modification of the damaged tissue.

Some evidence supports PRP's short-/medium-term effectiveness in relieving pain and improving function (de Vos et al., 2010; Peerbooms et al., 2010; Gosens et al., 2011), while some reviews have concluded that there was no significant benefit at all (Moraes et al., 2014; Keene et al., 2016).

A 2014 Cochrane review included 19 single-centre randomised trials (1088 participants) that compared PRP with placebo, whole blood, dry needling, or no treatment, for eight different soft tissue injuries. This was either as a direct treatment (for elbow lateral epicondylitis, patellar tendinopathy, and Achilles tendinopathy) or as an adjunct to surgery (anterior cruciate ligament reconstruction grafts and donor sites, rotator cuff repair, subacromial decompression, and Achilles rupture repair) (Moraes et al., 2014). Comparison with other active treatments was not included.

Most trials were judged to be at high risk of bias, with lack of standardisation of the PRP preparation. Overall, there was no clinically significant improvement in pain and function with PRP. The authors of the Cochrane review concluded that there was insufficient evidence to support the use of PRP (Moraes et al., 2014).

From another review of a further 10 randomised controlled trials (476 participants) by Keene et al. (2016), a similar conclusion of limited efficacy of PRP was drawn. In summary, the efficacy of PRP therapy has yet to be established.

However, there have been no major complications reported and it is generally a safe treatment option (de Vos et al., 2010; Peerbooms et al., 2010; NICE, 2013a, 2013b), with fewer side-effects compared to corticosteroid injection and surgery.

Many practitioners feel that PRP therapy is safe, given its autologous nature and long-term usage without any reported major complications. For this reason, in addition to its ready availability and ease of use in the clinical setting, it has become a popular choice in the musculoskeletal and sports medicine community.

Clinically, PRP can be considered for those patients who fail to improve with conservative treatment, especially in tendinopathy, or for those who want to avoid the potential side effects from (repeated) corticosteroid injections.

Practitioners should apply clinical reasoning and inform patients of the current evidence, possible risks, benefits and expected outcomes during the shared decision-making process, to allow them to make an informed decision about their care.

> **CLINICAL TIP**
>
> PRP can be considered for those patients who fail to improve with conservative treatment, especially in tendinopathy, or for those who want to avoid the potential side effects from (repeated) steroid injections.

Prolotherapy (Sclerosant Therapy)

The aim of prolotherapy is to increase ligament or tendon mass and ligament-to-bone or tendon-to-bone strength. Experiments have shown a statistically significant increase in collagen fibril diameter (Liu et al., 1983), suggesting that the sclerosing (fibrous tissue

> **USES OF PROLOTHERAPY IN MUSCULOSKELETAL MEDICINE**
> - Recurrent or chronic episodes of low back pain, with or without leg pain
> - Recurrent sacroiliac joint subluxation
> - Other conditions associated with ligamentous laxity such as subluxing capitate bone

forming) solution has an influence on connective tissue at the insertion sites.

Prolotherapy alone is not an effective treatment for chronic low-back pain but as part of a treatment package including spinal manipulation and exercise, prolotherapy may improve chronic low-back pain and disability.

Sclerosant solutions include hypertonic dextrose and sodium morrhuate and most practitioners are now using hypertonic dextrose in local anaesthetic. Occasionally, phenol is injected in conjunction with dextrose and glycerol.

The sclerosant causes an intense inflammatory reaction at the site of injection. The intention in producing such an intense inflammatory reaction is to stimulate the formation of new collagen fibres that are gradually incorporated into the existing ligament.

The immature fibres laid down are encouraged to contract and shorten by avoiding movement and stress during the repair and remodelling phases.

The intense reaction causes considerable pain. It would not be rational to use anti-inflammatory medication following prolotherapy, but simple analgesics, such as paracetamol, can be advised. A series of three to six injections at weekly intervals is usually required.

Unwanted Side Effects of Prolotherapy

Strong phenol, if used, penetrates the nerve endings, producing a local anaesthetic effect (Goodman and Gilman, 1970) that is permanent. It is not known whether the very low concentrations used in prolotherapy have any effect other than antiseptic.

Table 4.6 provides a summary of the principles of musculoskeletal muscle treatment, as applied to soft tissue lesions.

TABLE 4.6   Summary of Principles of Musculoskeletal Medicine Treatment Applied to Soft Tissue Lesions

Acute muscle belly lesions	Apply the principles of treatment for acute soft tissue lesions in the early stages, leading on to progressive rehabilitation Transverse frictions in a shortened position Grade A mobilisation Increasing depth of transverse frictions and progressive Grade A mobilisation until the full range of movement is restored Ideally treat daily, or as often as possible, in the early phase
Chronic muscle belly lesions	Transverse frictions in shortened position Progressive Grade A mobilisation Progressive rehabilitation.
Musculotendinous lesions (usually chronic)	Transverse frictions in accessible position Progressive Grade A mobilisation Progressive rehabilitation
Acute tenosynovitis	Transverse frictions, tendon on slight stretch Grade A mobilisation Apply the principles of treatment for acute soft tissue lesions in the early stages (as for Chronic tenosynovitis coming next in the table): OR Corticosteroid injection, bolus technique between tendon and sheath Modified activities for 2 weeks following injection (Grade A mobilisation) and then progressive rehabilitation
Chronic tenosynovitis	Transverse frictions, tendon on a stretch Grade A mobilisation Progressive rehabilitation OR Corticosteroid injection, bolus technique between tendon and sheath Modified activities for 2 weeks following injection (Grade A mobilisation) and then progressive rehabilitation
Chronic tendinopathy, teno-osseous junction	Transverse frictions, Grade A mobilisation Mills' manipulation, special technique for tennis elbow, friction just to analgesia, then Grade C manipulation Progressive rehabilitation OR Corticosteroid injection, peppering technique Modified activities for 2 weeks following injection (Grade A mobilisation) and then progressive rehabilitation
Stage I capsulitis	Grade B mobilisation OR Corticosteroid injection, bolus technique Modified activities for 2 weeks following injection (Grade A mobilisation), progressing to increased mobilisation once pain settles
Stage II capsulitis	Corticosteroid injection, bolus technique Modified activities for 2 weeks following injection (Grade A mobilisation), progressing to increased mobilisation once pain settles OR Grade A mobilisation, distraction techniques
Stage III capsulitis	Grade B mobilisation

Continued

TABLE 4.6   Summary of Principles of Musculoskeletal Medicine Treatment Applied to Soft Tissue Lesions

Acute bursitis	Corticosteroid injection, bolus technique Modified activities for 2 weeks following injection (Grade A mobilisation)
Chronic bursitis	Corticosteroid injection, large volume local anaesthetic, low dose, ideally bolus, or peppering technique Modified activities for 2 weeks following injection (Grade A mobilisation)
Acute ligament lesion	Apply the principles of treatment for acute soft tissue lesions in the early stages, leading on to progressive rehabilitation Transverse frictions Grade A mobilisation Progressing to an increased depth of transverse frictions and progressive Grade A mobilisation until the full range of movement is restored Ideally treat daily, or as often as possible, in the early phase
Chronic ligament lesion	Transverse frictions Progressive Grade A mobilisation Manipulation applied to chronic medial collateral ligament sprain of the knee and lateral ligament sprain of the ankle following the application of sufficient transverse frictions to achieve analgesic effect Progressive rehabilitation
Ligamentous laxity	Prolotherapy (sclerosant therapy) Modified activities for 2 weeks following injection
Loose body	Grade A mobilisation applied under strong manual traction
Subluxed carpal/tarsal bone	Grade A mobilisation applied under strong manual traction
Acute cervical lesion	'Bridging' mobilisation technique Grade A mobilisation
Subacute/chronic cervical lesion	Mobilisation under manual traction, progressing to manipulation if necessary
Acute lumbar lesion	'Pretzel' mobilisation technique Grade A mobilisation
Subacute/chronic lumbar lesion	Mobilisation techniques Manipulation Traction Caudal epidural injection
Sacroiliac joint lesion	Manipulation Mobilisation techniques Exercise

REVIEW QUESTIONS

1. For what purpose is a Grade B mobilisation used in peripheral joints? Review key treatment principles.
2. Consider how a Grade A mobilisation may be progressed during the rehabilitation process.
3. What does graded transverse frictions mean?
4. What are the principles of applying a manipulation?
5. Corticosteroid injections impair the body's ability to fight infection: What are the implications of this to clinical practice?

REFERENCES

Akeson, W., 1990. The response of ligaments to stress modulation and overview of the ligament healing response. In: Daniel, D., Akeson, W.H., O'Connor, J.J. (Eds.), Knee Ligaments: Structure, Function, Injury and Repair. Lippincott, Williams & Wilkins, Philadelphia, pp. 315–327.

Akeson, W., Amiel, D., Abel, M.F., et al., 1986. Effects of immobilization on joints. Clin. Orthop. Relat. Res. 219, 28–37.

Akeson, W., Amiel, D., La Violette, D., 1967. The connective-tissue response to immobility: a study of chondroitin-4 and 6-sulfate and dermatan sulfate changes in periarticular connective tissue of control and immobilized knees of dogs. Clin. Orthop. Relat. Res. 51, 183–197.

Akeson, W., Amiel, D., Woo, S.L.-Y., 1980. Immobility effects on synovial joints, the pathomechanics of joint contracture. Biorheology 17, 95–110.

Akeson, W., Woo, S.L.-Y., Amiel, D., et al., 1973. The connective tissue response to immobility: biochemical changes in periarticular connective tissue of the immobilized rabbit's knee. Clin. Orthop. Relat. Res. 93, 356–362.

Algafly, A.A., George, K.P., 2007. The effect of cryotherapy on nerve conduction velocity, pain threshold and pain tolerance. Br. J. Sports Med. 41, 365–369.

Amis, A.A., 1985. Biomechanics of ligaments. In: Jenkins, D.H.R. (Ed.), Ligament Injuries and Their Treatment. Chapman and Hall, London, pp. 3–28.

Arem, A.J., Madden, J.W., 1976. Effects of stress on healing wounds, 1: intermittent noncyclical tension. J. Surg. Res. 20, 93–102.

Baltaci, G., Ergun, N., Tunay, V., 2001. Effectiveness of cyriax manipulative therapy and elbow band in the treatment of lateral epicondylitis. Eur. J. Sports Traumatol. Rel. Res. 23, 113–118.

Bannuru, R.R., Natov, N.S., Dasi, U.R., et al., 2011. Therapeutic trajectory following intra-articular hyaluronic acid injection in knee osteoarthritis–meta-analysis. Osteoarthritis Cartilage 19 (6), 611–619.

Bannuru, R.R., Schmid, C.H., Kent, D.M., et al., 2015. Comparative effectiveness of pharmacologic interventions for knee osteoarthritis: a systematic review and network meta-analysis. Ann. Intern. Med. 162, 46–54.

Bannuru, R.R., Osani, M., Vaysbrot, E.E., et al., 2016. Comparative safety profile of hyaluronic acid products for knee osteoarthritis: a systematic review and network meta-analysis. Osteoarthritis Cartilage 24 (12), 2022–2041.

Bannuru, R.R., Osani, M.C., Vaysbrot, E.E., et al., 2019. OARSI guidelines for the non-surgical management of knee, hip, and polyarticular osteoarthritis. Osteoarthritis Cartilage 27, 1578–1589.

Bannuru, R.R., Vaysbrot, E.E., Sullivan, M.C., et al., 2014. Relative efficacy of hyaluronic acid in comparison with NSAIDs for knee osteoarthritis: a systematic review and meta-analysis. Semin. Arthritis Rheum. 43 (5), 593–599.

Baumgarten, K.M., 2008. Current treatment of trigger digits in patients with diabetes mellitus. J. Hand Surg. Am. 33 (6), 980–981.

Bennell, K.L., Hunter, D.J., Paterson, K.L., 2017. Platelet-rich plasma for the management of hip and knee osteoarthritis. Curr. Rheumatol. Rep. 19 (5), 24.

Bialosky, J.E., Bishop, M.D., Robinson, M.E., et al., 2008. The influence of expectation on spinal manipulation induced

hypoalgesia: an experimental study in normal subjects. BMC. Musculoskelet. Disord. 9 (1), 1–9.

Bialosky, J.E., Bishop, M.D., Robinson, M.E., et al., 2009. Spinal manipulative therapy has an immediate effect on thermal pain sensitivity in people with low back pain: a randomized controlled trial. Phys. Ther. 89 (12), 1292–1303.

Bleakley, C.M., Costello, J.T., 2013. Do thermal agents affect range of movement and mechanical properties in soft tissues? A systematic review. Arch. Phys. Med. Rehabil. 94, 149–163.

Bleakley, C.M., Glasgow, P., MacAuley, D.C., 2012. PRICE needs updating, should we call the POLICE? Br. J. Sports Med 46, 220–221.

Bleakley, C.M., McDonough, S.M., MacAuley, D.C., 2006. Cryotherapy for acute ankle sprains: a randomised controlled study of two different icing protocols. Br. J. Sports Med. 40, 700–705.

Blonna, D., Bonasia, D.E., Mattei, L., et al., 2018. Efficacy and safety of subacromial corticosteroid injection in type 2 diabetic patients. Pain Res. Treat. 2018, 9279343.

Boruta, P.M., Bishop, J.O., Braly, W.G., et al., 1990. Acute lateral ankle ligament injuries: literature review. Foot Ankle 11, 107–113.

Boussakri, H., Bouali, A., 2014. Subcutaneous rupture of the extensor pollicis longus tendon after corticosteroid injections in DeQuervain stenosing tendovaginitis. Case Rep. Orthop. 2014, 934384.

Bowsher, D., 1994. Modulation of nociceptive input. In: Wells, P.E., Frampton, V., Bowsher, D. (Eds.), Pain Management by Physiotherapy, second ed. Butterworth Heinemann, Oxford, pp. 30–31.

Brandy, W.D., Irion, J.M., 1994. The effect of time on static stretch on the flexibility of the hamstring muscles. Phys. Ther 74 (9), 845–852.

Brandy, W.D., Irion, J.M., Briggler, M., 1997. The effect of time and frequency of static stretching on the flexibility of the hamstring muscles. Phys. Ther 77 (10), 1090–1096.

Braun, H.J., Wilcox-Fogel, N., Kim, H.J., et al., 2012. The effect of local anesthetic and corticosteroid combinations on chondrocyte viability. Knee Surg. Sports Traumatol. Arthrosc. 20 (9), 1689–1695.

Brosseau, L., Casimiro, L., Milne, S., et al., 2002. Deep transverse friction massage for treating tendinitis. Cochrane Database Syst. Rev (4), CD003528.

Brown Jr., E.M., Frain, J.B., Udell, L., et al., 1953. Locally administered hydrocortisone in the rheumatic diseases; a summary of its use in 547 patients. Am. J. Med. 15 (5), 656–665.

Brumagne, S., Cordo, P., Lysens, R., et al., 2000. The role of paraspinal muscle spindles in lumbosacral position sense in individuals with and without low back pain. Spine 25, 989–994.

Burke-Evans, E., Eggers, G.W.N., Butler, J.K., et al., 1960. Experimental immobilization and remobilization of rat knee joints. J. Bone Joint Surg 42A, 737–758.

Bush, K., 2012. When should you order an MRI scan before performing an epidural injection for lower back pain? Int. Musculoskelet. Med 34 (4), 131–132.

Bush, K., Hillier, S., 1991. A controlled study of caudal epidural injections of triamcinolone plus procaine for the management of intractable sciatica. Spine 16 (5), 572–575.

Campagnolo, A.M., Tsuji, D.H., Sennes, L.U., et al., 2010. Histologic study of acute vocal fold wound healing after corticosteroid injection in a rabbit model. Ann. Otol. Rhinol. Laryngol. 119 (2), 133–139.

Carreck, A., 1994. The effect of massage on pain perception threshold. Manip. Phys 26, 10–16.

Catalano III, L.W., Glickel, S.Z., Barron, O.A., et al., 2012. Effect of local corticosteroid injection of the hand and wrist on blood glucose in patients with diabetes mellitus. Orthopedics 35 (12), e1754–e1758.

Chamberlain, G.J., 1982. Cyriax's friction massage: a review. J. Orthop. Sports Phys. Ther. 4, 16–22.

Chartered Society of Physiotherapy, 2008. Chartered Society of Physiotherapy (CSP) Position Paper on the Mixing of Medicines in Physiotherapy Practice. CSP, London.

Chazaud, B., 2020. Inflammation and skeletal muscle degeneration: Leave it to the macrophages! Trends in Immunology 41 (6), 481–492.

Chesterton, L.S., Foster, N.E., Ross, L., 2002. Skin temperature response to cryotherapy. Arch. Phys. Med. Rehabil. 83, 543–549.

Childs, J.D., Fritz, J.M., Flynn, T.W., et al., 2004. A clinical prediction rule to identify patients with low back pain most likely to benefit from spinal manipulation: a validation study. Ann. Intern. Med. 141, 920–928.

Chunekamrai, S., 1989. Changes in articular cartilage after intraarticular injections of methylprednisolone acetate in horses. Am. J. Vet. Res. 50, 1733–1741.

Cleland, J.A., Fritz, J.M., Whitman, J.M., et al., 2006. The use of a lumbar spine manipulation technique by physical therapists in patients who satisfy a clinical prediction rule: a case series. J. Orthop. Sports Phys. Ther. 36, 209–214.

Cuellar, J.M., Dutton, R.C., Antognini, J.F., et al., 2005. Differential effects of halothane and isoflurane on lumbar dorsal horn neuronal windup and excitability. Br. J. Anaesth. 94, 617–625.

Cyriax, J., 1982. Textbook of Orthopaedic Medicine, eighth ed. Baillière Tindall, London.

Cyriax, J., 1984. Textbook of Orthopaedic Medicine, eleventh ed Baillière Tindall, London.

Cyriax, J., Cyriax, P., 1993. Cyriax's Illustrated Manual of Orthopaedic Medicine. Butterworth Heinemann, Oxford.

Dasm, P., 2012. Comparative analysis of cyriax approach versus mobilization with movement approach in the treatment of patients with lateral epicondylitis. Indian J. Phys. Occupat. Ther. 6 (1), 96–102.

Davidson, C., Ganion, L., Gehlsen, G., et al., 1997. Rat tendon morphologic and functional changes resulting from soft tissue mobilization. Med. Sci. Sports Exerc. 29 (3), 313–319.

Davis, A.M., MacKay, C., 2013. Osteoarthritis year in review: outcome of rehabilitation. Osteoarthr. Cartil. 21, 1414–1424.

de Bruijn, R., 1984. Deep transverse friction: its analgesic effect. Int. J. Sports Med. 5, 35–36.

de Vos, R.J., Weir, A., van Schie, H.T., et al., 2010. Platelet-rich plasma injection for chronic Achilles tendinopathy: a randomized controlled trial. JAMA. 303 (2), 144–149.

Donihi, A.C., Raval, D., Saul, M., et al., 2006. Prevalence and predictors of corticosteroid-related hyperglycemia in hospitalized patients. Endocr. Pract. 12 (4), 358–362.

Dragoo, J.L., Braun, H.J., Kim, H.J., et al., 2012. The in vitro chondrotoxicity of single-dose local anesthetics. Am. J. Sports Med. 40 (4), 794–799.

Drugs.com. https://www.drugs.com/mtm/triamcinolone-injection.html. Accessed 25 August 2021.

Dubois, B., Esculier, J.-F., 2020. Soft-tissue injuries simply need PEACE and LOVE. Br. J. Sports Med. 54 (2), 72–73.

Durmuş, M., Yapıcı, A.K., Eski, M., et al., 2016. Linear cutaneous atrophy development due to intralesional corticosteroid therapy: Case report and review of the literature. Turkish J. Plastic Surg 24 (2), 90–93.

Ebrall, P.S., Bales, G.L., Frost, B.R., 1992. An improved clinical protocol for ankle cryotherapy. J. Manual Med 6, 161–165.

El-Hakim, I.E., Abdel-Hamid, I.S., Bader, A., 2005. Temporomandibular joint response to intraarticular dexamethason injection following mechanical arthropathy: a histological study in rats. Int. J. Oral Maxillofac. Surg. 34, 305–310.

Enneking, W.F., Horowitz, M., 1972. The intra-articular effects of immobilization of the human knee. J. Bone Joint Surg 54, 973–985.

Evans, P., 1980. The healing process at cellular level: a review. Physiotherapy 66, 256–259.

Even, J.L., Crosby, C.G., Song, Y., et al., 2012. Effects of epidural steroid injections on blood glucose levels in patients with diabetes mellitus. Spine 37, 46–50.

Flynn, T., Fritz, J., Whitman, J., et al., 2002. A clinical prediction rule for classifying patients with low back pain who demonstrate short-term improvement with spinal manipulation. Spine 27, 2835–2846.

Friedman, D.M., Moore, M.E., 1980. The efficacy of intraarticular steroids in osteoarthritis: a double-blind study. J. Rheumatol 7 (6), 850856.

Gay, R.E., Bronfort, G., Evans, R.L., 2005. Distraction manipulation of the lumbar spine: a review of the literature. J. Manipulative Physiol. Ther. 28 (4), 266–273.

Gehlsen, G., Ganion, L., Helfst, R., 1998. Fibroblastic responses to variation in soft tissue mobilization pressure. Med. Sci. Sports Exerc. 31 (4), 531–535.

George, S.Z., Bishop, M.D., Bialosky, J.E., et al., 2006. Immediate effects of spinal manipulation on thermal pain sensitivity: an experimental study. BMC Musculoskelet. Disord. 7, 68.

Goats, G.C., 1994. Massage – the scientific basis of an ancient art, part 1: the techniques. Br. J. Sports Med 28, 149–152.

Goodman, L.S., Gilman, A., 1970. The Pharmacological Basis of Therapeutics, fourth ed. Macmillan, New York.

Goodsell, M., Lee, M., Latimer, J., 2000. Short-term effects of lumbar posteroanterior mobilization in individuals with low-back pain. J. Manipulative Physiol. Ther. 23(5), 332–342.

Gosens, T., Peerbooms, J.C., van Laar, W., et al., 2011. Ongoing positive effect of platelet-rich plasma versus corticosteroid injection in lateral epicondylitis: a double-blind randomized controlled trial with 2-year follow-up. Am. J. Sports Med. 39 (6), 1200–1208.

Gracies, J.-M., 2005. Pathophysiology of spastic paresis. I: paresis and soft tissue changes. Muscle Nerve 31, 535–551.

Gregory, M.A., Deane, M.N., Mars, M., 2003. Ultrastructural changes in untraumatised rabbit skeletal muscle treated with deep transverse friction. Physiotherapy 89 (7), 408–416.

Grillet, B., Dequeker, J., 1990. Intra-articular steroid injection: a risk benefit assessment. Drug Saf 5, 205–211.

Grishko, V., Xu, M., Wilson, G., et al., 2010. Apoptosis and mitochondrial dysfunction in human chondrocytes following exposure to lidocaine, bupivacaine and ropivacaine. J. Bone Jt. Surg. Am. 92, 609–618.

Guadilla, J., Fiz, N., Andia, I., et al., 2012. Arthroscopic management and platelet-rich plasma therapy for avascular necrosis of the hip. Knee Surg. Sports Traumatol. Arthrosc. 20 (2), 393–398.

Guan, Y., Borzan, J., Meyer, R.A., et al., 2006. Windup in dorsal horn neurons is modulated by endogenous spinal mu-opioid mechanisms. J. Neurosci. 26, 4298–4307.

Hadler, N.M., Curtis, P., Gillings, D.B., et al., 1987. A benefit of spinal manipulation as adjunctive therapy for acute low back pain: a stratified controlled trial. Spine 12, 703–706.

Hanai, F., 1998. C fiber responses of wide dynamic range neurons in the spinal dorsal horn. Clin. Orthop. Relat. Res., 256–267.

Hardy, M.A., 1989. The biology of scar formation. Phys. Ther. 69, 1014–1023.

Hardy, M., Woodall, W., 1998. Therapeutic effects of heat, cold and stretch on connective tissue. J. Hand Ther. 11 (2), 148–156.

Hauser, R.A., 2009. The deterioration of articular cartilage in osteoarthritis by corticosteroid injections. J. Prolotherapy 1 (2), 107–123.

Henrotin, Y., Raman, R., Richette, P., et al., 2015. Consensus statement on viscosupplementation with hyaluronic acid for the management of osteoarthritis. Semin. Arthritis Rheum. 45 (2), 140–149.

Hollander, J.L., Jessar, R.A., Brown Jr., E.M., 1961. Intra-synovial corticosteroid therapy: a decade of use. Bull. Rheum. Dis. 11, 239–240.

Ingham, B., 1981. Transverse friction massage for the relief of tennis elbow. Phys. Sports Med. 9, 116.

Iwatsuki, H., Ikuta, Y., Shinoda, K., 2001. Deep friction massage on the masticatory muscles in stroke patients increases biting force. J. Phys. Ther. Sci. 13 (1), 17–20.

Järvinen, M.J., Lehto, M.U.K., 1993. The effects of early mobilization and immobilization on the healing process following muscle injuries. Sports Med 15, 78–89.

Jayaram, P., Kennedy, D.J., Yeh, P., et al., 2019. Chondrotoxic effects of local anesthetics on human knee articular cartilage: a systematic review. PMR 11 (4), 379–400.

Jevsevar, D.S., Brown, G.A., Jones, D.L., et al., 2013. The American Academy of Orthopaedic Surgeons evidence-based guideline on: treatment of osteoarthritis of the knee, second ed. J. Bone Joint Surg. Am 95, 1885–1886.

Joseph, M.F., Taft, K., Moskwa, M., et al., 2012. Deep friction massage to treat tendinopathy: a systematic review of a classic treatment in the face of a new paradigm of understanding. J. Sport Rehabil 21, 343–353.

Karpie, J.C., Chu, C.R., 2007. Lidocaine exhibits dose- and time-dependent cytotoxic effects on bovine articular chondrocytes in vitro. Am. J. Sports Med. 35 (10), 1621–1627.

Kaux, J.F., Samson, A., Crielaard, J.M., 2015. Hyaluronic acid and tendon lesions. Muscles Ligaments Tendons 5 (4), 264–269.

Keene, D.J., Alsousou, J., Willett, K., 2016. How effective are platelet rich plasma injections in treating musculoskeletal soft tissue injuries? Br. Med. J. 352, i517.

Kelly, E., 1997. The effects of deep transverse frictional massage to the gastrocnemius muscle. J. Orthop. Med. 19, 3–9.

Knobloch, K., 2016. Drug-induced tendon disorders. Adv. Exp. Med. Biol 920, 229–238.

Kolasinski, S.L., Neogi, T., Hochberg, M.C., et al., 2019. American College of Rheumatology/Arthritis Foundation guideline for the management of osteoarthritis of the hand, hip, and knee. Arthritis Rheumatol 72, 220–233.

Larmer, P.J., Reay, N.D., Aubert, E.R., et al., 2014. Systematic review of guidelines for the management of osteoarthritis. Arch. Phys. Med. Rehabil. 95, 375–389.

Latourte, A., Lellouche, H., 2021. Update on corticosteroid, hyaluronic acid and platelet-rich plasma injections in the management of osteoarthritis. Joint Bone Spine 88 (6), 105204.

Lee, K.S., 2013. Platelet-rich plasma injection. Semin. Musculoskelet. Radiol. 17 (1), 91–98.

Lee, H.J., Kim, Y.S., Ok, J.H., et al., 2015. Effect of a single subacromial prednisolone injection in acute rotator cuff tears in a rat model. Knee Surg. Sports Traumatol. Arthroscop. 23 (2), 555–561.

Leibovich, S.J., Ross, R., 1975. The role of the macrophage in wound repair. A study with hydrocortisone and antimacrophage serum. Am. J. Pathol. 78 (1), 71–100.

Liu, Y.K., Tipton, C.M., Matthes, R.D., et al., 1983. An in situ study of the influence of a sclerosing solution in rabbit medial collateral ligaments and its junction strength. Connect. Tissue Res. 11, 95–102.

Lo, I.K., Sciore, P., Chung, M., et al., 2009. Local anesthetics induce chondrocyte death in bovine articular cartilage disks in a dose- and duration-dependent manner. Arthroscopy 25 (7), 707–715.

Long, B., Koyfman, A., Gottlieb, M., 2018. Evaluation and management of septic arthritis and its mimics in the emergency department. West J. Emerg. Med. 20, 331–341.

MacAuley, D., 2001. Ice therapy: how good is the evidence? Int. J. Sports Med. 22, 379–384.

Madson, T.J., Hollman, J.H., 2015. Lumbar traction for managing low back pain: a survey of physical therapists in the United States. J. Orthop. Sports Phys. Ther. 45, 586–595.

Maheu, E., Bannuru, R.R., Herrero-Beaumont, G., et al., 2019. Why we should definitely include intra-articular hyaluronic acid as a therapeutic option in the management of knee osteoarthritis: results of an extensive critical literature review. Semin. Arthritis Rheum. 48 (4), 563–572.

Maheu, E., Rannou, F., Reginster, J.-Y., 2016. Efficacy and safety of hyaluronic acid in the management of osteoarthritis: evidence from real-life setting trials and surveys. Semin. Arthritis Rheum. 45, S28–S33.

Malfait, A.-M., Schnitzer, T.J., 2013. Towards a mechanism-based approach to pain management in osteoarthritis. Nat. Rev. Rheumatol. 9, 654–664.

Marks, J.G., Cano, C., Leitzel, K., et al., 1983. Inhibition of wound healing by topical steroids. J. Dermatol. Surg. Oncol 9, 819–821.

Marx, R.E., Carlson, E.R., Eichstaedt, R.M., et al., 1998. Platelet-rich plasma: growth factor enhancement for bone grafts. Oral Surg. Oral Med. Oral Pathol. Oral Radiol. Endod. 85 (6), 38–646.

Mathews, J.A., Hickling, J., 1975. Lumbar traction: a double-blind controlled study for sciatica. Rheumatol. Rehabil. 14, 222–225.

Medicines for Human Use (Marketing Authorisation etc) Regulations, 1994. SI 1994/3144. HMSO, London. https://www.legislation.gov.uk/uksi/1994/3144/regulation/7/made. Accessed 3 September 2021.

Melzack, R., Wall, P.D., 1988. The Challenge of Pain, second ed. Penguin, Harmondsworth.

Middleton, K.K., Barro, V., Muller, B., et al., 2012. Evaluation of the effects of platelet-rich plasma (PRP) therapy involved in the healing of sports-related soft tissue injuries. Iowa Orthop. J 32, 150–163.

Mohamed, M., Patel, S., Plavnik, K., et al., 2019. Retrospective analysis of septic arthritis caused by intra-articular viscosupplementation and steroid injections in a single outpatient center. J. Clin. Med. Res. 11 (7), 480–483.

Mohammadian, P., Gonsalves, A., Tsai, C., et al., 2004. Areas of capsaicin-induced secondary hyperalgesia and allodynia are reduced by a single chiropractic adjustment: a preliminary study. J. Manipulative Physiol. Ther. 27, 381–387.

Moraes, V.Y., Lenza, M., Tamaoki, M.J., et al., 2014. Platelet-rich therapies for musculoskeletal soft tissue injuries. Cochrane Database Syst. Rev. 14 (4), CD010071. 24782334

Nagrale, A., Herd, C., Ganvir, S., et al., 2009. Cyriax physiotherapy versus phonophoresis with supervised exercise in subjects with lateral epicondylalgia: a randomized clinical trial. J. Man. Manip. Ther. 17 (3), 171–178.

Necas, J., Bartosikova, L., Brauner, P., et al., 2008. Hyaluronic acid (hyaluronan): a review. Veterinarni Medicina 53, 397–411.

National Institute for Health and Care Excellence (NICE). 2013a. Autologous Blood Injection for Plantar Fasciitis (interventional procedure guidance 437). www.nice.org.uk/guidance/ipg437. Accessed 3 September 2021.

National Institute for Health and Care Excellence (NICE). 2013b. Autologous Blood Injection for Tendinopathy (interventional procedure guidance 438). www.nice.org.uk/guidance/ipg438. Accessed 3 September 2021.

National Institute for Health and Care Excellence (NICE). 2020. Osteoarthritis: Care And Management. https://www.nice.org.uk/guidance/cg177. Accessed 3 September 2021.

Norris, C.M., 2004. Sports Injuries: Diagnosis and Management for Physiotherapists, third ed. Butterworth Heinemann, Oxford.

Park, S.K., Choi, Y.S., Kim, H.J., 2013. Hypopigmentation and subcutaneous fat, muscle atrophy after local corticosteroid injection. Korean J. Anesthesiol. 65 (Suppl. 6), S59.

Paungmali, A., O'Leary, S., Souvlis, T., et al., 2003b. Hypoalgesic and sympathoexcitatory effects of mobilization with movement for lateral epicondylalgia. Phys. Ther. 83, 374–383.

Paungmali, A., O'Leary, S., Souvlis, T., et al., 2004. Naloxone fails to antagonize initial hypoalgesic effect of a manual therapy treatment for lateral epicondylalgia. J. Manipulative Physiol. Ther. 27, 180–185.

Paungmali, A., Vicenzino, B., Smith, M., 2003a. Hypoalgesia induced by elbow manipulation in lateral epicondylalgia does not exhibit tolerance. J. Pain 4, 448–454.

Pekarek, B., Osher, L., Buck, S., et al., 2011. Intra-articular corticosteroid injections: a critical literature review with up-to-date findings. Foot (Edinb.) 21 (2), 66–70.

Peerbooms, J.C., Sluimer, J., Bruijn, D.J., et al., 2010. Positive effect of an autologous platelet concentrate in lateral epicondylitis in a double-blind randomized controlled trial: platelet-rich plasma versus corticosteroid injection with a 1-year follow-up. Am. J. Sports Med. 38 (2), 255–262.

Piper, S.L., Kramer, J.D., Kim, H.T., et al., 2011. Effects of local anesthetics on articular cartilage. Am. J. Sports Med. 39 (10), 2245–2253.

Ponec, M., de Haas, C., Bachra, B.N., et al., 1977. Effects of glucocorticosteroids on primary human skin fibroblasts. Arch. Dermatol. Res. 259 (2), 117–123.

Ritter, J.M., Flower, R.J., Henderson, G., et al., 2019. Rang & Dale's Pharmacology, ninth ed. Elsevier, Edinburgh.

Rusanen, M., 1986. Scanning electron microscopical study of the effects of crystalloid and water-soluble glucocorticoids on articular cartilage. Scand. J. Rheumatol. 15, 47–51.

Saunders, S., 2000. Orthopaedic Medicine Course Manual. Saunders, London.

Schultz, G.S., Davidson, J.M., Kirsner, R.S., et al., 2011. Dynamic reciprocity in the wound environment. Wound Rep. Reg. 19 (2), 134–148.

Sellam, J., Courties, A., Eymard, F., et al., 2020. Recommendations of the French Society of Rheumatology on pharmacological treatment of knee osteoarthritis. Joint Bone Spine 87, 548–555.

Sevier, T.L., Wilson, J.K., 1999. Treating lateral epicondylitis. Sports Med. 28 (5), 375–380.

Shapiro, P.S., Rohde, R.S., Froimson, M.I., et al., 2007. The effect of local corticosteroid or ketorolac exposure on histologic and biomechanical properties of rabbit tendon and cartilage. Hand (NY) 2, 165–172.

Shaw, N.E., Lacey, E., 1973. The influence of corticosteroids on normal and papain-treated articular cartilage in the rabbit. J. Bone Joint Surg. Br. 55B, 197–205.

Sherman, S.L., James, C., Stoker, A.M., et al., 2015. In vivo toxicity of local anesthetics and corticosteroids on chondrocyte and synoviocyte viability and metabolism. Cartilage 6 (2), 106–112.

Smidt, N., Windt, D., Assendelft, W., et al., 2002. Corticosteroid injections, physiotherapy, or a wait-and-see policy for lateral epicondylitis: a randomised controlled trial. Lancet 359, 657–662.

Smith, C., Patel, R., Vannabouathong, C., et al., 2019. Combined intra-articular injection of corticosteroid and hyaluronic acid reduces pain compared to hyaluronic acid alone in the treatment of knee osteoarthritis. Knee Surg. Sports Traumatol. Arthrosc. 27 (6), 1974–1983.

Snodgrass, S., Rivett, D., Chiarelli, P., et al., 2003. Factors relating to thumb pain in physiotherapists. Aust. J. Physiother. 49, 243–250.

Stasinopoulos, D., Johnson, M.I., 2007. It may be time to modify the Cyriax treatment of lateral epicondylitis. J. Bodyw. Mov. Ther. 11, 64–67.

Stepan, J.G., London, D.A., Boyer, M.I., et al., 2014. Blood glucose levels in diabetic patients following corticosteroid injections into the hand and wrist. J. Hand Surg. 39 (4), 706–712.

Sterling, M., Jull, G., Wright, A., 2001. Cervical mobilisation: concurrent effects on pain, sympathetic nervous system activity and motor activity. Man. Ther. 6, 72–81.

Syed, H.M., Gree, L., Bianski, B., et al., 2011. Bupivacaine and triamcinolone may be toxic to human chondrocytes: a pilot study. Clin. Orthop. Relat. Res 469 (10), 2941–2947.

Tan, T., Xu, C., Kuo, F.C., Ghanem, E., et al., 2021. Risk factors for failure and optimal treatment of total joint arthroplasty for septic arthritis. J. Arthroplasty 36 (3), 892–896.

Threlkeld, A.J., 1992. The effects of manual therapy on connective tissue. Phys. Ther 72, 893–902.

Timestra, J.D., 2012. Update on ankle sprains. Am. Fa. Phys. 85 (12), 1170–1176.

Tipton, C.M., Vailas, A.C., Matthes, R.D., 1986. Experimental studies on the influences of physical activity on ligaments, tendons and joints: a brief review. Acta Med. Scand 711 (Suppl), 157–168.

Trellu, S., Dadoun, S., Berenbaum, F., et al., 2015. Intra-articular injections in thumb osteoarthritis: A systematic review and meta-analysis of randomized controlled trials. Joint Bone Spine 82 (5), 315–319.

Trojian, T.H., Concoff, A.L., Joy, S.M., et al., 2016. AMSSM scientific statement concerning viscosupplementation injections for knee osteoarthritis: importance for individual patient outcomes. Clin. J. Sport. Med 26, 1–11.

Tuqan, A., Koretz, B., 2014. Septic arthritis after intra-articular steroid injection. Proceedings of UCLA Healthcare. 18.

Usuba, M., Akai, M., Shirasaki, Y., et al., 2007. Experimental joint contracture correction with low torque – long duration repeated stretching. Clin. Orthop. Relat. Res 456, 70–78.

Velnar, T., Bailey, T., Smrkolj, V., 2009. The wound healing process: an overview of the cellular and molecular mechanisms. J. Int. Med. Res. 37, 1528–1542.

Vernon, H., 2000. Qualitative review of studies of manipulation-induced hypoalgesia. J. Manip. Physiol. Ther. 23 (2), 134–138.

Vicenzino, B., Collins, D., Benson, H., et al., 1998. An investigation of the interrelationship between manipulative therapy-induced hypoalgesia and sympathoexcitation. J. Manipulative Physiol. Ther. 21, 448–453.

Vicenzino, B., Paungmali, A., Buratowski, S., et al., 2001. Specific manipulative therapy treatment for chronic lateral epicondylalgia produces uniquely characteristic hypoalgesia. Man. Ther. 6, 205–512.

Videman, T., 1986. Connective tissue and immobilization: key factors in musculoskeletal degeneration? Clin. Orthop. 221, 26–32.

Viswas, R., Ramachandra, R., Anantkumar, P., 2012. Comparison of effectiveness of supervised exercise program and cyriax physiotherapy in patients with tennis elbow (lateral epicondylitis): a randomized clinical trial. ScientificWorld J. 2012, 939645.

Wang, A.A., Hutchinson, D.T., 2006. The effect of corticosteroid injection for trigger finger on blood glucose level in diabetic patients. J. Hand Surg. 31 (6), 979–981.

Warren, C.G., Lehmann, J.F., Koblanski, J.N., 1971. Elongation of the rat tail tendon: effect of load and temperature. Phys. Med. Rehabil 52, 465–474.

Watson, T., 2009. Tissue Repair Phases and Timescale. http://www.electrotherapy.org. Accessed 3 September 2021.

Wells, P., 1994. Manipulative procedures. In: Wells, P.E., Frampton, V., Bowsher, D. (Eds.), Pain Management by Physiotherapy, second ed. Butterworth Heinemann, Oxford, pp. 187–212.

Wieting, J.M., Cugalj, A.P., 2004. Massage, traction and manipulation. J. Pain Symptom Manag 28 (3), 244–249.

Wiggins, M.E., Fadale, P.D., Barrach, H., et al., 1994. Healing characteristics of a type I collagenous structure treated with corticosteroids. Am. J. Sports Med. 22 (2), 279–288.

Winter, B., 1968. Transverse frictions. S. Afr. J. Physiother 24, 5–7.

Wittkowski, H., Foell, D., af Klint, E., et al., 2007. Effects of intra-articular corticosteroids and anti-TNF therapy on neutrophil activation in rheumatoid arthritis. Ann. Rheum. Dis. 66 (8), 1020–1025.

Woo, S.L.-Y., 1982. Mechanical properties of tendons and ligaments, II: the relationship of immobilization and exercise on tissue remodelling. Biorheology. 19 (3), 385–408.

Woo, S.L.-Y., Matthews, J., Akeson, W., et al., 1975. Connective tissue response to immobility: correlative study of the biomechanical and biochemical measurements of normal and immobilised rabbit knees. Arthritis Rheum 18, 257–264.

Woo, S.L.-Y., Wang, C.W., Newton, P.O., et al., 1990. The response of ligaments to stress deprivation and stress enhancement. In: Daniel, D., Akeson, W.H., O'Connor, J.J. (Eds.), Knee Ligaments: Structure, Function, Injury and Repair. Lippincott, Williams & Wilkins, Philadelphia, pp. 337–349.

Woodman, R.M., Pare, L., 1982. Evaluation and treatment of soft tissue lesions of the ankle and forefoot using the Cyriax approach. Phys. Ther 62, 1144–1147.

Wright, A., 1995. Hypoalgesia post-manipulative therapy: a review of a potential neurophysiological mechanism. Man. Ther. 1, 11–16.

Young, P., Homlar, K.C., 2016. Extreme postinjection flare in response to intra-articular triamcinolone acetonide (Kenalog). Am. J. Orthop. (Belle Mead NJ) 45 (3), E108–E111.

Practice of Musculoskeletal Medicine

INTRODUCTION TO SECTION 2

Section 2 adopts a regional approach, comprising the shoulder, elbow, wrist and hand, cervical spine, thoracic spine, hip, knee, ankle and foot, lumbar spine and sacroiliac joint. Anatomy, assessment, common conditions and their management are discussed in turn for each region.

Throughout this book, functional anatomy is presented on a 'need to know' basis, being confined to clinically relevant information in the context of musculoskeletal medicine. It is not intended that detailed anatomy can be learned through its presentation here, however, and practitioners are advised to refer to anatomy textbooks alongside this text, to refresh their knowledge of musculoskeletal anatomy.

This text offers a framework for clinical reasoning and the development of practical skills. The guides to surface marking and palpation sections are provided to enhance skills in clinical diagnosis and to encourage accuracy in the application of techniques.

Practitioners will be able to draw on options available to them through their clinical experience and in their individual clinical setting, using clinical reasoning to guide the management of the conditions presented. It is expected that other approaches will be integrated into the musculoskeletal medicine approach.

It has been our experience in teaching musculoskeletal medicine that students gain confidence and competence more rapidly if they can at first be guided step by step through the techniques with feedback on their performance. It is strongly advised that practitioners should attend a foundation course in musculoskeletal medicine where they can learn and practise assessment procedures and treatment techniques in a supportive environment. Notwithstanding, although unable to provide feedback, this book aims to enable students to check their skills through reflective self-evaluation and to help them to develop their competency from there.

The Shoulder

SUMMARY

The shoulder is the most common site for upper extremity pain, with onset usually being gradual. Diagnosis can be difficult if conditions coexist and lesions are often grouped under the broader, non-specific headings of 'subacromial pain syndrome', 'rotator cuff related pain', 'instability' or 'frozen shoulder'.

It is not uncommon to find a tendinopathy or bursitis in conjunction with a secondary capsulitis. Reference of pain from the cervical region may mimic that from the shoulder and both areas are examined to establish the origin of symptoms. Shoulder pain can also be due to pathology in the chest and visceral structures, making thorough assessment essential.

Knowledge of anatomy and the use of selective tension aid the incrimination of the causative structure. Palpation then identifies the specific site of the lesion to which effective treatment can be applied.

This chapter outlines the relevant anatomy of the shoulder region with guidelines for palpation. The assessment procedure follows, incorporating the pertinent elements of the history and examination towards the identification of shoulder lesions.

The lesions are discussed, and treatments are suggested based on the principles of the theory and practice of the musculoskeletal medicine approach. The treatment techniques discussed in this chapter should be integrated into clinical practice alongside techniques drawn from other modalities. The importance of addressing the cause as well as the symptoms cannot be over-stressed.

ANATOMY

In the shoulder region, simultaneous coordinated movements occur at articulations between the scapula, humerus, clavicle and sternum. There are three synovial joints (glenohumeral, sternoclavicular and acromioclavicular joints) and two physiological joints (scapulothoracic and subacromial joints).

This section begins by pointing out the relevant features of the scapula, humerus, clavicle and sternum before describing the articulations between them and their associated ligaments and bursae.

Inert Structures

The large, flat *scapula* (Fig. 5.1) is suspended by its muscles against the posterolateral thoracic wall and overlies the second to seventh ribs in the neutral position. It is attached to the strut-like clavicle at the acromioclavicular joint (Fig. 5.2) and together they position, steady and brace the shoulder laterally, to allow the arm to clear the trunk.

The inferior junction of the medial and lateral borders of the scapula forms the *inferior angle*, which lies over the seventh rib and is crossed by latissimus dorsi.

The *lateral border* provides the origins of teres major below and teres minor above. The *medial border* is long, providing attachment for the levator scapulae and the rhomboid muscles; it joins the short superior border at the *superior angle*.

The suprascapular notch lies at the junction of the superior border with the coracoid process. This notch is converted by the superior transverse scapular ligament into a foramen for the passage of the suprascapular nerve. The suprascapular vessels pass above it.

The dorsal surface of the scapula is divided by the spine of the scapula into fossae above and below. The smaller upper *supraspinous fossa* gives origin to the supraspinatus muscle, and the lower, larger *infraspinous fossa* gives origin to infraspinatus. The two fossae communicate laterally at the spinoglenoid notch.

The costal surface shows a slight hollowing for the origin of subscapularis, and its medial border is roughened for the insertion of serratus anterior.

The lateral angle of the scapula is broadened to form the pear-shaped *glenoid fossa* (cavity) that articulates

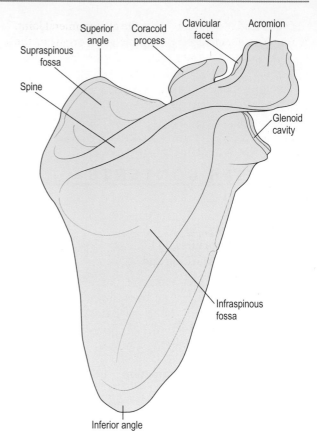

Fig. 5.1 Scapula—dorsal aspect. (From Gray's Anatomy) (Standring, 2015).

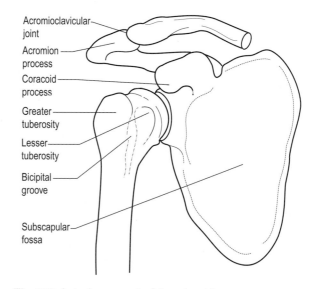

Fig. 5.2 Anterior aspect of the shoulder.

with the head of the humerus at the glenohumeral joint. A roughened *supraglenoid tubercle* gives origin to the long head of biceps, and a roughened *infraglenoid tubercle* gives origin to the long head of triceps.

The *spine of the scapula* is subcutaneous and, having arisen from the upper dorsal surface of the scapula, it widens laterally, projecting forwards to form the distinctive *acromion process*. When the acromion is viewed laterally it may be observed to be flat, slightly curved or to have an anterior hook-like process.

The lower border of the crest of the spine of the scapula is continuous with the lateral border of the acromion and forms a useful palpable bony landmark, the *posterior angle of the acromion*. The anteromedial border of the acromion shows an oval facet for articulation with the clavicle at the acromioclavicular joint.

Just above the glenoid fossa, the prominent hook-like *coracoid process* springs up and forwards to lie below the outer clavicle. With the arm in the anatomical position, the coracoid points directly forwards to form a prominent palpable bony landmark.

The long *humerus* extends from the shoulder to the elbow. The upper part of the humerus expands to bear a head and the greater and lesser tuberosities. The *head of the humerus* is approximately hemispherical and provides an articulating surface that is much greater than its scapular counterpart, the glenoid fossa.

Surrounding the head of the humerus is a slight constriction that represents the *anatomical neck* and separates the head from the two tuberosities. The head of the humerus joins the shaft at the *surgical neck*, which is so called because it is the common site of fracture of the humerus.

The *greater tuberosity* is large and quadrilateral and is the most lateral palpable bony landmark at the shoulder. Projecting laterally under the acromion, it is covered by the deltoid muscle and is continuous with the shaft of the humerus below (Fig. 5.2).

Three articular facets *sit* on its superior and posterior surface for the attachment of supraspinatus, infraspinatus and teres minor. Supraspinatus inserts into the highest or superior facet, infraspinatus into the middle facet and teres minor into the lower or inferior facet.

The sharp medial edge of the greater tuberosity forms the lateral lip of the *bicipital groove (intertubercular sulcus)*, which receives the insertion of pectoralis major.

The *lesser tuberosity* is a bony projection that lies below and lateral to the coracoid process. It receives the insertion of subscapularis on its medial aspect, and its sharp lateral edge forms the medial lip of the bicipital groove that receives the insertion of teres major.

The *clavicle* is subcutaneous, running horizontally between the acromion process of the scapula and the manubrium sterni, with which it articulates. On its lateral aspect is a small oval facet that articulates with the acromion at the acromioclavicular joint.

Inferiorly and laterally is a rounded conoid tubercle from which a roughened trapezoid line runs forwards and laterally. Both give attachment to the separate parts of the coracoclavicular ligament, which fastens the clavicle firmly to the scapula via the coracoid process (see below).

The *sternum* is a flat bone lying in the midline of the anterior chest where it provides attachment for the rib cage and clavicles on either side. Divided into three parts – the manubrium, body and xiphoid process – the upper part, the manubrium, is concave on its superior aspect, producing a depression called the jugular notch. On either side of the notch is a large cartilage-lined fossa which articulates with the medial end of the clavicle on each side.

The *acromioclavicular joint* is a synovial plane joint with fibrocartilage covering its articular surfaces. A wedge-shaped fibrocartilaginous disc drops down from the superior aspect, producing a partial division of the joint.

The articular facet on the lateral aspect of the clavicle is directed inferolaterally, and the corresponding facet on the medial border of the acromion is directed superomedially, producing a tendency for the clavicle to override the acromion. The plane of the joint tends to be variable, but usually slants slightly obliquely, sloping medially from superior to inferior.

The acromioclavicular joint is surrounded by a fibrous capsule that is thickened superiorly and inferiorly by the parallel fibres of the capsular ligaments running between the two bones (Fig. 5.3). The stability of the joint is provided by the strong accessory coracoclavicular ligament.

The clavicle acts as a strut or brace and allows the scapula to rotate and glide forwards and backwards. The movements at the acromioclavicular joint are passive, in the same way as those of the sacroiliac joint, in that no muscles act directly to move the joint. The small amount of movement available makes it impossible to determine a capsular pattern, although as a synovial joint it can be affected by arthritis.

The *coracoclavicular ligament* is separate from the acromioclavicular joint, but in strongly binding

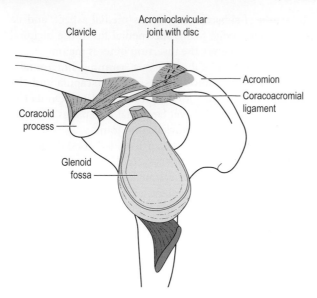

Fig. 5.3 Acromioclavicular joint, showing joint capsule, intra-articular disc and ligaments.

the scapula to the clavicle via the coracoid process, it provides a stabilising component to the joint. The ligament has two parts – the *trapezoid and conoid ligaments* – which are separate anatomically and functionally.

The more horizontal trapezoid ligament acts as a hinge for scapular motion, while the more vertical conoid ligament acts as a longitudinal axis for scapular rotation. Together, the ligaments prevent medial displacement of the acromion under the clavicle.

The *sternoclavicular joint* is a synovial joint between the medial end of the clavicle and a fossa on the superolateral aspect of the manubrium sterni. A fibrocartilaginous disc is positioned between the joint surfaces. It is an important joint as it is the point of attachment of the upper limb to the axial skeleton.

The clavicle transmits the weight of the upper limb to the axial skeleton via the coracoclavicular ligament and costoclavicular ligament, which attach the clavicle medially to the upper surface of the first rib and costal cartilage (Shah and Routal, 2015).

The *glenohumeral joint* is a synovial ball-and-socket joint between the head of the humerus and the glenoid fossa of the scapula, deepened by the fibrocartilaginous glenoid labrum (Fig. 5.4).

It is the most mobile joint in the body and forms the first link in a mechanical chain of levers that allows the arm to be positioned in space.

The two articular surfaces of the glenohumeral joint are incongruent, with the relatively large head of the humerus providing a surface area three to four times that of the glenoid fossa (Hulstyn and Fadale, 1995). This allows for the joint's immense range of movement but leads to its inherent instability. Movement at the spinal joints affects the range of movement available at the glenohumeral joint (Nordin and Frankel, 2020).

With little inherent bony stability available, stability is primarily dependent upon the static effects of the capsuloligamentous structures and the dynamic effects of the surrounding muscles. The muscle forces, mainly produced by the rotator cuff, stabilise the joint and produce a combination of shearing and compression forces, maintaining the humeral head in the glenoid fossa (Speer, 1995). There is also a negative pressure within the joint, leading to a suction effect that keeps the humeral head in place (Felstead and Ricketts, 2017).

The *glenohumeral joint capsule*, lined with synovium, is thin and spacious with a large volume, normally between 15 and 30 mL (Cailliet, 1991; Halder and An, 2000). It attaches to the edge of the glenoid fossa medially and surrounds the anatomical neck of the humerus laterally, except for its inferomedial part that descends to attach to the shaft of the humerus, approximately 1 cm below the articular margin.

The inferomedial portion of the capsule forms a loose axillary pouch, or fold, and consists of randomly organised collagen fibres (Hulstyn and Fadale, 1995). Although this arrangement facilitates movement, this part of the capsule is relatively weak, as it is not supported by muscles, and is often subject to strain.

The capsular fibres are mainly horizontal and are reinforced anteriorly by three capsular ligaments, the *superior, middle and inferior glenohumeral ligaments*, which are more clearly visible from inside the capsule (Fig. 5.5). The three bands together reinforce the anterior capsule (Standring, 2015).

The inferior glenohumeral ligament plays a major stabilising role in supporting the humeral head in a hammock or broad sling, particularly during abduction (Hulstyn and Fadale, 1995; Speer, 1995).

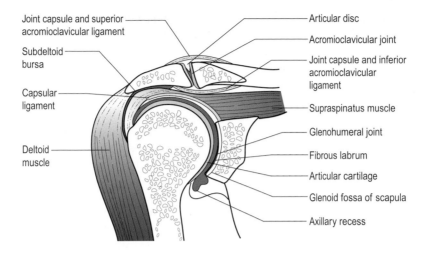

Joint capsule and superior acromioclavicular ligament

Subdeltoid bursa

Capsular ligament

Deltoid muscle

Articular disc

Acromioclavicular joint

Joint capsule and inferior acromioclavicular ligament

Supraspinatus muscle

Glenohumeral joint

Fibrous labrum

Articular cartilage

Glenoid fossa of scapula

Axillary recess

Fig. 5.4 Cross-section of glenohumeral joint showing internal structure.

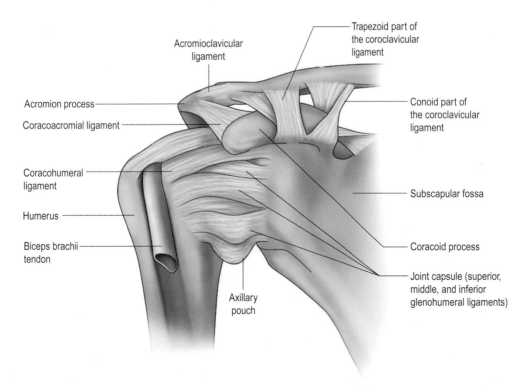

Acromioclavicular ligament

Trapezoid part of the coroclavicular ligament

Acromion process

Coracoacromial ligament

Conoid part of the coroclavicular ligament

Coracohumeral ligament

Humerus

Biceps brachii tendon

Subscapular fossa

Coracoid process

Joint capsule (superior, middle, and inferior glenohumeral ligaments)

Axillary pouch

Fig. 5.5 Anterior view of glenohumeral joint showing axillary pouch and capsular ligaments.

All three bands of the glenohumeral ligaments are taut in lateral rotation, and abduction stresses the middle and inferior bands. This may be significant in the development of the capsular pattern of the shoulder joint. The supraspinatus, infraspinatus, teres minor and subscapularis muscles (rotator cuff) also act as extensible ligaments to support the capsule, assisted by the long heads of triceps and biceps.

Much of the capsule is less than 1 mm thick, but it is thickened to between 1 and 2 mm near its humeral attachment where it receives the rotator cuff tendon fibres (Hulstyn and Fadale, 1995).

The *rotator interval* is a fibrous gap between the supraspinatus and subscapularis tendons and forms part of the rotator cuff. It is composed of fibres from supraspinatus and subscapularis together with the coracohumeral ligament, the superior glenohumeral ligament and parts of the capsule.

The key structure of the rotator interval is the *coracohumeral ligament*, which attaches between the dorsolateral aspect of the base of the coracoid and the greater, and to some extent, the lesser, tuberosities. It appears to be important for inferior stability of the glenohumeral joint and in limiting lateral rotation (Jost et al., 2000). It possibly contributes to the capsular pattern if the interval becomes reduced.

The *coracoacromial ligament* is an accessory ligament of the shoulder joint, forming an osseoligamentous arch over the superior aspect of the shoulder joint. It is triangular in shape and approximately 1 cm wide. Its apex attaches to the anterior aspect of the acromion and its base to the lateral aspect of the coracoid process.

The coracoacromial arch is separated from the underlying tendons by the subacromial bursa. The coracoacromial ligament is unusual in that it attaches to two parts of the same bone, probably functioning as a buffer. It provides stability for the head of the humerus against upwards displacement and protects it from direct vertical trauma (Petersilge et al., 1997).

Several bursae are associated with the shoulder joint (Fig. 5.6). An anterior *subscapular bursa* lies between the tendon of subscapularis and the anterior capsule, consistently communicating with the joint. A bursa, which occasionally communicates with the joint, may be present between the tendon of infraspinatus and the posterior capsule. Bursae may also be found on the superior aspect of the acromion, between the coracoid process and the capsule and associated with muscles and tendons crossing the joint.

Codman (1934) described the *subacromial bursa* as the largest and most complicated bursa at the shoulder

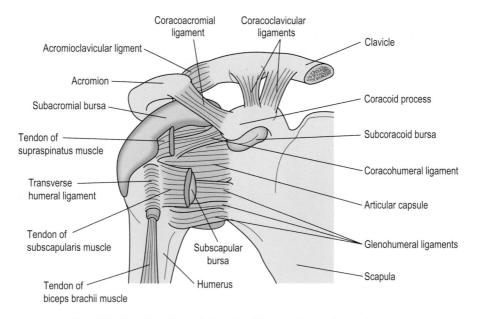

Fig. 5.6 Anterior view of the shoulder to show primary bursae.

(and in the body), forming a secondary scapulohumeral joint (Beals et al., 1998). It is independent of the shoulder joint and normally does not communicate with it. It therefore has a special role in the biomechanics of the shoulder joint and can be a cause of pain.

The subacromial bursa is a smooth synovial sac containing variable thin bands, or plicae, and is surrounded by fatty areolar tissue (Hulstyn and Fadale, 1995). Beals et al. (1998) identified by cadaver studies that only the anterior half of the under-surface of the acromion is contained within the subacromial bursal cavity. For injection access, a lateral approach is needed, to be able to reach and infiltrate the bursa.

The bursa's deep layer lies over the rotator cuff tendons and the head of the humerus (Cooper et al., 1993). Medially it extends under the acromion to the acromioclavicular joint line, and laterally it caps the greater tuberosity, separating it from the overlying deltoid muscle.

The *subacromial space* is approximately 7 to 14 mm deep (Frame, 1991) and is occupied by the subacromial bursa, the supraspinatus tendon, the superior part of the capsule of the shoulder joint and the tendon of the long head of biceps. The tightly packed structures move constantly in relation to one another and there is the potential for pathology and age-related changes.

The subacromial space can be considered to be a 'physiological' joint (Pratt, 1994; Kapandji, 2019). It is not a true articulation but is critical to shoulder movement. As supraspinatus pulls the greater tuberosity superiorly and medially, the walls of the subacromial bursa glide over one another, allowing the head of the humerus to slide (Netter, 1987).

Inflammation, the shape of the acromion or age-related changes of the acromioclavicular joint can all contribute to a reduction of the vertical proportions or stenosis of the subacromial space. A lesion in the space may produce a painful arc between 60 and 120 degrees of abduction.

The wide *range of movement* available at the glenohumeral joint consists of flexion, extension, abduction, adduction, medial and lateral rotation that all combine to provide circumduction. The range of elevation can be up to 180 degrees and may occur through flexion in the sagittal plane or abduction through the coronal plane.

The most functional movement is abduction in the plane of the scapula, known as *scaption*. This is not a fixed plane but occurs 30 to 40 degrees anteriorly to the coronal plane of the humerus (Frame, 1991). It places deltoid and supraspinatus in an optimal position to elevate the arm (Nordin and Frankel, 2020). Abduction is accompanied by lateral rotation in the coronal plane, which allows the greater tuberosity to clear the acromion; scaption does not involve this element of concomitant lateral rotation (Frame, 1991).

Active elevation (through abduction) consists of abduction from 0 to 60 occurring at the glenohumeral joint, 60 to 120 degrees occurring at the scapulothoracic joint and 120 to 180 degrees occurring at the glenohumeral and scapulothoracic joints, together with side flexion of the trunk to the opposite side (Kapandji, 2019).

With the inferior angle of the scapula fixed, approximately 90 degrees of passive glenohumeral abduction can be achieved. The normal range of passive lateral rotation is 80 to 90 degrees and medial rotation 100 to 110 degrees, with full range of medial rotation achieved by taking the arm behind the back.

Rolling and translational (gliding) movements also occur, and the glenohumeral joint surfaces can be separated by distraction.

Cameron (1995) looked at the shoulder as a weight-bearing joint. Although this joint is traditionally considered to be non-weight-bearing, he applied simple physical principles showing this not to be the case. With the weight of the adult arm estimated to be approximately 5 kg, forces equivalent to three times body weight are transmitted through the shoulder during simple daily activities.

The nerve supply to the glenohumeral joint is mainly from the C5 segment.

Contractile Structures

Four short muscles (supraspinatus, infraspinatus, teres minor and subscapularis) pass from the scapula to the head of the humerus. These tendons are not separate and interdigitate at their insertions to form a fibrous thickening of the capsule, known as the *rotator cuff*.

Supraspinatus (suprascapular nerve C4–C6) takes origin from the medial two-thirds of the supraspinous fossa. The bipennate fibres converge to pass under the acromion, blending with the capsule of the shoulder joint and adjacent tendon fibres of subscapularis and infraspinatus, and inserting into the upper of the three facets on the greater tuberosity (Fig. 5.7).

As the tendon passes to its insertion, it appears to be reinforced by the coracohumeral ligament that

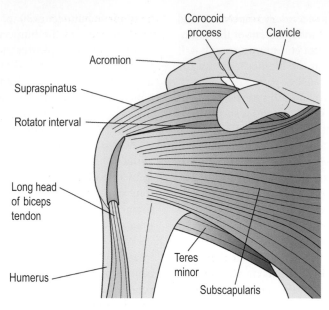

Fig. 5.7 Anterior aspect of the shoulder to show tendons and anterior interval.

runs parallel and is firmly adherent to it (Clark and Harryman, 1992). Supraspinatus compresses, abducts and provides a small amount of external rotation to the glenohumeral joint (Escamilla et al., 2009).

Together with the other rotator cuff muscles, supraspinatus stabilises the glenohumeral joint, providing horizontal compression and reducing vertical displacement. At lower scaption angles, activity in supraspinatus increases to provide additional compression of the humeral head to counter the superior translatory movements produced by deltoid activity (Escamilla et al., 2009).

Supraspinatus is considered to be responsible for initiating abduction before deltoid takes over at approximately 20 degrees (Pratt, 1994; Soames and Palastanga, 2018). However, both supraspinatus and deltoid have been shown to be active throughout the range of abduction, with an early rise in tension in supraspinatus fixing the humeral head and enabling deltoid to work at a better mechanical advantage (Cailliet, 1991; Frame, 1991).

Infraspinatus (suprascapular nerve C4–C6) is a thick triangular muscle that takes origin from the medial two-thirds of the infraspinous fossa. Its fibres converge to form a broad, thick tendon, passing over the posterior joint capsule, with which it blends, and inserting into

the middle of the three facets on the greater tuberosity of the humerus. Some of its fibres interdigitate with the adjacent supraspinatus.

Together with teres minor, with which it is sometimes fused, infraspinatus produces lateral rotation of the glenohumeral joint and is more effective in the lower range of abduction than at higher angles of elevation (Escamilla et al., 2009).

Teres minor (axillary nerve C5–C6) takes origin from the upper two-thirds of the lateral border of the scapula, above the origin of teres major. It inserts into the lowest of the three facets on the posterior aspect of the greater tuberosity, blending with the posterior capsule as it passes over it. It acts with infraspinatus to produce lateral rotation of the glenohumeral joint.

Subscapularis (upper and lower subscapular nerve C5–C6) takes origin from the medial two-thirds of the subscapular fossa on the costal surface of the scapula and inserts by a broad, thin, membranous tendon into the lesser tuberosity of the humerus (Fig. 5.7). It reinforces the anterior capsule from which it is partially separated by a bursa that communicates with the joint.

Subscapularis produces medial rotation of the glenohumeral joint, and both the upper and lower fibres are more effective in the lower range of abduction than at higher angles (Escamilla et al., 2009). Fibres from subscapularis and supraspinatus blend together to contribute to the rotator interval (Fig. 5.7).

As described above, the rotator cuff muscles are particularly important to the function of the shoulder, working together as extensible ligaments to provide dynamic stability, maintaining and centralising the head of the humerus in the glenoid fossa.

Shoulder movement, particularly elevation, is governed by force couples that involve the interaction of deltoid and the rotator cuff muscles (Nordin and Frankel, 2020). The rotator cuff muscles stabilise the glenohumeral joint in multiple shoulder positions. They help to elevate the arm and compress and centre the humeral head within the glenoid fossa during movement.

In early humeral elevation, the rotator cuff muscles are particularly important in resisting superior translatory movement due to deltoid activity (Escamilla et al., 2009), which would lead to functional instability.

As the rotator cuff tendons insert into the head of the humerus, they blend with the capsule of the joint forming a thickened common tendinous cuff. Fibres from subscapularis and infraspinatus interdigitate with those of supraspinatus in their deep layer, facilitating the distribution of forces directly or indirectly over a wider area (Clark and Harryman, 1992).

The tendon of the long head of biceps exits the capsule through a reinforced foramen at the junction of the insertions of supraspinatus and subscapularis onto the humerus (Hulstyn and Fadale, 1995). These tendons are frequently a source of pain through age-related changes or change in use.

Trapezius (spinal accessory nerve XI and ventral rami of C3–C4) is a large, flat triangular muscle forming a trapezium with its opposite number. It has a long line of attachment from the superior nuchal line, external occipital protuberance, ligamentum nuchae, the spinous processes and intervening supraspinous ligament from C7 to T12. The upper fibres descend to the posterior border of the lateral third of the clavicle, the middle fibres pass horizontally to the medial border of the acromion and the lower fibres pass upwards to the crest of the spine of the scapula.

In conjunction with other muscles, trapezius stabilises the scapula to allow functional movement of the arm, and the individual portions of the muscle help other muscles to produce primary movement. The upper fibres of trapezius and levator scapulae suspend the scapula against the thoracic cage and are constantly active during ambulation (Paine and Voight, 1993). Trapezius, together with serratus anterior, forms a force couple to rotate the scapula on the thoracic wall (Frame, 1991).

Rhomboids, major and minor (rhomboid branch of the dorsal scapular nerve C4–C5), form a line of attachment from the lower ligamentum nuchae and the spines of C7–T5 and pass to the medial border of the scapula to assist in its stabilisation against the thoracic cage. The rhomboids are active in scapular retraction, which is essential for overhead throwing movements and swimming strokes (for example, front crawl) (Paine and Voight, 1993).

Levator scapulae (C3–C5) descends from the transverse processes of the atlas and axis to the medial upper scapular border. Together with the rhomboids it controls and positions the scapula.

Latissimus dorsi (thoracodorsal nerve C6–C8) has an extensive origin from the lumbar spine, thoracolumbar fascia and thorax. The fibres converge towards the humerus, attaching to the inferior angle of the scapula as they pass by. The tendinous fibres twist through an angle of 180 degrees before inserting into the floor of the bicipital groove. At the shoulder, latissimus dorsi extends, adducts and medially rotates the humerus.

Teres major (lower subscapular nerve C6–C7) passes from the lower dorsal aspect of the scapula near the inferior angle to insert into the medial lip of the bicipital groove. It acts together with latissimus dorsi to adduct and medially rotate the humerus and together they form the posterior fold of the axilla. In conjunction with pectoralis major, teres major stabilises the shoulder joint.

Deltoid (axillary nerve C5–C6) is a large multipennate muscle that gives the shoulder its rounded contour. The muscle has three sets of fibres that all converge to insert into the deltoid tubercle in the middle of the lateral aspect of the shaft of the upper humerus.

Deltoid is the main abductor of the glenohumeral joint but it also assists other actions at the shoulder. The anterior fibres attach to the anterior border of the lateral third of the clavicle and work with pectoralis major to produce flexion and medial rotation. The middle fibres attach to the acromion and are strong abductors, helped by supraspinatus. The posterior fibres attach to the lower lip of the crest of the spine of the scapula and act with latissimus dorsi and teres major to produce extension and lateral rotation.

Pectoralis major (lateral and medial pectoral nerves, clavicular part C5–C6, sternocostal part C7–C8, T1) is a thick triangular muscle, originating as two separate clavicular and sternocostal parts from the anterior chest wall, to insert into the lateral lip of the bicipital groove. As the fibres cross to the arm, they twist to form the anterior axillary fold.

The two parts of the muscle are both powerful adductors and medial rotators of the humerus and the clavicular part also produces flexion. Together with latissimus dorsi, pectoralis major acts in climbing activities and is involved in pushing and throwing.

Pectoralis minor (both pectoral nerves C6–C8) passes from the upper ribs to the coracoid process. In conjunction with other muscles that anchor the scapula, pectoralis minor protracts, depresses, rotates and tilts the scapula.

Serratus anterior (long thoracic nerve C5–C7, descending on its external surface) has an extensive origin from the side of the thorax, passing around the thoracic cage to insert into the medial border of the costal surface of the scapula. It is responsible for stabilising the scapula during elevation and protraction of the scapula, in the functional activities of reaching and pushing. Loss of its nerve supply leads to winging of the scapula.

Movement of the scapula on the thoracic cage occurs at the scapulothoracic joint between two fascial planes, the most superficial of which lies between subscapularis and serratus anterior (Pratt, 1994; Kapandji, 2019). The surrounding muscles stabilise this joint and dynamically position the glenoid fossa to facilitate efficient glenohumeral movement (Paine and Voight, 1993).

Coracobrachialis (musculocutaneous nerve C5–C7) originates from the tip of the coracoid process where it forms a conjoint tendon with the short head of the biceps and inserts into the medial aspect of the middle of the shaft of the humerus. It adducts the humerus, and its position is analogous to the adductor group of muscles at the hip.

Biceps brachii (musculocutaneous nerve C5–C6) has a short head arising from the tip of the coracoid process and a long head originating from the supraglenoid tubercle and adjacent glenoid labrum, within the capsule of the glenohumeral joint. The intracapsular part of the tendon is surrounded by a double sheath, an extension of the synovial lining of the glenohumeral joint (Standring, 2015).

The long head passes through the subacromial space and exits the joint behind the transverse humeral ligament, emerging between the insertions of supraspinatus and subscapularis. It passes laterally with its synovial sheath, then turns a 90-degree angle into the bicipital groove. The two muscle bellies fuse to insert into the tuberosity of the radius via the biceps tendon.

Biceps has its main effect at the elbow where it is a powerful supinator and elbow flexor. The long head also assists forward flexion of the shoulder and exerts a stabilising effect on the superior aspect of the shoulder joint, which may be important for rehabilitation if the shoulder becomes less stable (Itoi et al., 1994).

Triceps (radial nerve C6–C8) originates by three heads. The long head arises from the infraglenoid tubercle of the scapula and the glenoid labrum, where it exerts a stabilising effect on the shoulder joint. It also assists adduction and extension movements of the humerus from the flexed position. The lateral head originates from the humerus above and lateral to the spiral groove and the medial head from the posterior humerus below the spiral groove. The three heads come together to insert into the olecranon process. The main action of the triceps is to extend the elbow.

GUIDE TO SURFACE MARKING AND PALPATION

Posterior Aspect

Palpate the *inferior angle of the scapula*, which, in most people, can be grasped between the index finger and thumb (Fig. 5.8). Abducting the arm may make the inferior angle easier to locate as it advances around the chest wall.

Palpate along the medial and lateral borders of the scapula. The lower medial border is subcutaneous and more readily palpable, lying parallel to, and approximately three fingers' width, from the spinous processes.

Visualise the position of *latissimus dorsi*, as it crosses the inferior angle, and track the *teres major* and *minor*

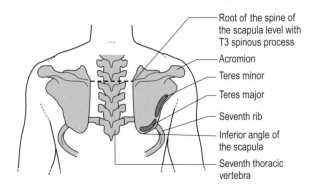

Fig. 5.8 Posterior aspect of the shoulder.

Root of the spine of the scapula level with T3 spinous process
Acromion
Teres minor
Teres major
Seventh rib
Inferior angle of the scapula
Seventh thoracic vertebra

muscles that take origin from the lateral border of the scapula. Teres major originates below teres minor.

The *crest of the spine of the scapula* may be visible and readily palpable. Feel it sloping down medially to meet the medial border of the scapula at the level of the spinous process of T3.

Palpate the lateral end of the spine of the scapula and follow the lower border around until it joins the lateral border of the acromion. A sharp 90-degree angle is formed here – the *posterior angle of the acromion* – which is a useful bony landmark.

Palpate the flat upper surface of the *acromion*, which is subcutaneous and forms the summit of the shoulder, lying just lateral to the acromioclavicular joint. Palpate the anterior edge of the acromion with an index finger and the posterior angle with a thumb, to appreciate its width.

Lateral Aspect

Palpate the lateral edge of the acromion. Note its depth and visualise the position of the subacromial bursa beneath it. Follow the anterior and posterior portions of the *deltoid muscle* down onto its insertion into the deltoid tubercle.

Anterior Aspect

Palpate the *clavicle*, which is usually visible and palpable throughout its length in most people (Fig. 5.2). Start at the medial end and follow the anterior curve as it lies over the first rib, then the reverse curve that produces a hollow at the lateral end of the clavicle. Below this hollow, between deltoid and pectoralis major, lies the infraclavicular fossa.

Palpate the *acromioclavicular joint* line that lies approximately a finger's width medial to the lateral border of the acromion. The clavicular end of the joint may project a little higher than the acromion since it overrides it slightly, and this may produce a slight step down between the clavicle and acromion.

If this is not obvious, palpate laterally along the anterior surface of the clavicle until a small, V-shaped depression is found that indicates the anterior joint line. It may also be found by palpating approximately one finger's width medially from the lateral border of the acromion.

Once identified, the joint line should be palpable from above. Apply a downwards pressure on the lateral end of the clavicle and ask the model to flex and extend the shoulder to feel movement at the joint. Palpate the anterior edge of the acromion.

Below the junction of the lateral third and the medial two-thirds of the clavicle, in the lateral infraclavicular fossa, feel the prominent *coracoid process* that forms an anterior projection when the arm is resting at the side. This is covered by the anterior deltoid and deep palpation, which may be uncomfortable, is necessary. With a finger on the coracoid process, abduct the arm. The coracoid should move out from under your palpating finger.

Moving slightly downwards and laterally from the coracoid process, palpate the *lesser tuberosity* of the humerus. Immediately lateral to it is the *bicipital groove* and further laterally still the *greater tuberosity*.

The *greater tuberosity* can be located easily as it lies in line with, and above, the lateral epicondyle of the humerus. It can be grasped with the thumb, index and middle fingers placed on its anterior, superior and posterior surfaces. Note its width. The greater tuberosity is slightly wider from anterior to posterior than the acromion process. Try to visualise its three facets for the insertions of supraspinatus, infraspinatus and teres minor.

Place the arm in the anatomical position and feel the greater tuberosity lying laterally and the lesser tuberosity lying anteriorly on either side of the bicipital groove. Relax the arm, allowing it to fall into the more functional position with some medial rotation, and feel the greater tuberosity lying more anteriorly and the lesser tuberosity medially.

Insertions of the Rotator Cuff Tendons

To palpate *supraspinatus*, the greater tuberosity must be brought forwards from under the acromion to expose its superior facet. Position the patient sitting at an angle of about 45 degrees against the couch. Medially rotate and extend the arm to position it behind the back.

Palpate for the anterior edge of the acromion and drop downwards onto the greater tuberosity. The tendon of supraspinatus is running directly forwards between the two bony points (remember that you have turned the greater tuberosity to lie more anteriorly). The tendon of insertion is approximately one finger's width and is easier to locate if you turn your finger to palpate across the tendon, with the side of your finger still in contact with the anterior edge of the acromion (Fig. 5.9).

To palpate *infraspinatus*, the greater tuberosity must be brought backwards from under the acromion to expose its middle facet. Position the patient in side-lying with the head raised on two pillows (or one folded). Rest the patient's hand on the cheek, or on the pillow alongside the face. The forearm should be free to allow the elbow to drop, to produce adduction and lateral rotation at the shoulder (Fig. 5.10).

Palpate for the posterior angle of the acromion and locate the greater tuberosity. The tendon of infraspinatus runs parallel to the spine of the scapula to insert into the greater tuberosity, immediately below the posterior angle of the acromion. The tendon of insertion is approximately two fingers wide. Together with the insertion of *teres minor* the tendon is three fingers wide.

To locate *subscapularis*, position the arm with the humerus in the anatomical position. Either palpate the coracoid process and move laterally and slightly downwards or identify the bicipital groove and move directly medially to find the sharp lateral lip of the lesser tuberosity (Fig. 5.11).

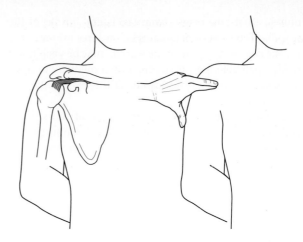

Fig. 5.9 Position of the arm for palpation of the supraspinatus tendon.

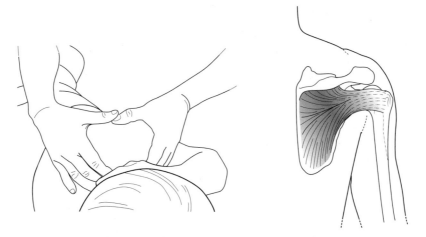

Fig. 5.10 Position of the arm for palpation of the infraspinatus tendon.

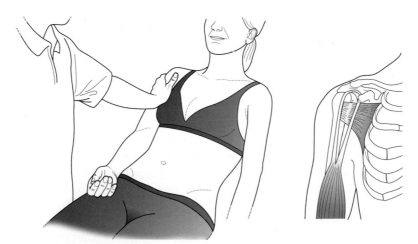

Fig. 5.11 Position of the arm for palpation of the subscapularis tendon.

Follow around onto the medial aspect of the lesser tuberosity to locate the insertion of subscapularis. The tendon itself cannot be felt and the underlying bone is tender to palpation. The tendon is approximately three fingers wide.

COMMENTARY ON THE EXAMINATION

The history at the shoulder is important, although it probably will not reveal a conclusive diagnosis. Cyriax (1982) considered the shoulder to be an 'honest' joint, but most clues are revealed in the examination rather than in the history.

Lesions may be complicated due to the many structures and wide range of movement at the shoulder. Pain can be associated with lesions inside or outside the shoulder joint, and it has a high prevalence with comorbidities (Kane et al., 2010; Wright et al., 2015). For instance, pain may be referred from cervical spine, secondary capsulitis can accompany bursitis or tendinopathy, and diabetic patients are five times more likely to develop frozen shoulder compared to non-diabetic patients (Zreik et al., 2016).

Observation

A general observation of the patient's *face, posture and gait* will alert the practitioner to abnormalities and serious illness. Acute subacromial bursitis, or resolving acute calcific tendinopathy, produce a constant severe pain that disturbs sleep and the patient can look tired. The acute shoulder is usually held in a position of comfort, which is normally in medial rotation with the elbow flexed and supported. An alteration in the rhythmical arm swing may be obvious.

Due to the many anatomical components that make up the shoulder region and the interrelationship between the function of each group, lesions can be subtle and complicated. Multiple lesions can exist and functional instability can produce secondary problems at the shoulder.

This text focuses on the differential diagnosis of specific lesions encountered in musculoskeletal medicine. For more detailed coverage of shoulder instability and its relationship to shoulder lesions the practitioner is referred to other texts that cover this subject.

History

The patient's *age, occupation, sports, hobbies and activities* may give clues to diagnosis. Functional instability is the main cause of shoulder symptoms in the younger patient. The younger patient engaged in physical work or active in sport may have a minor instability problem or a labral tear related to overload or injury, producing rotator cuff-related pain.

The working-aged patient may present with rotator cuff-related pain, chronic bursitis or capsulitis. In the older age group, degenerative rotator cuff lesions or tears with secondary capsulitis may occur (Table 5.1).

Overuse, unaccustomed use or underuse can be a common cause of pain felt at the shoulder, and the level of the patient's activity can be directly responsible for the condition. Knowledge of the patient's activity lifestyle is useful to be able to advise the patient on preventing recurrence.

Shoulder injuries are common in throwing sports, swimming and all overhead activities. Tennis strokes involve rotation, abduction and elevation, leading to repetitive loading of the tendons in the overhead position, possibly causing instability and pain that may be associated with a labral lesion (McCann and Bigliani, 1994).

It is relevant to know which arm is the patient's dominant arm. With the increasing use of imaging, diagnosis

TABLE 5.1 Lesions Suspected at Different Ages			
Lesion	Young	Middle	Old
Capsulitis	‡	***	*
Degeneration of glenohumeral joint	‡	*	**
Glenohumeral instability	***	*	‡
Trauma to acromioclavicular joint	***	**	*
Degeneration of acromioclavicular joint	‡	*	**
Bursitis	*	***	‡
Tendinopathy	‡	***	*
Calcific tendonitis	*	**	*
Tendon tears	‡	*	***
Fracture	**	*	***
Malignancy	*	*	*

Key: ***common; **less common; *rare; ‡highly unlikely.

of glenoid labral tears has become more common: notably, types of SLAP (superior labrum from anterior to posterior) lesion that occur more in the sporting population. The patient complains of a dull throbbing ache in the joint that can cause difficulty in sleeping. There is usually pain and a catching feeling as the arm is placed into the overhead position and compression of the joint may also produce pain, as in lying on the affected side.

The *site* of the pain does not reliably indicate the site of the lesion. The shoulder joint and its surrounding capsule, ligaments and muscles are mainly derived from the C5 segment. Lesions of any of these structures will cause the pain to be referred into the C5 dermatome that extends into the anterolateral aspect of the arm and forearm as far as the base of the thumb.

The most common point of referral for these structures is the area over the insertion of deltoid, sometimes referred to as the 'badge area' of the arm. The 'grasping sign', where the patient puts the whole hand over the deltoid area, to describe the area of pain, suggests a subacromial lesion.

The more irritable the lesion, the further the referral of pain into the C5 dermatome, such that the *spread* of pain will give an indication of the severity of the lesion. As a deep joint lying proximally in its dermatome, the glenohumeral joint has the potential to refer pain over a considerable distance into the upper limb.

The cervical spine can refer pain into the shoulder area, and further into the C5 dermatome, and will need to be excluded as a source of symptoms.

Other deeper structures, including visceral problems, can refer pain to the shoulder and the nature of the symptoms and other features will need to be considered as part of clinical reasoning.

The acromioclavicular joint and surrounding ligaments produce an accurate localisation of pain over the joint. This is because the acromioclavicular joint is a superficial joint giving little reference, in contrast to the glenohumeral joint. The patient might indicate this with the 'pointing sign', pointing with one finger to the acromioclavicular joint line.

The *onset* of the pain may be sudden or gradual. If the onset was sudden, it is important to know if there was any related trauma, with the possibility of fracture. A fall on the outstretched hand may initiate a traumatic shoulder joint capsulitis or, less commonly, chronic subacromial bursitis, tendon injury or acromioclavicular joint sprain.

Acromioclavicular lesions are usually associated with a traumatic onset. Degeneration of the joint in the working-aged to elderly may result from repeated trauma and provide an alternative cause of pain.

An acute subacromial bursitis or reabsorbing acute calcific tendinitis has a characteristic sudden onset with no apparent cause.

The common shoulder lesions of tendinopathy, bursitis or capsulitis present most typically with a gradual onset of pain due to change in use or unaccustomed use. A capsulitis may be precipitated by trauma, but this is often minor and the patient may not recall the incident. Stiffness and loss of functional movement are usually indicative of capsulitis. Tendinopathy may be provoked by change in use.

The *duration* of the symptoms gives an indication of the stage the lesion has reached in the inflammatory cycle.

The *symptoms and behaviour* need to be considered. The cervical spine can refer pain to the shoulder, the patient may complain of neck pain and there may be associated trigger points over the posterior aspect of the shoulder (Grubbs, 1993).

Visceral problems may mimic musculoskeletal lesions. Shoulder pain can be a manifestation of gastrointestinal, neurological, cardiological or rheumatological diseases (Lollino et al., 2012). Be prepared to explore the description of symptoms and to look for associated features such as nausea, cough and pain on breathing. General clinical deterioration such as unexplained weight loss and fever should be considered. The diaphragm is a C4 structure that will produce pain felt at the point of the shoulder if affected by adjacent conditions, such as pleurisy.

Non-specific shoulder pain may be associated with nerve entrapment or neuritis, which would be confirmed by signs of objective weakness but with no pain on shoulder movements (Biundo and Harris, 1993; Schulte and Warner, 1995).

The *behaviour* of the pain is relevant to diagnosis with the common lesions generally producing typical musculoskeletal pain on movement that is eased by rest. The patient should be asked if the pain is constant or only aggravated by movement, giving an indication of the irritability of the lesion.

Chronic tendinopathy or bursitis often produces a dull ache, although twinges of pain may be experienced during movement. An acute subacromial bursitis or reabsorbing acute calcific tendinitis produces severe pain that is constant and often unrelenting, preventing sleep.

A capsulitis shows increasing, worsening pain, referring further and further into the C5 dermatome. The inflammatory nature of the pain may be obvious with a description of pain and stiffness on waking. 'Catching' pain may be described on activities such as reaching for a seat belt or into the back of the car, or placing an arm in a coat sleeve, and can indicate a lesion within the subacromial space.

The behaviour can also help to assess the irritability of the lesion as well as distinguish it from a lesion that is referring pain into the shoulder area. If the patient is unable to lie on that side because the increase in pain disturbs sleep, the lesion is irritable. It may indicate a chronic subacromial bursitis, rotator cuff lesion or an irritable capsulitis.

> **THREE KEY QUESTIONS TO ASSESS IRRITABILTY OF SHOULDER LESIONS**
> - Does the pain spread below the elbow? (site and spread)
> - Can you lie on that side at night? (symptoms)
> - Is the pain constant? (behaviour)

A loss of functional activity, such as being unable to fasten a bra or reach into the back pocket, will indicate limitation of movement. There may be evidence of shoulder functional instability or labral tears in young, sporty patients complaining of 'clicking', 'snapping' or feeling as if the shoulder is 'coming out'.

To distinguish the lesion from one of cervical or thoracic origin, the patient should be questioned about the presence of paraesthesia and whether pain is increased on a cough, sneeze or deep breath. Heaviness, tiredness, puffiness, sweating or altered temperature may indicate associated or referred autonomic symptoms.

Assessment of *other joint involvement* could indicate generalised arthropathy, possibly degenerative or inflammatory. It is also interesting to note whether the patient has had previous shoulder problems since both 'frozen shoulder' (capsulitis) and acute subacromial bursitis often affect the other shoulder some years after the first occurrence.

The *medical history* will alert the practitioner to serious illness and operations experienced by the patient. The patient should be asked specifically about a history of thyroid problems, diabetes and cardiac conditions.

Hypothyroidism can lead to aching, tenderness and stiffness, especially in the shoulders and hips. There is a strong association between diabetes mellitus and the development of a frozen shoulder or tendinopathy (Owens-Burkhart, 1991; Clarnette and Miniaci, 1998; Zreik et al., 2016). Cardiac conditions can refer pain to the arm and shoulder (Arendt-Nielsen and Svensson, 2001).

The practitioner should listen for possible contraindications to treatment. An indication of the patient's current state of health is necessary, and the patient should be asked about recent unexplained weight loss. Tumours involving the shoulder area are rare but a history of primary tumour should raise the suspicion of metastatic disease as a possible diagnosis (Clarnette and Miniaci, 1998).

As well as past medical history, establish any ongoing conditions and treatment. Explore other previous or current musculoskeletal problems with previous episodes of the current complaint, any treatment given and the outcome of treatment.

Practitioners should *screen* routinely for psychosocial factors and consider relevant health comorbidities and lifestyle factors (see Chapter 1). These factors may contribute to the patient's presenting condition, or form a barrier to recovery and normal function, and should be addressed as an integral part of patient management.

Medications currently being taken by the patient should be determined to eliminate possible contraindications to treatment. The amount of analgesia and/or non-steroidal anti-inflammatory drug (NSAID) medication required by the patient gives an indication of the severity of the lesion.

From the history, the possible diagnoses are noted. If the eventual diagnosis is one of capsulitis, three key questions relating to the spread of pain and provocation factors asked during the history will give an indication of the severity of the lesion and act as a guide to treatment.

Inspection

The patient should undress sufficiently to allow the area to be inspected in a good light.

A general inspection will determine any *bony deformity*. Look at the position of the cervical spine and take an overall view of the spinal curvatures in general.

The general posture of the patient can be important, and any observations of asymmetry are recorded if they are relevant to the presenting condition. It has been suggested that abnormal cervical and thoracic posture, particularly an increased thoracic kyphosis, alters the resting position of the scapula and may be related to shoulder pain.

The position of the shoulders should be noted. Is one higher than the other or is the head of the humerus sitting more anteriorly? In a frozen shoulder, one shoulder may be held higher than the other due to pain, with the scapula elevated and retracted. There may be evidence of winging of the scapula and this is usually more obvious on movement.

Lumps, scars, bony prominences and bruising should be observed. A prominent bump at the end of the clavicle may signify an old fracture or dislocation of the acromioclavicular joint.

Colour changes and swelling are unusual findings at the shoulder unless associated with direct trauma.

Muscle wasting is suspected if the spine of the scapula is prominent, due to neuritis or rotator cuff injury/pathology. In chronic rotator cuff tendinopathy and/or degenerative tears, wasting of supraspinatus and infraspinatus may be obvious.

The 'popeye' deformity of a rupture of the long head of the biceps is usually obvious, but the patient does not particularly complain of pain. In deltoid atrophy, squaring of the shoulder occurs as deltoid is no longer rounded over the humeral head; this may be indicative of anterior dislocation (Clarnette and Miniaci, 1998).

State at Rest

Before any movements are performed, the state at rest is established to provide a baseline for subsequent comparison.

Examination by Selective Tension

The suggested sequence for examination of the shoulder will now be given, followed by a commentary including the reasoning in performing the movements and the significance of the possible findings. Comparison should always be made with the other side.

Examination of the shoulder should first exclude possible cervical lesions; therefore, six active cervical movements are performed, and if a pattern of signs emerges

implicating the cervical spine then a full assessment of this region should be conducted.

Three elevation tests are conducted for the glenohumeral joint. Active elevation indicates the patient's willingness to move the joint and provides an indication of pain, range and power. 'Willingness' can provide information on the level of pain but it can also be an indicator for 'yellow flags' (see Chapter 1). Cyriax described the shoulder as 'an emotional joint' and it is helpful to observe consistency in the range of movement and level of pain along with other findings as the examination proceeds.

Passive elevation is added to assess pain, range of movement and end-feel. The normal end-feel of passive

Eliminate the Cervical Spine
- Active cervical extension (Fig. 5.12a)
- Active right cervical rotation (Fig. 5.12b)
- Active left cervical rotation (Fig. 5.12c)
- Active right cervical side flexion (Fig. 5.12d)
- Active left cervical side flexion (Fig. 5.12e)
- Active cervical flexion (Fig. 5.12f)

Shoulder Elevation Tests
- Active elevation through flexion (Fig. 5.13)
- Passive elevation (Fig. 5.14)
- Active elevation through abduction for a painful arc (Figs 5.15 and 5.16a and b)

Passive Glenohumeral Movements
- Passive lateral rotation (Fig. 5.17)
- Passive abduction (Fig. 5.18)
- Passive medial rotation (Fig. 5.19)

Resisted Tests
- Resisted shoulder abduction (Fig. 5.20)
- Resisted shoulder adduction (Fig. 5.21)
- Resisted shoulder lateral rotation (Fig. 5.22)
- Resisted shoulder medial rotation (Fig. 5.23)
- Resisted elbow flexion (Fig. 5.24)
- Resisted elbow extension (Fig. 5.25)

Accessory Test for Acromioclavicular Joint or Lower Fibres of Subscapularis
- Passive shoulder flexion and adduction (scarf test) (Fig. 5.26)

Palpation
- Once a diagnosis has been made, the structure at fault is palpated for the exact site of the lesion

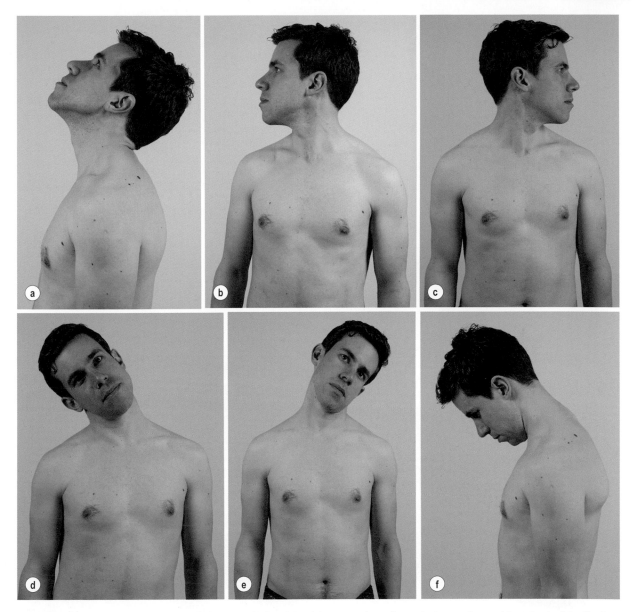

Fig. 5.12 Six active movements of the cervical spine: (a) extension; (b and c) rotations; (d and e) side flexions; (f) flexion.

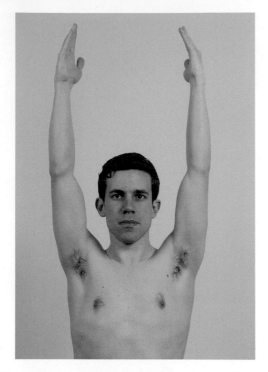

Fig. 5.13 Active shoulder elevation through flexion.

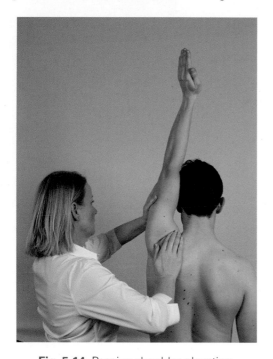

Fig. 5.14 Passive shoulder elevation.

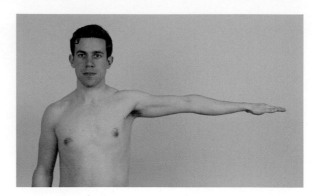

Fig. 5.15 Active elevation through abduction, looking for a painful arc.

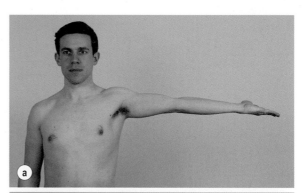

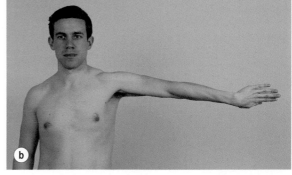

Fig. 5.16 Varying arm position to explore for a painful arc: (a) abduction with lateral rotation; (b) abduction with medial rotation.

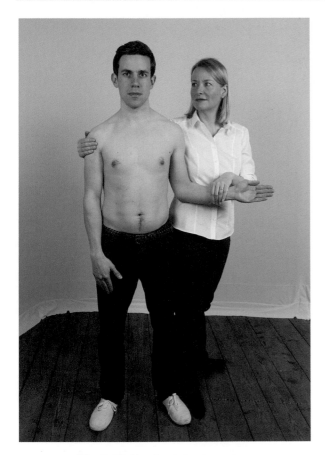

Fig. 5.17 Passive lateral rotation.

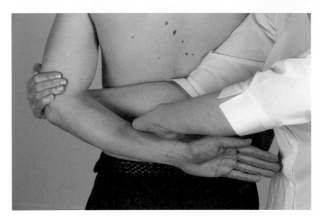

Fig. 5.19 Passive medial rotation.

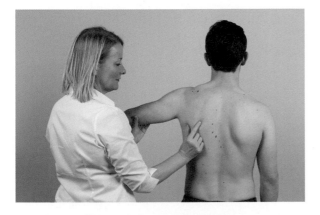

Fig. 5.18 Passive abduction.

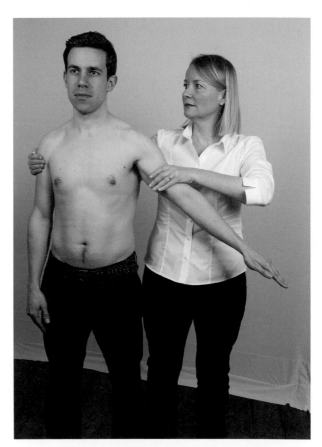

Fig. 5.20 Resisted abduction.

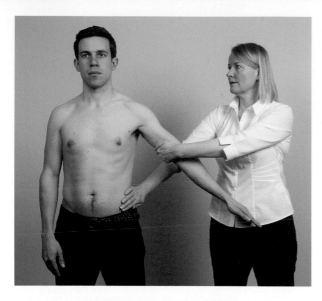

Fig. 5.21 Resisted adduction.

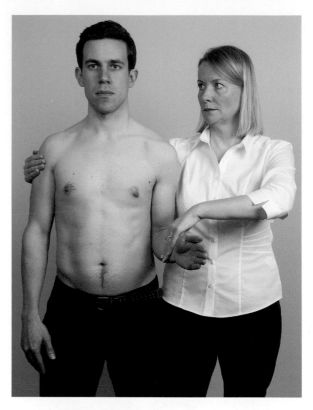

Fig. 5.23 Resisted medial rotation.

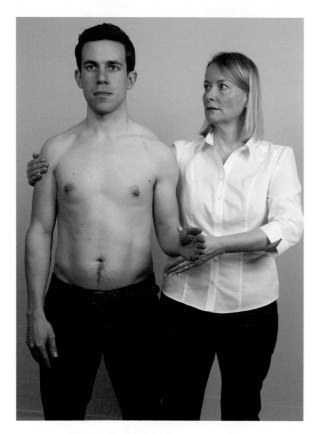

Fig. 5.22 Resisted lateral rotation.

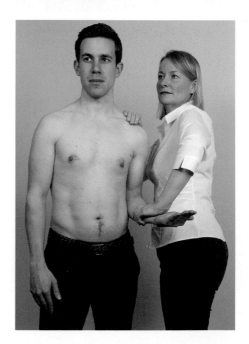

Fig. 5.24 Resisted elbow flexion.

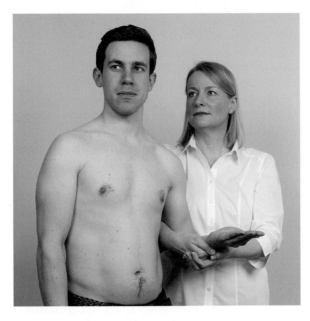

Fig. 5.25 Resisted elbow extension.

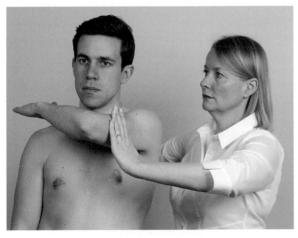

Fig. 5.26 The scarf test.

elevation is elastic. Any limitation of passive elevation suggests that the capsular pattern exists at the glenohumeral joint and this will be confirmed when the passive glenohumeral movements are assessed individually.

Active elevation through abduction is conducted in the coronal plane to assess for the presence of a painful arc. This involves abduction to 90 degrees followed by lateral rotation to enable the greater tuberosity to clear the coracoacromial arch. The test performed in this way is usually consistent with the patient's account of symptoms. However, functionally, the arm is more commonly lifted through scaption (see page 117).

A painful arc can indicate a lesion within the subacromial space. The specific structure will be revealed by completing the full examination procedure. An arc is more easily elicited on active movement as contraction of the muscle groups tends to raise the humeral head and reduce the space; it is generally found between 60 and 120 degrees of abduction.

Be prepared to explore for a painful arc, especially in light of findings later in the examination, remembering that a diagnosis is not made until the full examination has been completed. You may want to return to explore the painful arc later, and the position can be modified to place the rotator cuff tendons into a position where they are more vulnerable (see Figs 5.15 and 5.16a and b).

The passive glenohumeral movements are conducted looking for pain, range of movement and end-feel. Since variation in movement between individuals is probable, movements should always be compared with the other side. However, variation between sides may exist, for example, in tennis players or fast bowlers, who may have a greater range of one rotation at the expense of the other, on the dominant side.

Passive lateral and medial rotations have a normal elastic end-feel; passive abduction is assessed for range of movement only, by fixing the inferior angle of the scapula and assessing when it starts to move; it is not possible to appreciate the end-feel. Assessment of the passive glenohumeral movements may confirm the presence of the capsular pattern, indicating arthropathy.

As movements become limited in the capsular pattern they develop an abnormally 'hard' end-feel. The capsular pattern results in overall limitation of passive elevation. Limitation or pain at the end of range of lateral rotation only may be a sign of early capsulitis.

It may not be possible to fully assess the range of medial rotation in severe capsulitis since the accompanying limitation of abduction prevents the arm from being placed behind the patient's back. As a guide for subsequent comparison, measure the range of movement against certain landmarks that can be reached by the hand, such as the pocket, buttock, waist, inferior angle of scapula.

Subacromial bursitis provides a typical example of a non-capsular pattern of movement at the shoulder.

While the acromioclavicular joint does not demonstrate its own capsular pattern, it produces a non-capsular pattern of movement at the glenohumeral joint.

The resisted tests are conducted looking for pain and reduced power that will indicate a contractile lesion or possible neurological involvement.

Movement	Main muscles	'Assistors'
Flexion	Pectoralis major, anterior deltoid and coracobrachialis	Biceps brachii
Extension	Posterior deltoid, latissimus dorsi and teres major	
Abduction	Supraspinatus (0–15 degrees), middle fibres of deltoid (15–90 degrees), trapezius and serratus anterior (beyond 90 degrees)	
Adduction	Pectoralis major, latissimus dorsi and teres major	
Lateral Rotation	Infraspinatus	Teres minor
Medial Rotation	Subscapularis	Pectoralis major, latissimus dorsi, teres major, anterior deltoid

The resisted tests performed in the upright position apply a degree of upwards shear and compression to the glenohumeral joint in stabilising the head of the humerus. For this reason, the resisted tests may be accessory signs in subacromial bursitis or show involvement of the joint. To confirm diagnosis, the resisted tests may be repeated in lying, with some joint distraction, where the effect of compression and shear on the joint is reduced (Figs 5.27 and 5.28).

Resisted abduction tests mainly supraspinatus; resisted adduction tests latissimus dorsi and pectoralis major; resisted lateral rotation tests mainly infraspinatus and teres minor; resisted medial rotation tests mainly subscapularis; resisted elbow flexion tests biceps; and resisted elbow extension tests triceps.

The anatomical interdigitation of the tendinous insertions of the rotator cuff tendons means that the resisted tests described may not definitively incriminate one tendon; subsequent palpation of the structure implicated will help to identify the site of the lesion.

Painful weakness on resisted testing may indicate partial rupture, but it can be difficult to decide whether a test is producing real or apparent weakness since the patient is inhibited by pain from making a maximal effort (Pellecchia et al., 1996).

In athletes it may be difficult to produce positive findings, especially on resisted testing, as the symptoms may only be provoked during the athletic or sporting activity itself. It may be necessary for the patient to provoke the pain before the examination is carried out.

An accessory test, the 'scarf' test (as in putting a scarf over the opposite shoulder), may be performed to localise the lesion. This compresses the acromioclavicular joint or presses the lower fibres of the subscapularis tendon against the coracoid process. It may also be positive as part of the 'muddle' of signs of a chronic subacromial bursitis.

Palpation is conducted for the site of the lesion, but only along the structure determined to be at fault, since the shoulder is notorious for tender trigger points.

Based on the history and clinical examination, the practitioner should be able to establish the most likely diagnosis, using clinical reasoning and clinical judgement.

Additional special tests can be applied as necessary (see Hattam and Smeatham, 2020). For example, the musculoskeletal medicine approach does not investigate hypermobility at the shoulder with consequent instability, and the practitioner is recommended to employ provocative instability tests as appropriate.

Similarly, labral tears are difficult to diagnose clinically and to distinguish from other causes of pain. Several tests have been devised but none of them is highly sensitive or specific (Guanche and Jones, 2003; Dessaur and Magarey, 2008; Cook et al., 2012). However, there is a strong association between a labral tear and other shoulder symptoms such as impingement symptoms, recurrent anterior instability and functional instability, as in loading the arm in the elevated position and throwing (Liu et al., 1996; Hattam and Smeatham, 2020).

It tends to be a diagnosis by elimination but the 'gold standard' test for a labral tear is an MR arthrogram. Once diagnosed, onward referral for a surgical opinion is suggested in most cases.

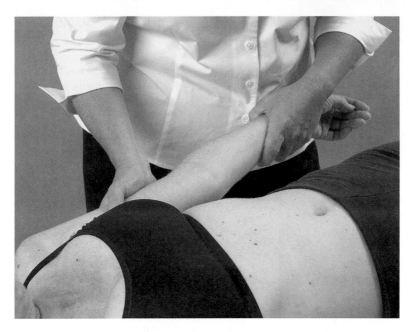

Fig. 5.27 Resisted shoulder abduction with distraction.

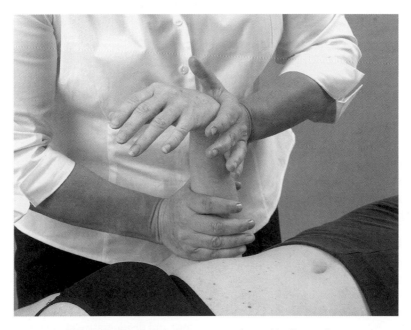

Fig. 5.28 Resisted elbow extension with distraction.

The examination of neural structures can also be incorporated into the procedure.

It is important to recognise potential serious pathology, such as infection, malignancy, fracture and inflammatory arthritis, and to make any appropriate onward referral in a timely manner. Should additional information be required to aid diagnosis or to add value to management, further investigations can be considered to inform decision making and planning.

If necessary, the practitioner may consider further investigations such as blood tests, radiological imaging and other diagnostic procedures (see Chapter 1). Investigations should be guided by suspected causes and differential diagnosis, as an extension to the clinical examination process. For example, X-ray can be considered if there is: a history of trauma, the patient is not improving with conservative treatment, symptoms have lasted for more than four weeks, movement is significantly restricted, severe pain, suspected significant arthritis or the presence of red flags (NICE, 2017). Ultrasound scanning can be considered with a suspected acute rotator cuff tear. Blood tests can be considered if malignancy, polymyalgia rheumatica, inflammatory arthritis or diabetes are suspected.

It is essential for practitioners to have a good level of understanding and interpretation of the results to be able to correlate clinical findings. It is also important to be familiar with local referral guidelines, referral pathways and the expertise of all members of the multidisciplinary team to optimise the integration of patient care.

CAPSULAR LESIONS

CAPSULAR PATTERN AT THE GLENOHUMERAL JOINT
- Most limitation of lateral rotation
- Less limitation of abduction
- Least limitation of medial rotation

Any restriction of the glenohumeral range of movement is demonstrated by an overall loss of shoulder elevation. The movements limited in the capsular pattern have a characteristic 'hard' end-feel, although this is less marked in the early stage.

Frozen Shoulder (Capsulitis)

The presence of the capsular pattern at the shoulder usually indicates 'frozen shoulder' or capsulitis, as discussed below. Less commonly, the shoulder can be affected by degenerative arthropathy, rheumatoid arthritis or any of the spondyloarthropathies.

The term 'frozen shoulder' is commonly used to describe any stiff or painful shoulder, but it is criticised for being an overused term, since it appears to avoid a more specific diagnosis. It is, however, an easy term to use and patients appear to understand it. It describes the functional restriction of both active and passive

movements in the capsular pattern, indicating involvement of the capsule of the shoulder joint, which is the key factor.

Frozen shoulder was described by Codman in 1934 and it is hard to better his original definition (Bunker, 2009). It provides an accurate picture of a condition that most musculoskeletal practitioners will recognise:

'This is a condition which comes on slowly with pain over the deltoid insertion, inability to sleep, painful incomplete elevation and external rotation, the restriction of movement being both active and passive, with normal radiograph, the pain being very trying and yet all patients are able to continue their daily habits and routines'.

Frozen shoulder is rare before the age of 40, with a peak incidence between 40 and 60. It is unusual in patients over 70 years (except secondary traumatic frozen shoulder) and in manual workers (Robinson et al., 2012).

The natural history of the condition is that it follows a pattern of increasing signs and symptoms (freezing), followed by a plateau stage (frozen) before a slow, spontaneous recovery of partial or complete function (thawing). Recovery tends to occur within 1 to 3 years (Wadsworth, 1986). A short painful period is associated with a short recovery period and a longer painful period with a longer period of recovery (Owens-Burkhart, 1991).

Abrassart et al. (2020) describe frozen shoulder as a 'disease' which often sees short-term improvement, but which bears a high chance of ongoing low-level restriction and pain'.

Robinson et al. (2012) support that observation, noting that up to 40% of patients may experience persistent symptoms with 50% of patients still having mild pain after seven years and 60% with persistent stiffness. It is estimated that 7% to 15% have some permanent loss of movement but there is usually little to no functional disability.

The cause of the condition is unknown. It is probably multifactorial, including a period of immobilisation due to pain, and may include local periarticular inflammatory and degenerative changes.

Some of the features are shared with other shoulder conditions but Bunker (2009) is clear that, provided the X-ray is normal, the one feature that distinguishes frozen shoulder from other conditions is the restriction of passive lateral rotation. He attributes this to the contracture of the capsular ligaments and puts forward a clear case for renaming the condition more accurately as 'contracture of the shoulder'.

Degenerative arthropathy and locked posterior dislocation are also associated with selective loss of lateral rotation, but both of these can be excluded with conventional X-rays (Robinson et al., 2012).

Association with other lesions has been reported, including cervical spine disorders, dysfunction of neural structures, thoracic spine immobility, thoracic or breast surgery, trauma, neurological disease, reflex sympathetic dystrophy, cardiovascular disease, stroke, systemic disease (in particular diabetes mellitus) and the presence of immunological factors, such as human leukocyte antigen (HLA)-B27 (Jeracitano et al., 1992; Anton, 1993; Grubbs, 1993; Stam, 1994; Zreik et al., 2016).

Schiefer et al. (2017) studied the prevalence of hypothyroidism in patients with frozen shoulder. They found that the prevalence was significantly higher in patients with frozen shoulder than in the control group.

Pathology of Frozen Shoulder

In a review of the literature, various authors observed and reported the following changes seen at arthrography, arthroscopy and surgery (Wadsworth, 1986; Owens-Burkhart, 1991; Wiley, 1991; Uhthoff and Sarkar, 1992; Anton, 1993; Grubbs, 1993; Uitvlugt et al., 1993; Stam, 1994; Bunker and Anthony, 1995; Bunker et al., 2000; Smith et al., 2001; Hanchard et al., 2011):

- Volumes of less than 10 mL, compared with the normal intra-articular volume, and a failure to fill the subscapularis bursa or biceps tendon sheath
- Inflammatory changes, formation of new blood vessels in the synovial membrane and capsule, adhesion formation, erythematous fibrinous pannus over the synovium and loss of the axillary fold
- Fibrosis, not inflammation, with changes similar to those seen in Dupuytren disease of the hand
- Retraction of the capsule away from the greater tuberosity, thickening of the coracohumeral ligament and subscapularis tendon and a loss of the normal interval between the glenoid and humeral head.

Frozen shoulder is usually associated with a spontaneous onset of gradually increasing shoulder pain, referring to the deltoid region, and forearm if severe, with an increasing limitation of movement.

Classification of conditions can be useful in deciding on appropriate management. Lundberg (1969) divided the syndrome into primary or secondary types and this simple classification has continued to apply:

- Primary frozen shoulder is idiopathic
- Secondary frozen shoulder occurs following a precipitating trauma or can arise from other causes, including post-surgery or diabetes.

Primary Frozen Shoulder

Primary (idiopathic) frozen shoulder appears to be the more common presentation with no detectable underlying cause for the symptoms (Robinson et al., 2012). The incidence ranges from 0.75% to 5% of the population. It is higher in diabetics (10% to 46%), where patients are prone to develop connective tissue disorders, and higher still in insulin-dependent diabetics.

Bunker and Anthony (1995) described the pathology as similar to Dupuytren disease with increased collagen, myofibroblast and fibroplasia. Tamai et al. (2014) also note the inflamed synovium, most often in the rotator interval region; thickened capsule with contracture; changes in the coracohumeral ligament; and an increase in type III collagen. Of the 50 patients with primary idiopathic frozen shoulder studied by Bunker and Anthony, 58% had Dupuytren disease elsewhere.

Although the condition is said to be fibrosing rather than inflammatory, once developed, the inflammatory drivers for Dupuytren disease and frozen shoulder are similar: TGF-β (transforming growth factor-beta) and PDGF (platelet-derived growth factor; Funk, 2008).

Secondary Frozen Shoulder

The incidence of secondary frozen shoulder is between 3% and 5% (Manske and Prohaska, 2008) and, as with primary frozen shoulder, it is much higher in diabetic patients, up to 30% higher (Zreik et al., 2016), with a tendency to more severe symptoms and resistance to treatment (Dias et al., 2005).

The patient's condition follows a typical pattern. The patient is usually between 40 and 70 years old; women are affected slightly more frequently than men (Dias et al., 2005; Kwaees and Charalambous, 2015); it can occur bilaterally (Chambler and Carr, 2003); the condition progresses slowly to spontaneous recovery over 1 to 3 years; and recurrence of the condition in the other shoulder within 2 to 5 years is common (Cyriax, 1982).

Causes of secondary frozen shoulder may include trauma, systemic illness or any condition that causes immobilisation of the shoulder (i.e. neurological conditions, fracture and pain associated with bursitis or tendinopathy, thyroid disease, cardiac disease, thoracic surgery, pulmonary disease, diabetes mellitus, postmenopausal hormonal changes or psychological factors such as depression, apathy and emotional stress) (Owens-Burkhart, 1991; Stam, 1994; Siegel et al., 1999; Zuckerman and Rokito, 2011; Lewis, 2015).

Diabetes is a risk factor for both primary and secondary frozen shoulder. It does not always follow the natural history of frozen shoulder and more often requires intervention. Diabetic frozen shoulder can be a difficult condition to manage, with a tendency to more severe symptoms and resistance to treatment (Dias et al., 2005) and is more likely to require operative management (Whelton and Peach, 2018).

Simplicity has always been at the heart of the musculoskeletal medicine approach. There have been attempts to introduce subcategories for frozen shoulder in relation to the conditions that may be associated, including rotator cuff tendon disorders, breast surgery, cerebral vascular accident, local fracture or systemic conditions (Zuckerman and Rokito, 2011) but these may not directly change the approach to treating the condition. The wider knowledge of conditions that may be associated with frozen shoulder does enhance clinical reasoning, however, and can have a role in clinical prognosis.

With respect to simplicity, Hanchard et al. (2011) were tasked to produce evidence-based guidelines for the diagnosis, assessment and 'standard' physiotherapy management of contracted (frozen) shoulder. The guidelines were intended to be accessible to a broad spectrum of practitioners, and, to that end, the classifications of 'pain predominant' and 'stiffness predominant' are used throughout the guidelines to provide comprehensive recommendations for management, based on the two presentations.

The pain- and stiffness-predominant classification is novel in that it has moved away from the traditional 'stages' of secondary frozen shoulder that are widely used to guide treatment and are described below. Time and review will tell if by simplifying the classification still further into the predominant symptoms and signs, clinical decision making for management will be facilitated and treatment outcomes enhanced.

Secondary frozen shoulder most frequently occurs following trauma. If precipitated by trauma, the incident may be minor and the initial pain usually settles.

Therefore, the patient may have difficulty recalling a traumatic incident or associating it with the onset of the pain.

A painful shoulder may be kept relatively immobile by involuntary muscle spasm, contributing to pain and stiffness, and the close proximity of other anatomical structures may also be relevant. The subacromial bursa, rotator cuff tendons and the long head of the biceps are all closely related to the capsule of the shoulder joint, and it may be possible for changes in these structures to have a secondary effect on the capsule.

As a guide, the condition can be classified into three stages (Cyriax and Cyriax, 1993; Beyers and Bonutti, 2012), each of which gives an indication of the irritability of the lesion and a suggested programme of treatment. As mentioned earlier, it can also be classified into two stages, as pain- or stiffness-dominant.

We shall refer to three stages here but whichever classification is used, the stages should be considered as a continuum, rather than abrupt, discrete changes as one stage changes to another.

The three special questions taken from the history (see next page) and the assessment of the degree of the capsular pattern, together with the end-feel of the passive movements, provide criteria to be able to judge the stage of the condition.

Stage 1. After the precipitating incident, the initial pain settles. Approximately 1 week later, pain develops and gradually increases. The pain is felt over the area of deltoid, but as inflammation increases, the pain can refer further into the C5 dermatome. The extent of reference of pain indicates the degree of severity of the condition. This stage develops over several weeks and pain is the key feature, not the limited movement.

Since the shoulder joint has a wide range of movement, the early developing capsular pattern may not affect function, and the patient may be oblivious to the loss of movement at this stage. Diagnosis in this early stage is not easy but it becomes conclusive once the capsular pattern of limited movement occurs. If treated early enough, it may be possible to abort the progressive cycle of the condition.

The assessment of the patient provides a set of signs and symptoms that classifies the patient as having stage 1 capsulitis and indicates an appropriate line of treatment.

From the history, the three key questions reveal that:

- The pain is usually above the elbow
- The pain is not usually constant
- The patient can usually sleep on that side at night.
  The examination shows that:
- A minor capsular pattern exists (this may involve lateral rotation only)
- The end-feel of passive movements remains relatively elastic, but is harder than the normal end-feel.

The history and examination indicate a relatively non-irritable joint capsule that may respond to peripheral Grade B mobilisation or corticosteroid injection. Any mobilising technique from a range of treatment approaches can be applied, and the treatment programme for each individual patient is formulated based on the practitioner's experience and the patient's preference. Musculoskeletal medicine treatment techniques will be described in the following pages.

Stage 2. Pain and loss of function are now the key features of the condition. The capsular pattern has developed to affect abduction and medial rotation adversely, and, subjectively, the latter is the most inconvenient functional movement for the patient to lose. As the pain gradually peaks and spreads, the patient notices an inability to reach into a back pocket, for example, or to do up a bra. The limitation of lateral rotation is apparent in that the patient is unable to comb their hair.

From the history, the three key questions reveal that:

- The pain usually spreads beyond the elbow
- The pain is usually constant
- The patient usually cannot sleep on that side at night.
  The examination shows that:
- A full capsular pattern is present
- The characteristic 'hard' end-feel of arthritis exists due to involuntary muscle spasm and capsular contracture.

The history and examination reveal an irritable joint capsule. The presence of the capsular pattern is marked. Adhesion formation in the axillary fold, tightness in the anterior capsular ligaments, shortening of subscapularis and contracture of the rotator interval combine to limit lateral rotation and abduction significantly, producing the capsular pattern.

At this stage, physical treatment alone may not be tolerated, or is of little benefit, although corticosteroid injection can be effective, combined with graded exercises (Dias et al., 2005). Relatively gentle pain-free mobilisation may be applied to restore accessory range. The musculoskeletal medicine treatment techniques will be described in the following pages.

Stage 3. If the patient progresses through the complete cycle of the condition, this represents the stage of recovery. The pain is settling and receding, and full functional movement is returning. However, the patient may be left with a degree of pain and some limited movement, especially lateral rotation and full elevation.

As mentioned, frozen shoulder is a self-limiting condition, including diabetic frozen shoulder, and is self-resolving, with or without treatment, in an average of 1 to 3 years (Wong et al., 2017).

Stage 3 shows similar signs and symptoms to stage 1, and the same treatment may be applied together with rehabilitation, including strengthening and stretching exercises, towards full function.

> **THREE KEY QUESTIONS TO ASSESS IRRITABILTY OF SHOULDER LESIONS**
> - Does the pain spread below the elbow? (site and spread)
> - Can you lie on that side at night? (symptoms)
> - Is the pain constant? (behaviour)

Differential diagnosis for frozen shoulder includes rotator cuff-related shoulder pain, subacromial bursitis, degenerative arthropathy and cervical spine disorders. It is important to consider red flags in the history and examination, including indicators of avascular necrosis, infection, tumour, fracture and posterior dislocation. Look for systemic signs including the patient appearing unwell and pyrexial, swelling and weight loss which might indicate more serious pathology (Table 5.2).

Management of Frozen Shoulder

There is no standard agreed treatment for frozen shoulder, despite many types of treatment having been used and studied. Guidelines and recommendations underpin clinical practice and interventions are usually

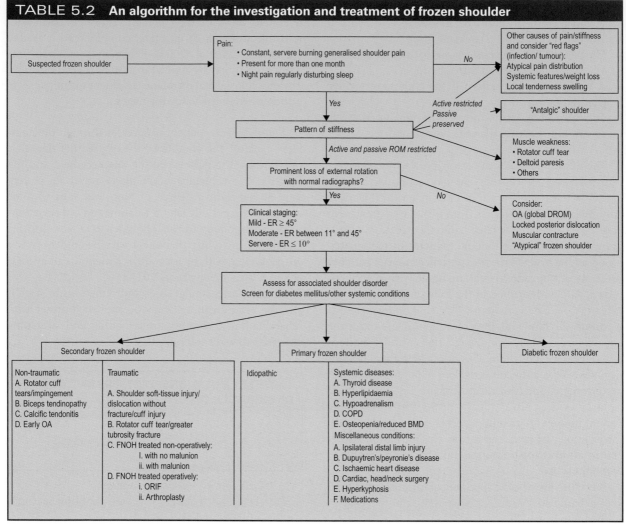

TABLE 5.2   An algorithm for the investigation and treatment of frozen shoulder

Suspected frozen shoulder

Pain:
• Constant, servere burning generalised shoulder pain
• Present for more than one month
• Night pain regularly disturbing sleep

No → Other causes of pain/stiffness and consider "red flags" (infection/ tumour): Atypical pain distribution / Systemic features/weight loss / Local tenderness swelling

Yes

Pattern of stiffness

Active restricted Passive preserved → "Antalgic" shoulder

Active and passive ROM restricted

→ Muscle weakness:
• Rotator cuff tear
• Deltoid paresis
• Others

Prominent loss of external rotation with normal radiographs?

Yes / No

No → Consider: OA (global DROM) / Locked posterior dislocation / Muscular contracture / "Atypical" frozen shoulder

Clinical staging:
Mild - ER ≥ 45°
Moderate - ER between 11° and 45°
Servere - ER ≤ 10°

Assess for associated shoulder disorder
Screen for diabetes mellitus/other systemic conditions

Secondary frozen shoulder / Primary frozen shoulder / Diabetic frozen shoulder

Non-traumatic
A. Rotator cuff tears/impingement
B. Biceps tendinopathy
C. Calcific tendonitis
D. Early OA

Traumatic
A. Shoulder soft-tissue injury/ dislocation without fracture/cuff injury
B. Rotator cuff tear/greater tubrosity fracture
C. FNOH treated non-operatively:
    I. with no malunion
    ii. with malunion
D. FNOH treated operatively:
    i. ORIF
    ii. Arthroplasty

Idiopathic

Systemic diseases:
A. Thyroid disease
B. Hyperlipidaemia
C. Hypoadrenalism
D. COPD
E. Osteopenia/reduced BMD
Miscellaneous conditions:
A. Ipsilateral distal limb injury
B. Dupuytren's/peyronie's disease
C. Ischaemic heart disease
D. Cardiac, head/neck surgery
E. Hyperkyphosis
F. Medications

From Robinson et al., 2012. *ROM*, range of movement; *ER*, external rotation; *FNOH*, fractured neck of humerus; *COPD*, chronic obstructive pulmonary; *OA*, osteoarthritis; *DROM*, decreased range of motion; *ORIF*, open reduction and internal fixation; *BMD*, bone mineral density.

adapted to the phase of the condition, the patient's presentation and shared decision making.

A stepped approach to the management of frozen shoulder is currently recommended (NICE, 2017; Hanchard et al., 2012). Less invasive treatments are generally offered first, including education/watchful wait, activity and work modification, simple analgesics and NSAIDs medication, physiotherapy (e.g. exercise,

mobilisation) and then injection therapy (e.g. corticosteroid, local anaesthetic, hyaluronic acid). If symptoms persist, more invasive treatments can be considered, such as hydrodilatation (Rymaruk and Peach, 2017), manipulation under anaesthetic (MUA) and arthroscopic or open surgery (Rangan et al., 2015, 2016).

Indications for surgery should be assessed on a case-by-case basis. General indications are persistent pain and restricted movements, despite a minimum of 3 to 6 months of non-surgical intervention (Neviaser and Neviaser, 2011; Kingston et al., 2018).

Levine et al. (2007), reported that patients with more severe initial symptoms, who were younger at the time of onset and had persistent restriction, are most likely to require surgery, despite 4 months of compliance with conservative treatment.

Studies on non-operative treatments for frozen shoulder have shown that physiotherapy (not defined) improves range of movement but does not necessarily provide pain relief. Corticosteroid injections have a benefit for short-term pain relief only (Haslan and Celiker, 2001; Ryan, 2005, both cited in Funk, 2007).

The aim of treatment in each of the measures listed previously, as in the use of musculoskeletal medicine techniques, is to relieve pain and restore function. For primary frozen shoulder, Cyriax (1982) suggested a course of intra-articular injections of corticosteroids to treat the pain. These are given over increasing intervals and, with the relief of pain, a gradual increase in movement occurs with recovery to full function.

For secondary frozen shoulder (i.e. traumatic arthritis), the practitioner has a choice of treatment dependent upon the stage of irritability, the techniques available and patient choice. Those recommended in musculoskeletal medicine will be described, but the practitioner is urged not to be limited to this choice, but to draw on experience of other mobilisation techniques that can be incorporated, to provide an individual treatment programme for each patient.

GRADE B MOBILISATION

(Saunders, 2000)

Peripheral Grade B mobilisation (see Chapter 4) is applied to the non-irritable joint only. The aim is to relieve pain and increase the range of movement. Heat may be used beforehand to assist the technique since heating enhances the viscoelastic properties of the capsule.

The condition, prognosis and treatment are explained carefully to the patient since the recovery time may be prolonged over many months, or even several years. The patient must be encouraged to continue the stretching techniques at home, eventually taking over treatment, with the practitioner remaining in a supervisory role for as long as necessary.

- Position the patient comfortably lying with the arm in as much elevation as possible (Fig. 5.29a and b).
- Place one hand on the sternum or scapula to stabilise the thorax and the other hand over the patient's raised elbow to apply a stretch into elevation.
- The principles of Grade B mobilisation are applied: heating (if possible), holding and repeating the stretch, working on the principles of creep (see Chapter 2), and returning the arm under some distraction for comfort (Fig. 5.30).

This technique is fairly firm and will cause a certain amount of post-treatment soreness. The pain may be aggravated for 2 to 4 hours and this should be explained to the patient. An increase in mobility is often reported before the reduction of pain but both are indications for continued treatment.

Distraction Techniques

These are a form of Grade A mobilisation since they occur within the pain-free range of movement. The aim is to restore the accessory range of movement to the joint.

The techniques can be applied together with Grade B mobilisation in the non-irritable joint, to settle the tissues after treatment, or alone in the more irritable joint, particularly if injection is not an option. Once the end-feel of the limited movements regains some elasticity, the joint is deemed to be non-irritable and techniques can be progressed, adding Grade B mobilisation.

LATERAL DISTRACTION

(Cyriax, 1984; Cyriax and Cyriax, 1993)

- Position the patient comfortably in supine lying close to the edge of the couch, which is raised to approximately hip height.
- Place a pillow under and around the arm to support it in the more comfortable position of adduction and some medial rotation.
- Place a hand into the axilla to apply the lateral distraction while simultaneously applying counterpressure to the patient's elbow, resting against your hip (Fig. 5.31).
- The distraction is held for as long as possible and repeated often.

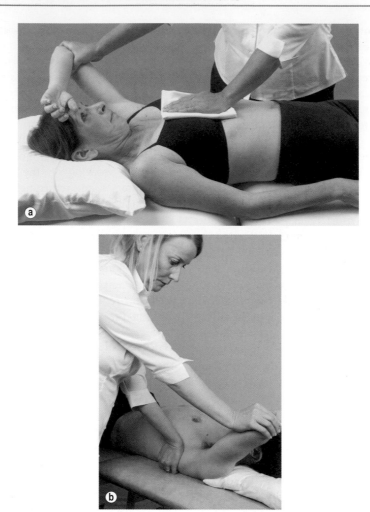

Fig. 5.29 Grade B mobilisation of the glenohumeral joint: (a) stabilising the sternum; (b) alternative, technique, stabilising the scapula.

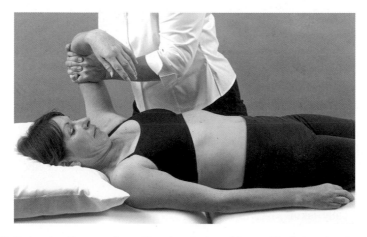

Fig. 5.30 Returning the arm from the elevated position, with distraction for comfort.

CAUDAL DISTRACTION

- Position the patient as described for lateral distraction.
- Hook your forearm into the crook of the patient's flexed elbow (Fig. 5.32).
- Apply sustained and repeated caudal distractions.

A 'seat belt' can be used to aid the distraction techniques, but the practitioner is referred to courses and texts on 'seat belt therapy' for the description of its use.

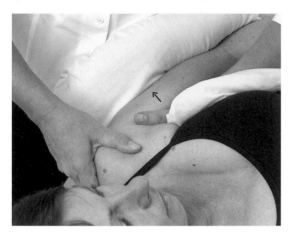

Fig. 5.31 Lateral distraction.

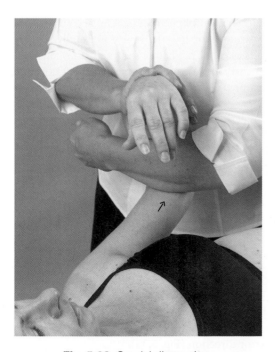

Fig. 5.32 Caudal distraction.

Other mobilising techniques can also be incorporated into this regime.

INJECTION OF THE GLENOHUMERAL JOINT (CYRIAX, 1984; CYRIAX AND CYRIAX, 1993)
Suggested needle size: 21 G × 1½ in. (0.8 × 40 mm) or 2 in. (0.8 × 50 mm) green needle
Dose: 20–40 mg triamcinolone acetonide in a total volume of 3–5 mL

It is important to check with local protocols before injecting the glenohumeral joint, since some pathways stipulate X-ray prior to injection, to rule out alternative diagnoses, red flags and contraindications.

A posterior approach is preferred.

- Position the patient comfortably either prone-lying or sitting (Fig. 5.33).
- Place the affected arm to rest in medial rotation across the abdomen with the elbow flexed.
- Stand behind the patient and place your thumb on the posterior angle of the acromion and your index or middle finger on the coracoid process.
- Insert the needle 1 cm below your thumb placed on the acromion and direct it forwards towards the index finger placed on the coracoid process (Fig. 5.34).
- Once the needle rests against the articular surface, deliver the injection as a bolus, withdrawing slightly if there is resistance.

An explanation of the condition and prognosis is important. The principle is to give another injection if the pain begins to peak, which usually occurs at

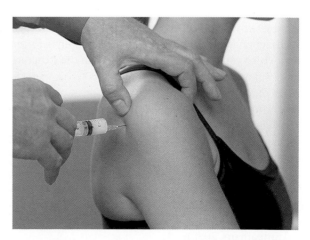

Fig. 5.33 Injection of the glenohumeral joint, sitting.

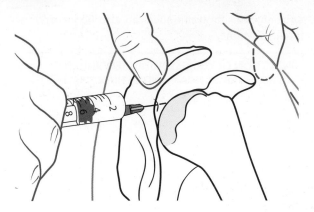

Fig. 5.34 Injection of the glenohumeral joint, showing direction of approach and needle position.

increasing intervals. Generally, not more than three or four injections are given in total, but it is important to check local policy.

The patient should minimise or modify activities for 2 weeks following injection.

NON-CAPSULAR LESIONS

Acromioclavicular Joint

The pain from the acromioclavicular joint is characteristically felt at the cap of the shoulder (epaulette region). The onset may be precipitated by trauma, either a fall on the outstretched hand or a direct blow such as a heavy fall against the wall while playing squash, in a rugby tackle or a touchdown.

Degenerative arthropathy affects the acromioclavicular joint, especially in those who have been extremely active in sport (Stenlund, 1993). Overload can provoke a traumatic arthritis of the degenerate joint. The degenerative changes cause narrowing and osteophyte formation, which can have a secondary effect on the structures in the subacromial space.

On examination, a non-capsular pattern of glenohumeral movement is present with pain felt at extremes of passive elevation, lateral and medial rotation; the acromioclavicular joint itself does not display a capsular pattern as such.

The diagnosis is confirmed by a positive scarf test (passive shoulder flexion and adduction (see Fig. 5.26) reproducing the pain by compressing and shearing the joint (Cyriax, 1982; Cyriax and Cyriax, 1993; Hattam and Smeatham, 2020).

Beitzel et al. (2014) proposed that acromioclavicular joint lesions associated with trauma may be difficult to diagnose correctly clinically, leading to poor clinical decisions and treatment outcomes.

Classification of injuries has been described by Cailliet (1991), and Hartley (1995) and Beitzel et al. (2014) discuss the most widely used Rockwood classification, albeit that it has the disadvantage of being purely radiographical. The Rockwood system describes six levels of classification but the most commonly encountered fall into the first three categories of type I to type III:

- Type I injury is a sprain of the acromioclavicular ligament with no radiographical abnormality.
- Type II injury involves disruption of the acromioclavicular ligaments and joint capsule; the coracoclavicular ligaments are sprained but intact; a vertical subluxation of up to 50% of the distal clavicle is observed.
- Type III injury involves a disruption of the acromioclavicular joint ligaments and joint capsule as well as the coracoclavicular ligaments; there is 100% superior displacement of the distal clavicle.

Beitzel et al. (2014) support the suggestion of the ISAKOS (International Society of Arthroscopy, Knee Surgery & Orthopaedic Sports Medicine) Upper Extremity Committee that type III lesions should be further classified into type IIIA (stable) and IIIB (unstable).

Treatment for type III injury is usually surgery but musculoskeletal medicine treatment may be useful in type I and II lesions. If the superior aspect of the capsular ligament is involved, it may be treated with transverse frictions as appropriate. In chronic lesions, corticosteroid injection of the joint may reduce symptoms.

TRANSVERSE FRICTIONS TO THE SUPERIOR ACROMIOCLAVICULAR CAPSULAR LIGAMENT

(Cyriax, 1984; Cyriax and Cyriax, 1993)

- Stand behind the seated patient and palpate the joint line.
- Using an index finger reinforced by a middle finger, thumb down on the scapula for counterpressure, direct the pressure down onto the tender ligament and impart the transverse frictions in an anteroposterior direction (Fig. 5.35).

- Maintain the technique for an appropriate time, according to the irritability of the lesion and stage of healing, to achieve analgesia and to mobilise the tissues.

Other mobilisation techniques can be incorporated into the treatment regime for acromioclavicular strain, and management may include strapping or taping the joint, particularly if the injury is type II.

- There is considerable variation in the size, shape and direction of the joint surfaces and if the joint is narrowed by degenerative changes it may be difficult to enter. The needle may have to be angled obliquely inferomedially and the presence of the articular disc may make entry difficult.
- Insert the needle into the joint and deliver the injection as a bolus, or pepper the superior ligament if needle entry proves to be difficult (Fig. 5.37).

The patient should minimise or modify activities for 2 weeks following injection.

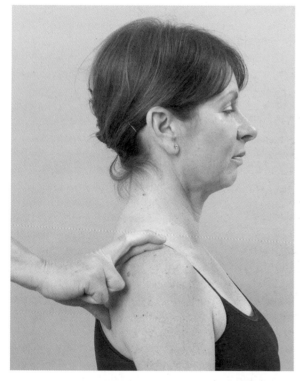

Fig. 5.35 Transverse frictions to the acromioclavicular joint.

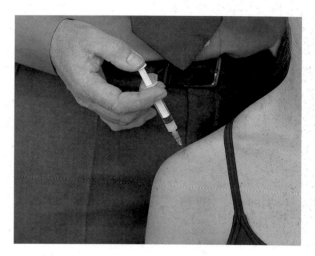

Fig. 5.36 Injection of the acromioclavicular joint.

INJECTION OF THE ACROMIOCLAVICULAR JOINT (CYRIAX, 1984; CYRIAX AND CYRIAX, 1993)
Suggested needle size: 23G × 1 in. (0.6 × 25 mm) blue needle or 25G × 5/8 in. (0.5 × 16 mm) orange needle
Dose: 10–20 mg triamcinolone acetonide in a total volume of 0.5–0.75 mL

- Position the patient comfortably sitting or in half-lying and palpate the superior aspect of the joint line (Fig. 5.36).

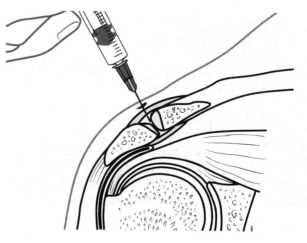

Fig. 5.37 Injection of the acromioclavicular joint showing direction of approach and needle position.

SUBACROMIAL PAIN SYNDROME/ ROTATOR CUFF-RELATED PAIN

The most common diagnosis of shoulder pain is 'subacromial pain syndrome' (SAPS), which is often referred to as 'rotator cuff-related pain' or 'shoulder impingement syndrome'. Each is a generic term to encompass pain associated with any lesion within a structure or structures within the subacromial space. These could include lesions within the rotator cuff tendons as well as the subacromial bursa. The prevalence of SAPS has been suggested to be 36% to 48% of all types of shoulder pain (Park et al., 2020).

Littlewood et al. (2015) referred to the range of diagnostic terms used to explain the problem and how they reflect the uncertainty around 'causative mechanisms, diagnosis, prognosis and the most effective treatments'.

The symptoms of SAPS have traditionally been associated with narrowing of the subacromial space and 'impingement' of structures against the underside of the acromion. Most of the clinical tests for the condition have been based on producing or detecting 'impingement' and examples include the Hawkins–Kennedy, Neer and 'empty can' tests, as well as the production of a painful arc during shoulder abduction.

More recently, there has been a move away from using the term 'impingement', due to the poor diagnostic accuracy of the individual impingement tests, the complexity of the possible mechanisms and pathologies associated with pain in the subacromial space and, importantly, the negligible reduction in pain with surgical acromiohumeral decompression in comparison to placebo (Park et al., 2020).

The rotator cuff, especially supraspinatus, maintains the subacromial space by depressing the head of the humerus, to prevent superior translation during abduction and elevation movements.

Repetitive use, fatigue or overload results in cumulative microtrauma, and the cuff muscles are unable to resist superior translation of the humerus, leading to subtle instability (Copeland, 1993).

Subtle or subclinical subluxation reduces the maximum congruency of the glenoid, and it appears that the supraspinatus and infraspinatus tendons are vulnerable in the posterosuperior labrum. The combination of instability and rotator cuff lesions should be considered in the younger athlete and the management directed at improving movement patterns to correct the instability (Iannotti, 1994).

In older patients, age-related changes occur in the subacromial space. Fatigue and degeneration of fibres may produce muscle weakness that leads to altered neuromuscular control and abnormal movement patterns. The humeral head is no longer effectively depressed and superior translation occurs, reducing the subacromial space (Copeland, 1993; Wilk and Arrigo, 1993; Greenfield et al., 1995). Di Mario and Fraracci (2005) found a correlation between a narrowed coracohumeral distance and subacromial pain.

Grimsby and Gray (2012) discuss an association with increased thoracic kyphosis and shoulder instability as a possible mechanism for the development of subacromial pain, especially in younger athletes (Hanchard et al., 2004; Brukner et al., 2017).

Subacromial pain syndrome can involve inflammation and oedema in the subacromial bursa in the first instance, and secondary thickening and fibrosis can then be followed by partial or full thickness tears of the rotator cuff. The tears are usually longitudinal and on the undersurface of the tendons, which may be relatively avascular compared with the bursal surface (Cailliet, 1991; Uhthoff and Sarkar, 1992; Copeland, 1993; Fukuda et al, 1994; McCann and Bigliani, 1994). Early tendon lesions may involve intrasubstance tears and calcific deposits can occur within the substance of the tendon (Meister and Andrews, 1993).

Positive signs of a subacromial lesion, or lesions, include painful or weak resisted abduction, external rotation or internal rotation and a painful arc, and there may be a combination of several signs if the subacromial bursa is involved. The pain is usually felt in the deltoid region.

Brukner et al., (2017) emphasise that a painful arc is a clinical sign, not a diagnosis, and is a finding in 44% to 66% of all complaints of shoulder pain (Michener et al., 2004).

Despite the poor diagnostic accuracy of the individual impingement tests (Park et al., 2020) the most sensitive tests for lesions within the subacromial space have been found to be the Hawkins–Kennedy, Neer and horizontal adduction tests and the tests with the highest specificity are the 'drop arm', Yergason and painful arc tests (Calis et al., 2000).

Johansson and Ivarson (2009) confirm further that the Neer sign, Hawkins–Kennedy test, Patte manoeuvre and Jobe test are highly reproducible and therefore reliable to use in clinical practice. The practitioner is referred to Hattam and Smeatham (2020) for a description of the tests.

Clinical testing is of use in early screening but a subacromial anaesthetic injection is more reliable in giving a definitive diagnosis of a lesion within the subacromial space (Alvarez-Nemegyei and Canoso, 2003).

Chronic Subacromial Bursitis

The subacromial bursa may be involved in subacromial pain syndrome, and subacromial bursitis is a relatively common cause of pain at the shoulder. However, it can present a challenge to diagnosis because of the muddled picture presented on examination.

The bursa's intimate relationship with the capsule, the rotator cuff tendons and the biceps tendon makes it difficult to diagnose definitively and treatment response can help to confirm or refute diagnosis.

Lesions can coexist, and a primary lesion can indirectly affect the structures closely related to it. In reviewing the anatomy, it will be seen that the lower synovial aspect of the bursa is also the upper aspect of the rotator cuff, the supraspinatus tendon in particular. They cannot be separated and a lesion of one may affect the other.

Prolonged inflammation can cause adhesion formation between the layers of the bursa and may produce a secondary frozen shoulder. In an unwell patient, subacromial abscess or infective bursitis should be suspected (Ward and Eckardt, 1993).

Subacromial bursitis has a gradual onset of pain, usually due to change in use. Together with rotator cuff lesions, bursitis is a common cause of pain in the working-aged active population where the arm is used in an overhead position, such as in racquet sports, stacking shelves, throwing activities of all kinds and swimming.

The patient complains of a low-grade ache over the insertion of deltoid and may not be able to sleep on that side at night. On examination, there is a non-capsular pattern of movement, often with pain felt at the end of range of passive elevation. A painful arc may be present and various resisted tests may also produce the pain.

The application of resisted tests produces some compression of the glenohumeral joint and subacromial space. This produces the characteristic muddle of signs associated with a bursitis. The pain may be on the application or release of resistance, or several positive signs may be produced, such as pain on resisted abduction, lateral rotation and elbow extension. The resisted tests may not be consistent and on reassessment of the patient a completely different set of resisted tests may be present.

A stepped approach to the management of chronic subacromial bursitis is currently recommended. Less invasive treatments are generally offered first, including education/watchful wait, activity and work modification, simple analgesics and NSAIDs medication, physiotherapy (e.g. exercise, mobilisation) and then injection. Mobilisation of the thoracic spine can also be included within the general management of SAPS (Meadows et al., 2020).

Injection consists of an injection of a large volume of low-dose local anaesthetic together with an appropriate amount of corticosteroid. A lateral insertion is used in the musculoskeletal medicine approach.

INJECTION OF CHRONIC SUBACROMIAL BURSITIS
Suggested needle size: 21 G × 1½ in. (0.8 × 40 mm) green needle
Dose: 20–40 mg triamcinolone acetonide in a total volume of 7 mL

- Position the patient comfortably in sitting with the arm hanging by the side.
- Locate the midpoint of the lateral border of the acromion and insert the needle just below, at an oblique angle upwards with respect to the acromion (Fig. 5.38).
- Insert the needle and deliver the injection as a bolus, having found the area, or areas, of less resistance (Fig. 5.39).

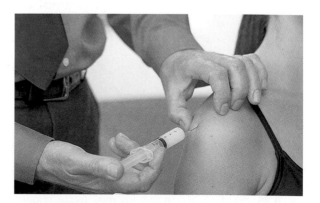

Fig. 5.38 Injection of the subacromial bursa.

- The synovial folds and adhesions within the bursa may present a resistance to the injection, and it may be necessary to deliver the injection by a series of horizontal withdrawals and reinsertions once the needle is in place.

The patient should minimise or modify activities for 2 weeks following injection.

As mentioned earlier, it may be difficult to distinguish subacromial bursitis from chronic rotator cuff tendinopathy, and injection into the subacromial space may be an appropriate choice of treatment when the dilemma occurs, since it can benefit both.

Attention should be paid to factors that could have led to the development of subacromial bursitis. An explanation is given to the patient, aiming to ensure normal shoulder movement and stability. Advice may be appropriate for activity modification.

Acute Calcific Tendinopathy (Acute Subacromial Bursitis)

This condition is likely to be the same, or similar to, the condition described by Cyriax (1982) and Cyriax and Cyriax (1993) as 'acute subacromial bursitis' and it is also referred to as 'acute calcific bursitis'. It is a completely separate entity from the 'chronic subacromial bursitis', described previously.

The condition appears to occur far more commonly in pre-menopausal women, but the cause of the condition is not completely understood. It appears to run through three stages during which calcium crystals are deposited and then resorbed. In the calcific stage, calcium crystals are deposited in the tendon which are then resorbed following macrophage activation. As the crystals are resorbed, oedema and leakage of the crystals into the subacromial bursa occur, leading to increased intratendinous pressure and pain (Albano et al., 2021).

The subacromial bursa itself has been described as a pro-inflammatory membrane (Baring et al., 2007) and it can also be implicated as a source of the pain in this acute condition, arising from the penetration of calcium deposits into the bursa itself. Imaging will confirm the presence of calcific deposits and/or inflammation in the subacromial space, as well as in the underlying rotator cuff, during the calcific stage (Figs 5.40 and 5.41).

As well as intrabursal migration, the calcific deposits may also extend to be intraosseous or intramuscular, where they can mimic infectious processes or malignancies and can lead to radiological diagnostic challenge and mistakes (Albano et al., 2021).

Acute calcific tendinopathy has a typical presentation of a rapid onset of pain for no apparent reason. The pain is felt in the shoulder area; it rapidly increases

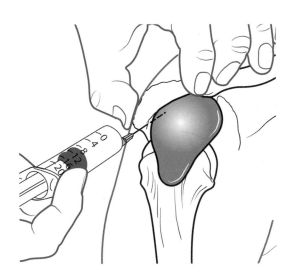

Fig. 5.39 Injection of the subacromial bursa showing direction of approach and needle position.

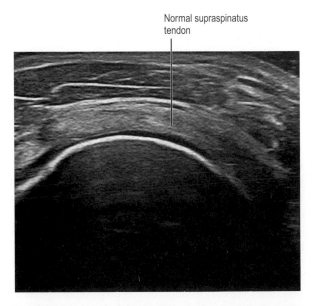

Normal supraspinatus tendon

Fig. 5.40 Ultrasound scan of normal supraspinatus tendon. (Provided by Kjetil Nord-Varhaug.)

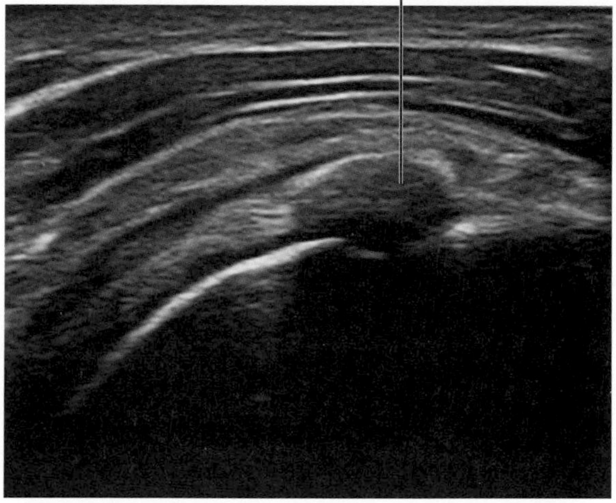

Calcific deposits in
supraspinatus tendon

Fig. 5.41 Ultrasound scan showing calcification within supraspinatus tendon. (Provided by Kjetil Nord-Varhaug.)

in severity and within hours the pain is referred into the whole C5 dermatome. The pain can be intense and generally does not respond to common pain-relieving and anti-inflammatory drugs. The patient may look tired and unwell as the condition is very painful and disturbs sleep.

The condition can be very distressing and patients frequently seek emergency help. Severe twinges of pain are experienced on attempted active movement, especially abduction, which compresses the painful bursa in the subacromial space.

It is important to consider serious pathology and onward referral should be made if the severe pain does not settle within 1 week. Otherwise, the condition is self-limiting and is usually very much better within 7 to 10 days, clearing completely within 6 weeks, although prone to recurrence (Cyriax, 1982).

On examination, a non-capsular pattern of limited movement is present. Usually, full lateral rotation can be coaxed, especially with a little distraction applied to the joint, but the range of abduction is severely limited by pain, indicating a non-capsular pattern.

Treatment does not alter the course of the condition but should take the form of an explanation to the patient and pain-relieving modalities. Oral administration of simple analgesics, with or without NSAIDs, is appropriate but a stronger prescription may be required.

Advice should also be given on sleeping position, suggesting that the arm should be well supported by pillows, bandaged to the side or supported inside a tight-fitting T-shirt to maintain comfort when the protective muscle spasm is lost during sleep.

If calcification is identified, a regime of 'watchful wait' is followed that may include injection for pain relief (see below). The calcification is usually absorbed spontaneously and, apart from addressing the pain of the condition, no further treatment is required.

If symptoms persist, the condition may be treated by barbotage of the tendon where the calcium deposits are punctured with a needle under image guidance, helping them to break up and dissolve. This technique is less invasive than surgery and provides good clinical results. Surgical resection is reserved for long-standing, refractory cases (Berg, 1997).

An injection of corticosteroid is usually helpful, although it may increase the pain initially as the bursa is already swollen and very painful. The technique is the same as for subacromial bursitis, but less volume is used.

Treatment consists of an injection of a small volume of low-dose local anaesthetic together with an appropriate amount of corticosteroid. General advice should be given on how to support the area whilst the symptoms settle and other pain-relieving modalities can be applied.

INJECTION OF ACUTE SUBACROMIAL BURSITIS
Suggested needle size: 21 G × 1½ in. (0.8 × 40 mm) green needle
Dose: 20 mg triamcinolone acetonide in a total volume of 3 mL

- Position the patient sitting comfortably with the arm hanging by the side.
- Locate the midpoint of the lateral border of the acromion and insert the needle just below, at an oblique angle upwards with respect to the acromion (see Figs 5.38 and 5.39).

The patient should minimise or modify activities for 2 weeks following injection.

CONTRACTILE LESIONS

The more common contractile lesions involved in subacromial pain syndrome involve the rotator cuff tendons, particularly supraspinatus. Rotator cuff lesions can vary from early-stage tendinopathy to degeneration and partial or complete thickness tears. The tendon of the long head of the biceps may also be involved and lesions may coexist with subacromial bursitis.

Tendinopathy can arise from change in use and usually has a gradual onset. Single traumatic incidents may produce tendinopathy, but this is unusual, and the trauma in this case is more likely to cause tearing of an already degenerate tendon.

Other causes can be abnormalities in the tendon itself or fatigue failure of muscles that provide support mechanisms for the humeral head in the glenoid. This can follow prolonged repetitive over-the-shoulder physical loads, poor posture and vibration (Alvarez-Nemegyei and Canoso, 2003). There can be associated instability, or lesions within the glenoid labrum.

September et al. (2007) also explored a genetic component, noting that, relative to a control group, siblings have more than twice the risk of developing rotator cuff tears and nearly five times the risk of experiencing symptoms.

Pain is localised to the deltoid area and, although the patient may be aware of a vague resting ache, the pain is increased markedly by movements such as reaching, pushing and pulling, and in particular with those activities using the hands above shoulder level.

On examination, passive movements should be full range with a normal end-feel, but occasionally the opposite passive movement or end-range passive elevation reproduces the pain by stretching or compressing the tendinous insertion, respectively.

Pain is reproduced on the appropriate resisted test and there may be localising signs of a painful arc and/or positive scarf test.

As discussed in the anatomy section, the rotator cuff tendons interdigitate and insert to form a tendinous cuff; it can be difficult to differentiate between the tendons and it may not be possible to make a definitive diagnosis. Resisted abduction implicates supraspinatus; resisted lateral rotation, infraspinatus and teres minor; and resisted medial rotation, subscapularis. Two or more resisted tests may be positive and subsequent palpation will determine the site of the lesion.

The resisted tests often reveal weakness as well as pain. This weakness may be due to tears or muscle inhibition due to pain. Weakness out of proportion to the pain experienced is likely to indicate a tear.

Tendinopathy can be associated with subacromial bursitis and can lead to secondary capsulitis through abnormal movement patterns due to pain. These conditions can 'muddy' the diagnosis. Several resisted tests may provoke pain and a capsular pattern can be superimposed on the non-capsular pattern of movement on examination.

Ultrasound scanning, MRI and MRI arthrograms are currently in common use to investigate and diagnose tendon lesions. MRI is used to identify suspected tears and MR arthrograms are used to identify labral lesions, as well as suspected tears. MRI is highly accurate in detecting full and partial thickness tears of the rotator cuff with a specificity as high as 95%. X-ray can be used to identify calcification in tendons.

Through clinical reasoning, it is important to link the findings of the investigations to the clinical findings, since scans can detect lesions that may be asymptomatic.

The aim of treatment for rotator cuff tendinopathy is to relieve pain and to restore full functional movement to the shoulder.

A stepped approach to the management of rotator cuff tendinopathy is currently recommended. Less invasive treatments are generally offered first, including education/watchful wait, activity and work modification, simple analgesics and NSAIDs medication, physiotherapy (e.g. exercise, mobilisation) and then injection therapy (e.g. corticosteroid, local anaesthetic, hyaluronic acid). If symptoms persist, more invasive treatments can be considered, such as barbotage therapy, subacromial decompression and acromioplasty and rotator cuff repair.

Early onset of tendinopathy may respond to conservative treatment. Progressive exercise is recommended as the first treatment of choice but there is little agreement on the optimal exercise programme to follow. A specific exercise programme is favoured over a non-specific exercise programme, with better long-term outcomes (Haik et al., 2016; Björnsson Hallgren et al., 2017). There is general agreement that the patient needs to commit to following the programme prescribed for at least 12 weeks to achieve a better outcome (Littlewood et al., 2015).

If the patient has pain that is affecting the quality of life, work and sleep, and/or the ability to engage with an exercise programme, then transverse frictions can be integrated into the programme, or a corticosteroid injection into the subacromial space can be considered once all the risks, benefits and side effects have been fully discussed and all contraindications ruled out.

Hanchard et al. (2004) were not convinced that there was sufficient good-quality evidence to support the use of injections in the general treatment of subacromial pain syndrome and, in light of the associated risks to the tendons, took the view that conservative treatment should precede the use of injections unless severe pain is present.

Currently, the whole question of tendinopathy is under debate with inflammation disputed as a component of the problem and degeneration of the tendon proposed as the cause. This leads to questions with regard to the prognosis for the patient.

An inflammatory problem is expected to resolve with treatment in up to approximately 3 weeks; a degenerative problem will take much longer (see discussion in Chapter 3). Furthermore, if the pathology of rotator cuff tendinopathy is degenerative, more questions are raised, such as why corticosteroid injection relieves pain.

Khan and Cook (2000) acknowledge that clinical experience and some studies show that corticosteroid injection does produce short-term relief of pain in tendon lesions but recognise that the mechanisms for this pain relief are currently not known.

Injection into the teno-osseous junctions of the individual tendons is controversial and a direct link with tendon rupture has been proposed but not proven at the time of writing. A consensus of opinion is hard to pin down, and practice appears to vary between those who continue to inject into the tendon itself in younger patients, where the good health of the tendon is assumed, and those who would always use an injection into the subacromial space to be able to bathe the intimately related tissues, whilst avoiding direct infiltration of the tendon structure.

An ultrasound scan of the tendons prior to injection of the teno-osseous junction, to establish the state of degeneration of the tendons, is common practice and is strongly recommended. However, to exercise caution, an injection into the subacromial space may be more appropriate, particularly if a lesion in the degenerate tendons produces inflammation in the subacromial space.

Injection of the individual tendons may occasionally be appropriate for a sub-group of patients, if a subacromial injection fails to achieve adequate pain relief, but the importance of checking with local policy cannot be over-stressed.

The outcome of treatment by injection under image guidance has been compared with outcomes following anatomically guided injections. Alvarez-Nemegyei and Canoso (2003) and Chen et al. (2006) reported successful treatment of rotator cuff tendinopathy with anatomically guided corticosteroid subacromial injection when compared with placebo, while Matthews and Glousman (2004) made a case for radiographically guided accurate steroid placement being associated with improved clinical benefit at a 2-week evaluation.

Bloom et al. (2012) based their Cochrane review of image-guided versus anatomically guided glucocorticoid injection for shoulder pain on 'moderate' evidence and found no advantage in pain, range of motion or safety of image-guided over anatomically guided injection. They further suggested that the benefits may arise from systemic rather than local effects.

Wu et al. (2015) focused on subacromial injection and conducted a systematic review and meta-analysis to assess the effectiveness of ultrasound-guided versus anatomically guided corticosteroid injection in adults with shoulder pain. Their findings were different from Bloom et al. (2012) and they concluded that the meta-analysis of their review provided evidence that ultrasound-guided injections did potentially offer a significantly greater clinical improvement.

Limitations of both reviews were acknowledged to be small sample sizes and the considerable clinical, methodological and statistical variation within the trials considered. However, access to ultrasound-guidance has become far more widespread and can be considered as an option where available.

Extracorporeal shock wave therapy (lithotripsy) has emerged as an appropriate treatment for calcific tendonitis and has also shown promise in the treatment of tendinopathies (Hsu et al., 2008; Scott et al., 2013). The mechanism of how lithotripsy is beneficial is not fully understood. It has been shown to enhance neovascularisation at the tendon–bone junction with early release of growth and proliferating factors that lead to improved blood supply and tissue regeneration.

Supraspinatus Tendinopathy

A lesion in supraspinatus produces pain on resisted abduction. Weakness may also be present which may be due to muscle inhibition because of the pain, or indicative of a partial or full thickness tear of the tendon, as mentioned previously.

A painful arc or pain at the end of range of passive elevation localises the lesion to the distal end of the tendon, usually at the teno-osseous junction. If pain is produced on resisted abduction only, without this localising sign, the lesion is more likely to be at the musculotendinous junction. Either way, palpation will confirm the exact site of the lesion and the treatments appropriate for each site are described below.

The following treatment techniques of transverse frictions and injection may be successful, but they do not stand alone and should be integrated into an individualised management plan, in which all components of the patient's problem are addressed, including eliminating the possible cause.

Joseph et al. (2012) found some evidence of benefit for the use of transverse frictions in the treatment of supraspinatus tendinopathy along with joint mobilisation. This supports the case for treating the rotator cuff tendons with frictions first, as part of a programme of musculoskeletal medicine management, and to leave injection as the second option rather than the 'treatment of choice'.

It is up to suitably qualified clinicians to exercise judgement based on current best practice and having checked with local policy.

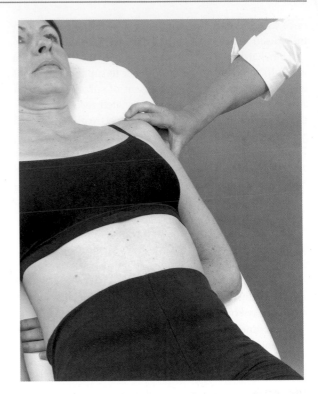

Fig. 5.42 Transverse frictions to the supraspinatus tendon, teno-osseous site.

TRANSVERSE FRICTIONS TO SUPRASPINATUS

(Cyriax, 1984; Cyriax and Cyriax, 1993)

Teno-osseous Junction

- Position the patient in sitting at an angle of 45 degrees, medially rotating the shoulder and placing the arm behind the back to expose the tendon insertion.
- Stand at the side of the patient and identify the area of tenderness.
- Place an index finger, reinforced by the middle finger, onto the tendon and direct the pressure down onto the insertion (Fig. 5.42).
- If the position is uncomfortable for the patient, an alternative position of side-lying, painful side uppermost and with the shoulder medially rotated and extended, can be adopted. Stand behind the patient in this position.
- Deliver the frictions transversely across the fibres, keeping the index finger parallel to the anterior edge

of the acromion process. The supraspinatus tendon is approximately one finger's width (1 cm).
- Maintain the technique for an appropriate time, according to the irritability of the lesion and stage of healing, to achieve analgesia and to mobilise the tissues.

Relative rest is advised where functional movements may continue but no overuse or stretching until pain-free on resisted testing. An appropriate progressive loading rehabilitation programme should be applied.

Musculotendinous Junction

- Position the patient in sitting with the painful shoulder abducted to 90 degrees and supported comfortably on the couch.
- Stand on the opposite side of the patient but facing forwards with your arm straight across and behind the patient's shoulders.
- Locate the musculotendinous junction in the 'V' created by the clavicle and the acromion process (Fig. 5.43).

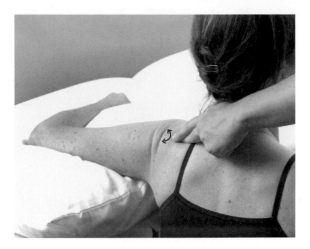

Fig. 5.43 Transverse frictions to the supraspinatus tendon, musculotendinous junction.

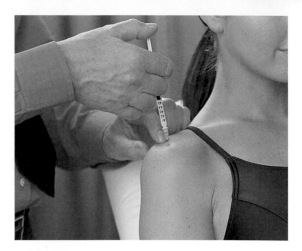

Fig. 5.44 Injection of the supraspinatus tendon.

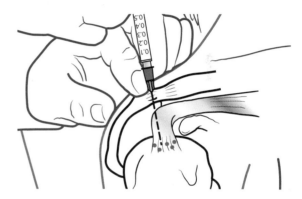

Fig. 5.45 Injection of the supraspinatus tendon showing direction of approach and needle position.

- Using the middle finger reinforced by the index finger, direct the pressure down onto the musculotendinous junction and deliver the transverse frictions by rotating the forearm.
- Maintain the technique for an appropriate time, according to the irritability of the lesion and stage of healing, to achieve analgesia and to mobilise the tissues.

Relative rest is advised where functional movements may continue but no overuse or stretching until pain-free on resisted testing.

> **INJECTION OF THE TENO-OSSEOUS JUNCTION OF SUPRASPINATUS (CYRIAX, 1984; CYRIAX AND CYRIAX, 1993)**
> Suggested needle size: 25 G × 5/8 in. (0.5 × 16 mm) orange needle or 23 G × 1 in. (0.6 × 25 mm) blue needle
> Dose: 10 mg triamcinolone acetonide in a total volume of 1 mL

- Position the patient as described for transverse frictions of the teno-osseous junction.
- Insert the needle perpendicular to the teno-osseous junction (Fig. 5.44) and deliver the injection using a peppering technique (Fig. 5.45).

The patient should minimise or modify activities for 2 weeks following injection. An appropriate progressive loading rehabilitation programme should be applied.

Infraspinatus Tendinopathy (± Teres Minor)

A lesion in infraspinatus and teres minor produces pain on resisted lateral rotation. A painful arc and pain at the end of range of passive elevation indicate that the lesion lies at the distal end of the tendon, usually at the teno-osseous junction. If no arc is present, the lesion is often a little further proximally in the body of the tendon. Palpation will confirm the exact site of the lesion.

TRANSVERSE FRICTIONS TO INFRASPINATUS

(Cyriax, 1984; Cyriax and Cyriax, 1993)

- Position the patient in side-lying with the head raised on two pillows (or one folded over), the hand resting on the cheek and the forearm free to allow the elbow to drop down below the shoulder. This laterally rotates and adducts the affected arm to expose the greater tuberosity (Fig. 5.46).

- Locate the area of tenderness and place a thumb on the area parallel to the direction of the tendon fibres; reinforce this with the other thumb.
- Standing back to apply body weight, press down onto the tendon and deliver a transverse sweep across the fibres, aiming to touch the posterior angle of the acromion with each stroke.
- The infraspinatus is two fingers (2 cm) wide; if teres minor is involved, the sweep should cover a width of three fingers (3 cm).
- If the lesion lies in the body of the tendon, the technique for transverse frictions is the same, but they are applied a little more proximally at the site of the lesion, as identified by palpation.
- Maintain the technique for an appropriate time, according to the irritability of the lesion and stage of healing, to achieve analgesia and to mobilise the tissues.

Relative rest is advised where functional movements may continue but no overuse or stretching until pain-free on resisted testing. An appropriate progressive loading rehabilitation programme should be applied.

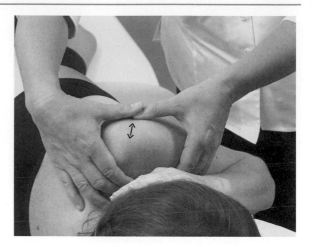

Fig. 5.46 Transverse frictions to the infraspinatus tendon (and position for injection).

> **INJECTION OF THE TENO-OSSEOUS JUNCTION OF INFRASPINATUS (CYRIAX, 1984; CYRIAX AND CYRIAX, 1993)**
> Suggested needle size: 23 G × 1 in. (0.6 × 25 mm) or 23 G × 1¼ in. (0.6 × 30 mm) blue needle or 21 G × 1½ in. (0.8 × 40 mm) green needle
> Dose: 10 mg triamcinolone acetonide in a total volume of 1 mL

- Position the patient as above for transverse frictions to infraspinatus (see Fig. 5.46).
- Locate the area of tenderness over the greater tuberosity, which now lies approximately two fingers' width below the posterior angle of the acromion.
- Insert the needle and deliver the injection by a peppering technique to the whole extent of the lesion, which may be up to 2 to 3 cm wide (Fig. 5.47).

The patient should minimise or modify activities for 2 weeks following injection. An appropriate progressive loading rehabilitation programme should then be applied.

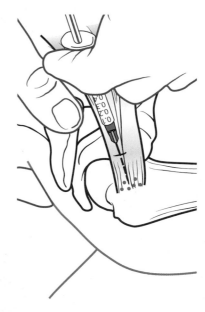

Fig. 5.47 Injection of the infraspinatus tendon showing direction of approach and needle position.

Subscapularis Tendinopathy

A lesion in subscapularis produces pain on resisted medial rotation. A painful arc indicates a lesion in the upper fibres; a positive scarf test indicates a lesion in the lower fibres. Palpation will confirm the exact site of the lesion, which may cover a large area of tendon, approximately three fingers wide.

TRANSVERSE FRICTIONS TO SUBSCAPULARIS

(Cyriax, 1984; Cyriax and Cyriax, 1993)

- Position the patient in sitting with the arm supported to allow the humerus to rest in the anatomical position (Fig. 5.48a).
- Locate the area of tenderness (upper fibres, lower fibres or both) on the medial aspect of the lesser tuberosity. The practitioner's position can be varied to give better access to the tendon (see Fig. 5.48a and b).
- Place the thumb perpendicular to the direction of the fibres, parallel to the shaft of the humerus and directed laterally
- Deliver the transverse frictions in a superoinferior direction transversely across the fibres.
- The subscapularis tendon is approximately three fingers wide (3 cm). If the full width of the tendon is affected, it may be necessary to divide the area into two sites for treatment as it is difficult to friction across the entire structure and a blister may be raised.
- Maintain the technique for an appropriate time, according to the irritability of the lesion and stage of healing, to achieve analgesia and to mobilise the tissues.

Relative rest is advised where functional movements may continue but no overuse or stretching until pain-free on resisted testing. An appropriate progressive loading rehabilitation programme should be applied.

> ### INJECTION OF SUBSCAPULARIS (CYRIAX, 1984; CYRIAX AND CYRIAX, 1993)
> Suggested needle size: 23 G × 1 in. (0.6 × 25 mm) or 23 G × 1¼ in. (0.6 × 30 mm) blue needle
> Dose: 10 mg triamcinolone acetonide in a total volume of 1 mL

- Position the patient as for transverse frictions of subscapularis (Fig. 5.49).
- Locate the lesser tuberosity
- Deliver the injection by peppering technique to the full width of the lesion at the insertion onto the lesser tuberosity (Fig. 5.50).

The patient should minimise or modify activities for 2 weeks following injection. An appropriate progressive loading rehabilitation programme should be applied.

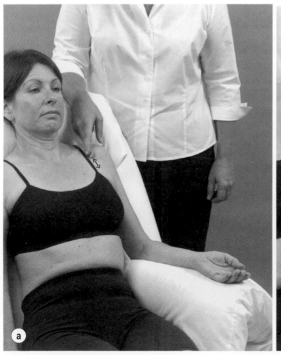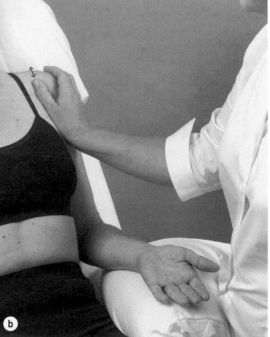

Fig. 5.48 (a and b) Positions for transverse frictions to the subscapularis tendon.

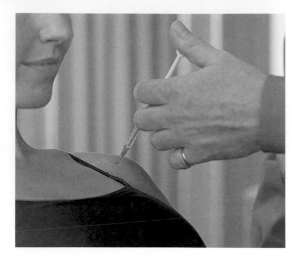

Fig. 5.49 Injection of the subscapularis tendon.

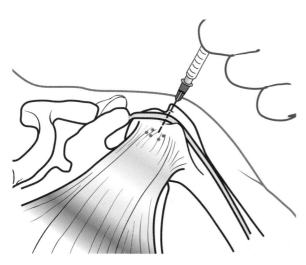

Fig. 5.50 Injection of the subscapularis tendon showing direction of approach and needle position.

Tendinopathy of the Long Head of Biceps

In its position in the subacromial space, the tendon of the long head of biceps may be involved in subacromial pain syndrome. It will produce pain felt at the shoulder on resisted elbow flexion, possibly with forward flexion at the shoulder.

A painful arc is usually present on forward flexion of the shoulder with a straight arm and the palm uppermost.

TRANSVERSE FRICTIONS TO THE LONG HEAD OF BICEPS

(Cyriax, 1984; Cyriax and Cyriax, 1993)

- Position the patient in sitting with the arm supported so that the humerus rests in the anatomical position (Fig. 5.51).
- Place a thumb parallel to the tendon in the groove, fingers wrapped around the arm for counterpressure.
- Deliver the transverse frictions by alternately rotating the arm into medial and lateral rotation. Alternatively, the practitioner may hold the patient's arm stationary and deliver the friction by abducting and adducting the thumb.
- Maintain the technique for an appropriate time, according to the irritability of the lesion and stage of healing, to achieve analgesia and to mobilise the tissues.

The long head of biceps is covered by a synovial sheath, but it can be difficult to apply the principle of stretch whilst being able to gain access to the rounded

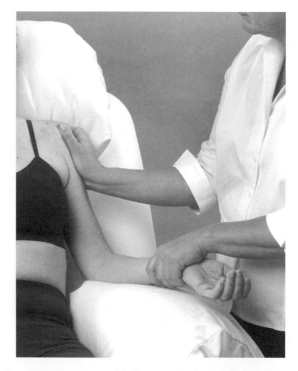

Fig. 5.51 Transverse frictions to the long head of biceps tendon.

tendon within the intertubercular groove. An element of shoulder extension can be included in either the sitting or side-lying (painful side uppermost) position and the technique adapted as necessary to be able to apply transverse frictions effectively across the full extent of the lesion.

> **INJECTION OF THE LONG HEAD OF THE BICEPS IN THE BICIPITAL GROOVE**
> Suggested needle size: 23 G × 1 in. (0.6 × 25 mm) or 23 G × 1¼ in. (0.6 × 30 mm) blue needle
> Dose: 10 mg triamcinolone acetonide in a total volume of 1 mL

Relative rest is advised where functional movements may continue but no overuse or stretching until pain-free on resisted testing.

- Position the patient as for the transverse frictions described earlier.

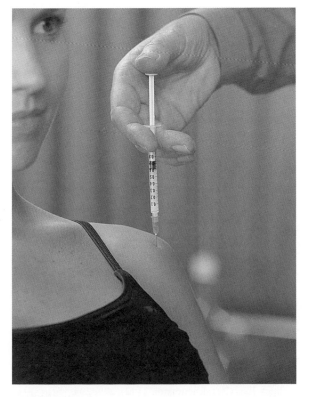

Fig. 5.52 Injection of the long head of biceps tendon.

- Locate the bicipital groove and slide the needle in, parallel to the groove (Fig. 5.52).
- Deliver the injection by a bolus technique alongside the tendon (Fig. 5.53).

The patient should minimise or modify activities for 2 weeks following injection.

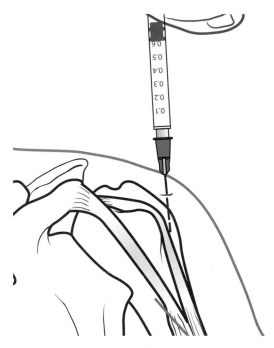

Fig. 5.53 Injection of the long head of biceps tendon showing direction of approach and needle position.

REVIEW QUESTIONS

1. Which structures can be implicated in subacromial pain syndrome?
2. How do you palpate for the supraspinatus tendon at its insertion onto the greater tuberosity?
3. Is there a way to differentiate between subacromial bursitis and rotator cuff tendinopathy?
4. Which treatment is appropriate for Stage 1 shoulder capsulitis? What clinical findings make it Stage 1?
5. What is the pain referral pattern for lesions around the shoulder?

CASE SCENARIOS

Case 1

History

- Sharon, a 43-year-old right-handed office worker, plays recreational tennis and has pain in her right deltoid region not spreading below the elbow. Gradual onset over last 2 months. Since moving office, her pain is getting worse. Intermittent pain, aggravated by overhead activity and tennis. She can lie on the right side and the pain eases with rest. No neurological considerations or neck symptoms, no previous shoulder problems. Good general health, taking occasional ibuprofen, no significant past medical history.

Examination

- Full and pain-free neck movements and normal reflexes/sensation. Pain end-range active shoulder elevation and has a painful arc through abduction. Pain end-range passive internal rotation, other passive movements full, pain-free and with normal end-feel. Pain on resisted abduction and lateral rotation: no obvious weakness. No specific tenderness on palpation.

Task

- Use clinical reasoning to consider differential diagnosis for this patient and any further tests you would wish to perform. Discuss treatment options for this patient.

Case 2

History

- Simon, a 25-year-old personal trainer, has a special interest in martial arts. He has pain over the right C4 dermatome with minimal referral into the upper trapezius. Sudden onset 1 week ago when thrown to ground by a colleague in a demonstration of self-defence moves, and he landed on tip of his shoulder. Pain is fairly constant and moving the shoulder actively is uncomfortable. He is unable to lie on that side. Neck feeling a little stiff in last couple of days. General health excellent, previous arthroscopy on left knee. Taking occasional paracetamol.

Examination

- Protecting shoulder with guarding, full range of neck movements with pain end-range right rotation. Active shoulder elevation to 100 degrees and abduction limited at 90 degrees. Passive lateral rotation full, limited internal rotation. Resisted tests full power with pain on resisted biceps. Tender on palpation over the acromioclavicular joint line.

Task

- What is the appropriate advice and treatment for this patient at this stage in the healing process? How would you adapt this for different grades of this injury?

Case 3

History

- Bryan, a 56-year-old brewery worker, is a keen fisherman. He is complaining of pain in left C5 dermatome spreading down as far as his forearm. Onset has been gradual over the last 3 months but now the pain has become unbearable and he is unable to lie on that side in bed. He cannot recall a specific injury except a fall onto that side a while before the pain commenced. Pain is constant and he struggles at work with lifting barrels. He has type II diabetes and is taking ibuprofen and statins.

Examination

- Capsular pattern of neck pain. Limited passive lateral rotation and pain end-range medial rotation of the left shoulder. End-feel is hard. Resisted shoulder movements pain-free.

Task

- Discuss differential diagnosis and appropriate treatment options for this patient.

REFERENCES

Abrassart, S., Kolo, F., Piotton, S., et al., 2020. 'Frozen shoulder' is ill-defined. How can it be described better? EFORT Open Rev. 5 (5), 273–279.

Albano, D., Coppola, A., Gitto, S., et al., 2021. Imaging of calcific tendinopathy around the shoulder: usual and unusual presentations and common pitfalls. Radiol. Med. 126 (4), 608–619.

Alvarez-Nemegyei, J., Canoso, J., 2003. Evidence-based soft tissue rheumatology. Part 1: Subacromial impingement syndrome. J. Clin. Rheumatol. 9 (3), 193–199.

Anton, H.A., 1993. Frozen shoulder. Can. Fam. Physician 39, 1773–1777.

Arendt-Nielsen, L., Svensson, P., 2001. Referred muscle pain: basic and clinical findings. Clin. J. Pain 17 (1), 11–19.

Baring, T., Emery, R., Reilly, P., 2007. Management of rotator cuff disease: specific treatment for specific disorders. Best Pract. Res. Clin. Rheumatol. 21 (2), 279–294.

Beals, T.C., Harryman, D.T., Lazarus, M., 1998. Useful boundaries of the subacromial bursa. J. Arthroscopic Relat. Surg. 14 (5), 465–470.

Beitzel, K., Mazzocca, A.D., Bak, K., et al., 2014. ISAKOS upper extremity committee consensus statement on the need for diversification of the Rockwood classification for acromio-clavicular joint injuries. Arthroscopy 30 (2), 271–278.

Berg, E., 1997. Calcific tendinitis of the shoulder. Orthop. Nurs. 16 (6), 68–69.

Beyers, M., Bonutti, P., 2012. Frozen shoulder. In: Donatelli, R. (Ed.), Physical Therapy of the Shoulder. Churchill Livingstone, Edinburgh.

Biundo, J.J., Harris, M.A., 1993. Peripheral nerve entrapment, occupation-related syndromes and sports injuries, and bursitis. Curr. Opin. Rheumatol. 5, 224–229.

Björnsson Hallgren, H.C., Adolfsson, L.E., Johansson, K., et al., 2017. Specific exercises for subacromial pain. Acta. Orthop. 88 (6), 600–605.

Bloom, J.E., Rischin, A., Johnston, R.V., et al., 2012. Image-guided versus blind glucocortoid injection for shoulder pain. Cochrane Database Syst. Rev. 15 (8), CD009147.

Brukner, P., Clarson, B., Cook, J., et al., 2017. Clinical Sports Medicine, vol. 1. Injuries, fifth ed. McGraw-Hill, Sydney.

Bunker, T., 2009. Time for a new name for frozen shoulder–contracture of the shoulder. Shoulder & Elbow 1, 4–9.

Bunker, T.D., Anthony, P.P., 1995. The pathology of frozen shoulder. J. Bone Joint Surg. 77B, 677–683.

Bunker, T.D., Reilly, J., Baird, K.S., et al., 2000. Expression of growth factors, cytokines and matrix metalloproteinases in frozen shoulder. J. Bone Joint Surg. 82B, 768–773.

Cailliet, R., 1991. Shoulder Pain, third ed. F A Davis, Philadelphia.

Calis, M., Kenan, A., Birtane, M., 2000. Diagnostic values of clinical diagnostic tests in subacromial impingement syndrome. Ann. Rheum. Dis. 59, 44–47.

Cameron, G., 1995. The shoulder is a weight-bearing joint: implications for clinical practice. J. Orthop. Med. 17, 46–50.

Chambler, A.F.W., Carr, A.J., 2003. Aspects of current management: the role of surgery in frozen shoulder. J. Bone Joint Surg. [Br] 85-B, 789–795.

Chen, M.J., Lew, H.L., Hsu, T.C., et al., 2006. Ultrasound-guided shoulder injections in the treatment of musculoskeletal disorders: current perspectives and future prospects. Clin. J. Pain. 17, 25–32.

Clark, J.M., Harryman, D.T., 1992. Tendons, ligaments and capsule of the rotator cuff. J. Bone Joint Surg. 74A, 713–725.

Clarnette, R.G., Miniaci, A., 1998. Clinical examination of the shoulder. Med. Sci. Sports Exerc. 30 (Suppl. 4), S1–S6.

Codman, E.A., 1934. The Shoulder: Rupture of the Supraspinatus Tendon and Other Lesions in or About the Subacromial Bursa. Miller & Company, Brooklyn: G.

Cook, C., Beaty, S., Kissenberth, M.J., et al., 2012. Diagnostic accuracy of five orthopedic clinical tests for diagnosis of superior labrum anterior posterior (SLAP) lesions. J. Shoulder Elbow Surg. 21 (1), 13–22.

Cooper, D.E., O'Brien, S.J., Warren, R.F., 1993. Supporting layers of the glenohumeral joint: an anatomic study. Clin. Orthop. Relat. Res. 289, 144–155.

Copeland, S., 1993. Throwing injuries of the shoulder. Br. J. Sports Med. 27 (4), 221–227.

Cyriax, J., 1982. Textbook of Orthopaedic Medicine, eighth ed. Baillière Tindall, London.

Cyriax, J., 1984. Textbook of Orthopaedic Medicine, eleventh ed. Baillière Tindall, London.

Cyriax, J., Cyriax, P., 1993. Cyriax's Illustrated Manual of Orthopaedic Medicine. Butterworth Heinemann, Oxford.

Dessaur, W.A., Magarey, M.E., 2008. Diagnostic accuracy of clinical tests for superior labral anterior posterior lesions: a systematic review. J. Orthop. Sports Phys. Ther. 38 (6), 341–352.

Dias, R., Cutts, S., Massoud, S., 2005. Frozen shoulder. Br. Med. J. 331 (7530), 1453–1456.

Di Mario, M., Fraracci, L., 2005. MR study of the intrinsic acromial angle in 74 symptomatic patients. Radiol. Med. 110 (3), 273–279.

Escamilla, R.F., Yamashiro, K., Paulos, L., et al., 2009. Shoulder muscle activity and function in common shoulder rehabilitation exercises. Sports Med. 39 (8), 663–685.

Felstead, A.J., Ricketts, D., 2017. Biomechanics of the shoulder and elbow. Orthop.Trauma. 31 (5), 300–305.

Frame, M.K., 1991. Anatomy and biomechanics of the shoulder. In: Donatelli, R.A. (Ed.), Clinics in Physical Therapy, Physical Therapy of the Shoulder. Churchill Livingstone, Edinburgh, pp. 1–18.

Fukuda, H., Hamada, K., Nakajima, T., et al., 1994. Pathology and pathogenesis of the intratendinous tearing of the rotator cuff viewed from en bloc histologic sections. Clin. Orthop. Relat. Res. 304, 60–67.

Funk, L., 2007. Frozen Shoulder. Online. https://www.shoulderdoc.co.uk/news/view/627. Accessed 3 September 2021.

Funk, L., 2008. Frozen shoulder. Int. Musculoskelet. Med. 31 (1), 36–39.

Greenfield, B., Catlin, P.A., Coats, P.W., et al., 1995. Posture in patients with shoulder overuse injuries in healthy individuals. J. Orthop. Sports Phys. Ther. 21, 287–295.

Grimsby, O., Gray, J., 2012. Interrelationship of the spine, rib cage, and the shoulder girdle. In: Donatelli, R. (Ed.), Physical Therapy of the Shoulder. Churchill Livingstone, Edinburgh, pp. 133–185.

Grubbs, N., 1993. Frozen shoulder syndrome – a review of the literature. J. Orthop. Sports Phys. Ther. 18, 479–487.

Guanche, C.A., Jones, D.C., 2003. Clinical testing for tears of the glenoid labrum. J. Arthroscopic Relat. Surg. 19 (5), 517–523.

Haik, M.N., Alburquerque-Sendin, F., Moreira, R.F.C., 2016. Effectiveness of physical therapy treatment of clearly defined subacromial pain: a systematic review of randomized controlled trials. Br. J. Sports Med. 50, 1124–1134.

Halder, A.M., An, K.-N., 2000. Anatomy and biomechanics of the shoulder. Orthop. Clin. N. Am. 31 (2), 159–176.

Hanchard, N., Cummins, J., Jeffries, C., 2004. Evidence-based Clinical Guidelines for the Diagnosis, Assessment and Physiotherapy Management of Shoulder Impingement Syndrome Chartered Society of Physiotherapy, London

Hanchard, N., Goodchild, L., Thompson, J., et al., 2011. Guidelines for the diagnosis, assessment and management of contracted (frozen) shoulder. https://www.csp.org.uk/publications/guidelines-diagnosis-assessment-management-contracted-frozen-shoulder. Accessed 4 September 2021.

Hanchard, N.C., Goodchild, L., Thompson, J., et al., 2012. Evidence-based clinical guidelines for the diagnosis, assessment and physiotherapy management of contracted (frozen) shoulder: quick reference summary. Physiotherapy 98 (2), 117–120.

Hartley, A., 1995. Practical Joint Assessment, Upper Quadrant, second ed. Mosby, London.

Hattam, P., Smeatham, A., 2020. Handbook of Special Tests in Musculoskeletal Examination, Second ed. Elsevier, Oxford.

Hsu, C.J., Wang, D.Y., Tseng, K.F., et al., 2008. Extracorporeal shock wave therapy for calcifying tendinitis of the shoulder. J. Shoulder Elbow Surg. 17 (1), 55–59.

Hulstyn, M.J., Fadale, P.D., 1995. Arthroscopic anatomy of the shoulder. Orthop. Clin. N. Am. 26, 597–612.

Iannotti, J.P., 1994. Evaluation of the painful shoulder. J. Hand Ther. 7, 77–83.

Itoi, E., Newman, S.R., Kuechle, D.K., et al., 1994. Dynamic anterior stabilizers of the shoulder with the arm in abduction. J. Bone Joint Surg. 76B, 834–836.

Jeracitano, D., Cooper, R., Lyon, L.J., et al., 1992. Abnormal temperature control suggesting sympathetic dysfunction in the shoulder skin of patients with frozen shoulder. Br. J. Rheumatol. 31, 539–542.

Johansson, K., Ivarson, S., 2009. Intra-and interexaminer reliability of four manual shoulder maneuvers used to identify subacromial pain. Man. Ther. 14, 231–239.

Joseph, M.F., Taft, K., Moskwa, M., et al., 2012. Deep friction massage to treat tendinopathy: a systematic review of a classic treatment in the face of a new paradigm of understanding. J. Sport Rehabil. 21, 343–353.

Jost, B., Koch, P., Gerber, C., 2000. Anatomy and functional aspects of the rotator interval. J. Shoulder Elbow Surg. 9 (4), 336–341.

Kane, S., Conus, S., Haltom, D., et al., 2010. A shoulder health survey: correlating behaviors and comorbidities with shoulder problems. Sports Health 2 (2), 119–134.

Kapandji, I.A., 2019. The Physiology of the Joints: Upper Limb, seventh ed. Handspring Publishing.

Khan, K.M., Cook, J.L., 2000. Overuse tendon injuries: where does the pain come from? Sports Med. Arthroscopy Rev 8, 17–31.

Kingston, K., Curry, E.J., Galvin, J.W., et al., 2018. Shoulder adhesive capsulitis; epidemiology and predictors of surgery. J. Shoulder Elbow Surg. 27 (8), 1437–1443.

Kwaees, T.A., Charalambous, C.P., 2015. Rates of surgery for frozen shoulder: an experience in England. Muscles Ligaments Tendons J. 5 (4), 276–279.

Levine, W.N., Kashyap, C.P., Bak, S.F., et al., 2007. Nonoperative management of idiopathic adhesive capsulitis. J. Shoulder Elbow Surg. 16 (5), 569–573.

Lewis, J., 2015. Frozen shoulder contracture syndrome. Aetiology, diagnosis and management. Man. Ther. 20 (1), 2–9.

Littlewood, C., Malliaras, P., Chance-Larsen, K., 2015. Therapeutic exercise for rotator cuff tendinopathy: a systematic review of contextual factors and prescription parameters. Int. J. Rehabil. Res. 38, 95–106.

Liu, S.H., Henry, M.H., Nuccion, S.L., 1996. A prospective evaluation of a new physical examination in predicting glenoid labral tears. Am. J. Sports Med. 24 (6), 721–725.

Lollino, N., Brunocilla, P.R., Poglio, F., et al., 2012. Non-orthopaedic causes of shoulder pain: what the shoulder expert must remember. Musculoskelet. Surg. 96 (1), 63–68.

Lundberg, B.J., 1969. The frozen shoulder. Acta Orthop. Scand. Suppl. 119, 1–59.

Manske, R.C., Prohaska, D., 2008. Diagnosis and management of adhesive capsulitis. Curr. Rev. Musculoskelet. Med. 1 (3–4), 180–189.

Matthews, P., Glousman, R., 2004. Accuracy of subacromial injection: anterolateral versus posterior approach. J. Shoulder Elbow Surg. 86A, 219–224.

McCann, P.D., Bigliani, L.U., 1994. Shoulder pain in tennis players. Sports Med. 17, 53–64.

Meadows, S., Smith, G., Vaswani, R., 2020. Physiotherapist survey: Increasing thoracic spine movement within the management of chronic subacromial impingement syndrome. J. Bodyw. Mov. Ther. 24 (1), 93–99.

Meister, K., Andrews, J.R., 1993. Classification and treatment of rotator cuff injuries in the overhead athlete. J. Orthop. Sports Phys. Ther. 18, 413–421.

Michener, L., Walsworth, M., Burnet, E., 2004. Effectiveness of rehabilitation for patients with subacromial impingement syndrome: a systematic review. J. Hand Ther. 17 (2), 152–163.

National Institute for Health and Care Excellence (NICE), 2017. Shoulder pain. https://cks.nice.org.uk/topics/shoulder-pain/. Accessed 3 September 2021.

Netter, F.H., 1987. Musculoskeletal System Part I. Ciba Collection of Medical Illustrations. Ciba-Giegy, New Jersey.

Neviaser, A., Neviaser, R.J., 2011. Adhesive capsulitis of the shoulder. J. Am. Acad. Orthop. Surg. 19 (9), 536–542.

Nordin, M., Frankel, V.H., 2020. Basic Biomechanics of the Musculoskeletal System, fifth ed. Wolters Kluwer, Philadelphia.

Owens-Burkhart, H., 1991. Management of frozen shoulder. In: Donatelli, R.A. (Ed.), Clinics in Physical Therapy, Physical Therapy of the Shoulder. Churchill Livingstone, Edinburgh, pp. 91–116.

Paine, R.M., Voight, M., 1993. The role of the scapula. J. Orthop. Sports Phys. Ther. 18, 386–391.

Park, S.W., Chen, Y.T., Thompson, L., et al., 2020. No relationship between the acromial distance and pain in adults with subacromial syndrome: a systematic review and meta-analysis. Sci. Rep. 10 (1), 20611.

Pellecchia, G.L., Paolino, J., Connell, J., 1996. Intertester reliability of the Cyriax evaluation in assessing patients with shoulder pain. J. Orthop. Sports Phys. Ther. 23, 34–38.

Petersilge, C.A., Witte, D.H., Sewell, B.O., et al., 1997. Normal regional anatomy of the shoulder. MRI Clin. N. Am. 5 (4), 667–680.

Pratt, N.E., 1994. Anatomy and biomechanics of the shoulder. J. Hand Ther. 7, 65–76.

Rangan, A., Goodchild, L., Gibson, J., et al., 2015. BESS/BOA patient care pathways: frozen shoulder. Shoulder Elbow 7 (4), 299–307.

Rangan, A., Hanchard, N., McDaid, C., 2016. What is the most effective treatment for frozen shoulder? Br. Med. J. 354, i4162.

Robinson, C.M., Seah, K.T.M., Chee, Y.H., et al., 2012. Frozen shoulder. J. Bone Joint Surg. Br. 94-B, 1–9.

Rymaruk, S., Peach, C., 2017. Indications for hydrodilatation for frozen shoulder. EFFORT Open Rev. 2 (11), 46208.

Saunders, S., 2000. Orthopaedic Medicine Course Manual. Saunders, London.

Schiefer, M., Teixeira, P.F.S., Fontanelle, C., et al., 2017. Prevalence of hypothyroidism in patients with frozen shoulder. J. Shoulder Elbow Surg. 26 (1), 49–55.

Schulte, K.R., Warner, J.J.P., 1995. Uncommon causes of shoulder pain in the athlete. Orthop. Clin. N. Am. 26, 505–528.

Scott, A., Docking, S., Vicenzino, B., et al., 2013. Sports and exercise-related tendinopathies: a review of selected topical issues by participants of the second International Scientific Tendinopathy Symposium (ISTS) Vancouver 2012. Br. J. Sports Med. 47, 536–544.

September, A.V., Schwellnus, M.P., Collins, M., 2007. Tendon and ligament injuries: the genetic component. Br. J. Sports Med. 41 (4), 241–246.

Shah, V.M., Routal, R.V., 2015. Structure of clavicle in relation to weight transmission. J. Clin. Diagnostic Res. 9 (7), AC01–AC04.

Siegel, L.B., Cohen, N.J., Gall, E.P., 1999. Adhesive capsulitis: a sticky issue. Am. Fam. Physician 59 (1), 1843–1852.

Smith, S.P., Devaraj, V.S., Bunker, T.D., 2001. The association between frozen shoulder and Dupuytren's disease. J. Shoulder Elbow Surg. 10 (2), 149–151.

Soames, R., Palastanga, N.R., 2018. Anatomy and Human Movement, seventh ed. Elsevier, Oxford.

Speer, K.P., 1995. Anatomy and pathomechanics of shoulder instability. Clin. Sports Med. 14, 751–760.

Stam, H.W., 1994. Frozen shoulder – a review of current concepts. Physiotherapy 80, 588–598.

Standring, S., 2015. Gray's Anatomy: The Anatomical Basis of Clinical Practice, forty-first ed. Churchill Livingstone, Edinburgh.

Stenlund, B., 1993. Shoulder tendinitis and osteoarthrosis of the acromioclavicular joint and their relation to sports. Br. J. Sports Med. 27, 125–130.

Tamai, K., Akutsu, M., Yano, Y., 2014. Primary frozen shoulder: a brief review of pathology and imaging abnormalities. J. Orthop. Sci. 19, 1–5.

Uhthoff, K.J., Sarkar, K., 1992. Periarticular soft tissue conditions causing pain in the shoulder. Curr. Opin. Rheumatol. 4, 241–246.

Uitvlugt, G., Detrisac, D.A., Johnson, L.J., et al., 1993. Arthroscopic observations before and after manipulation of frozen shoulder. J. Arthrosc. Relat. Surg. 9, 181–185.

Wadsworth, C.T., 1986. Frozen shoulder. Phys. Ther. 66, 1878–1883.

Ward, W.G., Eckardt, J.J., 1993. Subacromial/subdeltoid bursa abscesses, an overlooked diagnosis. Clin. Orthop. Relat. Res. 288, 189–194.

Whelton, C., Peach, C.A., 2018. Review of diabetic frozen shoulder. Eur. J. Orthop. Surg. Traumatol. 28 (3), 363–371.

Wiley, A.M., 1991. Arthroscopic appearance of frozen shoulder. J. Arthrosc. Relat. Surg. 7, 138–143.

Wilk, K.E., Arrigo, C., 1993. Current concepts in the rehabilitation of the athletic shoulder. J. Orthop. Sports Phys. Ther. 18, 365–378.

Wong, C.K., Levine, W.N., Deo, K., et al., 2017. Natural history of frozen shoulder: fact or fiction? A systematic review. Physiotherapy 103 (1), 40–44.

Wright, A.R., Shi, X.A., Busby-Whitehead, J., et al., 2015. The prevalence of neck and shoulder symptoms and associations with comorbidities and disability: the Johnston County Osteoarthritis Project. Myopain 23 (1–2), 34–44.

Wu, T., Song, H.X., Dong, Y., Li, J.H., 2015. Ultrasound-guided versus blind subacromial–subdeltoid injection in adults with shoulder pain: a systematic review and meta-analysis. Sem. Arthritis Rheum. 45, 374–378.

Zreik, N.H., Malik, R.A., Charalambous, C.P., 2016. Adhesive capsulitis of the shoulder and diabetes: a meta-analysis of prevalence. Muscles Ligaments Tendons J. 6 (1), 26–34.

Zuckerman, J.D., Rokito, A., 2011. Frozen shoulder: a consensus definition. J. Shoulder Elbow Surg. 20, 322–325.

SUMMARY

This chapter begins by outlining the relevant anatomy of the elbow and provides guidelines for palpation. A commentary on the history and examination sequence follows, leading to a discussion of the lesions that may be encountered.

Tennis elbow is the most commonly encountered elbow problem in clinical practice and presents a challenge to management. A treatment approach is suggested, and other common and more unusual lesions are addressed.

ANATOMY

Together with the shoulder, the elbow functions to position the hand in space. Anatomically, the elbow consists of two articulations: the elbow joint and the superior radioulnar joint.

Inert Structures

On the distal anterior surface of the humerus sits the *radial* and *coronoid fossae*. In full elbow flexion, these accommodate the rims of the radial head and coronoid process of the ulna. In full elbow extension, the olecranon fossa of the humerus accepts the olecranon process of the ulna.

The *capitulum* is roughly hemispherical in shape and articulates with the radial head. The *trochlea* is pulley- or spool-shaped and extends from the anterior aspect of the distal end of the humerus to the olecranon fossa posteriorly. Its prominent medial ridge provides a valgus tilt that contributes to the carrying angle of the elbow joint. It articulates with the trochlear notch of the ulna.

The proximal end of the *radius* consists of a head, neck and tuberosity. The radial head is cup-shaped superiorly for articulation with the capitulum. The periphery of the head is an articulating surface for the superior radioulnar joint, articulating with the inner surface of the *annular ligament*. The *radial tuberosity* gives insertion to the biceps tendon.

At the proximal end of the *ulna* is the massive, hook-shaped *olecranon process*. Anteriorly, the coronoid process arises with the radial notch on its medial side for articulation with the radius at the superior radioulnar joint. A subcutaneous *olecranon bursa* separates the posterior surface of the olecranon process from the skin.

The *elbow joint* is a synovial hinge joint between the capitulum and trochlea at the distal end of the *humerus*, and the proximal ends of the radius and ulna. The *superior (proximal) radioulnar joint* is a uniaxial pivot joint between the radial notch of the ulna and the medial side of the radial head. Both joints are contained within the same joint capsule.

The *joint capsule* surrounds the articular margins, originating anteriorly around the coronoid and radial fossae of the humerus and inserting into the annular ligament and anterior border of the coronoid of the ulna. Posteriorly it attaches to the olecranon fossa of the humerus and the olecranon of the ulna.

In common with other synovial hinge joints, the relatively weak articular capsule is reinforced by strong collateral ligaments.

The *medial collateral ligament* fans out from the medial epicondyle, where it is closely related to the common flexor tendon and primarily resists valgus stresses.

The *lateral collateral ligament* is a strong triangular band fanning out from the lateral epicondyle, where it underlies and shares a close anatomical relationship with the common extensor tendon. It runs on to blend with the annular ligament below.

The *radial collateral ligament* stabilises the radial head, preventing varus stresses, and the annular ligament stabilises the superior radioulnar joint.

The elbow joint has just two axes of motion and thus greater inherent stability than the shoulder (Miyasaka, 1999). It permits flexion and extension coupled with a small amount of adjunct rotation (Standring, 2015). Approximately 160 degrees of passive flexion occurs as the bones become almost parallel. The normal end-feel of elbow flexion is soft due to approximation of the flexor muscles. Passive extension is achieved by locking the olecranon into the olecranon fossa; it corresponds to a 180-degree angle and has a hard end-feel due to bone contact.

The *superior (proximal) radioulnar joint* permits pronation and supination. These movements occur between the circumference of the radial head in the fibro-osseous ring created by the annular ligament and the radial notch of the ulna. The annular ligament is covered internally by a thin layer of articular cartilage.

Movement at the superior and inferior radioulnar joints is rotation of the radius around the ulna to produce pronation and supination. The range of passive pronation is approximately 85 degrees, and passive supination is 90 degrees, normally they both have an elastic end-feel.

The *carrying angle (cubitus valgus)* is evident in the anatomical position. The medial end of the distal humerus projects more distally and anteriorly than the lateral, pushing the ulna laterally to produce this valgus angle. It is approximately 10 to 15 degrees in men and 20 to 25 degrees in women (Soames and Palastanga, 2018).

The *cubital fossa* is situated on the anterior aspect of the elbow. Its proximal border is an imaginary line drawn between the two epicondyles of the humerus; its lateral border is brachioradialis, and its medial border is pronator teres.

On the floor of the fossa lie supinator and biceps, and the roof is formed by the overlying skin and fascia. The contents of the cubital fossa, from lateral to medial, are the tendon of the biceps in the centre, the brachial artery and the median nerve.

The elbow joint receives a nerve supply from the musculocutaneous, median and radial nerves anteriorly and the ulnar and radial nerves posteriorly (C5–C8).

Contractile Structures

Biceps brachii (musculocutaneous nerve C5–C6) has two heads of origin. The muscle ends in a stout tendon that attaches deeply to the posterior aspect of the radial tuberosity. As the tendon passes to its insertion, it twists so that its anterior surface comes to rest laterally.

The tendon is separated from the anterior aspect of the radial tuberosity by the subtendinous *bicipital bursa*. The *bicipital aponeurosis* arises anteromedially from the distal end of the tendon and sweeps medially to blend with the antebrachial fascia.

Biceps is a powerful elbow flexor. Its secondary action, due to its insertion on the medial aspect of the radius, is to assist supinator in supination of the forearm, particularly with the elbow joint in 90 degrees of flexion; it has no supinating action in the extended elbow.

Brachialis (musculocutaneous nerve C5–C6) takes origin from the anterior aspect of the lower half of the shaft of the humerus and inserts into the coronoid process of the ulna. As it crosses the elbow joint some of its deep fibres insert into the capsule of the elbow joint. Its action is to flex the elbow in either pronation or supination.

Brachioradialis (radial nerve C5–C7) passes from a long attachment on the upper two-thirds of the lateral supracondylar ridge of the humerus to the distal end of the radius, just above the radial styloid. It flexes the elbow, being most effective in the mid-pronation–supination position.

Triceps (radial nerve C6–C8) has three heads of origin above the elbow, with its tendon inserting into the olecranon process. It is the main elbow extensor and is involved in pushing and thrusting activities as well as raising body weight on semi-flexed elbows, as in getting up from a chair.

Pronator teres (median nerve C6–C7) has two heads of origin: a humeral head from just above the medial epicondyle, the coronoid process and the common flexor tendon, and an ulnar head from the medial side of the coronoid process. It passes down laterally to insert into a roughened area along the lateral aspect of the shaft of the radius. Its main action is to pronate the forearm, especially against resistance.

Supinator (posterior interosseous nerve C5–C6) has its proximal attachment from the supinator crest of the ulna, lateral epicondyle of the humerus and the radial collateral and annular ligaments. It wraps round the elbow obliquely, laterally and distally, to insert into the proximal third of the radius, and supinates the forearm, bringing the palm of the hand to face upwards, throughout the range of elbow flexion.

Extensor carpi radialis longus (radial nerve C6–C7) takes its main origin from the lower third of the lateral supracondylar ridge (see Fig. 6.1), partly deep to the origin of brachioradialis, with some origin from the common extensor tendon. It passes to the radial side of the base of the second metacarpal.

Extensor carpi radialis brevis (posterior interosseous nerve C7–C8) takes its main origin from the lateral epicondyle via the common extensor tendon (see Fig. 6.1), in part deep to extensor carpi radialis longus, and inserts into the radial side of the base of the third metacarpal. It is very commonly involved in tennis elbow.

Extensor carpi radialis longus and brevis extend the wrist and produce radial deviation. They work synergistically with the finger flexor tendons by holding the wrist in extension, allowing the finger flexors to form an effective grip (Soames and Palastanga, 2018).

Other muscles that share the origin from the common extensor tendon with extensor carpi radialis brevis, and are also responsible for wrist extension, are *extensor digitorum*, *extensor digiti minimi* (see Fig. 6.1) and *extensor carpi ulnaris* (which also produces ulnar deviation) (Not shown in Fig. 6.1). All of these muscles are supplied by the posterior interosseous nerve (C7–C8).

Flexor carpi radialis (median nerve C6–C7) arises from the medial epicondyle via the common flexor tendon and becomes tendinous above the wrist before passing through its own lateral compartment under the flexor retinaculum. It inserts into the bases of the second and third metacarpals.

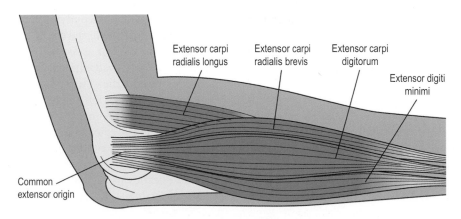

Fig. 6.1 Lateral aspect of the elbow in mid-position to show common extensor origin and tendons.

Palmaris longus (median nerve C7–C8), often absent, arises from the medial epicondyle via the common flexor tendon and passes over, not under, the flexor retinaculum, attaching to the distal flexor retinaculum and the palmar aponeurosis.

Flexor digitorum superficialis (median nerve C7–C8, T1) lies in a slightly deeper plane than the flexor muscles mentioned. It has a humeral head from the medial epicondyle, via the common flexor tendon, and a small radial head. It divides to pass under the flexor retinaculum before entering the fingers to attach to the middle phalanx of each.

Flexor carpi ulnaris (ulnar nerve C7–C8) has two heads of origin: a small humeral head from the medial epicondyle, via the common flexor origin, and an ulnar head from the ulna. It passes over the flexor retinaculum to pisiform.

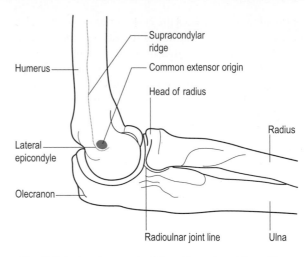

Fig. 6.2 Lateral aspect of the elbow in mid-position.

GUIDE TO SURFACE MARKING AND PALPATION

Lateral Aspect

Palpate the *lateral supracondylar ridge*, which is a subcutaneous sharp ridge, giving part origin to extensor carpi radialis longus and brachioradialis (Fig. 6.2).

The lateral supracondylar ridge terminates in the *lateral epicondyle*, a small bony projection that you will palpate more easily if the elbow is in mid-flexion.

Visualise the small facet on the anterolateral aspect of the lateral epicondyle that gives origin to the common extensor tendon of the superficial wrist extensor muscles. This facet faces anteriorly and is approximately the size of the patient's little fingernail. This appears to impose a mechanical disadvantage since large forces are transmitted through the *common extensor tendon* to this small site, leading to possible strain. The area may also be vulnerable to shearing stresses during all movements of the forearm.

Palpate the *head of the radius* on the lateral side of the extended forearm; it is located in a posterior depression just distal to the lateral epicondyle. Confirm the correct position by rotating the forearm to feel the radial head move under your finger.

Move a short distance proximally to palpate the *radiohumeral joint line*, just above the radial head. It can

also be palpated by dropping into the dimple on the posterolateral aspect of the olecranon.

The gap between the head of the radius and the capitulum of the humerus should be obvious; flex your elbow and feel the joint open, providing the most accessible point for an intra-articular injection. Flexion past 45 degrees tightens the joint capsule, making the joint line less apparent.

Identify *brachioradialis*, the most superficial forearm muscle on the lateral side of the forearm, by flexing the elbow against resistance in the mid-pronation–supination position.

Anterior Aspect

Palpate the *medial supracondylar ridge* that ends in the rounded knob of the *medial epicondyle* (Fig. 6.3). Identify the medial epicondyle, which is subcutaneous and most easily felt with the elbow in extension.

Palpate the anterior aspect of the medial epicondyle, which provides the attachment for the *common flexor tendon* of the superficial wrist flexor muscles.

Visualise the position of the superficial wrist flexor muscles by placing the thenar eminence of one hand onto the opposite medial epicondyle and spread the digits down the forearm to represent the following tendons (Fig. 6.4):

- Thumb: pronator teres
- Index: flexor carpi radialis
- Middle: palmaris longus

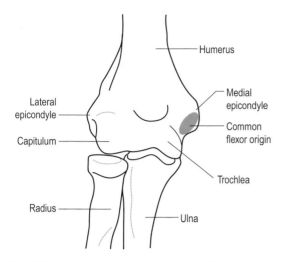

Fig. 6.3 Anterior aspect of the elbow in extension.

- Ring: flexor digitorum superficialis (deeper than the others and not so obvious)
- Little: flexor carpi ulnaris.

It is not possible to palpate the joint line of the elbow anteriorly because of the position of the flexor muscles, but it can be visualised approximately 1 cm below the elbow flexor crease that connects the medial and lateral epicondyles (Miyasaka, 1999; Soames and Palastanga, 2018).

Locate the tuberosity of the radius by flexing the elbow to make the biceps tendon more obvious. Follow the tendon down to its insertion onto the radial tuberosity. The tendon of the biceps will be easily palpable as it passes deep into the cubital fossa. The tuberosity is tender to deep palpation but it may not feel distinct to the palpating finger or thumb.

Place the arm in the anatomical position of elbow extension and supination and note the obvious valgus angle, known as the *carrying angle*. It should be symmetrical bilaterally.

Posterior Aspect

Palpate the proximal surface of the *olecranon process*, the point of the elbow, that is subcutaneous and most easily palpated when the elbow is flexed. The olecranon gives insertion to triceps and the subcutaneous olecranon bursa lies under the loose skin at the back of the elbow.

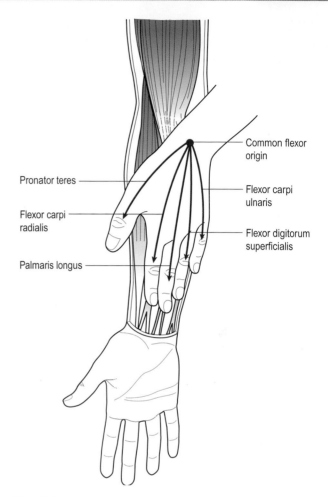

Fig. 6.4 The position of the muscles arising from the common flexor origin.

COMMENTARY ON THE EXAMINATION

Observation

Before proceeding with the history, a general observation of the patient's *face, posture and gait* will alert the practitioner to abnormalities and serious illness. The acute elbow joint with a history of recent trauma is usually held in a position of flexion and a degree of supination.

The more common lesions at the elbow are due to a change in use, i.e. tendinopathies, when abnormalities of posture are not usually apparent.

History

The patient's *age, occupation, sports, hobbies* and *activities* may give an indication of the nature of the onset and cause of the injury and can help the practitioner to reach a clinical diagnosis. They may also give an indication of whether the source of the problem is in the cervical spine.

Age may be relevant, as certain conditions affect particular age groups: for example, conditions such as 'pulled elbow' (a subluxation of the small radial head in the relatively immature annular ligament) affects children in the 1 to 4 years age group. Loose bodies can occur in adolescents, associated with osteochondritis dissecans, or in the working-aged/elderly group, associated with degenerative changes in the articular cartilage.

The lesions of tennis and golfer's elbow tend to be a problem of working age. Degenerative arthropathy generally affects the elderly, while rheumatoid arthritis may involve the elbow at any age.

The elbow joint and surrounding structures are situated within the C5–C7 and T1 dermatomes. However, the *site* of pain is usually well localised, indicating a superficial lesion. A *spread* of pain would indicate a more irritable lesion and possibly referral of pain from a deeper, more proximal structure.

Tennis or golfer's elbow may produce a diffuse reference of pain into the forearm as well as point tenderness over either the lateral or medial epicondyle, respectively. Olecranon bursitis produces local tenderness at the point of the elbow.

The *onset* of the symptoms may be sudden, due to trauma, or gradual, due to a change in use or arthropathy. If the onset is traumatic in nature, the mechanism of injury should be determined. Acute injuries include dislocations and fractures of the radial head, olecranon and distal humerus; distal biceps rupture; and posterolateral rotatory instability (Van Tongel et al., 2012).

Hyperextension injuries may cause a capsulitis, or a fall on the out-stretched hand may cause fracture (e.g. supracondylar, distal radius or ulna) and/or dislocation. Possible neurovascular complications, secondary to trauma, should be considered.

A sudden onset of pain associated with locking of the elbow could indicate a loose body.

The *duration* of the symptoms may be long-standing. The common presentation of tennis or golfer's elbow is pain of weeks' or even months' duration, while the less common loose body has recurrent episodes of twinging, often resolving spontaneously. Degenerative arthropathy is characterised by recurrent episodes of exacerbation of symptoms and has usually been present for months or years.

The duration of symptoms suggests the stage of the lesion in the healing process and will also give an indication for the likely length of treatment, with more chronic lesions usually taking longer to resolve.

The *symptoms and behaviour* need to be considered. Symptoms described by the patient can include twinges of pain with locking of the elbow, usually just short of full extension, which would indicate a possible loose body. A twinge of pain in the forearm on gripping is also associated with a tennis elbow, causing the patient to drop the object and giving an apparent feeling of muscle weakness. The elbow is affected in 20% to 50% of patients with rheumatoid arthritis and swollen and painful elbow joints, with significant stiffness in the morning, may indicate the condition (Mansat, 2001).

Paraesthesia may be indicative of nerve involvement and the exact location of these symptoms should be ascertained. Paraesthesia may be referred distally and in a dermatomal distribution from the cervical spine. The ulnar nerve lies in an exposed location behind the medial epicondyle, where it is occasionally subject to direct trauma and can produce paraesthesia in the nerve's distribution.

The behaviour of the pain indicates the nature of the lesion. Mechanical lesions are eased by rest and aggravated by repeated movements, particularly those involved in the mechanism of the lesion. For example, tennis elbow gives an increase of pain on gripping activities – simple things such as lifting a cup or opening jars. Patients often report that knocking the lateral aspect of the elbow can give excruciating pain and it is very tender to touch.

An indication of *medical history, other joint involvement* and *medications* will establish whether contraindications to treatment exist, or whether the lesion is part of an ongoing or new onset of inflammatory arthritis, for example. As well as past medical history, establish any ongoing conditions and treatment.

Explore other previous or current musculoskeletal problems with previous episodes of the current complaint, any treatment given and the outcome of treatment.

Practitioners should *screen* routinely for psychosocial factors and consider relevant health co-morbidities and lifestyle factors (see Chapter 1). These factors may contribute to the patient's presenting condition, or form a barrier to recovery and normal function, and should be addressed as an integral part of patient management.

Inspection

An inspection is conducted with the patient standing, with the upper limb resting in the anatomical position, if this can be achieved.

Assess the overall posture from above down, looking for any *bony deformity*, noting the position of the head, the lordosis in the cervical spine, the position of both shoulders and the scapulae. Assess the carrying angle in the anatomical position, comparing it with the other side for symmetry.

Inspect for *colour changes*, including bruising and abrasions associated with direct trauma. These may be located at the point of the elbow or over either epicondyle. Bruising over the biceps or triceps muscles can occur in contact sports where a direct blow is possible. Abrasions may be a site of entry for bacteria, with septic olecranon bursitis being a possible outcome.

Muscle wasting may be evident in the forearm if a patient has a long or recurrent history of tennis elbow. Other muscle wasting would be unusual and would probably be a neurological sign associated with cervical pathology.

Swelling is usually associated with trauma. It may be diffuse, engulfing the elbow area, in which case the elbow will be fixed in the position of ease, to accommodate the swelling with minimal pain. The dimples seen at the back of an extended elbow are obliterated if swelling is present, as here the capsule is lax and accommodates excess fluid. The 'popeye' sign of the ruptured long head of biceps can appear as a swelling in the lower arm.

Immediate swelling indicates bleeding and a possible haemarthrosis. Swelling developing 6 to 24 hours after trauma indicates synovial irritation and capsular involvement. Direct trauma can result in local swelling and a localised soft, boggy, fluctuating swelling may be seen over the point of the elbow, indicative of an olecranon bursitis.

Palpation

Since the elbow is a peripheral joint, the joint is palpated for signs of activity. *Heat* indicates joint activity which could be due to an inflammatory condition or infection (Fig. 6.5). S*ynovial thickening* has a similar cause and is most easily palpable over the radial head in chronic inflammatory conditions (Fig. 6.6).

Swelling is usually most apparent in the dimples at the back of the elbow and may be palpated in that area. Other swellings, such as that associated with olecranon bursitis, or nodules, can also be palpated to assess whether they are hard or soft.

State at Rest

Before any movements are performed, the state at rest is established to provide a baseline for subsequent comparison.

Examination by Selective Tension

The suggested sequence for the examination will now be given, followed by a commentary including the reason

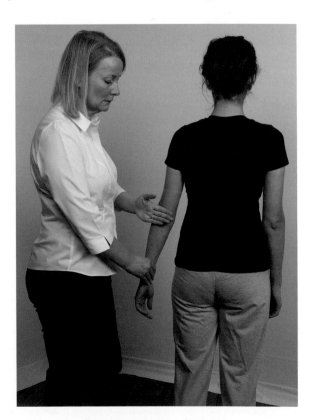

Fig. 6.5 Palpation for heat.

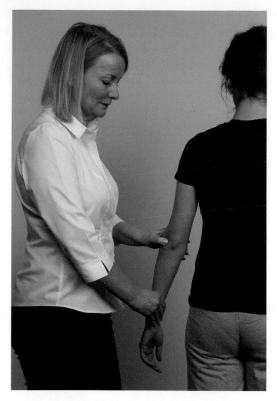

Fig. 6.6 Palpation for synovial thickening.

for performing the movements and the significance of the possible findings. Comparison should always be made with the other side.

It is important to screen other joints that may refer symptoms to the region. The 5th, 6th and 7th cervical dermatomes pass over the elbow joint region, and symptoms of cervical and/or shoulder origin should be considered and ruled out as necessary. Consider too the widespread area of referral associated with cardiac pathology.

The elbow joint and the superior radioulnar joint are assessed by four passive movements looking for pain, range and end-feel. Passive flexion normally has a 'soft' end-feel and passive extension has a 'hard' end-feel. At the superior radioulnar joint, passive pronation and supination have an 'elastic' end-feel. The signs elicited will establish whether the capsular pattern exists.

A loose body in the elbow joint produces a non-capsular pattern of movement with either limitation of passive flexion, or extension, but not usually both. The limited movement has an abnormal 'springy' end-feel.

Elbow and Superior Radioulnar Joints
- Passive elbow flexion (Fig. 6.7)
- Passive elbow extension (Fig. 6.8)
- Passive pronation of the superior radioulnar joint (Fig. 6.9)
- Passive supination of the superior radioulnar joint (Fig. 6.10)
- Resisted elbow flexion (Fig. 6.11)
- Resisted elbow extension (Fig. 6.12)
- Resisted pronation (Fig. 6.13a–c)
- Resisted supination (Fig. 6.13a–c)

Pain Provocation Tests for Tennis and Golfer's Elbow
- Resisted wrist extension for tennis elbow (Fig. 6.14)
- Resisted wrist flexion for golfer's elbow (Fig. 6.15)

Palpation
- Once a diagnosis has been made, the structure at fault is palpated for the exact site of the lesion

The resisted tests are conducted for the muscles around the elbow, looking for pain and power. Resisted elbow flexion tests biceps and resisted elbow extension tests triceps. Resisted pronation tests pronator quadratus and pronator teres, but since pronator teres takes origin from the common flexor tendon, this may be an accessory sign in golfer's elbow. Resisted supination tests biceps, since it is assessed with the elbow flexed, and supinator.

Movement	Main Muscles	'Assistors'
Flexion	Biceps brachii	Brachialis, brachioradialis
Extension	Triceps brachii	Anconeus
Pronation	Pronator teres	Pronator Quadratus
Supination	Supinator	Biceps brachii

Two provocative resisted tests are conducted at the wrist to assess the common extensor and common flexor tendons for tendinopathy. Resisted wrist extension and resisted wrist flexion are assessed with the elbow joint fully extended. Since they are not required to stabilise the elbow in this close packed or locked position, they contract strongly to resist the wrist movements and allow minor lesions to be detected.

To provoke pain, further provocative tests can be applied for tennis elbow, such as passive wrist flexion, resisted wrist extension from the flexed position

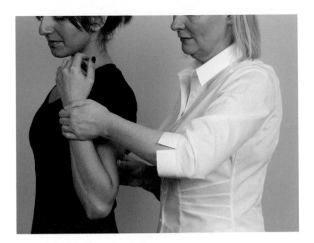

Fig. 6.7 Passive elbow flexion.

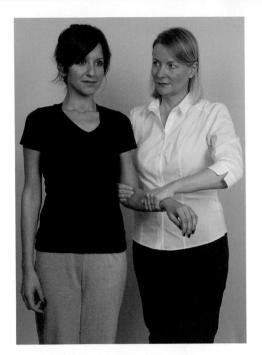

Fig. 6.9 Passive pronation.

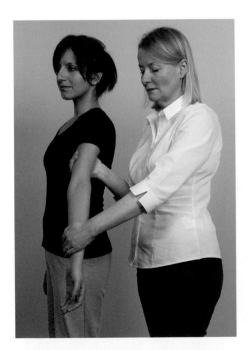

Fig. 6.8 Passive elbow extension.

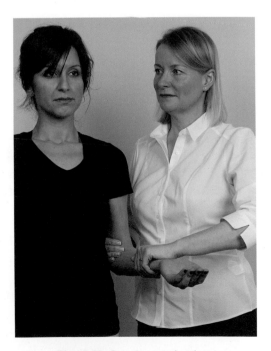

Fig. 6.10 Passive supination.

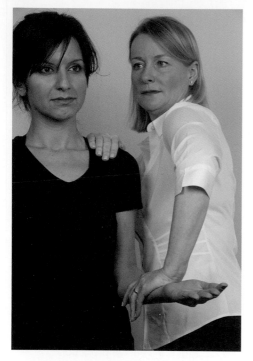

Fig. 6.11 Resisted elbow flexion.

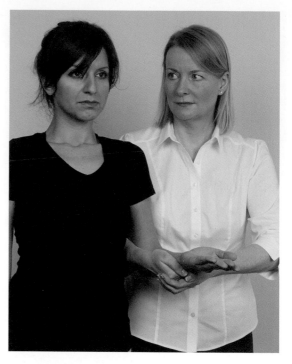

Fig. 6.12 Resisted elbow extension.

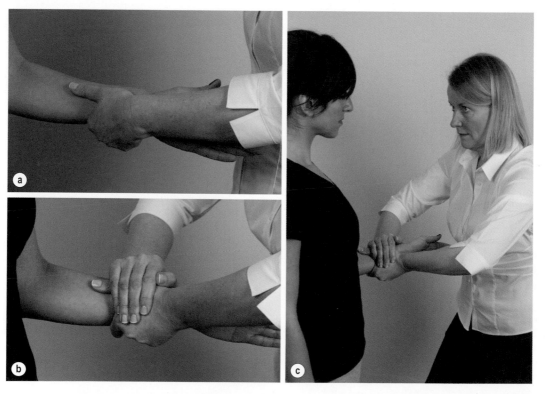

Fig. 6.13 (a–c) Hand and body positioning for resisted pronation and supination.

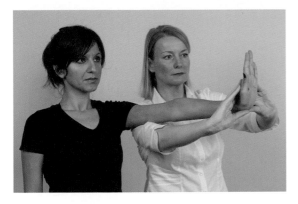

Fig. 6.14 Resisted wrist extension.

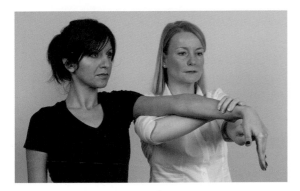

Fig. 6.15 Resisted wrist flexion.

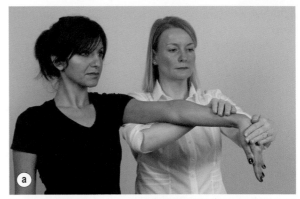

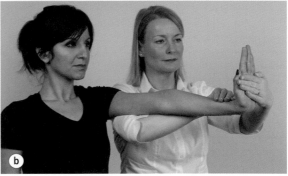

Fig. 6.16 Examples of further provocative tests: (a) resisted wrist extension from the flexed position; (b) resisted wrist flexion from the extended position.

(Fig. 16.6a), resisted radial deviation and resisted middle finger extension. For golfer's elbow, resisted wrist flexion can be assessed from the extended position (Fig. 16.6b).

Based on the history and clinical examination, the practitioner should be able to establish the most likely diagnosis, using clinical reasoning and clinical judgement.

It is important to recognise potential serious pathology, such as infection, malignancy, fracture and inflammatory arthritis, and to make any appropriate onward referral in a timely manner. Should additional information be required to aid diagnosis or to add value to management, further investigations can be considered to inform decision making and planning.

The practitioner may consider further investigations such as blood tests, radiological imaging, and other diagnostic procedures as an extension to clinical examination and to aid differential diagnosis (see Chapter 1). Investigations should be guided by suspected causes and are an extension to clinical examination.

Investigations are not usually performed routinely in a straightforward case of lateral elbow pain. However, in longstanding cases, plain X-ray of the elbow may show osteochondritis dissecans, degenerative joint changes or evidence of heterotopic calcification (Brukner et al., 2017). Ultrasound scanning is useful in assessing the degree of tendon damage as well as the presence of a bursitis. Electromyography (EMG) is used to rule out peripheral nerve compression.

CAPSULAR LESIONS

CAPSULAR PATTERN OF THE ELBOW JOINT
- More limitation of flexion than extension

CAPSULAR PATTERN OF THE SUPERIOR RADIOULNAR JOINT
- Pain at the end of range of both rotations

The capsular pattern indicates arthropathy, which at the elbow could be degenerative, inflammatory or traumatic. The history will direct you to the most likely cause. Differential diagnosis of elbow arthropathy includes osteomyelitis, septic arthritis, osteochondritis dissecans, intra-articular loose bodies and malignancy.

A stepped approach to management is currently recommended (NICE, 2020a). Less invasive treatments are generally offered first, including education/watchful wait, activity and work modification, simple analgesics and non-steroidal anti-inflammatory drugs (NSAIDs) medication, physiotherapy (e.g. exercise, mobilisation) and then injection therapy (e.g. corticosteroid, local anaesthetic, hyaluronic acid). If symptoms persist, more invasive treatments can be considered such as lateral elbow resurfacing or total elbow replacement.

The injection technique described affects both the elbow and superior radioulnar joint, which share the same joint capsule.

INJECTION OF THE ELBOW JOINT

Suggested needle size: 25G × 5/8 in. (0.5 × 16 mm) orange needle

Dose: 20–40 mg triamcinolone acetonide in a total volume of 3–4 mL

- Sit the patient with the elbow flexed to approximately 45 degrees and the forearm pronated (Fig. 6.17).
- Locate the radiohumeral joint line on the posterolateral aspect of the elbow.
- Insert the needle between the head of the radius and the capitulum (Fig. 6.18).
- Once intra-articular, deliver the injection as a bolus.

The patient should minimise or modify activities for 2 weeks following injection.

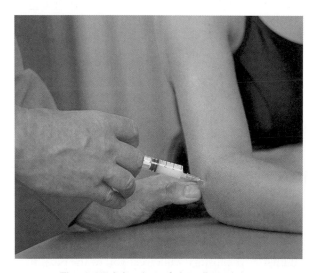

Fig. 6.17 Injection of the elbow joint.

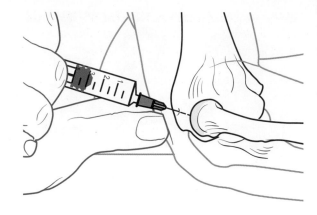

Fig. 6.18 Injection of the elbow joint, showing direction of approach and needle position.

Traumatic arthritis can be treated with other physiotherapy modalities to help with pain relief, and Grade A mobilisations and exercises can be given to increase the range of movement progressively within the limits of pain.

NON-CAPSULAR LESIONS

Loose Body

Osteochondritis dissecans occurs in adolescents and can give rise to loose body formation, particularly with activities such as gymnastics, throwing and racquet sports. Repeated compressive forces cause microtrauma between the radial head and capitulum and focal degeneration results in fragmentation and the formation of loose bodies (Patten, 1995; Steinbach et al., 1997). Surgical removal is advisable in this age group.

Loose bodies can also be encountered in the working-aged or elderly group. They are often associated with degenerative changes of the elbow joint (Saotome et al., 2006; Adla and Stanley, 2011). They may be a fragment or fragments of cartilage or bone, or both (osteochondral). They can be stable, fixed in a synovial recess or bursa, or attached to synovial membrane, where they tend not to be displaced.

Unstable loose bodies can move freely in the joint where they can become trapped at irregular intervals between the articular bone ends, causing intermittent symptoms and joint derangement (Bianchi and Martinoli, 1999; Adla and Stanley, 2011).

Characteristically, the patient complains of a history of twinging pain, with the elbow giving way under pressure or locking, usually just short of full elbow extension. The history alone may be the only diagnostic evidence available. Diagnostic imaging is usually necessary to identify and localise loose bodies before arthroscopic removal. Magnetic resonance imaging (MRI) is more sensitive than radiography for loose bodies, especially if the loose bodies are nonossified, and they are more readily identified if an effusion is present (Simonson et al., 2010).

Differential diagnosis of loose bodies at the elbow includes fracture, osteochondritis dissecans and joint arthropathy.

On examination, a non-capsular pattern may exist with either a small degree of limitation of flexion or extension, but not usually both. The end-feel of the limited movement is abnormally springy.

The treatment of choice to reduce a loose body is strong traction together with Grade A mobilisation, theoretically aiming to shift the loose body to another part of the joint, where it can be accommodated, and to restore full, pain-free movement.

The technique described below can also be useful for mobilising stiff joints, where traction is the key component for increasing mobility, while avoiding the extremes of each movement.

There are two possible techniques, both working towards elbow extension. The choice of which technique to choose is arbitrary. It may be necessary to try both and repeat the more successful technique, although sometimes one or more applications of the first technique selected is sufficient. As with all mobilisation techniques, the patient is reassessed after each one and a decision is made about the next, based on the outcome.

- Step forwards, taking the elbow joint towards extension (not full range), while simultaneously rotating the forearm with several flicking movements towards supination (Fig. 6.20).
- The technique is easier to perform if you begin the rotation from a position of some pronation.

Towards Extension and Pronation

- The patient's position is the same.
- Face the movement of pronation, placing the thumbs on the extensor surface of the forearm over the radius (Fig. 6.21).
- Establish the traction as above and step backwards, simultaneously rotating the forearm with several flicking movements towards pronation (Fig. 6.22).
- The technique is easier to perform if you begin the rotation from a position of some supination.

If the treatment couch is not suitable for the technique, an alternative standing position may be used with the patient's arm fixed against the edge of a door frame and with padding between the arm and the frame (Fig. 6.23). The technique is then applied as described above.

The patient may need to be reviewed to assess the success of the treatment. Generally speaking, the technique is usually successful, but the condition may recur. Excessive recurrences of the condition may need referral for a surgical opinion.

Olecranon Bursitis

Swelling and inflammation of the olecranon bursa can arise from repeated pressure and friction or to direct

MOBILISATION FOR LOOSE BODY IN THE ELBOW JOINT

(Saunders, 2000)

Towards Extension and Supination

- Position the patient against the raised head of a couch, with the arm resting against a pillow and the elbow in approximately 90 degrees of flexion.
- Use a butterfly grip with the thumbs placed on the flexor surface of the forearm over the radius (Fig. 6.19).
- Face the direction of the supination movement and lift the leg furthest from the patient off the ground, leaning out to establish traction with straight arms.

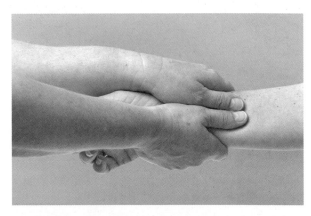

Fig. 6.19 Hand position for mobilisation for loose body in the elbow joint, towards extension and supination.

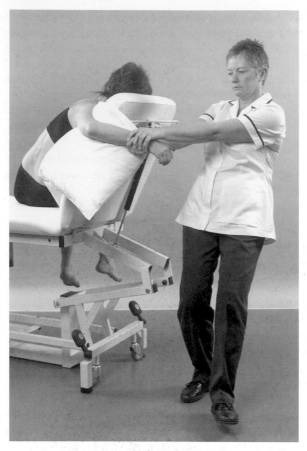

Fig. 6.20 Body position for mobilisation for loose body in the elbow joint, towards extension and supination: step forwards.

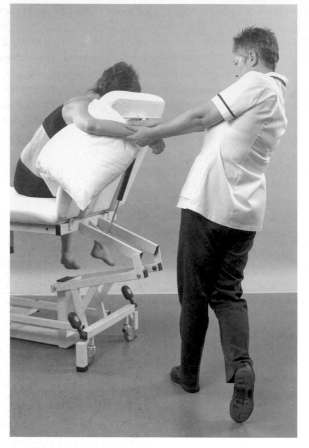

Fig. 6.22 Body position for mobilisation for loose body in the elbow joint, towards extension and pronation: step backwards.

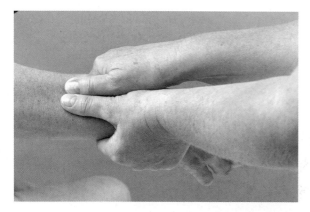

Fig. 6.21 Hand position for mobilisation for loose body in the elbow joint, towards extension and pronation.

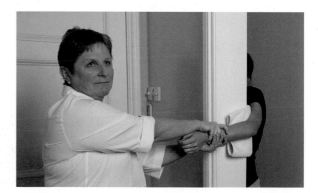

Fig. 6.23 Alternative position for mobilisation for loose body in the elbow joint.

trauma to the bursa. The bursa is vulnerable to trauma on the posterior surface of the elbow, and septic bursitis is not uncommon (Nicola, 1992; Hoppmann, 1993).

The patient may present with an obvious swelling over the olecranon that is boggy and fluctuant.

A stepped approach to management is currently recommended. Less invasive treatments are generally offered first, including ice, compression bandage, activity and work modification, simple analgesics and NSAIDs medication. If the practitioner is confident that the bursitis is not septic and the effusion is causing pain with impaired function, then aspiration with or without corticosteroid injection can be considered (NICE, 2021). This procedure is usually performed under image guidance.

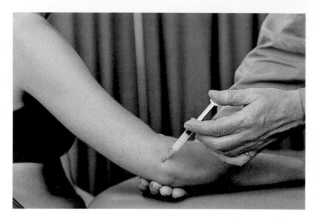

Fig. 6.24 Injection of olecranon bursitis.

INJECTION OF OLECRANON BURSITIS (KESSON ET AL., 2003)

Suggested needle size: 21 G × 1½ in. (0.8 × 40 mm) green needle

Dose: 10 mg triamcinolone acetonide in a total volume of 2 mL

- Seat the patient with the elbow supported in a degree of flexion.
- Palpate the obvious swollen bursa and mark a convenient point for inserting the needle.
- Insert the needle into the bursa (Figs 6.24 and 6.25).
- Aspirate first to check for the presence of infection and, if clear, the injection can be delivered as a bolus.

The patient should minimise or modify activities for 2 weeks following injection.

Pulled Elbow

This condition usually presents to the general practitioner's surgery or the Emergency Department.

Typically, the child is between 1 and 4 years old and has a sudden onset of pain in the arm followed by a reluctance to use the arm. The child is unhappy and holds the arm in elbow flexion and pronation. The arm is pain-free provided it is not moved.

There may be a history of the child stumbling or falling, or it may occur if the child grabs the cot rails or other stationary object while falling. Frequently, the child is accompanied by an embarrassed parent if the cause was pulling a resistant toddler or lifting the child by the hands and swinging him or her in play.

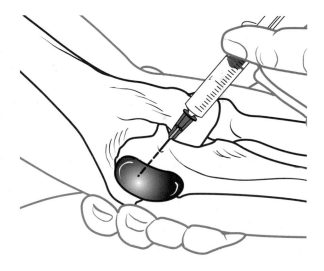

Fig. 6.25 Injection of olecranon bursitis, showing direction of approach and needle position.

The mechanism is thought to be a distal subluxation of the radial head through the annular ligament (Hardy, 1978; Kohlhaas and Roeder, 1995); however, X-rays taken before and after reduction show no evidence of displacement (Hardy, 1978). An X-ray is therefore of little value unless the nature of the trauma is significant when a fracture dislocation of the elbow must be ruled out (Brukner et al., 2017) and they can be missed. Kraus et al. (2010) reported that there were 11 cases of fractures misdiagnosed as pulled elbow over a 36-month period in a Paediatric Emergency Department.

To Reduce a Pulled Elbow

- Support the child's elbow with one hand, feeling the radial head. Provide axial compression towards the elbow joint with the other hand placed on the distal forearm.
- Quickly pronate the forearm through a small range while maintaining axial compression until a click is felt.
- The reduction is confirmed by immediate use of the arm by the child, to the subsequent relief of the parent.

CONTRACTILE LESIONS

Tennis Elbow

Tennis elbow is the most common cause of lateral sided elbow pain. The term 'tennis elbow' is not entirely appropriate for the condition, but it is still widely used (Keijsers et al., 2019).

Tendinopathy is the more appropriate term as a generic descriptor (Khan and Cook, 2000). The condition involves the superficial extensor carpi radialis brevis tendon in 95% of cases (Keijsers et al., 2019), and it is by far the most common lesion treated at the elbow, being five to eight times more common than golfer's elbow (Coonrad and Hooper, 1973; Gellman, 1992; Gabel, 1999).

Tennis elbow is common in the general population and affects people of working age (20 to 65 years), especially those in the 40 to 50 age group (Keijsers et al., 2019). Of all diagnosed cases, 35% to 64% are associated with work-related activities, with tennis players representing just 8% of the total diagnosed. Competitive tennis players are susceptible to tennis elbow though, with 50% experiencing at least one episode (Noteboom et al., 1994).

Occupation, repetitive loading and unaccustomed activity do appear to be factors, with heavier activities such as waitressing and manual labour bringing on the condition, as well as low-load activities, such as keyboarding, being the cause in a large proportion of patients.

In common with other tendinopathies, the aetiology is not fully understood. Cook et al. (2016) suggest a continuum model from disrepair to degeneration, with abnormal tendon structure and neovascularisation (Cook et al., 2016, Keijsers et al., 2019) (see Chapter 3).

The severity of symptoms is associated with changes observed on ultrasound scanning, including intra-tendinous calcification, tendon thickening and diffuse heterogeneity (Keijsers et al., 2019).

The dominant arm is usually affected and the patient complains of a gradually increasing pain felt on the lateral aspect of the elbow and posterior aspect of the forearm, sometimes referred to the wrist and into the dorsum of the hand. The condition is so common that patients often make the diagnosis themselves.

There can be a constant ache and the pain is aggravated by repeated gripping actions, together with rotation of the forearm. The pain is often worse in the morning and can fluctuate according to the previous day's activity.

Point tenderness is present over the lateral epicondyle, and patients will usually experience excruciating pain when the elbow is knocked – which they often report happens more frequently – possibly due to altered proprioception.

An apparent muscle weakness may be reported, as pain is often accompanied by a severe twinge that causes the patient to drop relatively light objects (e.g. coffee cup). Pienimäki et al. (2002) demonstrated similar subjective pain reports in tennis and golfer's elbow, but a greater reduction in grip strength was associated with tennis elbow.

Several factors can contribute to the condition and problems can coexist within the elbow joint and surrounding neural structures. Pain may restrict the range of active movement, and the relative immobilisation may produce an associated capsular pattern at the elbow joint.

Dysfunction at one site can cause dysfunction at others, and adverse neural tension can be a primary or associated cause of tennis elbow (Yaxley and Jull, 1993). A cervical lesion can refer pain into the forearm and mimic tennis elbow, or cervical syndromes can coexist with a lesion at the elbow.

Nerve entrapment at the elbow may also be a complication (Noteboom et al., 1994; Hartley, 1995). The posterior interosseous nerve (passing between the two heads of supinator) is susceptible to muscular compression. The upper edge of the superficial head of supinator is a thickened fibrous band forming a firm arch known as the arcade of Frohse, which provides a possible site for nerve entrapment. This may complicate the clinical presentation of tennis elbow and may be a reason for poor response to treatment.

On examination, there is usually a full range of pain-free movement at the elbow joint with pain on resisted wrist extension. Most authors and practitioners agree that pain on resisted extension of the wrist and tenderness to palpation over the lateral epicondyle at the insertion of extensor carpi radialis brevis are pathognomonic of the condition. Imaging is rarely needed in the initial workup of patients with lateral elbow pain (Keijsers et al., 2019).

Palpation determines the site of the lesion. Of the cases of tennis elbow encountered, most (1 in 10) involve the teno-osseous junction of the common extensor tendon with the remaining cases involving the body of the tendon, the extensor carpi radialis longus attachment on the supracondylar ridge or the muscle bellies (Fig. 6.26) (Cyriax, 1982).

Differential diagnosis of tennis elbow includes calcific tendinopathy, elbow arthropathy, radial nerve entrapment, osteochondritis dissecans of the capitulum and cervical radiculopathy (NICE, 2020b)

Treatment of Tennis Elbow

A stepped approach to management is currently recommended. Less invasive treatments are generally offered first, including education/watchful wait, activity and work modification, simple analgesics and NSAIDs medication, elbow clasp, physiotherapy (e.g. exercise, mobilisation) and then injection therapy (e.g. corticosteroid, platelet-rich plasma [PRP] or autologous blood

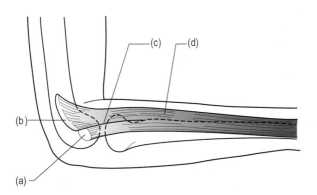

Fig. 6.26 Four possible sites of tennis elbow: (a) teno-osseous junction (enthesis); (b) supracondylar ridge; (c) body of the common extensor tendon; (d) the muscle bellies.

injection). If symptoms persist, more invasive treatments can be considered, such as open or arthroscopic debridement of tendinosis and/or release or repair of the damaged extensor tendon insertion (NICE, 2020b)

Treatment of tennis elbow should always look to address the causative factors. A full explanation should be given so that the patient shares in decisions on appropriate management and is responsible for modifying activities that may have caused or are aggravating the condition.

For example, lifting should be performed with the forearm supinated rather than pronated (Gellman, 1992), and various counterforce elbow or forearm supports are available to alter the stress on the common extensor origin or to rest the wrist to avoid strain.

With current knowledge that tendinopathy is more likely to be due to degenerative change than inflammation, educating the patient in terms of prognosis becomes important. Patients need to understand that a minimum of 3 to 6 months may be required to resolve their problem (Gabel, 1999).

In most cases, tennis elbow is self-limiting and with watchful wait and avoidance of aggravating activities, 80% resolve within 6 months and 90% after 1 year (Keijsers et al., 2019).

Definitive evidence for the treatment of tennis elbow remains elusive. Details of physiotherapy programmes are often hard to discern from studies, and the lack of standardisation of injection protocols makes it hard to make comparisons between the treatments applied.

Greenfield and Webster (2002) identified 24 different treatment modalities that, in the absence of evidence for the treatments, demonstrated that physiotherapists use judgement largely based on past experience when choosing treatment for tennis elbow. Progressive strengthening and stretching were identified as popular treatments, and 67.5% and 64.4% of respondents used transverse frictions and Mills' manipulation.

On balance, there tends to be little evidence that better outcomes are achieved with physiotherapy and rehabilitation if patients are willing to 'wait and see' (Smidt et al., 2002a; Nimgade et al., 2005; Bisset et al., 2006).

The manual approach to the treatment of tennis elbow in musculoskeletal medicine is Mills' manipulation, after transverse frictions to achieve analgesia, and with the approach being used by so many practitioners (Greenfield and Webster, 2002), the lack of evidence to support the technique is frustrating. Joseph et al. (2012) did find some weak evidence of benefit of transverse frictions for tennis elbow in combination with Mills' manipulation, but the lack of standardisation made it difficult to come to a firm conclusion.

The stages in the development of tendinopathy have now been proposed to guide treatment, with the application of progressive loading as a key component of rehabilitation, alongside other treatment modalities (Cook and Purdam, 2009) (see Chapter 3).

The earlier stages of tennis elbow may respond to a progressive loading programme (Cook and Purdam, 2009), but the more degenerative stage may respond to a combination of eccentric strengthening and stretching exercises, alongside other treatment modalities that aim to stimulate cell activity, increase protein production and restructure the matrix (Cook and Purdam, 2009).

The outcome of treating tennis elbow can be disappointing. The condition may be resistant to treatment and is prone to recurrence. Some recalcitrant cases can persist for more than 2 years (Keijsers et al., 2019).

The musculotendinous, neural, neurological and articular components should all be assessed in the resistant tennis elbow, although there is little evidence in the literature to confirm that addressing all possible components gives any better results.

Some cases of tennis elbow come to surgery, as a last resort, involving tenotomy of the extensor tendons at the lateral epicondyle. A review by Bateman et al. (2019) concluded that surgical interventions are no more effective than non-surgical and sham interventions, but they acknowledged that the studies reviewed were generally of poor methodological quality.

Cyriax (1982) and Cyriax and Cyriax (1993) describe four possible sites of the lesion:

- Teno-osseous junction – mainly extensor carpi radialis brevis
- Supracondylar ridge – origin of extensor carpi radialis longus
- Body of the common extensor tendon
- The muscle bellies.

Tennis Elbow at the Teno-Osseous Junction

Cyriax (1982) and Cyriax and Cyriax (1993) describe the teno-osseous junction as the most common tennis elbow lesion.

Pain is localised to the common extensor tendon at the teno-osseous junction, mainly affecting the extensor carpi radialis brevis on the anterolateral aspect of the lateral epicondyle of the humerus.

Treatment at this site is by Mills' manipulation, with transverse frictions being used to gain some analgesia prior to the technique. An injection can be considered as an alternative.

G. Percival Mills described his technique for the treatment of tennis elbow in the *British Medical Journal* in 1928. On examining patients with tennis elbow, he found that on combined pronation and wrist and finger flexion, the elbow joint could not achieve full extension. He suggested that forcing the restricted movement (now known as Mills' manipulation) could be curative.

The aim of the manipulation is to elongate the scar tissue by mobilising adhesions within the teno-osseous junction, thus making the area mobile and pain-free.

For the Mills' manipulation to be performed, the patient needs to have full passive elbow extension. This should have been revealed during the clinical examination, but it is wise to check again before proceeding. If the patient does not have full passive elbow extension on examination, the manipulative thrust will affect the elbow joint, rather than the common extensor tendon, possibly causing a traumatic arthritis. In this case, transverse frictions can be used alone, without the manipulation, applying the principles for chronic tendon lesions to provide pain relief for subsequent progressive loading exercises.

Before the Mills' manipulation is performed, the teno-osseous junction is prepared by transverse frictions to produce an analgesic effect in preparation for the manipulative technique.

When palpating for the facet for attachment of the common extensor tendon, remember that it faces anteriorly and is approximately the size of the patient's little fingernail.

MILLS' MANIPULATION
(Cyriax, 1984; Cyriax and Cyriax, 1993)

Preparation for the Mills' Manipulation

- Position the patient comfortably in sitting with the elbow fully supinated and in 90 degrees of flexion; this exposes the tendon by allowing it to run directly forward from the anterior aspect of the epicondyle.
- Locate the anterolateral aspect of the lateral epicondyle and identify the area of tenderness (Fig. 6.27).

- The site of the lesion should first be prepared by deep transverse frictions to produce an analgesic effect before applying the technique.
- Apply transverse frictions with the side of the thumb tip, applying the pressure backwards onto the teno-osseous junction (Fig. 6.28).
- Maintain this pressure while imparting transverse frictions in a direction towards your fingertips, which should be positioned around the posteromedial side of the elbow for counterpressure.
- Continue until the patient reports a 'numbing' effect (analgesia) at the site.

The Mills' manipulation is performed immediately after the numbing effect of the transverse frictions has been achieved (see the following section).

> **CLINICAL TIP**
> When performing a Grade C peripheral manipulation for appropriate chronic lesions, the transverse frictions are ONLY applied to gain some analgesia and should not be continued after the numbing effect, as when used in isolation.

Application of the Mills' Manipulation

- Ensure that the patient has full passive elbow extension.
- Position the patient on a chair with a back rest. Stand behind the patient:
- Support the patient's arm under the crook of the elbow with the shoulder joint abducted to 90 degrees and medially rotated. The forearm will automatically fall into pronation (Fig. 6.29).
- Place the thumb of your other hand in the web space between the patient's thumb and index finger and fully flex the patient's wrist and pronate the forearm (Fig. 6.30a–c).
- Move the hand supporting the crook of the elbow onto the posterior surface of the elbow joint, and while maintaining full wrist flexion and pronation, extend the patient's elbow until you feel all the slack has been taken up in the tendon.

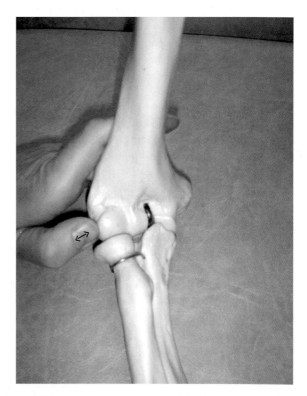

Fig. 6.28 Transverse frictions for tennis elbow, teno-osseous site, showing site of anterolateral facet on the lateral epicondyle of the humerus and the direction of application.

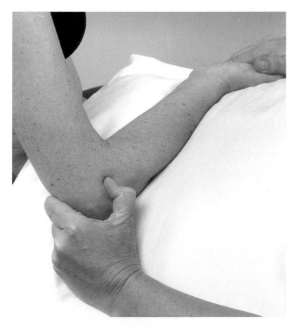

Fig. 6.27 Transverse frictions for tennis elbow, teno-osseous site.

- Step sideways to stand behind the patient's head, taking care to prevent the patient from leaning away either forwards or sideways, which would reduce the tension on the tendon (Fig. 6.31). Straighten your arm if possible, but be careful not to lose the wrist flexion.
- Apply a minimal amplitude, high-velocity thrust (Grade C manipulation) by simultaneously side-flexing your body away from your arms and pushing smartly downwards with the hand over the patient's elbow.

Rade et al. (2012) looked at myoelectric activity in the pre-manipulative stretch position for Mills' manipulation. They proposed that changes observed in myoelectric activity were in a pattern that suggested that muscle and neural mechanisms may be an integral part of the manipulation.

Cervical side flexion, towards the painful side, reduced activity in the peripheral nerves and biceps brachii and brachioradialis (the muscles that restrain the manipulation movement of elbow extension), thus allowing for a more comfortable technique and allowing the manipulative thrust to fall more specifically on the common extensor tendon.

However, with the mechanism of the benefit of applying the Mills' manipulation not fully understood, it is interesting to consider that neural tension may be a necessary and desirable component of the procedure. More work is needed to test this hypothesis.

There should be no reproduction of paraesthesia during the technique and, as discussed above, side-flexing the neck towards the painful side and moving the arm forwards a little may help to reduce neural tension (Rade et al., 2012; M. Rade, Nov 2013, personal correspondence) and alleviate this symptom.

One effective technique is conducted at each treatment session since it is not a comfortable procedure for the patient and the effects of treatment often become fully apparent over the following few days.

Between sessions, the patient is instructed to continue stretching the tendon to maintain length and mobility. An appropriate progressive loading rehabilitation programme should be applied.

Corticosteroid injection can be provided as part of the package of care for short-term relief if pain remains severe and function is significantly affected.

Several studies have concluded that corticosteroid injection is more effective for relief of pain in the short term (Assendelft et al., 1996; Verhaar et al., 1996; Smidt et al., 2002b; Barr et al., 2009; Gaujoux-Viala et al., 2009; Coombes et al., 2010). Corticosteroid injection alone may not give better outcomes at 1 year follow-up, however (Coombes et al., 2013), and a high rate of recurrence has been reported (Bisset et al., 2006).

Corticosteroid injections can produce more adverse responses than all other conservative interventions, including fat atrophy, skin depigmentation and rupture (Coombes et al., 2010; Chesterton et al., 2011). It should also be considered that corticosteroids can be potentially harmful to tendon tissue, and they should not be the first line of treatment (Keijsers et al., 2019).

Corticosteroid injection should only be considered when the patient requires pain relief, when they provide a

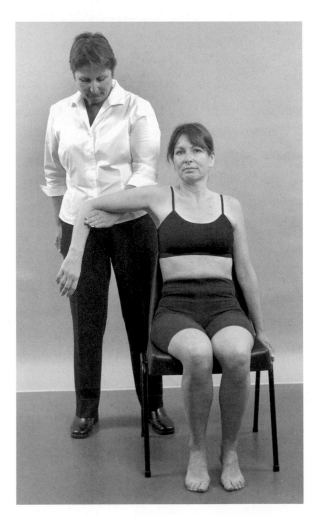

Fig. 6.29 Mills' manipulation, starting position.

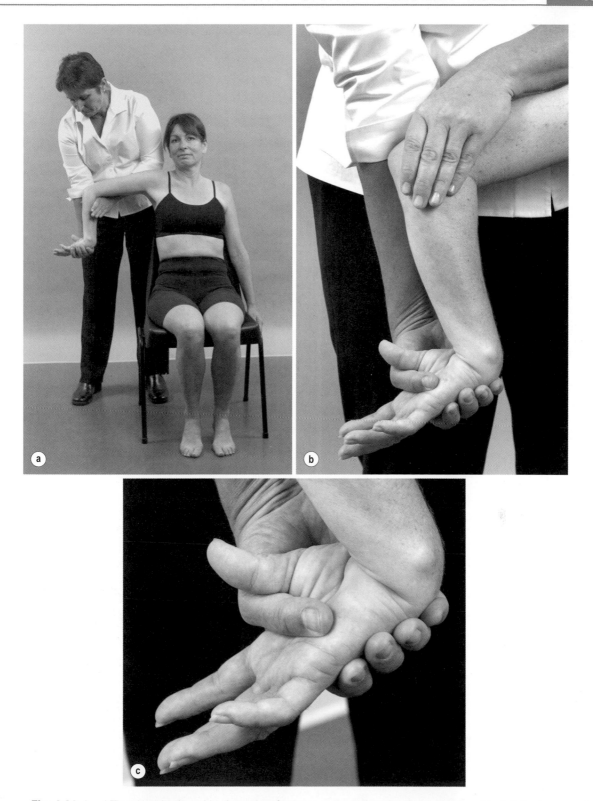

Fig. 6.30 (a–c) The thumb placed in the palm, forearm pronated and wrist maintained in full flexion.

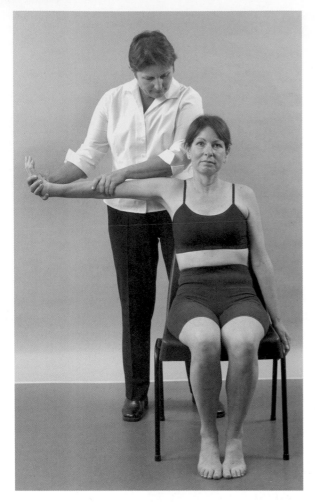

Fig. 6.31 Positioning of hand on posterior aspect of extended elbow for application of the Grade C manipulation.

window of opportunity to address causative factors and to introduce progressive loading towards full rehabilitation.

INJECTION OF TENNIS ELBOW, TENO-OSSEOUS SITE

Suggested needle size: 25 G × 5/8 in. (0.5 × 16 mm) orange needle

Dose: 10 mg triamcinolone acetonide in a total volume of 1 mL

- Support the patient with the forearm resting on a pillow, the elbow flexed to approximately 90 degrees and fully supinated (Fig. 6.32).

- Identify the area of tenderness over the teno-osseous junction of the common extensor tendon with the anterolateral aspect of the lateral epicondyle.
- Insert the needle from an anterior direction, perpendicular to the facet, and deliver the injection by a peppering technique (Fig. 6.33).

The patient should minimise or modify activities for 2 weeks following injection. An appropriate progressive loading programme should be applied

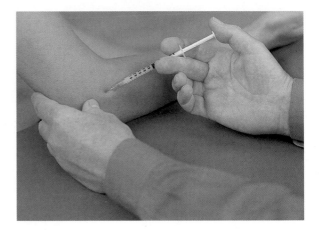

Fig. 6.32 Injection of tennis elbow, teno-osseous site.

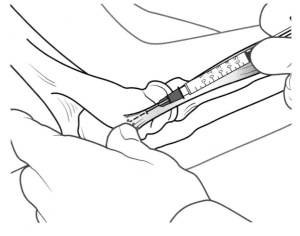

Fig. 6.33 Injection of tennis elbow, teno-osseous site, showing direction of approach and needle position.

TRANSVERSE FRICTIONS TO THE ORIGIN OF EXTENSOR CARPI RADIALIS LONGUS FROM THE SUPRACONDYLAR RIDGE

(Cyriax, 1984; Cyriax and Cyriax, 1993)

Transverse frictions are the recommended treatment at this site.

- Position the patient with the elbow supported in 90 degrees of flexion.
- Sit facing the patient, and place the pad of your thumb against the lower third of the lateral supracondylar ridge (Fig. 6.34).
- Direct the pressure back against the ridge and impart the transverse frictions in a superior inferior direction.
- Maintain the technique for an appropriate time, according to the irritability of the lesion and stage of healing, to achieve analgesia and to mobilise the tissues.

An appropriate progressive loading rehabilitation programme should be applied.

TRANSVERSE FRICTIONS TO THE BODY OF THE COMMON EXTENSOR TENDON

(Cyriax, 1984; Cyriax and Cyriax, 1993)

This site of tennis elbow is less common. The area of tenderness is located in the region of the radial head. Injection of the tendon is controversial and treatment is preferably by transverse frictions.

- Position the patient with the elbow supported in 90 degrees of flexion and the forearm supported in pronation (Fig. 6.35).
- Locate the body of the tendon over the radial head.
- Impart transverse frictions across the fibres.
- Maintain the technique for an appropriate time, according to the irritability of the lesion and stage of healing, to achieve analgesia and to mobilise the tissues.

An appropriate progressive loading rehabilitation programme should be applied.

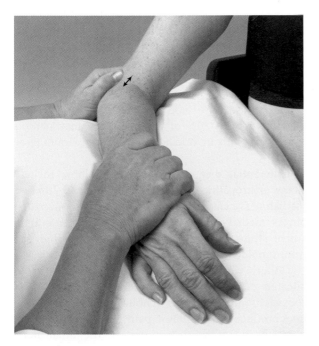

Fig. 6.34 Transverse frictions for tennis elbow, supracondylar ridge.

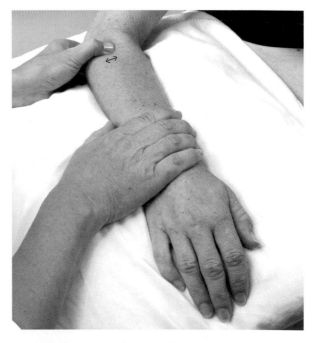

Fig. 6.35 Transverse frictions for tennis elbow, body of the tendon.

TRANSVERSE FRICTIONS TO THE MUSCLE BELLIES

(Cyriax, 1984; Cyriax and Cyriax, 1993)

The lesion is in the bellies of the common extensor muscles lying deep to the brachioradialis. This tends to present as an acute lesion following unaccustomed activity, but pain may also refer into the area from an acute lesion at the common extensor origin. Treatment with transverse frictions is usually successful and the lesion settles quickly.

- Position the patient with the forearm supported with the elbow flexed to 90 degrees and the forearm in the mid- position (Fig. 6.36).
- Palpate for the site of the lesion deep to brachioradialis.
- Grasp the affected muscle fibres between a finger and thumb and impart the transverse frictions using a pinching pressure applied up and down in a superior inferior direction.
- Maintain the technique for an appropriate time, according to the irritability of the lesion and stage of healing, to achieve analgesia and to mobilise the tissues.

The transverse frictions should be followed by Grade A mobilisation which can be continued and progressed as a home exercise.

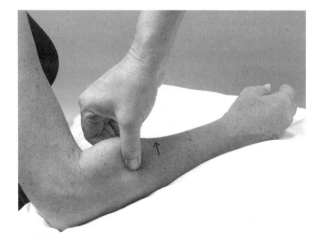

Fig. 6.36 Transverse frictions for tennis elbow, muscle bellies.

Golfer's Elbow

Although not as common as tennis elbow, golfer's elbow has a similar presentation, aetiology, disease process and management.

Golfer's elbow is believed to be due to the stress of repeated muscle contraction of the flexor-pronator muscle group which may also be combined with an associated valgus force such as when swinging or throwing (when swinging a golf club, tennis, archery, bowling or throwing overhead). Non-sporting activities, such as carpentry, knitting and embroidery, in which repetitive wrist flexion and pronation are performed may also be associated with this condition (McMurtrie and Watts, 2012; Kiel and Kaiser, 2021).

In the degenerative process of golfer's elbow, tendinosis is evident rather than the acute inflammatory changes of tendinopathy (Bennett, 1994; Patten, 1995; Kiel and Kaiser, 2021).

The patient presents with a gradual onset of pain on the medial aspect of the arm. This may radiate distally, but, in general, it does not refer as far as the pain experienced in tennis elbow.

The pain is aggravated by use and the elbow is often stiff after rest.

On examination, resisted wrist flexion with the elbow extended reproduces the patient's pain. There is usually pain and tenderness at the anterior facet of the medial epicondyle on palpation.

Diagnosis of golfer's elbow is primarily clinical (Amin et al., 2015). X-rays are usually normal and are more useful to rule out other causes of elbow pain. In 20% to 30% of patients, they may demonstrate periostitis or calcific tendinopathy (Kane et al., 2014).

Differential diagnosis for golfer's elbow includes elbow arthropathy, C6 or C7 radiculopathy, ulnar or median nerve entrapment, synovitis, loose body, osteophytes, medial epicondyle avulsion, ulnar collateral ligament strain, biceps tendinopathy, and referred pain from shoulder or cervical spine.

Golfer's elbow, generally speaking, is a less complicated condition to treat than tennis elbow, but coexistent ulnar neuritis (cubital tunnel syndrome) may produce medial elbow pain with tenderness and paraesthesia in the distribution of the ulnar nerve (Kurvers and Verhaar, 1995; O'Dwyer and Howie, 1995). The median nerve passes between the two heads of pronator teres and may also be subject to muscular compression.

Treatment of Golfer's Elbow

A stepped approach to the management of golfer's elbow is currently recommended. Less invasive treatments are generally offered first, including education/watchful wait, activity and work modification, elbow clasp, simple analgesics and NSAIDs medication, physiotherapy (e.g. exercise, mobilisation) and then injection therapy (e.g. corticosteroid, local anaesthetic, hyaluronic acid). If symptoms persist, more invasive treatments can be considered, such as surgical release of the common flexor tendon at the epicondyle and debridement of pathological tissue (Vinod and Ross, 2015).

There are two sites for the lesion: teno-osseous site and musculotendinous site. The common flexor tendon takes origin from the anterior aspect of the medial epicondyle – the teno-osseous site – and the musculotendinous site is just below. Palpation will identify the site of the lesion.

In the musculoskeletal medicine approach, treatment may be by either transverse frictions or corticosteroid injection for the teno-osseous site or transverse frictions alone for the musculotendinous site.

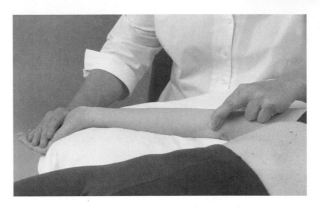

Fig. 6.37 Transverse frictions for golfer's elbow, teno-osseous site.

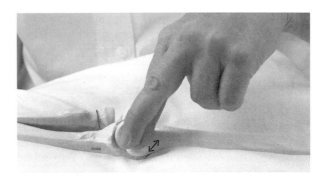

Fig. 6.38 Transverse frictions for golfer's elbow, teno-osseous site, to give an indication of the direction of application.

TRANSVERSE FRICTIONS FOR GOLFER'S ELBOW, TENO-OSSEOUS SITE

(Cyriax, 1984; Cyriax and Cyriax, 1993)

- Position the patient in supine lying with the elbow supported in extension and locate the area of tenderness on the anterior aspect of the medial epicondyle (Fig. 6.37).
- Using an index finger reinforced by the middle finger, and thumb for counterpressure, impart the transverse frictions by applying the pressure downwards onto the anterior aspect and sweeping transversely across the fibres (Fig. 6.38).
- Maintain the technique for an appropriate time, according to the irritability of the lesion and stage of healing, to achieve analgesia and to mobilise the tissues.

Relative rest is advised where functional movements may continue. It is important to maintain the length of the tissue, but there should be no overuse or stretching until pain-free on resisted testing.

An appropriate progressive loading rehabilitation programme should be applied.

TRANSVERSE FRICTIONS FOR GOLFER'S ELBOW, MUSCULOTENDINOUS SITE

- Position yourself and the patient as above and, using the index finger, move 1 cm distally to palpate the musculotendinous junction at the inferior edge of the medial epicondyle (Fig. 6.39).
- Maintain the pressure against the bone and impart the frictions transversely across the fibres.
- Maintain the technique for an appropriate time, according to the irritability of the lesion and stage of healing, to achieve analgesia and to mobilise the tissues.

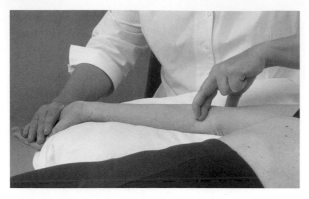

Fig. 6.39 Transverse frictions for golfer's elbow, musculotendinous junction.

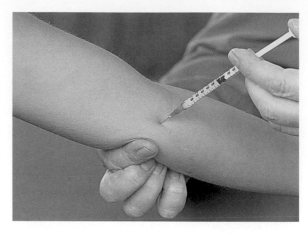

Fig. 6.40 Injection of golfer's elbow, teno-osseous site.

Relative rest is advised where functional movements may continue. It is important to maintain the length of the tissue but there should be no overuse or stretching until pain-free on resisted testing.

Corticosteroid injection can be provided as part of the package of care for a short-term relief if pain remains severe and function is significantly affected. As with tennis elbow, corticosteroid injections for golfer's elbow lead to short-term improvement but have a high rate of recurrence and are no better than other options in the long term (Stahl, 1997; Coombes et al., 2010; Krogh et al., 2013; Küçükşen et al., 2013; Mardani-Kivi et al., 2013). There is also a potential risk of fat atrophy, skin pigmentation and rupture.

Therefore, corticosteroid injection should only be considered when patients require pain relief and a window of opportunity to begin rehabilitation. The technique is described here.

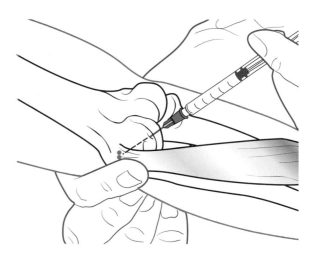

Fig. 6.41 Injection of golfer's elbow, teno-osseous site, showing direction of approach and needle position.

INJECTION OF GOLFER'S ELBOW, TENO-OSSEOUS SITE (CYRIAX, 1984; CYRIAX AND CYRIAX, 1993)

Suggested needle size: 25 G × 5/8 in. (0.5 × 16 mm) orange needle or 23 G × 1 in. (0.6 × 25 mm) blue needle
Dose: 10 mg triamcinolone acetonide in a total volume of 1 mL

- Position the patient with the elbow supported in extension and fully supinated.
- Locate the anterior aspect of the medial epicondyle and identify the area of tenderness.

- Insert the needle perpendicular to the facet (Fig. 6.40) and deliver the injection by a peppering technique (Fig. 6.41). Bear in mind the position of the ulnar nerve behind the medial epicondyle.

An alternative position for the injection is shown in Fig. 6.42.

The patient should minimise or modify activities for 2 weeks following injection. An appropriate progressive loading rehabilitation programme should be applied.

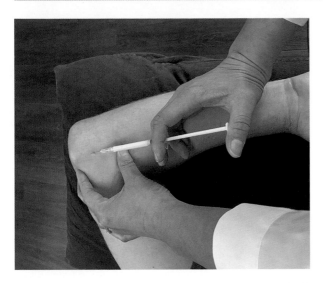

Fig. 6.42 Injection of golfer's elbow (alternative position).

Biceps

At the elbow, the lesion lies either at the insertion onto the radial tuberosity or in the muscle belly. It usually arises from a change in use and can be difficult to differentiate from inflammation of the subtendinous bursa at this site. The patient complains of pain at the elbow on resisted elbow flexion and resisted supination of the flexed elbow. Passive stretching into elbow extension can also cause pain.

A stepped approach to the management of biceps tendinopathy is currently recommended. Less invasive treatments are generally offered first, including education/watchful wait, activity and work modification, simple analgesics and NSAID medication, physiotherapy (e.g. exercise, mobilisation) and then injection therapy (e.g. corticosteroid, PRP injection). Surgical intervention is rarely indicated. It may be appropriate for partial rupture of tendons and is usually performed early (under 6 weeks) in a sub-group of patients.

Transverse frictions may be applied to the lesion at either site. The lesion at the insertion at the radial tuberosity is deep for access, and an injection of corticosteroid is an alternative treatment, preferably under image guidance.

Excessive friction may cause inflammation of the subtendinous biceps bursa, and differential diagnosis from bicipital tendinopathy may be difficult. A muddled presentation of signs is found, confirming the diagnosis of bursitis. Pain may be reproduced on resisted elbow flexion, passive elbow extension and passive elbow pronation, as the bursa is squeezed against its insertion.

A stepped approach to management is appropriate to treat the bursitis but injection is more likely to resolve the symptoms than transverse frictions.

TRANSVERSE FRICTIONS TO THE INSERTION OF BICEPS AT THE RADIAL TUBEROSITY

(Cyriax, 1984; Cyriax and Cyriax, 1993)

- Position the patient with the elbow joint flexed to 90 degrees and supinated.
- With your thumb, locate the insertion of biceps at the radial tuberosity and apply pressure against it, deeply and laterally (Fig. 6.43).
- Wrap your fingers around the forearm to provide counterpressure.
- Deliver the transverse frictions by alternately rotating the patient's forearm between pronation and supination while maintaining the pressure against the radial tuberosity.
- Maintain the technique for an appropriate time, according to the irritability of the lesion and stage of healing, to achieve analgesia and to mobilise the tissues.

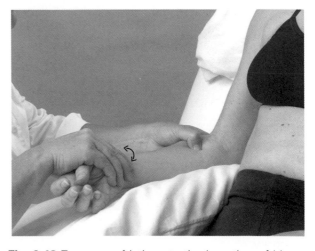

Fig. 6.43 Transverse frictions to the insertion of biceps at the radial tuberosity.

The injection technique is described here.

INJECTION OF THE INSERTION OF BICEPS AT THE RADIAL TUBEROSITY (CYRIAX, 1984; CYRIAX AND CYRIAX, 1993)

Suggested needle size: 23 G × 1 in. (0.6 × 25 mm) blue needle

Dose: 10 mg triamcinolone acetonide in a total volume of 1 mL

- Position the patient in prone lying in the anatomical position.
- Without changing the position of the glenohumeral joint, carefully pronate the extended forearm keeping your thumb in contact with the radial head to confirm your position.
- Insert the needle between the radius and ulna approximately 2 cm distal to the radiohumeral joint line until the resistance of the tendon insertion is felt (Fig. 6.44).
- Deliver the injection by a peppering technique to the tendon and adjacent area if the bursa is also involved (Fig. 6.45).

The patient should minimise or modify activities for 2 weeks following injection.

If the lesion lies in the muscle belly, the general principles of treatment can be applied (see Chapter 4).

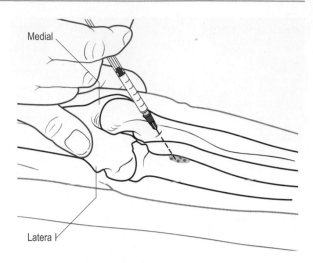

Fig. 6.45 Injection of biceps insertion at the radial tuberosity, showing direction of approach and needle position.

REVIEW QUESTIONS

1. Describe the technique of Mills' manipulation.
2. What is a pulled elbow? What would be the key clinical findings and differential diagnosis?
3. How do you treat a loose body of the elbow?
4. Palpate the two sites of golfer's elbow: consider the rehabilitation of a reactive tendinopathy.
5. What other factors do you need to consider when managing a chronic tennis elbow?

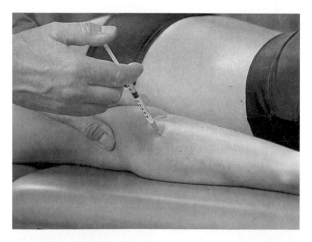

Fig. 6.44 Injection of biceps insertion at the radial tuberosity.

CASE SCENARIOS

Case 1

History

- Joanna, a 47-year-old receptionist, is a keen equestrian. She is complaining of fairly constant pain over the left lateral epicondyle following a fall off her horse 3 weeks ago when the horse dragged her by the reins along the ground for 10 m. The pain has gotten worse. Pain is aggravated by gripping, the arm feels weak and the bone sensitive. Pain is worse in the morning and especially after a busy day at work filing. General health good, previous left Achilles tendinopathy.

Examination

- Protecting the left elbow and not willingly moving the arm. Pain and limited elbow extension with a springy end-feel. Full and pain-free elbow flexion. Pain on resisted wrist extension with some apparent weakness. Tender over the common extensor origin.

Task

- Consider differential diagnosis and any investigations you may consider for this patient. Plan a treatment approach.

Case 2

History

- Susannah, a 55-year-old physical education teacher has a 3-month history of pain over the right lateral epicondyle following a sponsored volleyball match, where she played for 8 h without a break. Pain is aggravated by lifting and clenching her fist. The elbow feels stiff first thing in the morning.

Examination

- No obvious bony abnormality, full elbow movements with pain on resisted wrist extension. Tender over the common extensor origin.

Task

- Mills' manipulation is an appropriate treatment for this patient. Review the anatomy of the wrist extensor tendons at the elbow. What are the indications/contraindications for Mills' manipulation and the purpose of transverse friction massage?

Case 3

History

- Alison, a 45-year-old artist, has a 3-month history of pain over the left medial epicondyle. The onset was gradual, and she associates it with playing table tennis with her children. The pain is twingy in nature and is aggravated by lifting her large canvasses at work. She has had previous neck pain but is currently pain-free.

Examination

- Pain-end-range passive elbow extension and end-feel hard, pain on resisted wrist flexion and palpation of the common flexor origin.

Task

- Review the anatomical structures that originate on the medial epicondyle. Consider an appropriate treatment regime, home exercises and advice. When would it be appropriate to inject this lesion?

REFERENCES

Adla, D.N., Stanley, D., 2011. Primary elbow osteoarthritis: an updated review. Shoulder Elbow 3, 41–48.

Amin, N.H., Kumar, N.S., Schickendantz, M.S., 2015. Medial epicondylitis: evaluation and management. J. Am. Acad. Orthop. Surg. 23 (6), 348–355.

Assendelft, W.J.J., Hay, E.M., Adshead, R., et al., 1996. Corticosteroid injections for lateral epicondylitis: a systematic overview. Br. J. Gen. Pract. 46, 209–216.

Barr, S., Cerisola, F.L., Blanchard, V., 2009. Effectiveness of corticosteroid injections compared with physiotherapeutic interventions for lateral epicondylitis: a systematic review. Physiotherapy 95 (4), 251–265.

Bateman, M., Littlewood, C., Rawson, B., Tambe, A.A., 2019. Surgery for tennis elbow: a systematic review. Shoulder Elbow 11 (1), 35–44.

Bennett, J.B., 1994. Lateral and medial epicondylitis. Hand Clin. 10, 157–163.

Bianchi, S., Martinoli, C., 1999. Detection of loose bodies in joints. Radiol. Clin. N. Am. 37 (4), 679–690.

Bisset, L., Beller, E., Jull, G., et al., 2006. Mobilisation with movement and exercise, corticosteroid injection or wait and see for tennis elbow: randomised trial. Br. Med. J. 333 (7575), 939.

Brukner, P., Clarson, B., Cook, J., et al., 2017. Clinical Sports Medicine, vol. 1: Injuries, fifth ed. McGraw-Hill, Sydney.

Chesterton, L.S., Mallen, C.D., Hay, E.M., 2011. Management of tennis elbow. Open Access. J. Sports Med. 2, 53–59.

Cook, J.L., Purdam, C.R., 2009. Is tendon pathology a continuum? A pathology model to explain the clinical presentation of load-induced tendinopathy. Br. J. Sports Med. 43, 409–416.

Cook, J.L., Rio, E., Purdam, C.R., Docking, S.I., 2016. Revisiting the continuum model of tendon pathology: what is its merit in clinical practice and research? Br. J. Sports Med. 50, 1187–1191.

Coombes, B.K., Bisset, L., Brooks, P., et al., 2013. Effect of corticosteroid injection, physiotherapy, or both on clinical outcomes in patients with unilateral lateral epicondylalgia. JAMA 5, 461–469.

Coombes, B.K., Bisset, L., Vicenzino, B., 2010. Efficacy and safety of corticosteroid injections and other injections for management of tendinopathy: a systematic review of randomised controlled trials. Lancet 376 (9754), 1751–1767.

Coonrad, R.W., Hooper, W.R., 1973. Tennis elbow: its course, natural history, conservative and surgical management. J. Bone Joint Surg. 55A, 1177–1182.

Cyriax, J., 1982. Textbook of Orthopaedic Medicine, eighth ed. Baillière Tindall, London.

Cyriax, J., 1984. Textbook of Orthopaedic Medicine, eleventh ed. Baillière Tindall, London.

Cyriax, J., Cyriax, P., 1993. Cyriax's Illustrated Manual of Orthopaedic Medicine. Butterworth Heinemann, Oxford.

Gabel, G.T., 1999. Acute and chronic tendinopathies at the elbow. Curr. Opin. Rheumatol. 11 (2), 138–143.

Gaujoux-Viala, C., Dougados, M., Gossec, L., 2009. Efficacy and safety of steroid injections for shoulder and elbow tendonitis: a meta-analysis of randomised controlled trials. Ann. Rheum. Dis. 68 (12), 1843–1849.

Gellman, H., 1992. Tennis elbow lateral epicondylitis. Orthop. Clin. N. Am. 23, 75–82.

Greenfield, C., Webster, V., 2002. Chronic lateral epicondylitis: survey of current practice in the outpatient departments in Scotland. Physiotherapy 88 (10), 578–594.

Hardy, R.H., 1978. Pulled elbow. J. R. Coll. Gen. Pract. 28, 224–226.

Hartley, A., 1995. Practical Joint Assessment, Upper Quadrant, second ed. Mosby, London.

Hoppmann, R.A., 1993. Diagnosis and management of common tendinopathy and bursitis syndromes. J. S. C. Med. Assoc. 89, 531–535.

Joseph, M.F., Taft, K., Moskwa, M., et al., 2012. Deep friction massage to treat tendinopathy: a systematic review of a classic treatment in the face of a new paradigm of understanding. J. Sport Rehabil. 21, 343–353.

Kane, S.F., Lynch, J.H., Taylor, J.C., 2014. Evaluation of elbow pain in adults. Am. Fam. Physician 89 (8), 649–657. Apr 15

Keijsers, R., de Vos, R.-J., Kuijer, P.P.F.M., et al., 2019. Tennis elbow. Shoulder Elbow 11 (5), 384–392.

Kesson, M., Atkins, E., Davies, I., 2003. Musculoskeletal Injection Skills. Butterworth Heinemann, Oxford.

Khan, K.M., Cook, J.L., 2000. Overuse tendon injuries: where does the pain come from? Sports Med. Arthrosc. Rev. 8, 17–31.

Kiel, J., Kaiser, K., 2021. Golfers Elbow. StatPearls Publishing. https://www.ncbi.nlm.nih.gov/books/NBK519000/. Accessed 20 August 2021.

Kohlhaas, A.R., Roeder, J., 1995. Tee shirt management of nursemaid's elbow. Am. J. Orthop. (Belle Mead NJ) 24 (1), 74.

Kraus, R., Dongowski, N., Szalay, G., Schnettler, R., 2010. Missed elbow fractures misdiagnosed as radial head subluxations. Acta Orthop. Belg. 76 (3), 312–315.

Krogh, T.P., Bartels, E.M., Ellingsen, T., et al., 2013. Comparative effectiveness of injection therapies in lateral epicondylitis: a systematic review and network meta-analysis of randomized controlled trials. Am. J. Sports Med. 41 (6), 1435–1446.

Küçükşen, S., Yilmaz, H., Salli, A., et al., 2013. Muscle energy technique versus corticosteroid injection for management of chronic lateral epicondylitis: randomized controlled trial with 1-year follow-up. Arch. Phys. Med. Rehabil. 94 (11), 2068–2074.

Kurvers, H., Verhaar, J., 1995. The results of operative treatment of medial epicondylitis. J. Bone Joint Surg. 77A, 1374–1379.

McMurtrie, A., Watts, A.C., 2012. Tennis elbow and Golfer's elbow. Orthop. Trauma 26 (5), 337–344.

Mansat, P., 2001. Surgical treatment of the rheumatoid elbow. Joint Bone Spine 68, 198–210.

Mardani-Kivi, M., Karimi-Mobarakeh, M., Karimi, A., Akhoondzadeh, N., Saheb-Ekhtiari, K., Hashemi-Motlagh, K., 2013. The effects of corticosteroid injection versus local anesthetic injection in the treatment of lateral epicondylitis: a randomized single-blinded clinical trial. Arch. Orthop. Trauma Surg. 133 (6), 757–763.

Mills, G.P., 1928. Treatment of tennis elbow. Br. Med. J. 1 (3496), 12–13.

Miyasaka, K.C., 1999. Anatomy of the elbow. Orthop. Clin. N. Am. 30 (1), 1–13.

National Institute for Health and Care Excellence (NICE)., 2020a. Osteoarthritis: care and management. NICE. https://www.nice.org.uk/guidance/cg177. Accessed 3 September 2021.

National Institute for Health and Care Excellence (NICE)., 2020b. Tennis elbow. https://cks.nice.org.uk/topics/tennis-elbow/. Accessed 3 September 2021.

National Institute for Health and Care Excellence (NICE)., 2021. Olecranon bursitis. https://cks.nice.org.uk/topics/olecranon-bursitis/. Accessed 4 September 2021.

Nicola, T.L., 1992. Elbow injuries in athletes. Prim. Care. 19, 283–302.

Nimgade, A., Sullivan, M., Goldman, R., 2005. Physiotherapy, steroid injections, or rest for lateral epicondylosis? What the evidence suggests. Pain Pract. 5 (3), 203–215.

Noteboom, T., Cruver, R., Keller, J., et al., 1994. Tennis elbow: a review. J. Orthop. Sports Phys. Ther. 19, 357–366.

O'Dwyer, K.J., Howie, C.R., 1995. Medial epicondylitis of the elbow. Int. Orthop. 19, 69–71.

Patten, R.M., 1995. Overuse syndromes and injuries involving the elbow: MR imaging findings. Am. J. Roentgenol. 164, 1205–1211.

Pienimäki, T.T., Siira, P.T., Vanharanta, H., 2002. Chronic medial and lateral epicondylitis: a comparison of pain, disability and function. Arch. Phys. Med. Rehabil. 83, 317–321.

Rade, M., Shacklock, M., Peharec, S., et al., 2012. Effect of cervical spine position on upper limb myoelectric activity during pre-manipulative stretch for Mills manipulation: a new model, relations to peripheral nerve biomechanics and specificity of Mills manipulation. J. Electromyogr. Kinesiol. 22, 363–369.

Saotome, K., Tamai, K., Osada, D., et al., 2006. Histologic classification of loose bodies in osteoarthrosis. J. Orthop. Sci. 11 (6), 607–613.

Saunders, S., 2000. Orthopaedic Medicine Course Manual. Saunders, London.

Simonson, S., Lott, K., Major, N.M., 2010. Magnetic resonance imaging of the elbow. Semin. Roentgenol. 45 (3), 180–193.

Smidt, N., van der Windt, D.A., Assendelft, W.J., 2002a. Corticosteroid injections, physiotherapy or wait-and-see policy for lateral epicondylitis. Clin. J. Sport Med. 12 (6), 403–404.

Smidt, N., Assendelft, W.J., van der Windt, D.A., et al., 2002b. Corticosteroid injections for lateral epicondylitis: a systematic review. Pain 96 (1–2), 23–40. 2

Soames, R., Palastanga, N., R., 2018. Anatomy and Human Movement, seventh ed. Elsevier, Oxford.

Stahl, S., Kaufman, T., 1997. The efficacy of an injection of steroids for medial epicondylitis. A prospective study of sixty elbows. J. Bone Joint Surg. Am. 79 (11), 1648–1652.

Standring, S., 2015. Gray's Anatomy: The Anatomical Basis of Clinical Practice, forty-first ed. Churchill Livingstone, Edinburgh.

Steinbach, L.S., Fritz, R.C., Tirman, P.F.J., et al., 1997. Magnetic resonance imaging of the elbow. Europ. J. Radiol. 25, 223–241.

Van Tongel, A., Macdonald, P., Van Riet, R., Dubberley, J., 2012. Elbow arthroscopy in acute injuries. Knee Surg. Sports Traumatol. Arthrosc. 20, 2542–2548.

Verhaar, J.A.N., Walenkamp, G.H.I.M., van Mameren, H., et al., 1996. Local corticosteroid injection versus Cyriax-type physiotherapy for tennis elbow. J. Bone Joint Surg. 78B, 128–132.

Vinod, A.V., Ross, G., 2015. An effective approach to diagnosis and surgical repair of refractory medial epicondylitis. J. Shoulder Elbow Surg. 24 (8), 1172–1177.

Yaxley, G.A., Jull, G.A., 1993. Adverse neural tension in the neural system: a preliminary study of tennis elbow. Aust. J. Physiother. 39, 15–22.

The Wrist and Hand

CHAPTER CONTENTS

SUMMARY

This chapter takes a pragmatic approach to the identification of specific lesions at the wrist and hand and suggests localised treatment that can form a component of overall management. It begins with a description of the relevant anatomy to enable accurate treatment to the lesions presented.

ANATOMY

The bones of the wrist and hand comprise the distal ends of the radius and ulna, proximal and distal rows of carpal bones, metacarpals, and phalanges (Fig. 7.1).

The following paragraphs describe the articulations between them.

Inert Structures

The *distal radioulnar joint* is a pivot joint between the head of the ulna and the ulnar notch of the radius. Linked mechanically to the superior radioulnar joint, it is responsible for the movements of pronation (85 degrees) and supination (90 degrees).

A *triangular fibrocartilaginous articular disc complex* closes the distal radioulnar joint inferiorly and is the

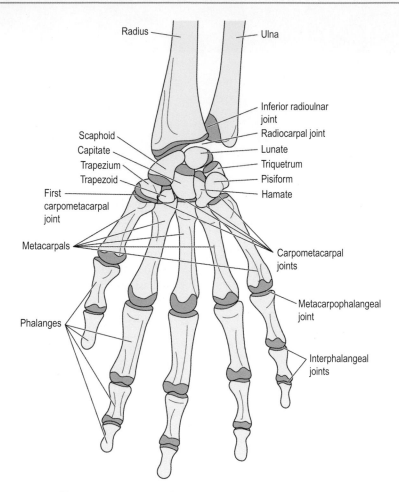

Fig. 7.1 Bones of the wrist and hand – palmar aspect.

main structure uniting the radius and ulna (Soames and Palastanga, 2018). It lies in a horizontal plane, attaching to the ulnar styloid and to the lower edge of the ulnar notch of the radius.

The disc articulates with the lunate when the hand is in ulnar deviation. It adds to the stability of the joint and acts as an articular cushion for the ulnar side of the carpus, absorbing compression, traction, and shearing forces but being prone to degenerative changes (Livengood, 1992; Rettig, 1994; Wright et al., 1994; Steinberg and Plancher, 1995). The disc itself has no nerve supply, suggesting that pain associated with traumatic and degenerative disc lesions at the wrist must have other causes (Unglaub et al., 2012).

The movements of pronation and supination rotate the radius around the ulna. Supination is stronger;

hence the thread of nuts and screws that are tightened by supination in right-handed people.

The *wrist joint*, or radiocarpal joint, is a biaxial, ellipsoid joint between the distal end of the radius and the articular disc and the proximal row of bones within the *carpus*.

The wrist joint is surrounded by a fibrous capsule lined with synovial membrane and reinforced by collateral ligaments. Both collateral ligaments pass from the appropriate styloid process to the carpal bones on the medial and lateral sides of the carpus. A fibrocartilaginous *meniscus* projects into the joint from the ulnar collateral ligament.

Within the carpus, there are two rows of carpal bones (Fig. 7.2). On the palmar aspect, from the radial to the ulnar side, they are:

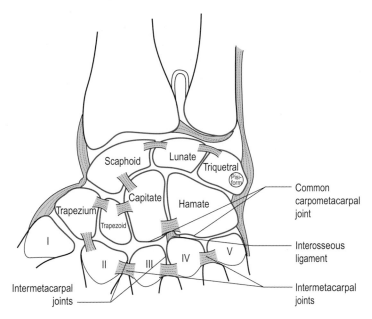

Fig. 7.2 Carpal bones. (From Soames and Palastanga, 2018. Reprinted by permission of Elsevier Ltd.)

- Proximal row: *scaphoid, lunate, triquetral, pisiform*
- Distal row: *trapezium, trapezoid, capitate, hamate.*

The wrist joint complex includes the *midcarpal joint*, between the two rows of carpal bones, and has mobility as well as stability, which is important for the function of the hand.

The carpal bones all articulate with their neighbours, except pisiform, which is a separate sesamoid bone that sits on the palmar aspect of triquetral. The intercarpal joints are all supported by intercarpal ligaments.

Movements at the wrist are extension (passive, 85 degrees), flexion (passive, 85 degrees), ulnar deviation (passive, 45 degrees), radial deviation (passive, 15 degrees) and circumduction. The close-packed position of the wrist joint is full extension.

There are five *carpometacarpal joints* between the carpus and the metacarpals. The *first carpometacarpal joint (trapeziometacarpal joint)* is a saddle joint with a loose articular capsule and extensive joint surfaces, giving it a wide range of movement.

The first metacarpal has been rotated medially for the movement of opposition. Flexion and extension occur in a plane parallel to the palm of the hand, while abduction and adduction occur in a plane at right angles to the palm of the hand (Fig. 7.3a–d).

The close-packed position of the first carpometacarpal joint is strong opposition when great force is transmitted to the joint. The functionally opposed thumb is subjected to compressive stresses that make the joint vulnerable to degenerative arthropathy.

The *metacarpophalangeal joints* are normally considered to be ellipsoid, but irregularities on the metacarpal heads can lead to their classification as bicondylar; the *interphalangeal joints* are hinge joints. Both are supported by palmar and collateral ligaments, and the extensor tendons and digital expansions support the dorsal surfaces of the joints.

The *flexor retinaculum*, a strong fibrous band across the carpus, creates a fibro-osseous passage, the *carpal tunnel*, through which pass the flexor tendons of the digits, the median nerve and vessels. The flexor retinaculum has four points of attachment: the pisiform and hook of hamate medially and the tuberosity of the scaphoid and ridge of trapezium laterally (Fig. 7.4). Its attachment onto the trapezium splits to form a separate compartment for the tendon of flexor carpi radialis.

The *median nerve* enters the carpal tunnel deep to palmaris longus. It shares its compartment of the carpal tunnel with nine tendons comprising the four tendons of flexor digitorum superficialis, the four tendons of flexor digitorum profundus, and flexor pollicis longus.

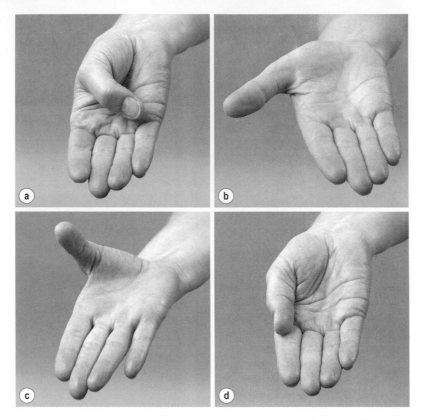

Fig. 7.3 Movements of the metacarpophalangeal joint of the thumb: (a) flexion; (b) extension; (c) abduction; (d) adduction.

On leaving the carpal tunnel, the median nerve supplies the thenar muscles before dividing into four or five digital branches.

The wrist and hand joints receive a nerve supply from branches of the radial, median and ulnar nerves (C6, 7 and 8).

Contractile Structures

Pronator quadratus (median nerve C8, T1) binds the lower part of the radius and ulna and is the principal pronator of the forearm.

Palmaris longus (median nerve C7–C8) passes over, not under, the flexor retinaculum, to attach to the distal part of the flexor retinaculum and the palmar aponeurosis.

The flexor muscles on the palmar aspect of the wrist are presented here first, followed by the wrist and finger extensors, the thumb tendons, and then the small muscles of the hand.

At the palmar aspect of the wrist and in the hand, the flexor tendons described below pass under the flexor retinaculum and are contained within synovial sheaths (Standring, 2015; Fig. 7.5).

Flexor carpi radialis (median nerve C6–C7) is the most lateral superficial flexor tendon. It passes through its own fibro-osseous compartment on the lateral side of the carpal tunnel to insert into the base of the second and third metacarpals.

Flexor digitorum superficialis (median nerve C7–C8, T1) lies medial to palmaris longus but is not as visible as it lies in a slightly deeper plane. In the carpal tunnel, the four tendons of the muscle are contained within the same synovial sheath, with tendons to the third and fourth fingers lying superficial to those to the second and fifth. Each tendon divides to provide a passage for the flexor digitorum profundus tendons before continuing to insert at either side of the middle phalanx.

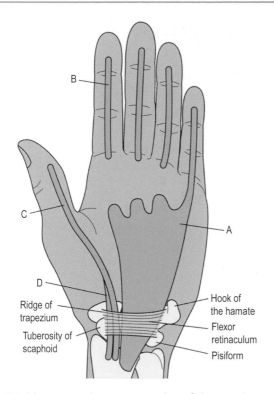

B

C

A

D

Ridge of trapezium

Tuberosity of scaphoid

Hook of the hamate

Flexor retinaculum

Pisiform

Fig. 7.4 Diagrammatic representation of the attachment of the flexor retinaculum and adjacent synovial sheaths of A - flexors digitorum superficialis and profundus, B – Flexor tendon in the fingers, C – Flexor pollicis longus, D – Flexor carpi radialis. (From Soames and Palastanga, 2018. Reprinted by permission of Elsevier Ltd.)

Flexor digitorum profundus (medial part supplied by the ulnar nerve; lateral part supplied by the median nerve C8, T1) divides into four tendons that lie deep to flexor digitorum superficialis in the carpal tunnel. They pass through tunnels created by superficialis and attach to the distal phalanx of each finger.

Flexor carpi ulnaris (ulnar nerve C7–C8) is the most medial superficial flexor tendon and can be traced easily onto its insertion into pisiform. The tendon sends slips onwards as the pisohamate and pisofifth-metacarpal ligaments. The pisohamate ligament converts the space between pisiform and the hamate into a tunnel (tunnel of Guyon) for the passage of the ulnar vessels and nerves. This tendon does not pass under the carpal tunnel and is not contained within a synovial sheath.

Extensor carpi radialis longus (radial nerve C6–C7) and *extensor carpi radialis brevis* (posterior interosseous nerve C7–C8) pass deep to the tendons of abductor pollicis longus and extensor pollicis brevis, under the extensor retinaculum, to attach to the radial side of the base of the second and third metacarpals, respectively.

Extensor digitorum (posterior interosseous nerve C7–C8) divides into four tendons that pass under the extensor retinaculum to insert into the dorsal digital expansions of the fingers.

Extensor carpi ulnaris (posterior interosseous nerve C7–C8) lies in a groove between the head of the ulna and the styloid process under the extensor retinaculum. It attaches to the medial side of the base of the fifth metacarpal.

Extensor digiti minimi (posterior interosseous nerve C7–C8) inserts into the dorsal digital expansion of the little finger.

Extensor indicis (posterior interosseous nerve C7–C8) joins the ulnar side of the extensor digitorum tendon, passing to the index finger.

Flexor pollicis longus (median nerve C8, T1) passes through the lateral side of the carpal tunnel and inserts into the palmar aspect of the base of the distal phalanx of the thumb.

Abductor pollicis longus and *extensor pollicis brevis* (posterior interosseous nerve C7–C8) become tendinous and superficial in the lower forearm where they cross the tendons of extensor carpi radialis longus and brevis at an intersection point, a site of potential friction (Fig. 7.6). They occupy the same synovial sheath in the first compartment of the extensor retinaculum and form the lateral border of the anatomical snuffbox.

The abductor pollicis longus inserts into the base of the first metacarpal and extensor pollicis brevis into the base of the proximal phalanx. Because of its position, abductor pollicis longus has also been considered both anatomically and functionally to be a radial deviator of the wrist (Elliott, 1992a).

Extensor pollicis longus (posterior interosseous nerve C7–C8) deviates around the ulnar side of the dorsal tubercle of the radius to pass to the base of the distal phalanx of the thumb. It forms the medial border of the anatomical snuffbox (Fig. 7.6).

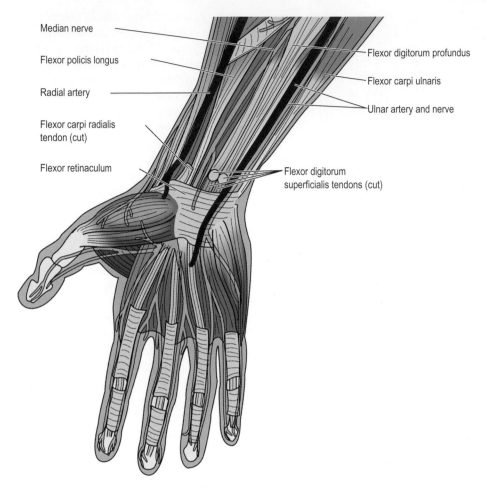

Median nerve

Flexor policis longus

Radial artery

Flexor carpi radialis tendon (cut)

Flexor retinaculum

Flexor digitorum profundus

Flexor carpi ulnaris

Ulnar artery and nerve

Flexor digitorum superficialis tendons (cut)

Fig. 7.5 Palmar aspect of the wrist showing position of the flexor retinaculum, its adjacent tendons and nerves.

The *radial artery* passes under abductor pollicis longus and extensor pollicis brevis, crossing the snuff-box obliquely towards the first dorsal interosseous muscle. Its position should be noted so that it can be avoided when injecting the first carpometacarpal joint (Fig. 7.6).

The *lumbricals* are four small muscles that arise from the flexor digitorum profundus tendons and pass to the radial side of the dorsal digital expansions of each finger. With attachments that link flexor and extensor tendons, they function by flexing the metacarpophalangeal joints and extending the interphalangeal joints. The first two lumbricals are supplied by the median nerve, and the third and fourth by the ulnar nerve, C8, T1.

The *dorsal interossei* (ulnar nerve C8, T1) are four bipennate muscles arising from adjacent sides of the metacarpal bones and inserting into the dorsal digital expansion and base of the proximal phalanx of the appropriate finger. They abduct the fingers from the midline of the middle finger.

The *palmar interossei* (ulnar nerve C8, T1) are four smaller muscles originating from the palmar aspect of the metacarpal bones and inserting into the dorsal digital expansions of the appropriate finger. They are responsible for adducting the fingers towards the middle finger.

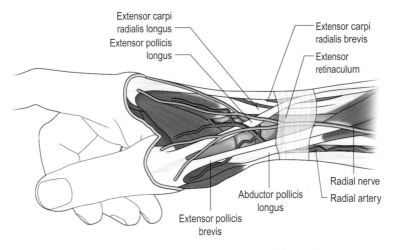

Fig. 7.6 Tendons at the lateral aspect of the wrist.

Labels in figure:
Extensor carpi radialis longus
Extensor pollicis longus
Extensor carpi radialis brevis
Extensor retinaculum
Radial nerve
Radial artery
Abductor pollicis longus
Extensor pollicis brevis

GUIDE TO SURFACE MARKING AND PALPATION

Palmar Aspect

Look for three creases (not distinct in everyone) on the palmar aspect of the lower forearm:

- The distal wrist crease joins pisiform and the tubercle of the scaphoid at the heel of the hand (Backhouse and Hutchings, 1990), marking the proximal border of the flexor retinaculum.
- The middle crease joins the two styloid processes, marking the position of the wrist joint line.
- The proximal crease (if present) marks the proximal extent of the flexor tendon sheaths.

Palpate the *radial and ulnar styloid processes* at the wrist; the radial styloid extends slightly more distally than the ulnar styloid.

Consider the position of the bones that make up the two rows of carpal bones (Fig. 7.2). From the radial to the ulnar side, an easy way to remember the order is:

simply **l**earn **t**he **p**arts	**s**caphoid, **l**unate, **t**riquetral, **p**isiform
that **t**he **c**arpus **h**as	**t**rapezium, **t**rapezoid, **c**apitate, **h**amate

Palpate *pisiform*, the pea-shaped sesamoid bone, which lies at the base of the hypothenar eminence, giving insertion to flexor carpi ulnaris.

Move your thumb approximately 1.5 cm distally and diagonally from pisiform, in the direction of the index finger. Lying roughly in line with the ring finger is the *hook of hamate.* Palpate deeply, and tenderness will confirm its presence.

Radially deviate the wrist to make the *tuberosity of the scaphoid* more prominent. It lies at the base of the thenar eminence, close to the tendon of flexor carpi radialis.

Move your thumb from the tuberosity of the scaphoid, diagonally and distally approximately 1 cm, to lie in line with the index finger, and feel the *ridge of the trapezium* through the bulk of the thenar eminence. It is best felt with the wrist joint in extension and is tender to deep palpation.

Joining the four points described – pisiform, hook of hamate, tuberosity of scaphoid and ridge of trapezium – gives the position of the *flexor retinaculum*, which is approximately the size of your thumb when placed horizontally across the proximal palm (see Fig. 7.4).

Identify the superficial forearm flexor tendons as they cross the palmar aspect of the wrist from the radial to ulnar side.

Flexor carpi radialis is the most lateral tendon. *Palmaris longus* passes over the flexor retinaculum and can be brought into prominence by opposing the thumb and little finger with the wrist flexed. *Flexor digitorum superficialis*, lying in a deeper plane, may not be readily palpable, but *flexor carpi ulnaris* can be followed down to its insertion onto pisiform.

Palpate for the *radial pulse* on the palmar aspect of the lower radius lateral to flexor carpi radialis. The *ulnar pulse* can be palpated on the lower ulna, lateral to flexor carpi ulnaris.

Consider the position of the *median nerve* as it enters the carpal tunnel deep to palmaris longus. If palmaris longus is absent, oppose the thumb and little finger and the midline crease produced gives the position of the median nerve.

Dorsal Aspect

Pronate the forearm and the *head of the ulna* can be seen as a rounded elevation in the distal forearm (Fig. 7.7). Palpate to the ulnar side of the head and feel the tendon of *extensor carpi ulnaris* in the groove between the head of the ulna and the *styloid process.*

Palpate the *inferior radioulnar joint* line, which lies approximately 1.5 cm laterally from the ulnar styloid. Confirm its presence by passively gliding the head of the ulna against the radius and feeling the joint line.

On the lower end of the radius, palpate the *dorsal tubercle (of Lister)* lying roughly in line with the index finger. The tubercle is grooved on either side by the passing tendons. *Extensor carpi radialis longus* and *brevis* pass on its lateral side, while *extensor pollicis longus* passes on its medial side before taking a 45-degree turn laterally, where it can be traced to its insertion into the base of the distal phalanx of the thumb.

The *capitate* is the largest carpal bone and is roughly the size of the patient's thumbnail. It is wider dorsally and is roughly peg-shaped. It is situated in the centre of the carpus, articulating mainly with the third metacarpal distally, trapezoid laterally, hamate medially and the concavity formed by the scaphoid and lunate proximally (Steinberg and Plancher, 1995; Standring, 2015).

To locate the position of the capitate, run your finger proximally down the shaft of the third metacarpal with the wrist in slight flexion and drop over the end into the shallow depression where the capitate sits.

Place the wrist in flexion with the thumb relaxed, to allow the tendon of extensor pollicis longus to fall out of the way and to expose the base of the metacarpals. Now palpate the insertions of *extensor carpi radialis longus* and *brevis* onto the radial side of the base of the second and third metacarpals, respectively. Palpate the insertion of extensor carpi ulnaris onto the medial side of the base of the fifth metacarpal.

Lateral Aspect

Pronate the forearm and make a fist. The fleshy elevation seen at the distal end of the radius is formed by the musculotendinous junctions of *abductor pollicis longus* and *extensor pollicis brevis* as they wind around the lower radius, crossing over the tendons of extensor carpi radialis longus and brevis at the intersection point (Fig. 7.6).

Locate the *anatomical snuffbox* (by extending the thumb), which is bordered by the tendons of abductor pollicis longus and extensor pollicis brevis laterally and by extensor pollicis longus medially. Palpate the *radial styloid* at the proximal end of the anatomical snuffbox and the first carpometacarpal joint at the distal end.

Locate the tendons of abductor pollicis longus and extensor pollicis brevis; you can sometimes feel a V-shaped gap between the two.

Move the wrist into ulnar deviation and the scaphoid can be palpated distal to the radial styloid; it moves with the hand, where the radial styloid does not. The scaphoid can be grasped between your thumb posteriorly in the base of the snuffbox and your index finger anteriorly.

Move distally to palpate the trapezium, lying between the scaphoid and the base of the first metacarpal.

Palpate the *first carpometacarpal joint* line by running a thumb down the shaft of the first metacarpal into the anatomical snuffbox. Flex and extend the joint to check its location.

Palpate the *first dorsal interosseous muscle* in the web between index finger and thumb; it can be made more prominent by resisting abduction of the index finger.

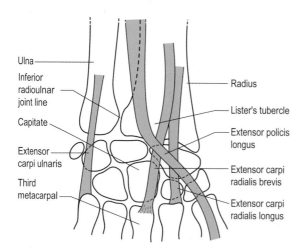

Ulna
Inferior radioulnar joint line
Capitate
Extensor carpi ulnaris
Third metacarpal

Radius
Lister's tubercle
Extensor policis longus
Extensor carpi radialis brevis
Extensor carpi radialis longus

Fig. 7.7 Dorsal aspect of the wrist.

COMMENTARY ON THE EXAMINATION

Observation

Before proceeding with the history, a general observation of the patient's *face, posture and gait* will alert the practitioner to serious abnormalities or injuries. The painful hand may be held in an antalgic position. The arm swing may be absent from the gait pattern, and the hand may be held stiffly against the side or across the body. Difficulty with fine movements may be observed during undressing, indicating a problem with dexterity.

History

The patient's *age, occupation, sports, hobbies* and *activities* may give an indication of the cause and a possible diagnosis since most problems in the lower forearm involve arthropathy, trauma or change in use. Mobile phone texting and the use of handheld gaming devices have joined the more traditional causative factors of keyboards and knitting.

The specific activities required in an occupation should be explored to expose the precise movements required of the upper limb, often repetitively for several hours a day. For example, racquet sports, golf, and hockey can all give rise to symptoms in the wrist and hand resulting from the impact forces and positioning of the upper limb.

The *site* of pain is usually well localised by the patient with little *spread* since these are peripheral joints and structures lying at the end of their respective dermatomes, have little scope for reference.

The presence of paraesthesia or any apparent reference of pain may suggest a more proximal lesion, and all proximal joints must be examined, including the cervical spine.

A fractured scaphoid gives localised pain and point tenderness in the anatomical snuffbox, while X-ray investigation may not show evidence of the fracture for several weeks (Livengood, 1992). Most occult fractures are visible at 2 weeks, but 2% to 5% of scaphoid fractures are missed on initial presentation. Magnetic resonance imaging (MRI) and/or a bone scan should be considered early on to confirm diagnosis (Pillai and Jain, 2005).

The *onset* of the symptoms may be sudden, if due to trauma, or more gradual if associated with a change in use or arthropathy. If the onset is traumatic in nature, the possibility of fracture should be eliminated. Frequently, a direct injury involving a fall on the outstretched hand may cause fracture of the scaphoid or subluxation of the capitate or lunate bones and may also cause traumatic arthritis with soft-tissue swelling and contusion. Indirect injury can also occur from a rotational force or maximal effort in racquet sports (Rettig, 1994).

Most injuries at the wrist and hand develop from a change in use. Tendinopathy may come on gradually if associated with prolonged over- or underuse or more quickly if associated with sudden trauma or unaccustomed activity. De Quervain's tenosynovitis and carpal tunnel syndrome (see pages 219 and 215) may be associated with more proximal lesions, such as nerve entrapment or lesions of the cervical spine. They will tend to have a gradual onset.

A hyperextension injury to the thumb is a relatively common sporting injury, producing a traumatic arthritis of sudden onset, in either the first carpometacarpal joint or the metacarpophalangeal joint. This may occur in skiing (skier's thumb) or sports that involve catching a ball, such as volleyball, netball or goalkeeping in soccer.

Arthropathy in the hand may be inflammatory, degenerative or traumatic, with the latter having a sudden onset. Rheumatoid arthritis comes on gradually over weeks or months or even years. It is common in the smaller joints and therefore readily affects the joints of the wrist and hand where deformity is characteristic; it is usually bilaterally symmetrical (NICE, 2020a). Any synovial space can be involved, including the tendon sheaths and bursae, as well as the joints. Juvenile idiopathic arthritis has less symmetrical joint involvement than adult rheumatoid arthritis.

Degenerative arthropathy comes on gradually over months or years and affects the first carpometacarpal joints and the distal interphalangeal joints more readily. These joints are subjected to stress in the functional position and are used through all extremes of range, predisposing them to arthropathy. Degenerative arthropathy can affect any joint in the wrist and hand.

The *duration* of symptoms can help with differential diagnosis and can also help to indicate the stage of the lesion in the healing process. Although they are long-term conditions, rheumatoid arthritis and acute episodes of degenerative arthropathy tend to have periods of remission and exacerbation, while traumatic lesions may be of fairly short duration. Overuse syndromes have a gradual onset with symptoms present for many months.

The *symptoms and behaviour* need to be considered. The nature of the pain is important: Is it localised or vaguely diffuse, deep or superficial, sharp, burning or aching? An accurate description of other symptoms, especially paraesthesia, is relevant to be able to trace the source of pressure or nerve entrapment. The distribution of pins and needles and whether they possess edge and/or aspect helps to determine their origin.

Stiffness of the hand may be relevant to arthritis or ligamentous lesions, and it is therefore appropriate to know the daily pattern of the symptoms. Rheumatoid arthritis is also associated with persistent synovitis, including pain that is worse at rest, swelling around the joints, and significant early morning stiffness, which usually lasts over an hour (NICE, 2020a). Heat, coldness, sweating, dryness and other sensory changes may also be relevant, suggesting the vasomotor changes of Raynaud's syndrome or complex regional pain syndrome.

The behaviour of the pain indicates the nature of the lesion, with mechanical lesions normally eased by rest and aggravated by activity. Are the symptoms constant or intermittent, getting worse or better, or staying the same? Many lesions are aggravated by repetition of the causative trauma.

An indication of *medical history, other joint involvement and medications* will establish whether contraindications to treatment techniques exist. As well as past medical history, establish any ongoing conditions and treatment. Family history may be relevant to inflammatory or degenerative conditions.

Explore other past or current musculoskeletal problems with previous episodes of the current complaint, any treatment given and the outcome of treatment.

Practitioners should *screen* routinely for psychosocial factors and consider relevant health co-morbidities and lifestyle factors (see Chapter 1). These factors may contribute to the patient's presenting condition or form a barrier to recovery and normal function and should be addressed as an integral part of patient management.

Inspection

Fracture or dislocation commonly occurs with a fall on the outstretched hand and shows obvious *bony deformity* and *swelling*. Subluxation, for example of the capitate, may be seen as a bump on the dorsum of the hand with the wrist in flexion.

Deformities of the fingers are commonly associated with rheumatoid arthritis or may result from forced hyperextension injuries, as in wicketkeeping, for example. If an extensor tendon is avulsed or torn from the distal phalanx, a mallet finger occurs with flexion of the distal interphalangeal joint. This can be associated with sporting injuries or may simply occur if the finger is caught forcibly, while making the bed, for example.

A bony swelling of the distal interphalangeal joint is a characteristic deformity known as a Heberden's node, associated with degenerative arthropathy. Degenerative arthropathy of the first carpometacarpal joint produces a capsular pattern that may draw the thumb into a position of flexion and medial rotation with obvious bony osteophytes at the base of the thumb.

Dupuytren's contracture is a deformity with contraction of the palmar fascia, causing flexion of principally the ring and little fingers. Clubbed fingers may be indicative of systemic vascular or respiratory disease.

Colour changes, which may indicate circulatory involvement, should be further investigated by palpating for the arterial pulses. The fingers, in particular, can give clues to serious underlying pathology, and the colour and shape of the fingers and nails should be noted. Bruising may be apparent, resulting from direct trauma, and may be associated with abrasions on the palm due to a fall on the outstretched hand.

Muscle wasting may be obvious in the flattening of the thenar muscles, producing the ape-like hand with the thumb moving back in line with the other fingers. This indicates involvement of the median nerve in the carpal tunnel or possibly cervical nerve root compression. Similarly, ulnar nerve or lower cervical nerve root compression involve the hypothenar eminence, and if the intrinsic muscles are involved a claw hand develops. Involvement of the radial nerve affects the wrist extensors and produces a dropped wrist.

Swelling indicates joint activity, and the wrist may be fixed in the mid-position due to the presence of a joint effusion. Contusions with swelling are due to direct trauma. Rheumatoid arthritis usually presents with persistent swelling around the joints, and hard, firm swellings (rheumatoid nodules) over the extensor surface of the wrist are observed in over a third of people with rheumatoid arthritis (NICE, 2020a).

Ganglia are mucus-filled cysts, which are commonly seen around the wrist, particularly on the dorsum of the hand (70%) (Kuliński et al., 2019; Gregush and Habusta, 2020), and approximately 20% on the palmar side (Gregush and Habusta, 2020). Ganglion cysts account for 60% to 70% of soft-tissue masses found in the hand

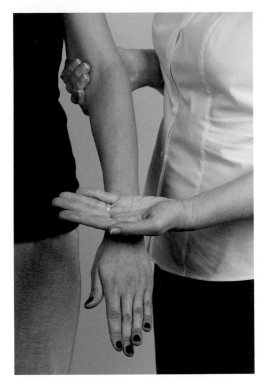

Fig. 7.8 Palpation for heat.

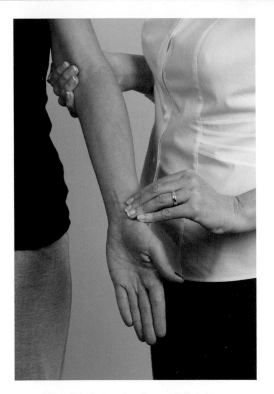

Fig. 7.9 Palpation for radial pulse.

and wrist. Although they can form at any age, they are most commonly found in women between the ages of 20 and 50.

Palpation

Since these are peripheral joints, palpation for signs of activity is conducted. Temperature changes are assessed. *Heat* indicates joint activity, while cold may indicate circulatory problems (Fig. 7.8). It may be appropriate to palpate the ulnar and/or radial pulse (Fig. 7.9). *Synovial thickening* is usually palpated on the dorsum of the wrist (Fig. 7.10). *Swelling* is usually observed around the wrist as well, where it may be fusiform or diffuse. Other swellings, such as nodules or ganglia, can be palpated to assess whether they are hard or soft. With rheumatoid arthritis, swelling around the joints usually gives a 'boggy' feeling on palpation (NICE, 2020a).

State at Rest

Before any movements are performed, the state at rest is established to provide a baseline for subsequent comparison.

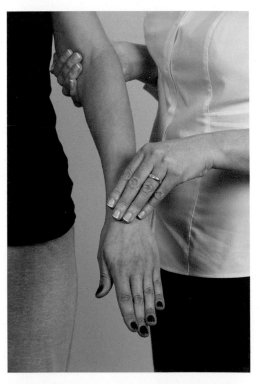

Fig. 7.10 Palpation for synovial thickening.

Examination by Selective Tension

The suggested sequence for the examination will now be given, followed by a commentary including the reason for performing the movements and the significance of the possible findings. Comparison should always be made with the other side.

Inferior Radioulnar Joint
- Passive pronation (Fig. 7.11)
- Passive supination (Fig. 7.12)

Wrist Joint
- Passive flexion (Fig. 7.13)
- Passive extension (Fig. 7.14)
- Passive ulnar deviation (Fig. 7.15)
- Passive radial deviation (Fig. 7.16)
- Resisted flexion (Fig. 7.17)
- Resisted extension (Fig. 7.18)
- Resisted ulnar deviation (Fig. 7.19)
- Resisted radial deviation (Fig. 7.20)

First Carpometacarpal Joint
- Passive extension and adduction (Fig. 7.21)
- Resisted flexion (Fig. 7.22)
- Resisted extension (Fig. 7.23)
- Resisted abduction (Fig. 7.24)
- Resisted adduction (Fig. 7.25)

Interossei
- Resisted finger abduction for dorsal interossei (Fig. 7.26)
- Resisted finger adduction for palmar interossei (Fig. 7.27)

Palpation
- Once a diagnosis has been made, the structure at fault is palpated for the exact site of the lesion

Fingers
- Passive and resisted testing of the fingers is not performed routinely

---

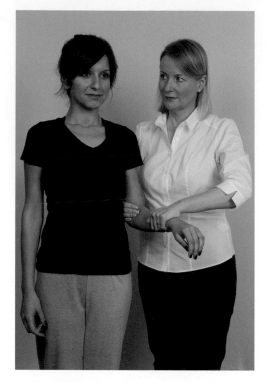

Fig. 7.11 Passive pronation.

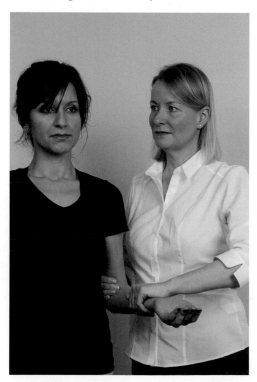

Fig. 7.12 Passive supination.

The inferior radioulnar joint gives pain felt at the wrist and is assessed using two passive movements, passive pronation and supination, looking for pain, range of movement, end-feel and the presence of the capsular pattern. Both rotations normally have an elastic end-feel.

The wrist joint is then assessed by four passive movements, looking for pain, range of movement and end-feel. Passive flexion normally has an elastic end-feel due to tissue tension and passive extension a hard

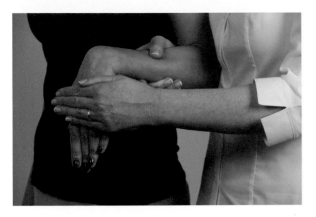

Fig. 7.13 Passive flexion.

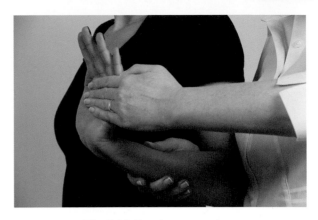

Fig. 7.14 Passive extension.

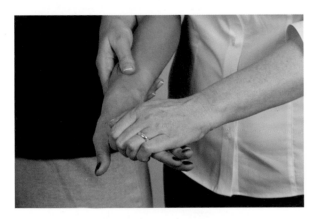

Fig. 7.15 Passive ulnar deviation.

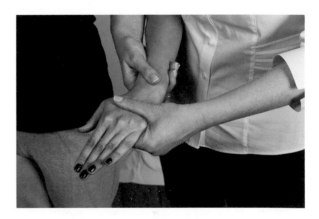

Fig. 7.16 Passive radial deviation.

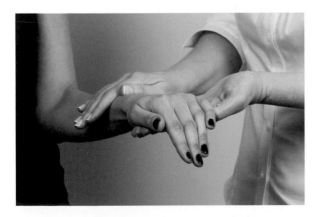

Fig. 7.17 Resisted flexion.

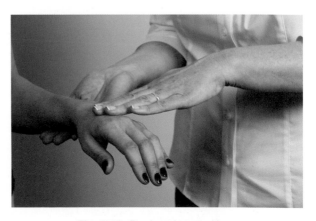

Fig. 7.18 Resisted extension.

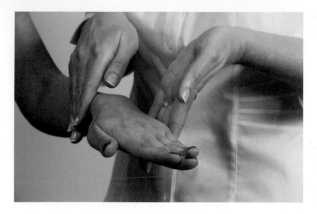

Fig. 7.19 Resisted ulnar deviation.

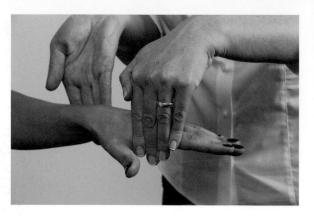

Fig. 7.20 Resisted radial deviation.

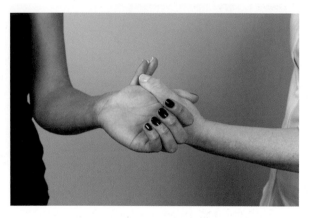

Fig. 7.21 Passive extension and adduction of the thumb.

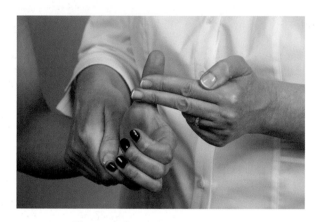

Fig. 7.22 Resisted thumb flexion.

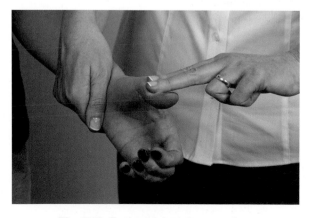

Fig. 7.23 Resisted thumb extension.

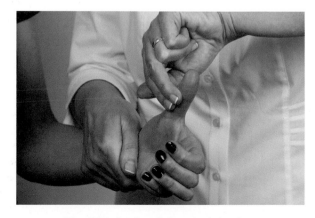

Fig. 7.24 Resisted thumb abduction.

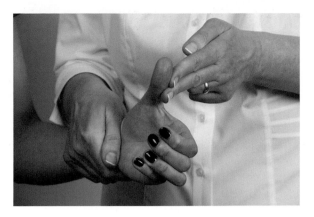

Fig. 7.25 Resisted thumb adduction.

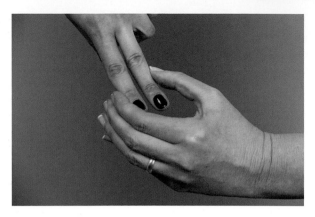

Fig. 7.26 Resisted finger abduction for dorsal interossei.

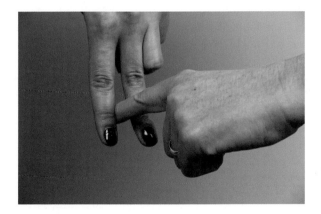

Fig. 7.27 Resisted adduction for palmar interossei.

Movement	Main Muscles	'Assistors'
Wrist flexion	Flexor carpi ulnaris, flexor carpi radialis	Flexor digitorum superficialis
Wrist extension	Extensor carpi radialis longus and brevis, extensor carpi ulnaris	Extensor digitorum
Wrist ulnar deviation	Flexor carpi ulnaris, extensor carpi ulnaris	
Wrist radial deviation	Extensor carpi radialis, flexor carpi radialis	
Thumb flexion	Flexor pollicis longus	Flexor pollicis brevis
Thumb extension	Extensor pollicis longus	Extensor pollicis brevis, abductor pollicis brevis
Thumb abduction	Abductor pollicis brevis	
Thumb adduction	Adductor pollicis	
Finger abduction	Dorsal interossei	
Finger adduction	Palmar interossei	

end-feel, while both deviations normally display an elastic end-feel. The presence of the capsular pattern indicates arthritis; the non-capsular pattern may be due to a subluxed carpal bone (e.g. the capitate) or collateral ligament sprain.

The contractile structures at the wrist are assessed by resisted tests looking for pain and power. A positive finding requires palpation of the appropriate anatomical structure to establish the exact site of the lesion.

The first carpometacarpal joint is assessed by passive application of one combined movement, passive extension and adduction, which is always painful if the capsular pattern is present.

The contractile structures around the thumb are assessed by resisted tests looking for pain and power. Resisted flexion assesses flexor pollicis longus, resisted extension assesses extensor pollicis longus and brevis, resisted abduction assesses abductor pollicis longus and resisted adduction assesses adductor pollicis.

The interossei are assessed by two resisted tests looking for pain and power. Resisted finger abduction assesses the dorsal interossei and resisted finger adduction assesses the palmar interossei.

Passive and resisted movements of the fingers are not part of the routine examination but are included if necessary. Passive movements may establish the capsular patterns described as follows.

Based on the history and clinical examination, the practitioner should be able to establish the most likely diagnosis, using clinical reasoning and clinical judgement. Should additional information be required to aid diagnosis or to add value to management, further investigations can be considered to inform decision making and planning.

Practitioners may consider further investigations such as blood tests, radiological imaging, and other diagnostic procedures (see Chapter 1). Investigations should be guided by suspected causes and are an extension to clinical examination. For example, if a specific underlying cause is suspected, such as diabetes, hypothyroidism or a ganglion, blood tests or ultrasound scanning may be appropriate. Blood tests can also be considered if vitamin B12 deficiency, peripheral neuropathy and inflammatory arthritis are suspected. Depending on local pathways, nerve conduction studies and electromyography (EMG) may be required prior to onward referral for a surgical opinion.

It is important to recognise potential serious pathology, such as infection, malignancy, fracture, new onset of paraesthesia after injury, and inflammatory arthritis, and to make any appropriate onward referral in a timely manner.

If a fracture is suspected, the validated Amsterdam wrist rules, developed in 2015, can inform clinical decision making in determining which patients need radiographic imaging for wrist pain following trauma. The aim is to reduce unnecessary imaging and patient exposure to radiation, and this outcome was confirmed in a subsequent evaluation study (Mulders et al., 2020).

CAPSULAR LESIONS

The presence of the capsular pattern at the joints indicates an arthropathy. Rheumatoid arthritis more readily affects the smaller joints and is seen as symmetrical involvement of the joints in the wrist and hand with deformity characteristic of the condition.

Degenerative arthropathy affects the first carpometacarpal and distal interphalangeal joints more readily. The thumb may be flexed towards the palm of the hand by the contracted anterior joint capsule, and the distal interphalangeal joints of the fingers may show the characteristic Heberden's nodes.

Trauma may produce traumatic arthritis and fracture should be eliminated.

A stepped approach to the management of capsular lesions in the wrist and hand is currently recommended (NICE, 2020b). Less invasive treatments are generally offered first, including education/watchful wait, activity and work modification, wrist or thumb splint, simple analgesics and non-steroidal anti-inflammatory drugs (NSAIDs) medication and physiotherapy (e.g. exercise, mobilisation). Injection therapy (e.g. corticosteroid, local anaesthetic, hyaluronic acid) may then be considered for severe pain and significant functional impairment.

Consider referral to occupational therapy for advice and assessment on assistive devices for daily activities to reduce repetitive high load to the wrist and hand joints, if indicated. If symptoms persist, more invasive treatments can be considered, such as trapeziectomy and joint replacement surgery (Wajon et al., 2015; NICE, 2020b). This management approach is consistent with the European League Against Rheumatism (EULAR) recommendations for the management of hand osteoarthritis (Kloppenburg et al., 2019).

Grade B mobilisation is appropriate for the limitation of movement associated with degenerative arthropathy. An alternative treatment for the first carpometacarpal joint is described as follows.

Arthropathy in the wrist and hand responds to corticosteroid injection as part of the stepped approach.

Inferior (Distal) Radioulnar Joint

CAPSULAR PATTERN OF THE INFERIOR RADIOULNAR JOINT
- Pain at end of range of both rotations

The inferior radioulnar joint is most commonly affected by rheumatoid arthritis.

INJECTION OF THE INFERIOR RADIOULNAR JOINT (CYRIAX, 1984; CYRIAX AND CYRIAX, 1993)

Suggested needle size: 25 G × 1 in. (0.6 × 25 mm) blue needle

Dose: 10–20 mg triamcinolone acetonide in a total volume of 0.5 mL

- Position the patient with the forearm supported in full pronation.
- Identify the inferior radioulnar joint line and insert the needle, which may need to be angled, into the joint (Fig. 7.28).
- Give the injection as a bolus once the needle is intracapsular (Fig. 7.29).

The patient should minimise or modify activities for 2 weeks following injection.

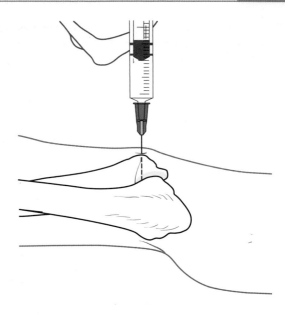

Fig. 7.29 Injection of the inferior radioulnar joint showing direction of approach and needle position.

Wrist Joint

CAPSULAR PATTERN OF THE WRIST JOINT
- Equal limitation of flexion and extension
- Eventual fixation in the mid-position

The wrist joint is most commonly affected by rheumatoid arthritis and traumatic arthritis.

INJECTION OF THE WRIST JOINT

Suggested needle size: 23 G × 1 in. (0.6 × 25 mm) blue needle

Dose: 20–30 mg triamcinolone acetonide in a total volume of 3 mL

- Position the patient with the wrist supported and the forearm in full pronation (Fig. 7.30).
- Locate a point of entry, which may be at either side of the extensor carpi radialis brevis tendon.
- Give the injection as a bolus once the needle is intracapsular (Fig. 7.31).
- Alternatively, in the rheumatoid wrist, or if degeneration is sufficient to prevent access to the joint, make two or three needle insertions and pepper the area of synovial thickening with a series of withdrawals and reinsertions. This technique is not comfortable for the patient.

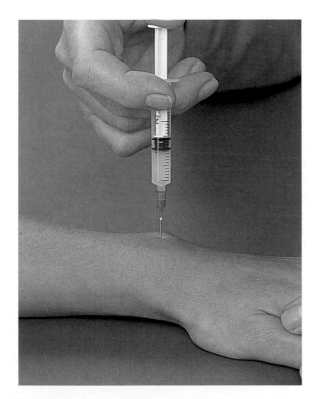

Fig. 7.28 Injection of the inferior radioulnar joint.

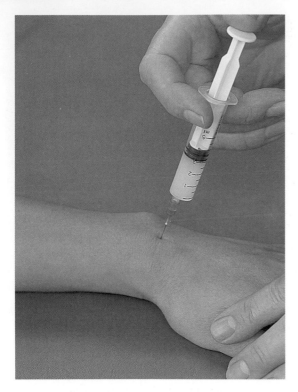

Fig. 7.30 Injection of the wrist joint.

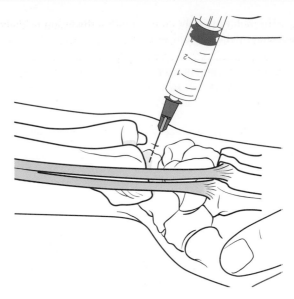

Fig. 7.31 Injection of the wrist joint showing direction of approach and needle position.

The patient should minimise or modify activities for 2 weeks following injection.

First Carpometacarpal Joint

> **CAPSULAR PATTERN OF THE FIRST CARPOMETACARPAL JOINT.**
> • Most limitation of extension

Degenerative arthropathy of the first carpometacarpal joint is a common arthropathy, particularly in post-menopausal women (Ahern et al., 2018).

The 'Eaton and Glickel grading system' is based on radiological findings and is the most commonly used system for classifying the severity of the stages of degeneration. The classification ranges from Stage I to IV according to the changes in joint space and features associated with degeneration. It is recognised that the changes may not reliably correlate with the severity of symptoms, but it can act as a guide to determine appropriate conservative or surgical management (Anakwe and Middleton, 2011; Ahern et al., 2018).

The patient complains of pain and tenderness at the base of the thumb and on using the thumb under compression (e.g. when writing or gripping).

Confirmation of the capsular limitation can be made by asking the patient to put the hands into the prayer position and spreading the thumbs into extension, comparing the two sides.

An axial compression test applies longitudinal pressure down the shaft of the first metacarpal with rotation of the thumb to grind the articular surfaces together. If positive, a sudden sharp pain is usually reproduced at the base of the thumb as compression is applied and occasionally crepitus may be noted. The test confirms the diagnosis of osteoarthropathy (Anakwe and Middleton, 2011; Choa et al., 2014; Hattam and Smeatham, 2020) and differentiates the condition from de Quervain's tenosynovitis (see page 219). Care should be taken not to use excessive flexion of the thumb as this may stretch the extensor pollicis brevis, bringing on pain associated with de Quervain's tenosynovitis and resulting in a false-positive result (Choa et al., 2014).

The musculoskeletal medicine approach relies on the clinical presentation, and an elastic end-feel on testing the limited movements indicates that the lesion is likely to respond to frictions and stretches to the joint. A harder end-feel indicates that injection would be appropriate.

In the persistence of pain with severe limitation of function, an orthopaedic opinion can be sought and surgery may be indicated.

TRANSVERSE FRICTIONS TO THE ANTERIOR CAPSULAR LIGAMENT OF THE FIRST CARPOMETACARPAL JOINT

(Cyriax, 1984; Cyriax and Cyriax, 1993)

- Place the patient's thumb comfortably into extension and adduction.
- Apply transverse frictions with the thumb or index finger reinforced by the middle finger (Fig. 7.32).
- Direct the frictions down onto the anterior capsular ligament and apply the sweep transversely across the fibres.
- Maintain the technique for an appropriate time, according to the irritability of the lesion and stage of healing, to achieve analgesia and to mobilise the tissues.

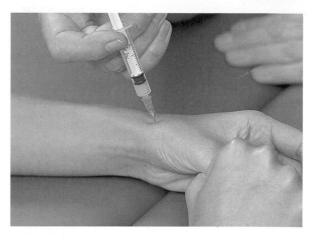

Fig. 7.33 Injection of the first carpometacarpal joint.

The principles for stretching capsular adhesions can be applied, i.e. Grade B mobilisation, and distraction is also a useful technique to apply to this joint.

> **INJECTION OF THE FIRST CARPOMETACARPAL JOINT (CYRIAX, 1984; CYRIAX AND CYRIAX, 1993)**
> Suggested needle size: 25 G × 5/8 in. (0.5 × 16 mm) orange needle
> Dose: 10–20 mg triamcinolone acetonide in a total volume of 0.5–0.75 mL

- Position the patient with the hand resting comfortably. The patient can apply a degree of distraction to the affected thumb (Fig. 7.33).
- Identify the joint line by running your thumb down the first metacarpal into the anatomical snuffbox to locate the joint line.
- Insert the needle into the joint and give the injection as a bolus (Fig. 7.34).
- Alternatively, if the thenar eminence is flattened, identify the joint line anteriorly. In either case, osteophyte formation may make the injection difficult.

The patient should minimise or modify activities for 2 weeks following injection.

Finger Joints

> **CAPSULAR PATTERN OF THE FINGER JOINTS**
> - Slightly more limitation of flexion than extension

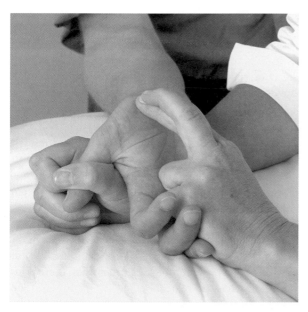

Fig. 7.32 Transverse frictions to the anterior capsular ligament of the first carpometacarpal joint.

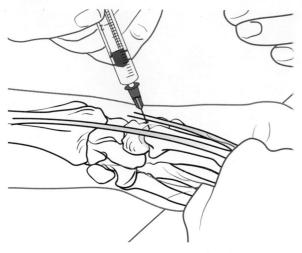

Fig. 7.34 Injection of the first carpometacarpal joint showing direction of approach and needle position.

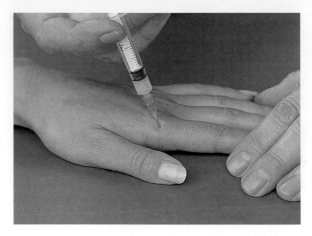

Fig. 7.35 Injection of the metacarpophalangeal joint.

INJECTION OF THE FINGER JOINTS
Suggested needle size: 25 G × 5/8 in (0.5 × 16 mm) orange needle
Dose: 5–10 mg triamcinolone acetonide in a total volume of 0.5–0.75 mL

- Identify the affected joint.
- With knowledge of the position of the tendons and ligaments around it, find a point of convenient access, usually on the dorsal aspect avoiding the digital expansions (Figs 7.35 and 7.36).
- Angle the needle obliquely and, once intra-articular, give the injection as a bolus (Figs 7.37 and 7.38).

The patient should minimise or modify activities for 2 weeks following injection.

NON-CAPSULAR LESIONS

Subluxed Carpal Bone

The capitate is particularly prone to dorsal subluxation or displacement because it is roughly peg-shaped, with its dorsal surface slightly wider than its palmar surface. The lunate sits between scaphoid and triquetral and the lower end of the radius and the articular disc and may displace anteriorly when the wrist is forced into extension (Norris, 2004). Posterior displacements may also occur.

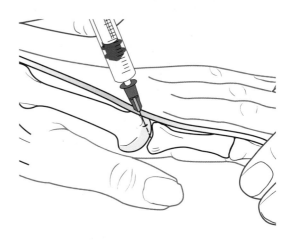

Fig. 7.36 Injection of the metacarpophalangeal joint showing direction of approach and needle position.

Either bone may displace, but it is commonly the capitate. The mechanism of injury involves a fall on the outstretched hand or repeated compression through the extended wrist, as occurs in gymnastics, for example, causing the capitate to displace dorsally.

The patient may complain of pain and limited movement and may be concerned about the bump seen on the dorsum of the hand. Occasionally, a subluxed capitate may have been present for a long time, when there is less chance of successful relocation.

On examination, there is a non-capsular pattern. Passive extension is painful and limited by a bony block. Passive flexion can usually achieve full range, but the

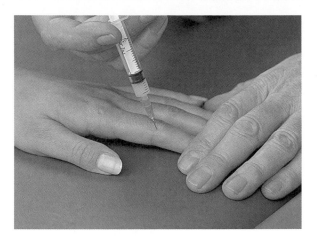

Fig. 7.37 Injection of the interphalangeal joint.

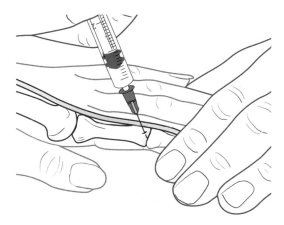

Fig. 7.38 Injection of the interphalangeal joint showing direction of approach and needle position.

REDUCTION OF THE CAPITATE
(Saunders, 2000)

- Locate the capitate by running a thumb down the shaft of the third metacarpal to its base and onto the adjacent displaced capitate (Fig. 7.39).
- Place the tip of one thumb, reinforced by the other, on top of the capitate, and wrap your fingers comfortably around the patient's thenar and hypothenar eminences (Fig. 7.40).
- Placing your little finger into the web between the patient's thumb and index finger will prevent you from flexing the patient's wrist during the technique (Fig. 7.41).

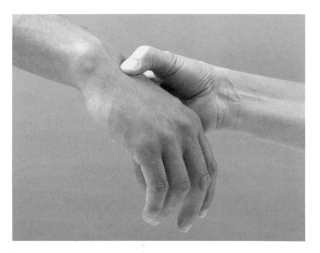

Fig. 7.39 Palpating for the capitate bone at the base of the third metacarpal.

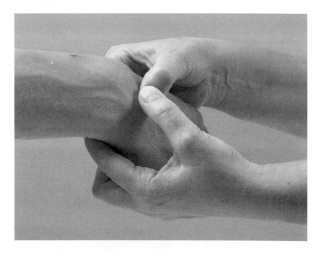

Fig. 7.40 Thumb position for the reduction of the capitate.

patient experiences pain at the end of range. A bony bump may be obvious on passive flexion, but this should not be confused with the base of the third metacarpal, which is also prominent. Diagnosis is dependent upon the appropriate history and the presence of the non-capsular pattern.

The principle of treatment applied here is to relocate the capitate under strong traction. It should be emphasised that this is a Grade A mobilisation technique performed under strong traction, not a manipulation at the end of range.

The technique for the capitate mobilisation will be explained here, but it can be adapted if another carpal bone is displaced.

- Position the patient's proximal row of carpal bones level with the edge of the couch. Instruct an assistant to fix this proximal row of carpal bones with the web of the hand parallel to the edge of the couch, reinforced with the other hand, to give counterpressure (Fig. 7.42).
- Place your feet directly under the patient's hand and lean back to apply strong traction (Fig. 7.43).
- Allow this traction to establish for a few seconds to separate the two rows of carpal bones.

- Apply a sharp downwards movement, aiming to relocate the capitate.
- The technique may also be applied with the patient seated alongside the couch (Fig. 7.44).
- Re-examine the patient to assess the results and repeat if necessary.

If pain persists after relocation, the ligaments surrounding the capitate may be treated with transverse frictions (Fig. 7.45a and b).

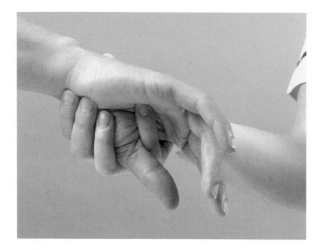

Fig. 7.41 Finger position for the reduction of the capitate.

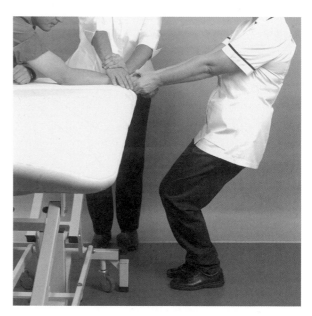

Fig. 7.43 Body position for the reduction of the capitate.

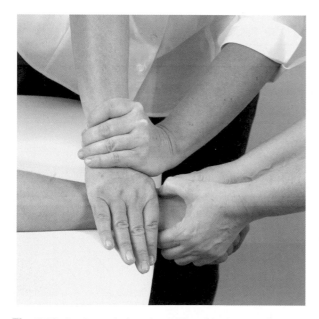

Fig. 7.42 Assistant's hand position for the reduction of the capitate.

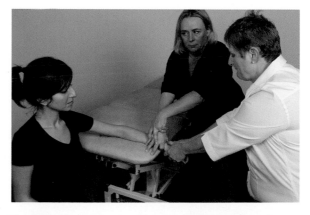

Fig. 7.44 Alternative position for reduction of capitate

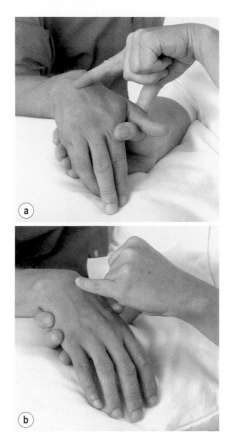

Fig. 7.45 Transverse frictions to the capitate ligaments: (a) horizontally for vertical fibres and (b) vertically for horizontal fibres.

Collateral Ligaments at the Wrist Joint

The collateral ligaments may be injured by a traumatic overstretching of the wrist joint or by repetitive micro-trauma due to unaccustomed activity. The condition may also be associated with rheumatoid arthritis.

The patient complains of localised pain and the ligament is tender to palpation. Stretching the ligament by passive movement in the opposite direction reproduces the pain. Radial collateral ligament sprain produces pain on passive ulnar deviation, and a sprained ulnar collateral ligament produces pain on passive radial deviation.

Either lesion may be treated by applying the principles of transverse frictions, having placed the hand in a suitable position to gain access to the ligament (Figs 7.46 and 7.47).

Carpal Tunnel Syndrome

The mechanism of the lesion is uncertain but involves some compression of the median nerve in the carpal tunnel. Mechanical and vascular factors are believed to be involved, with inflammation increasing the size of structures lying within the tunnel, causing swelling and compression, or with scarring affecting the perineural circulation (Anderson and Tichenor, 1994).

The muscles of the thenar eminence may be affected by denervation, abductor pollicis brevis in particular, causing the thumb to fall back into line with the other digits and flattening of the thenar eminence.

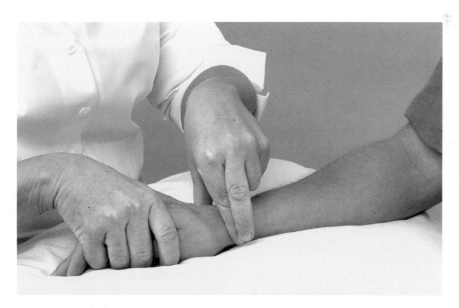

Fig. 7.46 Transverse frictions to the radial collateral ligament.

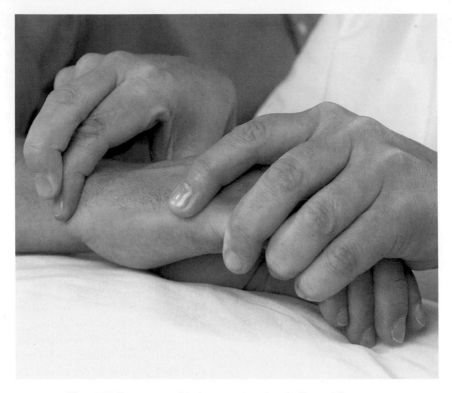

Fig. 7.47 Transverse frictions to the ulnar collateral ligament.

Anything that reduces the already tight space in the tunnel compresses the nerve. Intrinsic factors include inflammation and swelling of any structure within the tunnel, or reduction of the size of the tunnel itself, including tenosynovitis, hypothyroidism, diabetes mellitus, pregnancy, obesity, rheumatoid arthritis and acromegaly (Keith et al., 2009; Feather et al., 2020).

External factors include trauma, pressure, repetitive occupational or leisure activities, repeated gripping or squeezing, excessive vibration from heavy machinery, keyboard use, knitting, woodworking, using power tools, or racquet sports. Carpal tunnel syndrome is also found in association with coexistent cervical radiculopathy and polyneuropathy (Keith et al., 2009).

Bland (2007) refers to a strong genetic predisposition to carpal tunnel syndrome. It occurs more commonly in women between the ages of 40 and 60, peaking in the late 50 s (Norris, 2004; Bland, 2007).

The presenting signs and symptoms of carpal tunnel syndrome are variable. They can include aching, a burning sensation and tingling or numbness of the fingertips of the radial three and a half digits on the palmar surface (Phalen, 1966).

About 70% of patients experience numbness at night, and 40% complain of pain radiating proximally into the lower forearm with simultaneous paraesthesia felt in the fingers (Smith and Wernick, 1994). The symptoms may wake patients, and they can usually gain relief by shaking or rubbing the hands (Cailliet, 1990). Patients may complain of a loss of dexterity and sensitivity, with clumsiness of hand function.

On examination, flattening of the thenar eminence may be observed if median nerve compression has occurred. Objective sensory loss may be found in prolonged cases of compression with weakness of the thenar muscles, especially abductor pollicis brevis, if the motor branch is involved.

Bland (2007) observes that Tinel's sign and Phalen's test are the most widely used and recognised tests for confirming the diagnosis, although it should be recognised that these tests are not perfect diagnostic indicators (Hattam and Smeatham, 2020). Nerve conduction studies show diminished nerve velocity across the wrist in 90% of patients who go on to have proven nerve compression at surgery (Smith and Wernick, 1994).

Tinel's sign for median nerve compression in the carpal tunnel involves tapping the flexor retinaculum. It is positive if pins and needles are elicited in the radial three and a half digits (Hoppenfeld, 1976; Hartley, 1995; Ekim et al., 2007).

Phalen's test applies compression to the median nerve in the carpal tunnel, achieved by maintaining maximum wrist flexion. The test is positive if pins and needles are reproduced. A normal hand would develop tingling if this position were maintained for 10 minutes or more; a patient with carpal tunnel syndrome will report the onset of pain, numbness and tingling within 1 to 2 min. If symptoms are not reproduced within 3 min, the test may be considered to be negative (Hoppenfeld, 1976; Cailliet, 1990; Vargas Busquets, 1994; Hartley, 1995; Ekim et al., 2007; Hattam and Smeatham, 2020).

There is also a *Reverse Phalen's* test. The patient maintains a position of full wrist and finger extension for 2 minutes. The pressure on the carpal tunnel increases after 10 seconds (compared to 20 to 30 seconds for the standard Phalen test). The longer the position is held, the greater the pressure on the wrist and carpal tunnel.

In a study comparing the changes in pressure between Phalen and Reverse Phalen's tests, it was noted that the average pressure change for Phalen's test was 4 mm Hg in 2 minutes, versus 34 mm Hg at 1 minute and 42 mm Hg at 2 minutes for the Reverse Phalen test. The Reverse Phalen's test may therefore be a more appropriate clinical test for truly compressing the carpal tunnel and provoking symptoms of carpal tunnel syndrome. (Physiopedia, 2021)

The '*link test*' can be applied to assess muscle strength; the thumb and individual fingers are opposed in turn and the examiner attempts to break the link, which should not be possible if the patient possesses normal muscle power.

Examination of the cervical spine and neural tension testing should be conducted if there is any suspicion that the lesion lies more proximally.

Differential diagnosis for carpal tunnel syndrome is cervical radiculopathy (especially C6/7), vibration white finger, degenerative arthropathy of the first carpometacarpal joint, peripheral neuropathy, diabetes and hypothyroidism.

Treatment of Carpal Tunnel Syndrome

A stepped approach to the management of carpal tunnel syndrome is currently recommended. Less invasive treatments are generally offered first, including education/watchful wait, activity and work modification, splinting, simple analgesics, physiotherapy (e.g. mobilisation, neural gliding techniques) and then corticosteroid injection therapy. Surgery is an option when there is clinical evidence of median nerve denervation. If symptoms persist, more invasive treatments can be considered, such as surgical release (Keith et al., 2009).

The causative factors should be discussed with the patient and attempts made to avoid aggravating activities. The patient may be fitted with a wrist support splint to wear at night, to avoid flexion, especially during pregnancy.

Symptomatic relief may be gained from a corticosteroid injection, but it is important to check with local guidance and policy before injecting.

Three high-quality Cochrane studies evaluated treatment for carpal tunnel syndrome and consistently showed strong and moderate evidence for the effectiveness of corticosteroids (oral or injection) (Connor et al., 2003; Marshall et al, 2007; Verdugo et al., 2008). Corticosteroid injection seems to be the most effective non-surgical management in short term and medium term, compared to oral corticosteroid (Wong et al., 2001; Verdugo et al., 2008) and placebo (Marshall et al., 2007; Verdugo et al., 2008; Atroshi et al., 2013).

Corticosteroid injections can be considered for patients with carpal tunnel syndrome who wish to avoid or delay surgical treatment (Celiker et al., 2002; Peters-Veluthamaningal et al., 2010; Atroshi et al., 2013;). However, up to half of patients who have had corticosteroid injection have symptom recurrence (Peters-Veluthamaningal et al., 2010).

A systematic review by Huisstede et al. (2010a) also supported the short- and medium-term effectiveness of corticosteroid injection, but the benefit was not maintained in the long term, and it was not as beneficial as surgery, which is the most effective treatment compared to all non-surgical options (Huisstede et al., 2010b).

If injection is unsuccessful, or symptom relief is short term only, surgical release of the flexor retinaculum may be considered. Significant weakness and wastage of the thenar muscles, or nerve conduction tests demonstrating significant loss of conduction velocity, will usually be indications for surgery.

INJECTION OF THE CARPAL TUNNEL (CYRIAX, 1984; CYRIAX AND CYRIAX, 1993)

Suggested needle size: 23 G × 1 in or 1¼ in. (0.6 × 25/30 mm) blue needle
Dose: 20 mg triamcinolone acetonide

- Position the patient with the wrist supported in extension.
- Choose a point of entry between the distal and middle wrist creases on the ulnar side of palmaris longus. If palmaris longus is absent, oppose the thumb and little finger to produce a midline crease as a guide and keep to the ulnar side (Fig. 7.48).
- Angle the needle parallel to and between the flexor tendons until it is under the flexor retinaculum. Be careful to check that there is no paraesthesia before injecting to avoid injury to the median nerve.
- Give the injection as a bolus within the tunnel (Fig. 7.49).

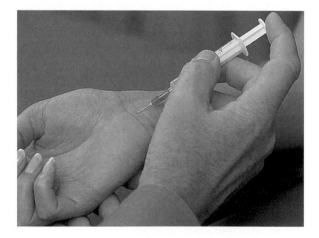

Fig. 7.48 Injection of the carpal tunnel.

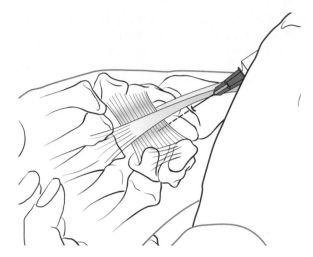

Fig. 7.49 Injection of the carpal tunnel showing direction of approach and needle position.

The patient should minimise or modify activities for 2 weeks following injection.

Fibrocartilage Tears and Meniscal Lesions

A triangular fibrocartilaginous disc complex is related to the distal radioulnar joint inferiorly, and a fibrocartilaginous meniscus projects into the wrist joint from the ulnar collateral ligament. These intra-articular structures are prone to degenerative changes, tears and occasionally displacement.

Trauma, such as a fall on the outstretched hand or repetitive joint overloading, can cause degeneration and tears. Central or radial tears are the most common (Rettig, 1994; Al-Shihabi et al., 2015). A mechanical lesion involving a tear or displacement of any part of the intra-articular complex presents with pain and clicking felt on the ulnar side of the wrist.

On examination, the clicking may be appreciated by the practitioner while palpating the wrist and simultaneously pronating and supinating the forearm. Passive ulnar deviation may reproduce the pain, and point tenderness may be felt just distal to the ulnar styloid.

To confirm the diagnosis of a mechanical lesion of the intra-articular complex, the wrist is placed into extension and ulnar deviation, and axial compression is applied to the ulnar side of the wrist while the wrist is passively circumducted (Fig. 7.50). A positive test produces localised pain at the ulnar side of the wrist joint and/or a click or crepitus on movement.

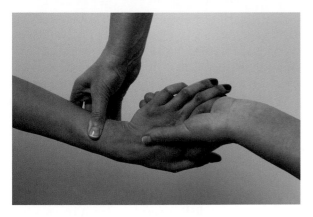

Fig. 7.50 Test for fibrocartilage tears and meniscal lesions.

Treatment involves strong distraction to reduce possible displacement, or the patient may be referred for arthroscopy and excision.

CONTRACTILE LESIONS

Tendinopathy at the teno-osseous junction of a tendon and tenosynovitis affecting the tendon in its sheath, as it runs under either the flexor or extensor retinacula, are common lesions found at the wrist and hand.

A change in use or being more sedentary can cause the lesion, which may be tendinopathy or tenosynovitis of a single unit, or part of an overall more complex syndrome.

A stepped approach to the management of tendinopathy or tenosynovitis is currently recommended. Less invasive treatments are generally offered first, including education/watchful wait, wrist or thumb splint, activity and work modification, simple analgesics and NSAIDs medication, physiotherapy (e.g. exercise, mobilisation) and then injection therapy (e.g. corticosteroid, local anaesthetic, platelet-rich plasma [PRP] injection). If symptoms persist, more invasive treatments can be considered, such as tenotomy and tendon repair.

In the musculoskeletal medicine approach, tendinopathy at the teno-osseous junction can be treated by transverse frictions or injection, in some circumstances.

Tenosynovitis is treated by transverse frictions, which are applied with the tendon on a stretch, to restore the gliding function of the tendon sheath, and are graded according to the irritability or severity of the lesion. Injection is delivered as a bolus between the tendon and its sheath.

All sites are subjected to relative rest from aggravating factors following treatment.

The more common contractile lesions will now be discussed.

De Quervain's Tenosynovitis

This common condition, originally described in 1895, is tenosynovitis involving the tendons of abductor pollicis longus and extensor pollicis brevis in the first extensor compartment at the wrist (Elliott, 1992a; Livengood, 1992; Rettig, 1994; Klug, 1995).

Uncomplicated inflammation of the shared synovial sheath is known as de Quervain's tenosynovitis. If the shared sheath is thickened due to scarring associated with chronic inflammation it becomes stenotic (Marini et al., 1994); it is then known as de Quervain's stenosing tenosynovitis. Occasionally, a ganglion is associated with the condition, especially if it is chronic (Tan et al., 1994; Klug, 1995).

Women are more commonly affected and the condition may be bilateral in up to 30% of patients (Klug, 1995). Onset is occasionally due to direct trauma but more typically due to repetitive occupational or leisure activities. Shea et al. (1991) reported a case of de Quervain's tenosynovitis associated with repeated gear-shifting in a mountain biker. Gout or rheumatoid arthritis may be associated conditions.

Pain is felt on the radial side of the wrist with point tenderness over the radial styloid. Pain is aggravated by movements into ulnar deviation, forced flexion/adduction of the thumb and wringing movements of the hand, especially into ulnar deviation. Crepitus may be audible during movements of the wrist.

On examination, a local, thickened swelling may be obvious, especially to palpation (Anderson and Tichenor, 1994), with the pain reproduced on resisted thumb abduction and extension.

Passive movements of the thumb also reproduce the pain as the tendon is pushed or pulled through the thickened, inflamed sheath. The axial grind test for arthritis of the first carpometacarpal joint should be negative in de Quervain's tenosynovitis.

Finkelstein's test, placing the patient's thumb in the palm of the hand and positioning the hand into ulnar deviation, produces excruciating pain over the radial styloid. If positive, it is pathognomonic of de Quervain's tenosynovitis (Livengood, 1992; Elliott, 1992b; Rettig, 1994; Hattam and Smeatham, 2020).

Treatment may be by transverse frictions or by corticosteroid injection.

TRANSVERSE FRICTIONS FOR DE QUERVAIN'S TENOSYNOVITIS

- Place the thumb into flexion and ulnar deviation at the wrist, to put the tendons on as much the stretch as can be tolerated (Fig. 7.51).
- Direct the frictions down onto the tendons using two fingers side by side and sweep transversely across the fibres.
- Maintain the technique for an appropriate time, according to the irritability of the lesion and stage of healing, to achieve analgesia and to mobilise the tissues.

Relative rest is advised where functional movements may continue but no overuse or stretching until pain-free on resisted testing. A splint to support the thumb in the resting position may be helpful.

Shin et al. (2020) conducted a prospective randomised study and showed that pain and clinical outcomes significantly improved after corticosteroid injection at 3 months. They also found that the incidence and severity of skin pigmentation or atrophy was not significantly different between image-guided and anatomically-guided corticosteroid injection. According to Peters-Veluthamaningal et al. (2009), the beneficial effects of steroid injections for symptoms were maintained during the follow-up after 12 months.

Several authors have explored the effectiveness of combined treatments for de Quervain's tenosynovitis. Weiss et al. (1994) compared the use of corticosteroid and lidocaine with splinting alone in the treatment of de Quervain's syndrome and established better results in the injection group. Mardani-Kivi et al. (2014) found that a combination of corticosteroid injection and thumb spica casting was more effective than injection alone in terms of pain relief and functional outcomes at 6 months follow-up.

As de Quervain's tenosynovitis is a chronic lesion, it may form part of a syndrome involving occupational overuse, and a full examination of the cervical spine and upper limb may be required, including neural tension. All components of the condition should be treated appropriately.

INJECTION FOR DE QUERVAIN'S TENOSYNOVITIS
Suggested needle size: 25 G × 5/8 in. (0.5 × 16 mm) orange needle
Dose: 10 mg triamcinolone acetonide in a total volume of 1 mL

- Position the patient sitting, with the wrist supported, holding the thumb in a degree of flexion and the wrist in ulnar deviation and slight extension.
- Identify the tendons of abductor pollicis longus and extensor pollicis brevis and the V-shaped gap between them at the base of the first metacarpal.
- Insert the needle between and parallel to the two tendons (Fig. 7.52).
- Give the injection as a bolus into the shared sheath (Fig. 7.53).
- If the injection has been correctly placed, a slight swelling will be seen around the tendons.

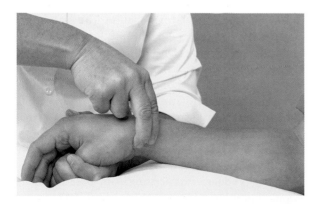

Fig. 7.51 Transverse frictions for de Quervain's tenosynovitis.

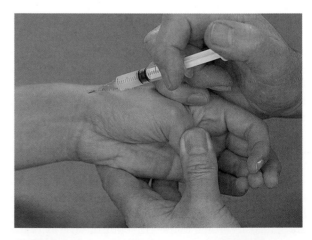

Fig. 7.52 Injection for de Quervain's tenosynovitis.

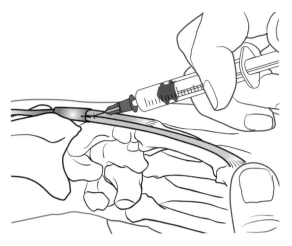

Fig. 7.53 Injection for de Quervain's tenosynovitis showing direction of approach and needle position.

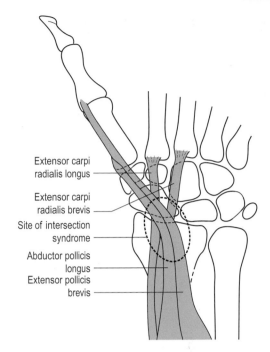

Extensor carpi radialis longus

Extensor carpi radialis brevis

Site of intersection syndrome

Abductor pollicis longus

Extensor pollicis brevis

Fig. 7.54 Site of intersection syndrome.

The patient should minimise or modify activities for 2 weeks following injection.

Intersection Syndrome or Oarsman's Wrist

The intersection, or crossover, point between the two sets of tendons (abductor pollicis longus/extensor pollicis brevis and extensor carpi radialis longus/brevis) occurs at a point on the radius and can extend up to approximately 4 cm proximal to the wrist (Livengood, 1992; Klug, 1995) (Fig. 7.54).

This is a point of potential friction between the structures as they exert tension in different directions. This can lead to tenosynovitis where the tendons pass under the extensor retinaculum or, more commonly, inflammation of the musculotendinous junction in the lower forearm.

The condition is provoked by overuse, and the patients usually present with acute pain and the classical signs of inflammation, heat, redness, swelling and disturbed function. Crepitation is usually audible on movement, but pain makes objective testing difficult.

TRANSVERSE FRICTIONS FOR INTERSECTION SYNDROME

Treatment begins immediately with protection, rest and ice to control pain and inflammation. Gentle transverse frictions are given, ideally on a daily basis,

to give pain relief, and the patient usually recovers relatively quickly.

- Position the patient comfortably on a pillow.
- Identify the area of tenderness, which is obvious on the lower radial aspect of the forearm.
- Place a thumb along the length of the painful tendons and by abduction and adduction of the thumb or pronation and supination of your forearm, impart the frictions transversely across the fibres (Fig. 7.55).
- Alternatively, all four finger pads can be placed at right angles across the tendons to impart the frictions transversely across the fibres.
- Maintain the technique for an appropriate time, according to the irritability of the lesion and stage of healing, to achieve analgesia and to mobilise the tissues.

Relative rest is advised where functional movements may continue within the pain-free range but no overuse or stretching until pain-free on resisted testing.

This condition is commonly provoked again by a change in use, and the patient will need advice on manual handling tasks and activity modification.

Extensor Carpi Ulnaris Tendinopathy

After de Quervain's, tenosynovitis of extensor carpi ulnaris is the next most common tenosynovitis at the

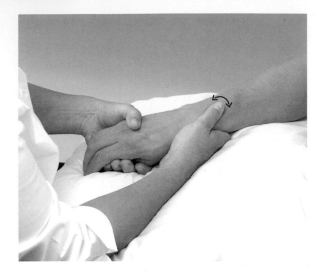

Fig. 7.55 Transverse frictions for intersection syndrome.

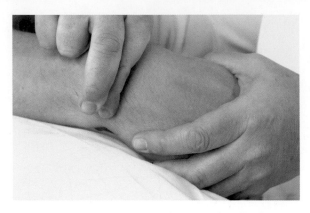

Fig. 7.56 Transverse frictions for extensor carpi ulnaris tenosynovitis.

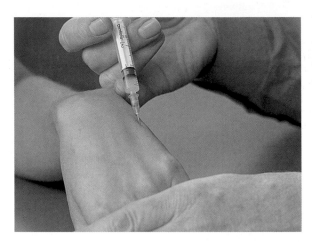

Fig. 7.57 Injection for extensor carpi ulnaris at teno-osseous site.

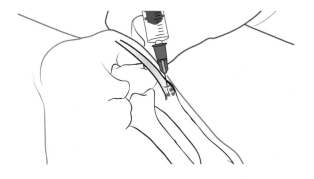

Fig. 7.58 Injection for extensor carpi ulnaris at teno-osseous site showing direction of approach and needle position.

wrist (Klug, 1995). Tenosynovitis or tendinopathy at the teno-osseous junction is usually due to a change in use, sometimes occurring in the non-dominant hand of the tennis player who uses a double-handed backhand when the 'take back' involves an extreme position of ulnar deviation (Rettig, 1994).

Direct trauma may cause subluxation of the tendon from the groove between the head of the ulna and the styloid process (Livengood, 1992; Rettig, 1994). The patient complains of pain and clicking on the ulnar side of the wrist. When the extended wrist is actively taken from radial to ulnar deviation, the subluxation of the tendon can be observed, and this will help differentiate the condition from a triangular fibrocartilage complex or meniscal lesion.

Transverse frictions can be used with the tendon on a stretch in tenosynovitis (Fig. 7.56) and against the insertion for the teno-osseous junction.

Alternatively, the principles of corticosteroid injection are applied, either injecting between the tendon and sheath in tenosynovitis or peppering the insertion at the base of the fifth metacarpal (Figs 7.57 and 7.58).

INJECTION FOR EXTENSOR CARPI ULNARIS TENOSYNOVITIS OR TENDINOPATHY

Suggested needle size: 25G × 5/8 in. (0.5 × 16mm) orange needle

Dose: 10mg triamcinolone acetonide in a total volume of 1mL given as a bolus between the tendon and its sheath given by peppering technique at the teno-osseous junction

Extensor Carpi Radialis Longus and Brevis Tendinopathy

The lesion is usually at the teno-osseous junction where it is due to overuse or it may be associated with a bony metacarpal protuberance (Rettig, 1994; Bergman, 1995). Pain is felt on resisted wrist extension and resisted radial deviation.

The principles of transverse frictions or corticosteroid injection are applied to treat the lesion.

TRANSVERSE FRICTIONS FOR EXTENSOR CARPI RADIALIS LONGUS AND BREVIS TENDINOPATHY

For treatment with transverse frictions:

- Position the patient with the wrist in flexion to expose the base of the metacarpals and to allow the long extensor tendon to the thumb to fall out of the way.
- Identify the site of the lesion by palpation at the radial side of the base of either the second or third metacarpals (Fig. 7.59).
- Direct the transverse frictions down onto the insertion and sweep transversely across the fibres.
- Maintain the technique for an appropriate time, according to the irritability of the lesion and stage of healing, to achieve analgesia and to mobilise the tissues.

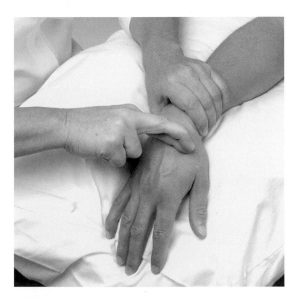

Fig. 7.59 Transverse frictions to extensor carpi radialis longus or brevis tendons at teno-osseous site.

Alternatively, the principles of corticosteroid injection are applied, using a peppering technique Figs 7.60 and 7.61.

INJECTION FOR EXTENSOR CARPI RADIALIS LONGUS AND BREVIS TENDINOPATHY

Suggested needle size: 25G × 5/8 in. (0.5 × 16 mm) orange needle
Dose: 10 mg triamcinolone acetonide in a total volume of 1 mL given by peppering technique at the teno-osseous junction

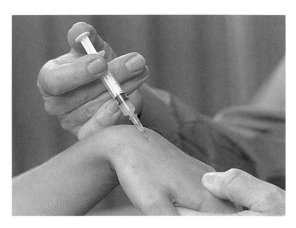

Fig. 7.60 Injection for extensor carpi radialis longus or brevis tendons at teno-osseous site.

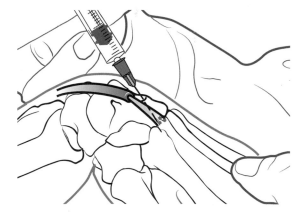

Fig. 7.61 Injection for extensor carpi radialis longus or brevis tendons at teno-osseous site showing direction of approach and needle position.

Flexor Carpi Ulnaris Tendinopathy

Insertional tendinopathy can occur at the proximal or distal teno-osseous junctions at the pisiform.

Treatment consists of transverse frictions or cortico-steroid injection.

TRANSVERSE FRICTIONS FOR FLEXOR CARPI ULNARIS TENDINOPATHY

- Flex the patient's little finger to relax the hypothenar eminence.
- If applying transverse frictions at the proximal site, rotate your finger as you apply some downward pressure on the edge of the palm to apply your finger pad against the proximal aspect of pisiform (Fig. 7.62).
- Similarly, press into the palm and rotate your thumb to apply pressure against the pisiform for transverse frictions to the distal site (Fig. 7.63).
- Sweep transversely across the fibres at either site. The use of either thumb or finger is not crucial, and it may be easier for you to swap between them. The point is to direct your pressure against the proximal or distal aspects of pisiform to be able to apply the transverse friction to the specific site of the lesion.
- Maintain the technique for an appropriate time, according to the irritability of the lesion and stage of healing, to achieve analgesia and to mobilise the tissues.

The corticosteroid injection is delivered by a peppering technique into the lesion (Figs 7.64 and 7.65). Remember the position of the ulnar nerve, lying just laterally to the tendon, so that you can avoid it when injecting.

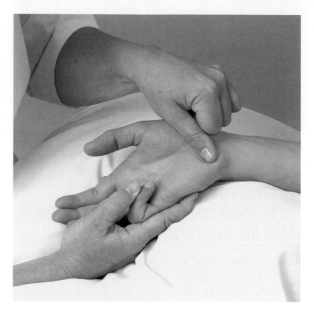

Fig. 7.63 Transverse frictions to flexor carpi ulnaris tendinopathy, distal site.

INJECTION FOR FLEXOR CARPI ULNARIS TENDINOPATHY

Suggested needle size: 25 G × 5/8 in. (0.5 × 16 mm) orange needle

Dose: 10 mg triamcinolone acetonide in a total volume of 1 mL given by peppering technique at the teno-osseous junction

---

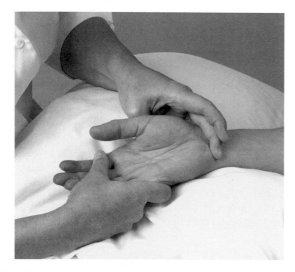

Fig. 7.62 Transverse frictions to flexor carpi ulnaris tendinopathy, proximal site.

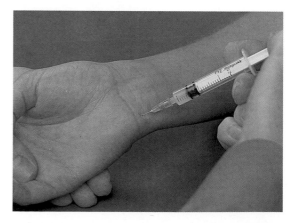

Fig. 7.64 Injection for flexor carpi ulnaris tendinopathy, proximal site.

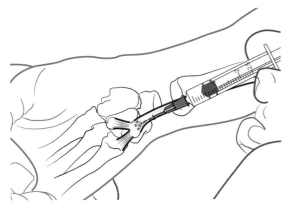

Fig. 7.65 Injection for flexor carpi ulnaris tendinopathy, proximal site, showing direction of approach and needle position.

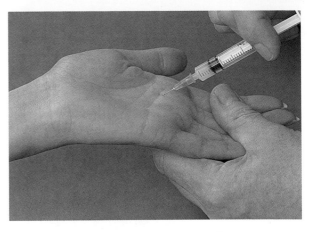

Fig. 7.66 Injection for trigger finger.

Trigger Finger or Thumb

Flexor tendons in the hand are contained within fibrous sheaths that have thickened areas known as pulleys. These may provide a restriction to movement, producing 'trigger finger' or 'trigger thumb'.

Trigger finger, or thumb, is a snapping phenomenon producing a painful catch as a flexor tendon is caught at a pulley during flexion and then released during forced extension (Smith and Wernick, 1994; Murphy et al., 1995).

Palmar trauma or irritation can cause thickening of the tendon, sheath or pulley and a palpable nodule may exist. Some 35% of cases involve the flexor pollicis longus tendon and 50% involve the middle or ring finger flexor tendons (Smith and Wernick, 1994).

The condition may be secondary to systemic disease such as rheumatoid arthritis or diabetes mellitus.

Treatment by corticosteroid injection can be curative, restoring painless, smooth full range of movement to the digit (Murphy et al., 1995).

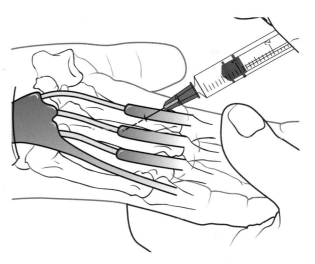

Fig. 7.67 Injection for trigger finger showing direction of approach and needle position.

> **INJECTION OF TRIGGER FINGER OR THUMB**
> Suggested needle size: 25G × 5/8 in. (0.5 × 16 mm) orange needle
> Dose: 10 mg triamcinolone acetonide in a total volume of 0.5 mL

- Insert the needle towards the thickened nodule of the affected tendon on the palmar surface.

- Angle the needle approximately 45 degrees, distally or proximally, with the bevel of the needle parallel to the tendon.
- Avoid injecting into the tendon and nodule itself by withdrawing back from the substance of the tendon slightly until a loss of resistance is appreciated.
- Deliver the injection slowly as a bolus (Figs 7.66 and 7.67).

The patient should minimise or modify activities for 2 weeks following injection.

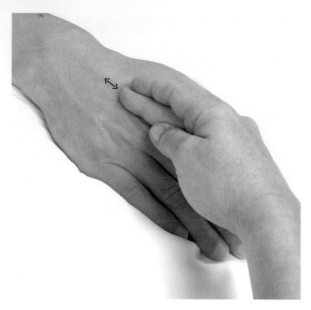

Fig. 7.68 Transverse frictions to the dorsal interossei.

Interosseous Muscle Lesions

Strain of the dorsal interossei more commonly affects musicians and tennis players, for example. The patient presents with a vague pain at the metacarpophalangeal joint or between the metacarpals, which is exacerbated by repeated gripping (Rettig, 1994). Pain will be reproduced by resisted abduction of the appropriate finger or fingers.

The treatment of choice is transverse frictions. Palpation will determine the site, but it is often from the origin of the interosseous muscle on one metacarpal.

TRANSVERSE FRICTIONS TO THE DORSAL INTEROSSEI

- Direct your pressure against the metacarpal and perform the sweep parallel to the shaft (Fig. 7.68).
- Maintain the technique for an appropriate time according to the irritability of the lesion and stage of healing, to achieve analgesia and to mobilise the tissues.

REVIEW QUESTIONS

1. How do you differentiate carpal tunnel syndrome from cervical nerve root compression?
2. Which tendons are involved in intersection syndrome?
3. Where does the radial artery cross the wrist joint?
4. Explain the principles for transverse frictions to tendons around the wrist.
5. Which tests would be positive with an articular disc injury at the wrist?

CASE SCENARIOS

Case 1

History

- Dave is a 36-year-old roofer who enjoys surfing. He has a 6-day history of pain over the dorsal aspect of his right wrist. There was a sudden onset of pain while falling off his surfboard when his hand hit the surfboard, forcing his wrist into extension. It hurts to push or pull himself up through roof hatches. No significant medical history, taking ibuprofen.

Examination

- No obvious bony deformity, but he has limited passive wrist extension and pain on full wrist flexion. Resisted tests are negative.

Task

- Consider differential diagnosis and any further testing that may be required. Where would you expect him to be tender on palpation? What are the treatment options for this man?

Case 2

History

- Erica is a 67-year-old retired schoolteacher with a passion for baking. She has recently taken up bread-making and enjoys kneading the dough. Following an intense day of baking for a local fete 6 weeks ago, she noticed pain at the base of her left thumb. The pain is intermittent and gets worse if she puts pressure through her thumb. It is not improving, and she has had to stop making bread. She is on statins and has had a left total knee joint replacement.

Task

- Consider differential diagnosis and how the examination findings would differ for the different pathologies.

Examination

- All passive and resisted wrist movements are negative. Pain is on passive thumb extension/adduction with limitation and a slightly harder end-feel. An awareness of pain on all thumb resisted tests, but power is normal. Tender on palpating the anterior first carpometacarpal joint line.

Task

- Have you come to a clinical diagnosis? What treatments are suitable to try for this lady? Is an X-ray necessary?

Case 3

History

- Simon is a 52-year-old banker with no hobbies except playing sudoku. He has noticed a catching sensation in the palm of his right hand that has occurred for no apparent reason. It is most prominent when he tries to straighten his fingers. This has been present for the last 2 months and is getting worse. He has recently been diagnosed with Type II diabetes, which is diet controlled.

Examination

- He has full pain-free passive and resisted movements of the finger joints, but active 4th finger flexion to extension has a twitch/catching sensation that is obvious to the eye. There is a nodule on palpation over the flexor tendon that is painful.

Task

- What is his likely diagnosis? Why does this condition occur, and what is the current evidence-based treatment choice for this?

REFERENCES

Ahern, M., Skylass, J., Wajon, A., Hush, J., 2018. The effectiveness of physical therapies for patients with base of thumb osteoarthritis: Systematic review and meta-analysis. Musculoskelet. Sci. Pract. 35, 46–54.

Al-Shihabi, L., Wysocki, R.W., Ruch, D.S., 2015. Management of Type 1A TFCC Tears. In: Geissler, W.B. (Ed.), Wrist and Elbow Arthroscopy. Springer, New York, pp. 59–65.

Anakwe, R.E., Middleton, S.D., 2011. Osteoarthritis at the base of the thumb. Br. Med. J. 343, d7122.

Anderson, M., Tichenor, C.J., 1994. A patient with de Quervain's tenosynovitis: a case study report using an Australian approach to manual therapy. Phys. Ther. 74, 314–326.

Atroshi, I., Flondell, M., Hofer, M., et al., 2013. Methylprednisolone injections for the carpal tunnel syndrome: a randomized, placebo-controlled trial. Ann. Intern. Med. 159 (5), 309–317.

Backhouse, K.M., Hutchings, R.T., 1990. A Colour Atlas of Surface Anatomy – Clinical and Applied. Wolfe Medical, London.

Bergman, A.G., 1995. Synovial lesions of the hand and wrist. Magn. Reson. Imaging Clin. N. Am. 3, 265–279.

Bland, J., 2007. Carpal tunnel syndrome. Br. Med. J. 335, 343–346.

Cailliet, R., 1990. Soft Tissue Pain and Disability, second ed. F A Davis, Philadelphia.

Celiker, R., Arslan, S., Inanici, F., 2002. Corticosteroid injection vs. nonsteroidal antiinflammatory drug and splinting in carpal tunnel syndrome. Am. J. Phys. Med. Rehabil. 81 (3), 182–186.

Choa, R.M., Parvizi, N., Giele, H.P., 2014. A prospective case-control study to compare the sensitivity and specificity of the grind and traction-shift (subluxation-relocation) clinical tests in osteoarthritis of the thumb carpometacarpal joint. J. Hand Surg. Eur. 39 (3), 282–285.

Connor, D., Marshall, S., Massy-Westropp, N., 2003. Non-surgical treatment (other than steroid injection) for carpal tunnel syndrome. Cochrane Database Syst. Rev. 2003 (1), CD003219.

Cyriax, J., 1984. Textbook of Orthopaedic Medicine, eleventh ed. Baillière Tindall, London.

Cyriax, J., Cyriax, P., 1993. Cyriax's Illustrated Manual of Orthopaedic Medicine. Butterworth Heinemann, Oxford.

Ekim, A., Armagan, O., Tascioglu, F., et al., 2007. Effect of low level laser therapy in rheumatoid arthritis patients with carpal tunnel syndrome. Swiss Med. Wkly. 137 (23–24), 347–352.

Elliott, B.G., 1992a. Abductor pollicis longus – a case of mistaken identity. J. Hand Surg. Br. 17B, 476–478.

Elliott, B.G., 1992b. Finkelstein's test: a descriptive error that can produce a false positive. J. Hand Surg. Br. 17B, 481–482.

Feather, A., Randall, D., Waterhouse, M., 2020. Kumar and Clark's Clinical Medicine, tenth ed. Elsevier, London.

Gregush, R.E., Habusta, S.F., 2020. Ganglion Cyst. StatPearls Publishing. https://www.ncbi.nlm.nih.gov/books/NBK470168/. Accessed 20 August 2021.

Hartley, A., 1995. Practical Joint Assessment – Lower Quadrant, second ed. Mosby, London.

Hattam, P., Smeatham, A., 2020. Handbook of Special Tests in Musculoskeletal Examination, second ed. Elsevier, Oxford.

Hoppenfeld, S., 1976. Physical Examination of the Spine and Extremities. Appleton Century Crofts, Norwalk, CT.

Huisstede, B.M., Hoogvliet, P., Randsdorp, M.S., et al., 2010a. Carpal Tunnel Syndrome. Part I: Effectiveness of Nonsurgical Treatments–A Systematic Review. Arch. Phys. Med. Rehabil. 91 (7), 981–1004.

Huisstede, B.M., Randsdorp, M.S., Coert, J.H., et al., 2010b. Carpal Tunnel Syndrome. Part II: Effectiveness of Surgical Treatments – A Systematic Review. Arch. Phys. Med. Rehabil. 91 (7), 1005–1024.

Keith, M.W., Masear, V., Amadio, P.C., et al., 2009. Treatment of carpal tunnel syndrome. J. Am. Acad. Orthop. Surg. 17 (6), 397–405.

Kloppenburg, M., Kroon, F.P., Blanco, 2019. 2018 update of the EULAR recommendations for the management of hand osteoarthritis. Ann. Rheum. Dis. 78 (1), 16–24.

Klug, J.D., 1995. MR diagnosis of tenosynovitis about the wrist. Magn. Reson. Imaging Clin. N. Am. 3, 305–312.

Kuliński, S., Gutkowska, O., Mizia, S., et al., 2019. Dorsal and volar wrist ganglions: The results of surgical treatment. Adv. Clin. Exp. Med. 28 (1), 95–102.

Livengood, L., 1992. Occupational soft tissue disorders of the hand and forearm. Wis. Med. J 91 (10), 583–584.

Mardani-Kivi, M., Mobarakeh, M.K., Bahrami, F., et al., 2014. Corticosteroid injection with or without thumb spica cast for de Quervain tenosynovitis. J. Hand Surg. Am. 39 (1), 37–41.

Marini, M., Boni, S., Pingi, A., et al., 1994. De Quervain's disease: diagnostic imaging. Chir. Organi. Mov. 79, 219–223.

Marshall, S., Tardif, G., Ashworth, N., 2007. Local corticosteroid injection for carpal tunnel syndrome. Cochrane Database Syst. Rev (2), CD001554.

Mulders, M.A.M., Walenkamp, M.M.J., Sosef, N.L., et al., 2020. The Amsterdam Wrist Rules to reduce the need for radiography after a suspected distal wrist fracture: an implementation study. Eur. J. Trauma Emerg. Surg. 46 (3), 573–582.

Murphy, D., Failla, J.M., Koniuch, M.P., 1995. Steroid versus placebo injection for trigger finger. J. Hand Surg. Am. 20A, 628–631.

National Institute for Health and Care Excellence (NICE)., 2020a. When should I suspect rheumatoid arthritis. https://cks.nice.org.uk/topics/rheumatoid-arthritis/diagnosis/when-to-suspect-ra/ Accessed 20 August 2021.

National Institute for Health and Care Excellence (NICE)., 2020b. Osteoarthritis: care and management. https://www.nice.org.uk/guidance/cg177. Accessed 20 August 2021.

Norris, C.M., 2004. Sports Injuries: Diagnosis and Management for Physiotherapists, second ed. Butterworth Heinemann, Oxford.

Palastanga, N., Field, D., Soames, R., 2012. Anatomy and Human Movement, sixth ed. Butterworth Heinemann, Edinburgh.

Peters-Veluthamaningal, C., Winters, J.C., Groenier, K.H., et al., 2009. Randomised controlled trial of local corticosteroid injections for de Quervain's tenosynovitis in general practice. BMC Muculoskeletal Disord 10, 131.

Peters-Veluthamaningal, C., Winters, J.C., Groenier, K.H., et al., 2010. Randomised controlled trial of local corticosteroid injections for carpal tunnel syndrome in general practice. BMC Fam. Pract. 11, 54.

Phalen, G.S., 1966. The carpal-tunnel syndrome. Seventeen years' experience in diagnosis and treatment of six hundred fifty-four hands. J. Bone Joint Surg. Am. 48 (2), 211–228.

Physiopedia, 2021. Phalen's test. https://www.physio-pedia.com/Phalen%E2%80%99s_Test#cite_note-Magee-1. Accessed 4 September 2021.

Pillai, A., Jain, M., 2005. Management of clinical fractures of the scaphoid: results of an audit and literature review. Eur. J. Emerg. Med. 12 (2), 47–51.

Rettig, A., 1994. Wrist problems in the tennis player. Med. Sci. Sports Exerc. 26, 1207–1212.

Saunders, S., 2000. Orthopaedic Medicine Course Manual. Saunders, London.

Shea, K.G., Shumsky, I.B., Shea, O.F., 1991. Shifting into wrist pain – de Quervain's disease and off-road mountain biking. Phys. Sports Med. 19, 59–63.

Shin, Y.H., Choi, S.W., Kim, J.K., 2020. Prospective randomized comparison of ultrasonography-guided and blind corticosteroid injection for de Quervain's disease. Orthop. Traumatol. Surg. Res. 106 (2), 301–306.

Smith, D.L., Wernick, R., 1994. Common nonarticular syndromes in the elbow, wrist and hand. Postgrad. Med. 95, 173–188.

Soames, R., Palastanga, N.R., 2018. Anatomy and Human Movement, seventh ed. Elsevier, Oxford.

Standring, S., 2015. Gray's Anatomy: The Anatomical Basis of Clinical Practice, forty-first ed. Churchill Livingstone, Edinburgh.

Steinberg, B.D., Plancher, K.D., 1995. Clinical anatomy of the wrist and elbow. Clin. Sports Med. 14, 299–313.

Tan, M.Y., Low, C.K., Tan, S.K., 1994. De Quervain's tenosynovitis and ganglion over first dorsal extensor retinacular compartment. Ann. Acad. Med. 23, 885–886.

Unglaub, F., Wolf, M.B., Dragu, A., et al., 2012. Nerve fiber staining investigations in traumatic and degenerative disc lesions of the wrist. J. Hand Surg. Am. 36A, 843–846.

Vargas Busquets, M.A.V., 1994. Historical commentary: the wrist flexion test Phalen's sign. J. Hand Surg. Am. 19, 521.

Verdugo, R.J., Salinas, R.A., Castillo, J.L., et al., 2008. Surgical versus non-surgical treatment for carpal tunnel syndrome. Cochrane Database Syst. Rev. 2008 (4), CD001552.

Wajon, A., Vinycomb, T., Carr, E., et al., 2015. Surgery for thumb (trapeziometacarpal joint) osteoarthritis. Cochrane Database Syst. Rev. 2008 (4), CD004631.

Weiss, A.P., Akelman, E., Tabatabai, M., 1994. Treatment of de Quervain's disease. J. Hand Surg. Am. 19A, 595–598.

Wong, S.M., Hui, A.C., Tang, A., et al., 2001. Local vs systemic corticosteroids in the treatment of carpal tunnel syndrome. Neurology 56, 1565–1567.

Wright, T.W., Del Charco, M., Wheeler, D., 1994. Incidence of ligament lesions and associated degenerative changes in the elderly wrist. J. Hand Surg. Am. 10A, 313–318.

The Cervical Spine

CHAPTER CONTENTS

SUMMARY

This chapter begins with a summary of the key points of cervical anatomy.

Differential diagnosis and the elements of clinical examination will be discussed. Patients who are suitable for the treatments described will be identified.

Safety is paramount in the application of manual techniques to the cervical spine. The contraindications to treatment will be emphasised and guidelines for safe practice will be provided since both are of vital importance. Clinical models will be presented to guide treatment choice.

ANATOMY

The spinal column is a series of motion segments, each of which consists of an interbody joint and its two adjacent facet joints. The structural arrangement of the cervical spine is designed principally for mobility. It is the most mobile region of the spine, although its mobility is arguably at the expense of stability.

Its wide range and combinations of movements are related to changes in the direction of vision, the positioning of the upper limbs and hands and locomotion. It is also an area of potential danger as it gives bony protection to major blood vessels that supply the brain and the spinal cord (Taylor and Twomey, 1994; Nordin and Frankel, 2001; Kerry and Taylor, 2006). It has a close neurophysiological connection to the vestibular and visual systems as well and can therefore be the source of many different symptoms (Kristjansson, 2005).

Cervical Joints

Anatomically and functionally, the cervical spine can be divided into two segments.

The *upper segment* consists of the atlas and the axis (C1 and C2). Its structure is designed for mobility, with approximately one-third of cervical flexion and extension and over half of axial rotation occurring at this level (Mercer and Bogduk, 2001).

The *atlas* (C1) is composed of two lateral masses, supporting articular facets, and their joining anterior and posterior arches. The superior facets articulate with the occipital bone of the cranium at the *atlanto-occipital joints* and their condylar shape facilitates nodding movements of the head (Netter, 1987; Mercer and Bogduk, 2001). The inferior facets articulate with the axis at the *atlantoaxial joints* where rotation is the principal movement.

The axis (C2) has broad superior articular facets, which support the lateral masses of the atlas. They bear the axial load of the head and atlas and transmit the load to the rest of the cervical spine.

The axis supports the *dens* or *odontoid process* on its superior surface, and the dens provides a pivot around which the atlas rotates at the synovial median atlantoaxial joint (Mercer and Bogduk, 2001). There is no intervertebral disc between the atlas and axis.

The internal *ligaments of the upper cervical segment* are particularly important to its stability (Fig. 8.1).

The *tectorial membrane* is a superior extension of the posterior longitudinal ligament that covers the dens and its ligaments, acting as protection for the junction of the spinal cord and the medulla in the brain.

The *alar ligaments* are strong rounded cords that pass from each side of the dens but not normally to the atlas (Osmotherly et al., 2013), and ascend laterally to attach to the medial sides of the occipital condyles. They relax in extension and limit flexion, as well as rotation to the contralateral side.

The *transverse ligament* of the atlas is a strong horizontal band with extensions passing vertically and horizontally from its midpoint to form a ligamentous complex called the *cruciform ligament*. This, together with the *apical ligament* of the dens, is responsible for keeping the dens in close contact with the atlas. Any instability in the upper cervical segment, such as that which can occur with rheumatoid arthritis, trauma, or

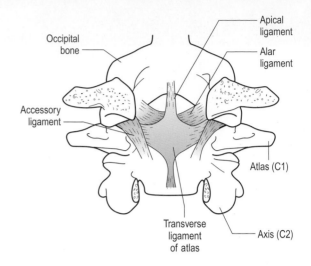

Fig. 8.1 Upper cervical internal ligaments. (From Middleditch and Oliver, 2005. Reprinted by permission of Elsevier Ltd.)

Down's syndrome, is a contraindication to musculoskeletal medicine techniques.

The *lower segment* contributes to overall mobility and consists of typical cervical vertebrae C3–C6 and the atypical C7, which is known as the *vertebra prominens* because of its long spinous process.

A typical cervical vertebra consists of a small, broad, weight-bearing *vertebral body* (Fig. 8.2), the superior surface of which is raised on each side, like a bucket seat, to form *uniform processes*. The unciform processes articulate with corresponding facets on the vertebra above to form the *uncovertebral joints* or *joints of Luschka*.

Two short *pedicles* lie posteriorly and two long, narrow *laminae* form the vertebral arch, which, together with the *vertebral body*, surrounds a large, triangular vertebral canal. The laminae come together to form a bifid *spinous process*.

Superior and inferior *articular processes*, at the junction of the pedicles and laminae, articulate at the synovial *facet joints*, which form an articular pillar on either side of the spine.

Short, gutter-shaped *transverse processes* slope anterolaterally to transport the emerging nerve root. The *foramen transversarium*, a distinctive feature in the

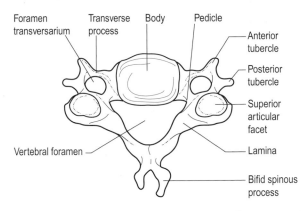

Fig. 8.2 Typical cervical vertebra. (From Soames and Palastanga, 2018. Reprinted by permission of Elsevier Ltd.)

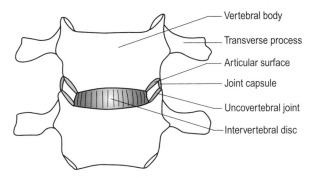

Fig. 8.3 Uncovertebral joints. (From Soames and Palastanga, 2018. Reprinted by permission of Elsevier Ltd.)

transverse processes on each side of the cervical vertebrae, houses the vertebral artery.

The *ligaments of the lower cervical segment* provide stability and allow mobility.

The *ligamentum nuchae* is a strong, fibroelastic sheet that protects the joints posteriorly and provides an intermuscular septum.

The *ligamentum flavum* is a highly elastic ligament linking adjacent laminae. In the cervical spine, it allows separation of the vertebrae during flexion and assists the neck's return to the upright posture. Its elastic properties also allow it to return to its original length, preventing buckling into the spinal canal where it could compromise the spinal cord.

The *posterior longitudinal ligament* passes from the axis to the sacrum and is at its broadest in the cervical spine, where it covers the entire floor of the cervical vertebral canal, supporting the disc and possibly preventing its posterior displacement. It is taut in flexion and relaxed in extension.

Mercer and Bogduk (1999) identified three distinct layers of the posterior longitudinal ligament. The deep layer, consisting of short fibres, spans each intervertebral joint and extends in an alar (wing-shaped) pattern as far as the posterior end of the base of the uncinate process, where it is thought to compensate for a deficient posterior annulus fibrosus.

The *anterior longitudinal ligament* protects the anterior aspect of the intervertebral joints and, with other anterior soft tissues, limits cervical extension.

The joints of the lower cervical segment consist of the interbody joint anteriorly and the two facet joints posteriorly. The interbody joint is made up of the intervertebral joint and the uncovertebral joints. When stacked, the joints can be considered to form three pillars in a triangular formation, the vertebral bodies and uncinate processes forming the anterior column and the two articular pillars formed by the facet joints arranged posteriorly (Mercer and Bogduk, 1999).

The *intervertebral joint* is a symphysis formed between the relatively avascular intervertebral disc and the adjacent vertebral bodies. The disc contributes to mobility, and as it ages, clefts forming from the uncovertebral joints provide translatory glide to the movements of flexion and extension.

The *uncovertebral joints* (joints of Luschka) are formed between the unciform processes and corresponding facets on the vertebral body above (Fig. 8.3), though their existence has been challenged (Mercer and Bogduk, 1999). They may be true synovial joints or adventitious fibrous joints that have developed through clefts or fissures in the lateral corners of the annulus fibrosis of the intervertebral disc, originally described by Hubert von Luschka in 1858 (Prescher, 1998).

These fissures are absent in young children and appear to develop in conjunction with the development of the unciform process. Once formed, the fissures in the annulus develop a pseudocapsule in which vascularised synovial folds have been seen.

As synovial 'joints', degenerative changes can lead to osteophyte formation on the uncinate process, predominantly in the lower cervical segments. Posterior osteophytes can encroach on the intervertebral canal, possibly leading to compression of the emerging spinal nerve root, and anterior osteophytes could compress the vertebral artery.

The uncovertebral joints contribute to mobility by providing a translatory gliding component to flexion and extension as well as stabilising the spine by limiting the amount of side flexion.

The *facet (zygapophyseal) joints* are synovial plane joints with relatively lax fibrous capsules to facilitate movement. The articular facets are angled at approximately 45 degrees to the vertical so that side flexion and rotation of the lower cervical spine occur as a coupled movement. This angle of inclination adds to translatory glide during flexion and extension (Taylor and Twomey, 1994; Jaumard et al., 2011). Together with the disc, the facet joints transfer load and guide and restrain movement in the spine (Jaumard et al., 2011).

The facet joints of the spine are well innervated by the medial branches of the dorsal rami (Bogduk et al., 1982). They have been shown to cause pain at all spinal levels in the neck, upper and mid back, and low back, with pain referring to the head or upper extremity, chest wall, and lower extremity in normal volunteers (Dwyer et al., 1990; Fukui et al., 1996).

A number of intra-articular structures have been described, particularly vascular synovial folds, as well as fat pads and meniscoid structures. All are highly innervated and can be a potential source of pain (Taylor and Twomey, 1994; Manchikanti et al., 2002a; Middleditch and Oliver, 2005).

As synovial joints, the facet joints are prone to degenerative changes and osteophyte formation may affect the size of the intervertebral foramen. Facet joints have been implicated as a cause of pain in 54% to 67% of patients with persistent neck pain (Barnsley et al., 1995; Lord et al., 1996; Manchikanti et al., 2002b).

Intervertebral Discs

There are six cervical intervertebral discs that facilitate and restrain movement as well as transmit loads from one vertebral body to the next (Fig. 8.4).

Cervical discs are approximately 5 mm thick (Soames and Palastanga, 2018) and the thinnest of all the intervertebral discs. Each forms part of the anterior wall of

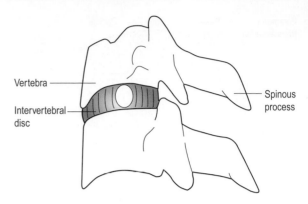

Fig. 8.4 Cervical vertebrae, interbody joint and posterior elements. (From Soames and Palastanga, 2018. Reprinted by permission of Elsevier Ltd.)

the intervertebral foramen and is thicker anteriorly, contributing to the cervical lordosis.

The intervertebral disc consists of an annulus fibrosus, nucleus pulposus, and transitional superior and inferior vertebral end-plates. Its intrinsic structure is unlike that of lumbar discs, however, and differs with age (Peng and Bogduk, 2019).

At birth, the *nucleus pulposus* of the cervical disc consists of no more than 25% of the entire disc, and it undergoes rapid degeneration with age such that by the age of 30, the nucleus is indistinguishable and forms a firm fibrocartilaginous plate (Mercer and Bogduk, 1999; Peng and Bogduk, 2019).

The structure of the *annulus fibrosus* is different anteriorly and posteriorly (Mercer and Bogduk, 1999). The *anterolateral annulus* forms a crescent shape when viewed from above, which is thicker medially and thinner laterally, tapering out to the unciform processes (Fig. 8.5). It consists of a thin paramedian band of collagen fibres that run longitudinally between the vertebral bodies to form a dense, anterior interosseous ligament.

Collagen fibres have been found 2 to 3 mm from the surface of the anterior annulus, embedded with proteoglycans and forming a fibrocartilaginous mass that has a pearly appearance. Moving more deeply, the core of the fibrocartilaginous mass becomes more homogeneous and forms the apparent nucleus of the disc.

Because the cervical discs lack a gelatinous nucleus that is constrained by a circumferential annulus fibrosus,

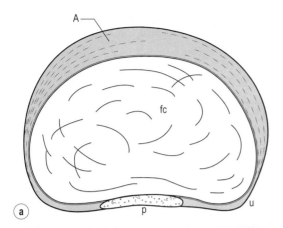

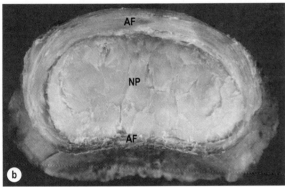

Fig. 8.5 Top views of a cervical disc. (a) Sketch showing how the anterior annulus (A) is crescentic, thik anteriorly, but tapering towards the uncinate region (u). It surrounds a central fibrocartilaginous core (fc). The posterior annulus (p) is limited to paramedian longitudinal fibres. (b) Photograph showing the top view of a 39-year-old cervical intervertebral disc. The annulus fibrosus (AF) is thick and fibrous, tapering posteriorly towards the uncinate region. Posteriorly, the thin AF is found only towards the midline. Centrally, the nucleus pulposus (NP) appears as a fibrocartilaginous core. (From Kristjansson, 2005. Reprinted by permission of Elsevier Ltd.)

posterior two-thirds of the disc in older specimens (bipartite disc). Strong shear forces are transmitted through the intervertebral disc, particularly during rotation and side flexion. C3–C5 are the most loaded segments, and it is at these levels that the fissures in the disc first appear.

The *posterior annulus* demonstrates features that are different from the anterior annulus. It consists of a thin layer of a set of vertically oriented collagen fibres, not more than 1 mm thick, passing between adjacent vertebrae and extending out as far as the unciform process on each side.

The deep layer of the posterior longitudinal ligament, with short fibres spanning each intervertebral joint, appears to compensate for the lack of annular fibres in the posterior part of the disc, supporting the nucleus posteriorly. Posterolaterally, the alar fibres of the posterior longitudinal ligament alone contain the nucleus. These may become torn or stretched by a herniated disc.

Degenerate cervical discs may herniate laterally at the uncovertebral region, reflected posterolaterally by the stronger median part of the posterior longitudinal ligament, to cause unilateral pressure on the dura, dural nerve root sleeve, and underlying nerve root in the intervertebral canal.

The *vertebral end-plate* offers protection by preventing the disc from bulging into the vertebral body. It acts as a semipermeable membrane, which, by diffusion, facilitates the exchange of nutrients between the vertebral body and the disc.

The triangular vertebral canal is the largest in the cervical spine and allows for posterior disc movement, even though the spinal cord is enlarged in this region. Posterolateral prolapse may encroach on the dural nerve root sleeve and underlying nerve root, and there is the possibility that degenerative changes can lead to compression of the spinal cord, leading to cervical myelopathy.

Arm pain does not appear to be as commonly associated with cervical disc lesions as leg pain is with lumbar disc lesions. Dural pressure due to a cervical disc herniation tends to produce central or unilateral scapular pain.

Nerve Supply to the Intervertebral Disc

The cervical discs receive innervation posteriorly from the cervical sinuvertebral nerves, laterally from the vertebral nerve, and anteriorly from branches of the

as in lumbar discs, they are not susceptible to internal disc disruption. They are also not loaded by approximately 50% of body weight, as are the lumbar discs. Conversely, their essentially ligamentous structure could make them more susceptible than lumbar discs to the equivalent of ligamentous injury (Peng and Bogduk, 2019).

Clefts extend into the fibrocartilaginous core laterally from the uncovertebral region; partially into the core in younger patients but totally transecting the cervical sympathetic trunks (Peng and DePalma, 2018; Peng and Bogduk, 2019). Mendel et al. (1992) found evidence of nerve fibres and mechanoreceptors in the posterolateral region of the annulus.

Pain can be due to the mechanical effect of secondary compression of pain-sensitive structures, and/or associated with the increased amounts of inflammatory cytokines in a degenerative disc. These upregulate nerve growth factor (NGF), messenger ribonucleic acid (mRNA) expression and the secretion of NGF protein, which is thought to make the disc 'painful' (Peng and DePalma, 2018).

Disc material is believed to undergo a process of degradation that contributes to its herniation. The stimulation of the nerve root by chemical pain mediators within the disc may also play a role in the pathophysiology of cervical radiculopathy. Herniated disc material may incite the production of various inflammatory cytokines, such as substance P, bradykinin, and prostaglandins and other pain mediators known to be involved in radiculopathy (Rhee et al., 2007).

The three most common ways that an exiting nerve root can be irritated or compressed are posterolateral herniation of a disc, a degenerative disc causing decreased height of the neural foramen, and cervical spondylosis, which can occur at the vertebral body, uncovertebral joint or facet joint (Yoon, 2011).

Cervical Spinal Nerves

There are eight cervical spinal nerves, each of which is approximately 1 cm long. Each nerve, together with the dorsal root ganglion, occupies a large, funnel-shaped intervertebral foramen (Fig. 8.6).

The *spinal nerve* is composed of one dorsal or posterior nerve root and one ventral or anterior nerve root, the ventral nerve root emerging more caudally from the dura mater (Tanaka et al., 2000). The dorsal nerve root carries sensory fibres, and the ventral nerve root carries motor fibres.

The spinal nerve occupies one-fourth to one-third of the intervertebral foramen diameter and carries with it an investment of the dura mater, the dural nerve root sleeve. The dural nerve root sleeve is sensitive to pressure and produces pain in a segmental distribution.

Cervical spinal nerves generally emerge horizontally, therefore the nerve roots are normally vulnerable to pressure only from the disc at that particular level, producing signs and symptoms in one segment only (Fig. 8.7).

However, Tanaka et al. (2000), in a cadaver study, showed that the roots below C5 reached their intervertebral foramen with increasing obliquity, making compression of more than one nerve root below this level possible. Indication of more than one nerve root involvement should be considered suspicious, however, until proven otherwise.

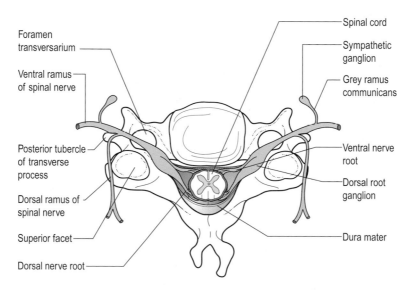

Foramen transversarium

Ventral ramus of spinal nerve

Posterior tubercle of transverse process

Dorsal ramus of spinal nerve

Superior facet

Dorsal nerve root

Spinal cord

Sympathetic ganglion

Grey ramus communicans

Ventral nerve root

Dorsal root ganglion

Dura mater

Fig. 8.6 Formation of a spinal nerve. (From Middleditch and Oliver, 2005. Reprinted by permission of Elsevier Ltd.)

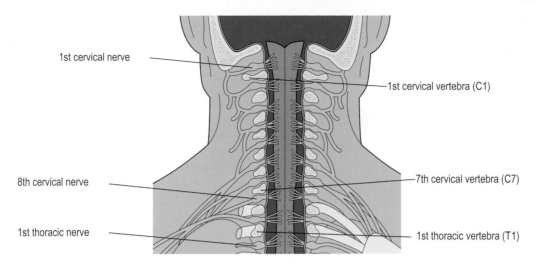

1st cervical nerve

8th cervical nerve

1st thoracic nerve

1st cervical vertebra (C1)

7th cervical vertebra (C7)

1st thoracic vertebra (T1)

Fig. 8.7 Horizontal direction of emerging nerve roots.

At the C7–T1 disc, 78% of specimens showed that the C8 nerve roots did not have any contact with the disc at the entrance of the intervertebral foramen, which could account for the low frequency of C8 radiculopathy.

Nerve root compression was found to occur at the entrance of the intervertebral foramen and was determined to be due to herniated discs and osteophytes in the uncovertebral region anteriorly, and to the superior articular process, ligamentum flavum and periradicular fibrous tissue posteriorly (Tanaka et al., 2000).

Motor impairment, therefore, is suggestive of anterior compression from a disc prolapse or degenerative changes in the uncovertebral region, whereas sensory change is indicative of compression due to changes in the posterior structures. A large disc prolapse or gross degenerative change, anteriorly or posteriorly, may compress both elements of the nerve root.

After it leaves the intervertebral foramen, the spinal nerve immediately divides into *ventral* and *dorsal rami*.

The *sinuvertebral nerve* is a mixed sensory and sympathetic nerve, receiving origin from the ventral ramus and the grey ramus communicans of the sympathetic system (Fig. 8.8). The nerve returns through the intervertebral foramen and gives off ascending, descending and transverse branches to supply structures at, above and below the segment (Middleditch and Oliver, 2005; Standring, 2015; Soames and Palastanga, 2018).

The sinuvertebral nerve supplies the dura mater, posterior longitudinal ligament and the outer part of the annulus of the intervertebral disc (Bogduk, 1994, 2023).

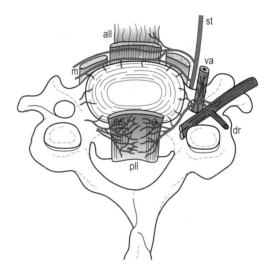

Fig. 8.8 A sketch of the innervation of the plexuses surrounding a cervical intervertebral disc (*based on Groen et al. 1990*). The sinuvertebral nerves form a dense plexus accompanying the posterior longitudinal ligament (pll). Anteriorly, branches of the sympathetic trunk (st) supply the front of the disc and form a plexus accompanying the anterior longitudinal ligament (all). *dr*, Dorsal ramus; *va*, vertebral artery; *m*, prevertebral muscles. (From Bogduk, 1994. Reprinted by permission of Elsevier Ltd.)

Cranial Nerves

Twelve pairs of cranial nerves are traditionally described that emerge directly from the brain (Table 8.1).

Apart from the optic nerve (II), which is considered to be part of the central nervous system, the cranial nerves form part of the peripheral nervous system, but their ganglia originate in the central nervous system.

It is important to test the cranial nerves if vascular pathology is suspected. The range of pathologies is presented in Table 8.2 on page 245 and the tests for the cranial nerves are described in Table 8.3 on page 259.

Cervical Arteries

In relation to the diagnosis and treatment of cervical lesions, the principal arteries for consideration are the vertebral and internal carotid arteries, each of which has a right and left artery in the cervical spine.

Anatomically, the *vertebral artery* is divided into the following four sections, which include two right-angled bends where it is vulnerable to internal and external factors, which could compromise blood flow (Fig. 8.9) (Middleditch and Oliver, 2005; Standring, 2015):

- Its origin from the subclavian artery
- Its passage through each foramen transversarium except C7. In this section, it gives off spinal branches that supply the spinal cord and its sheaths via the intervertebral foramen
- The first right-angled bend, turning medially to pass behind the lateral mass of the atlas
- The second right-angled bend, turning vertically to enter the foramen magnum to unite with the

TABLE 8.1	Cranial nerves	
Nerve		**Function/Muscles controlled**
I	Olfactory	Sense of smell
II	Optic	Vision
III	Oculomotor	Most eye muscles
IV	Trochlear	Superior oblique muscle
V	Trigeminal	Facial sensation; muscles of mastication
VI	Abducens	Lateral rectus
VII	Facial	Facial expression; taste
VIII	Vestibulocochlear	Hearing; balance
IX	Glossopharyngeal	Pharynx sensation
X	Vagus	Muscles of larynx and pharynx
XI	Accessory	Trapezius and sternocleidomastoid
XII	Hypoglossal	Tongue muscles

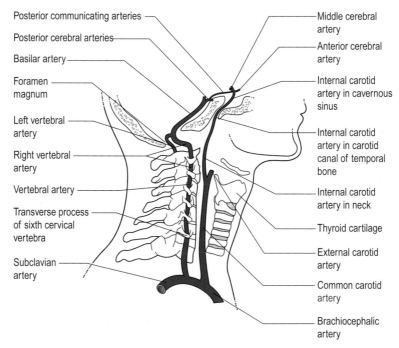

Fig. 8.9 Pathway of vertebrobasilar arteries. (From Soames and Palastanga, 2018. Reprinted by permission of Elsevier Ltd.)

opposite vertebral artery to form the basilar artery, which passes on to contribute to the circle of Willis.

The artery is elastic, particularly in its first and third sections, which allows it to accommodate movement. Anatomical anomalies and variations exist and commonly one vertebral artery is narrower than its partner.

Degenerative changes in the artery itself, in the intervertebral canal, uncovertebral joints and facet joints make it vulnerable to blockage as well as possibly distorting its pathway.

The *internal carotid artery* arises from the bifurcation of the common carotid artery in the anterior cervical spine (see Fig. 8.9). It supplies most of the ipsilateral cerebral hemisphere, the eye and accessory organs, the forehead and part of the nose. It ascends to enter the cranial cavity via the carotid canal and turns anteriorly to end by dividing into the anterior and middle cerebral arteries, which anastomose into the circle of Willis.

The internal carotid arteries together provide the most significant proportion of blood to the brain; 80%, compared with 20% passing through the posterior vertebral artery system. Blood flow is known to be influenced by neck movements, particularly extension and less so rotation (Rivett et al., 1999; Kerry and Taylor, 2006).

Muscles

Whiplash-associated disorder (WAD) is commonly encountered in the cervical spine, but the muscle anatomy of the cervical spine is not covered within this chapter because diagnosis and treatment are not described for individual cervical muscles within this approach. WAD is managed as the more general presentation of the 'acute' neck, described later in this chapter (page 260).

CLINICAL DIAGNOSIS AND MANAGEMENT AT THE CERVICAL SPINE

An understanding of the anatomy at the cervical spine, together with a detailed history and examination of the patient, will help with the selection of patients suitable for manual treatment and will contribute to safe practice.

The two main areas of concern in this region are the cervical arteries and the spinal cord, and certain signs and symptoms will become evident on examination that would exclude patients from manual treatment techniques and require timely onward referral. Similarly, there are other causes of neck pain in which manual

treatment techniques are either contraindicated or not appropriate.

The following section is divided into two parts:
- The first part defines non-specific neck pain and lists possible causes, incidence, risk factors, diagnosis, management and prognosis. (Assessment of the cervical spine is covered in detail in the next section, 'Commentary on the Examination'.)
- The second part looks at other causes of neck pain and associated signs and symptoms, diagnosis and management. Most of these conditions have a more specific or identifiable cause. On the whole, these patients are not appropriate for treatment with manual musculoskeletal medicine treatment techniques and require suitable referral.

The following categories and content are drawn from the National Institute for Health and Care Excellence (NICE) topics and British Medical Journal (BMJ) Best Practice Topics. Additional sources are referenced throughout.

Non-Specific Neck Pain

In practice, there is now less emphasis on specific diagnosis of mechanical lesions and, following rigorous assessment, patterns of presentation (clinical models) have been devised to guide treatment programmes. The clinical models used in the musculoskeletal medicine approach are outlined later in this chapter.

'Simple' or non-specific neck pain is pain or discomfort in the neck and/or shoulder girdle, with or without pain referred into the arm. Symptoms vary with physical activity and over time. In most cases, no specific cause can be found and it is usually multifactorial.

Degenerative changes, predominantly in the cervical discs, with osteophyte formation, may be apparent, with involvement of adjacent soft-tissue structures. However, many adults over the age of 30 demonstrate similar changes and the boundary between normal ageing and disease is difficult to establish.

As well as being a potential source of pain itself, herniation of the disc into the vertebral or intervertebral canal can have a secondary effect on any pain-sensitive structure lying within the canal.

A central herniation of cervical disc material produces central and/or bilaterally referred symptoms. A unilateral herniation produces unilaterally referred symptoms. Reference of pain arising from compression of the central structures is characteristically multisegmental (see Chapter 1). Involvement of the unilateral structures, dural nerve root sleeve and/or the nerve root produces segmentally referred signs and symptoms.

The anatomy of the facet joint with its intra-articular structures makes it susceptible to possible mechanical derangement. It is difficult to differentiate pathology in the absence of neurological signs or symptoms, and primary disc lesions and facet joint lesions appear to be similar in their presentation. There is usually minimal reference of pain into the arm from the facet joints (Cooper et al., 2007).

Non-specific neck pain is a common condition that causes significant disability and 40% to 70% of adults will experience a significant episode in their lifetime. In the UK population, it has been suggested that about one-fifth of adults report a new episode of neck pain occurring within the previous 12 months (Croft et al., 2001). Relapses are common, and up to 20% of acute neck pain will go on to become chronic neck pain. Neck pain increases from 18 to 30 years of age through to the age of 50 to 55.

Risk factors for non-specific neck pain include female gender, history of low back or neck disorders, high job demand, job insecurity, low social or work support, poor workstation design, poor work posture and sedentary work position, repetitive or precision work. It can also be associated with a history of mental stress, sleep disorders, sedentary lifestyle, smoking and trauma (NICE, 2018a).

Diagnosis of non-specific neck pain is clinical, and further investigation is not normally required.

For patients with acute neck pain (lasting less than 6 weeks) or subacute neck pain (lasting 6 to 12 weeks), management should include the following recommendations:
- Provide reassurance – non-specific neck pain is a common problem that usually resolves within a few weeks.
- Offer oral analgesics (e.g. ibuprofen, paracetamol or codeine). The choice depends on the severity of the pain, personal preference, tolerance and risk of adverse effects.
- Consider offering a topical nonsteroidal anti-inflammatory drug (NSAID).
- Encourage activity and a return to a normal lifestyle.
- Consider prescribing muscle relaxants.

- Consider a referral to physiotherapy for a multi-modal treatment strategy which may include stretching and strengthening exercise and a form of manual therapy.
- Consider referral to a psychologist if appropriate.
- Consider referral to occupational health for people with neck pain related to their job.

People with persistent neck pain (lasting more than 12 weeks) can be considered for referral to a pain clinic/team/specialist.

The majority of patients with non-specific neck pain will usually recover from their current episode within a few weeks (Hoving et al., 2004; Enthoven et al., 2004; NICE, 2018a). However, the clinical course may be similar to that of low back pain, with a pattern of intermittent episodes of pain and disability over a period of years (Croft et al., 2001).

A study of UK adults with neck pain demonstrated that approximately 48% of people continue to report persistent neck pain 12 months later (Croft et al., 2001) In the longer term (30 months), persistent neck pain can be expected in as many as 88% of the population with neck pain (Öberg et al., 2003).

Other Causes of Neck Pain

The differential diagnosis of neck pain is broad, including musculoskeletal lesions (rotator cuff tendinopathy and other shoulder pathologies), trauma, arthropathy, cervical radicular pain/radiculopathy, peripheral neuropathy and non-musculoskeletal conditions. Non-musculoskeletal conditions can be classified as neurological, inflammatory, vascular, malignant or infectious.

This part of the chapter considers the other causes of neck pain in turn, including serious non-musculoskeletal pathologies that have features and 'red flags' that should be listened for and looked out for in clinical examination.

Shoulder Pathologies

Cervical spine and shoulder pathologies frequently coexist, especially in the ageing population (Gumina et al., 2013). In some patients, persistent neck pain may be caused by shoulder pathologies such as shoulder capsulitis, subacromial bursitis, calcific tendinopathy and degenerative arthropathy of the acromioclavicular joint.

The difficulty in making this diagnosis is that the patient can appear to present with neck pain rather than with typical shoulder symptoms. Therefore, it is important to exclude the shoulder joint as a primary source of pain, as part of the examination of the cervical spine, and to conduct a full shoulder examination if indicated (see Chapter 5). Additional tests can be used to confirm diagnosis, such as the 'Arm Squeeze test', or diagnostic injection into the subacromial space.

Traumatic or Acute Neck Pain

Acute cervical spine trauma encompasses a wide range of potential injuries to ligaments, muscles, bones, and spinal cord that follow acute incidents ranging from a seemingly innocuous fall to a high-energy road traffic accident (more than 40 mph).

Patients may present immediately after a traumatic incident or days to weeks later. In all cases, careful investigation is required to ensure that the stability of the cervical spine has not been compromised, since, in extreme cases, cervical spine instability can lead to progressive neurological deficit, quadriplegia, and even death.

With *cervical fracture*, there is a history of trauma which could be a fall from height, axial loading of the head (e.g. diving), high-speed road traffic accident, bicycle collision. It can be associated with numbness, weakness and paralysis.

Neck movements should not be examined until clinical features which may indicate a fracture have been excluded.

Some presentations of WAD can also be classified as non-specific neck pain, but the condition will be dealt with within this traumatic neck pain section. Acute whiplash injury follows sudden or excessive hyperextension, hyperflexion or rotation of the neck and presents with neck pain and other symptoms.

Symptoms may be very severe, despite no specific abnormality being found on detailed clinical or radiological investigation. Soft-tissue injury is the most likely explanation. The practitioner is directed to the Quebec Task Force Classification of whiplash-associated disorders for further information.

The most common symptoms are:
- Neck pain, may be referred to the shoulder or arm (88% to 100% of people)
- Headache (55% to 66% of people)

There may also be a reduced range of neck movements, muscular spasm and stiffness, as well as other less common symptoms that include fatigue, dizziness, paraesthesia, deafness, tinnitus, dysphagia, nausea, memory loss and temporomandibular joint pain.

The prognosis is uncertain and personal, and societal factors have a large impact on the course of recovery.

Risk factors include (NICE, 2018b):
- Female gender, and multiple studies have indicated a higher frequency of whiplash injury in women than in men (0.5 to 3.0 incidence rate).
- Age 18 to 25 years: This age group is generally associated with higher-velocity injuries following road traffic accidents.
- Lack of preparation or awareness of collision: A more relaxed occupant is more likely to be injured in a collision.
- Head rotated at time of collision: The greater the rotation, the greater the unilateral loading force on the cervical zygapophyseal joints.
- Previous cervical spine trauma or surgery: Prior whiplash injury predisposes a person to a poorer prognosis following a second injury.

Initial assessment of whiplash injury includes assessment of any associated injuries; inspection of the skin; excluding other causes of neck pain; neurological examination; examining for 'Kernig's sign' and 'Brudzinski's sign' and palpating the neck for tenderness (NICE, 2018b).

With people under 65, the 'Canadian C-spine rule' is a useful tool to determine whether imaging of the cervical spine is required for fracture or dislocation. (A digital version of the C Spine Rule can be found at: https://www.mdcalc.com/canadian-c-spine-rule.)

The recommendations for management are:
- Provide reassurance that recovery from WAD and other traumatic injuries usually occurs within the first 2 to 3 months.
- Encourage early return to usual non-provocative, pre-accident activities and early mobilisation, and explain that:
  - Symptoms are a normal reaction to being injured.
  - Maintaining normal activities and staying active are important factors in recovery.
  - Restriction of activity may delay recovery.

- It is important to focus on improvements in function.
- Discourage rest, immobilisation, and the use of soft collars.
- Ensure optimal medication (e.g. ibuprofen, paracetamol or codeine) – the choice depends on the severity of pain, personal preferences, tolerance, and risk of adverse effects.
- Consider referral to physiotherapy for a multimodal treatment strategy, which may include range of motion exercises, strengthening and stretching exercises, and manual therapy.

Guidance for WAD specifically suggests that referral to a pain management service or pain-trained practitioners should be considered for people:

- Who are considered to have a poor expectation of recovery or a high expectation of ongoing disability.
- With symptoms of acute stress disorders (symptoms exhibited within 4 weeks of injury), symptoms of post-traumatic stress disorder (symptoms lasting at least 4 weeks); depressed mood or feelings of depression about pain; anxiety or fear about pain; high levels of frustration or anger about the pain; passive coping; kinesiophobia and avoiding activities due to fear of pain.

Torticollis (or wry neck) is a painful condition with signs and symptoms that can include spasm of neck muscles, abnormal neck movements and an awkward position of the head and neck. It is classified as congenital (which is not usually painful) or acquired, which may or may not be painful.

'Acute torticollis' is an acquired torticollis with a duration of less than 6 weeks.

Clinical features of acute torticollis include:

- Sudden onset of severe unilateral pain that may be referred to the head or shoulder, with deviation of the neck to one side.
- Restricted and painful neck movements.
- Diffuse tenderness on the affected side with palpable spasm, possibly with tender points of muscle spasm (trigger points).
- No history of trauma preceding the onset of pain, but there may be a history of exposure to cold, prolonged or unusual positioning of the neck.

The following points should be considered by the General Practitioner or other Primary Care Practitioner (NICE, 2018c):

- Optimise medication.
- Consider a referral for physiotherapy.
- Provide useful information and advice – see the 'Treatment of neck pain' section.
- Advise people to return for further assessment if their symptoms do not improve, or if they deteriorate.

The prognosis for acute torticollis is good. The condition is usually self-limiting, with symptoms resolving after 7 to 10 days (Cohen, 2015; Athanassacopoulos and Chiverton, 2016; Cohen and Hooten, 2017).

Arthropathy

Arthropathy in the cervical spine occurs in synovial joints and involves the facet and uncovertebral joints. The capsular pattern is demonstrated by the cervical spine as a whole.

The pattern of symmetrical limitation of the rotations

CAPSULAR PATTERN OF THE CERVICAL SPINE
- Equal limitation of rotations
- Equal limitation of side flexions
- Some limitation of extension
- Usually full flexion

---

and side flexions is distinctive, and the limited movements have the 'hard' end-feel of arthropathy. The history will indicate the type of arthropathy: degenerative, inflammatory or traumatic.

Degenerative arthropathy (cervical spondylosis) involves the spontaneous degeneration of the disc and/or facet joints, with osteophyte formation. It is commonly asymptomatic, even though cervical x-rays and magnetic resonance imaging (MRI) may show severe degeneration.

Symptoms include central (axial) neck pain, which includes reduced motion of the cervical spine in the capsular pattern, paraspinal muscle spasm, and referred pain. Stiffening of the neck is particularly evident on rotation when the patient may, for example, have difficulty reversing the car. Painful symptoms can occur during acute exacerbations of the condition, precipitated by trauma or overuse.

- *Cervical spondylotic radiculopathy* is a specific syndrome of radiating arm pain following a single cervical nerve root distribution. It arises from mechanical compression and/or chemical irritation of that specific nerve root, usually at its exit from the spinal canal.
- *Cervical spondylotic myelopathy* is a specific syndrome of neurological deficit in the upper and lower extremities resulting from spinal cord pressure in the cervical spine, due to degenerative changes in the disc and/or zygapophyseal joints (see 'Cervical myelopathy (neurological)').
- *Tinnitus and vertigo* may be associated symptoms of degenerative arthropathy of the cervical spine.
- *Matutinal headaches* may be due to ligamentous contracture around the upper two cervical joints, the atlanto-occipital and atlantoaxial joints, and may be associated with degenerative arthropathy. A condition called 'old man's matutinal headache' is described, where the patient, usually an elderly man, wakes every morning with a bilateral headache that eases after a few hours (Cyriax, 1982).

Central neck pain can be treated with manual traction, provided there are no contraindications, and the degenerative arthropathy itself does not present a contraindication to treatment. However, rotation under traction should be avoided due to the close proximity of the degenerate facet and uncovertebral joints to the course of the vertebral artery.

Tinnitus and vertigo can respond well to manual traction, but the vertebrobasilar system must be ruled out as the cause. Manual traction is also appropriate for the 'old man's matutinal headache' above, provided there are no contraindications.

Cervical Radicular Pain/Radiculopathy

Radicular arm pain describes pain in one or both arms, often secondary to compression or irritation of nerve roots in the cervical spine. The pain typically follows a specific dermatomal pattern.

Cervical radiculopathy describes a neurological deficit within the upper limb, in keeping with a single nerve root level. The hallmark clinical signs and symptoms of cervical radiculopathy are pain, sensory loss, motor weakness, and reflex deficit in the distribution of the affected nerve root. The most commonly affected nerve roots are C7 (50% to 70%), C6 (>20%), C8 (10%), and

C5 (2% to 10%) (Kuijper et al., 2009). It is most prevalent in people aged 50 to 54 years.

The most common examination findings of cervical radiculopathy are painful neck movements and muscle spasm. Diminished deep tendon reflex is the most common objective neurological finding, with triceps involvement being the most prevalent. Weakness is the second most common finding (Radhakrishnan et al., 1994).

Risk factors include white race, cigarette smoking and prior radiculopathy. Other risk factors include lifting heaving objects, driving a car or machinery that vibrates, and playing golf (Iyer and Kim, 2016).

In the absence of red flags, plain X-rays of the cervical spine are unlikely to help and may lead to false-positive findings. MRI is indicated in people with cervical radiculopathy, which has failed to improve after 4 to 6 weeks of conservative management and is significantly affecting the quality of life. Earlier MRI can be considered if clinically indicated by severe pain or objective neurological deficit.

If cervical radiculopathy has been present for less than 4 to 6 weeks and there are no objective neurological signs, conservative management should be provided. Most people with cervical radiculopathy will improve, regardless of the treatment, and approximately 88% of people improve within four weeks with conservative management. (Refer to the treatment approach suggested for Clinical Model 3, page 261.)

Surgery is usually restricted to people (8% to 33% of those with nerve root pain) who have persistent or debilitating pain combined with loss of power or sensation. Indications for surgery include:

- Signs and symptoms of cervical radiculopathy, and
- Cervical radiculopathy with unremitting radicular pain despite 6 to 12 weeks of conservative treatments or progressive motor weakness, and
- MRI that shows nerve root compression.

Some patients may wish for more conservative management for their radiculopathy, or may have too many risk factors to consider surgery. In that case, it may be appropriate to refer them to the local pain team/clinic/specialist for consideration for spinal injections, amongst other options.

Peripheral Neuropathy

There are a number of conditions that can present with cervical, shoulder and scapular signs and symptoms, and it is important to be aware of them for differential diagnosis.

Brachial neuritis is also known as neuralgic amyotrophy, Parsonage–Turner syndrome, brachial neuropathy, neuritis of the shoulder girdle and shoulder-girdle-syndrome, is a rare condition and typically affects young adults.

The aetiology is unknown, but it has been associated with various causative factors including trauma, infection, virus, heavy exercise, surgery, autoimmune conditions and vaccinations. It is the most common cause of brachial plexopathy, a form of peripheral neuropathy where there is damage or dysfunction in the brachial plexus.

Brachial neuritis characteristically presents with three stages:

- Acute onset of severe pain in the shoulder, which may refer both distally into the arm and proximally into the neck and may persist from days to weeks.
- Resolution of pain and the onset of painless paresis, atrophy and sensory impairment of the shoulder girdle and/or upper limb, due to involvement of the brachial plexus or its component nerves.
- Gradual recovery.

Presentation can vary greatly, depending on the predominant site of the lesion, that is, upper, lower or whole brachial plexus, or the uncommon involvement of a single peripheral nerve. Typically, the upper trunk of the plexus is affected with supraspinatus, infraspinatus serratus anterior and deltoid being particularly vulnerable.

Management is conservative and the prognosis is good with 75% of patients fully recovered at 2 years (Miller et al., 2000; Mamula et al., 2005; Hussey et al., 2007; Sumner, 2009).

Nerve entrapments and neuritis can present with similar signs and symptoms of neuropathy, but their aetiology is different. Nerve conduction studies and electromyography (EMG) are used to confirm the diagnosis of neuropathy and imaging may provide the source of compression as well as demonstrate other features (Duralde, 2000; Aldridge et al., 2001).

Nerve entrapments, or injuries, have a mechanical cause with persistent symptoms that may need surgical release if they do not settle. They can arise from direct trauma, repetitive or forceful scapular movement or space-occupying lesions, or they can be idiopathic.

Suprascapular, long thoracic and spinal accessory neuritis usually present with pain in the scapula and upper arm that settles in approximately three weeks. The cause may be due to trauma or it may follow a viral infection. There is weakness of the muscles supplied by the affected nerve that usually settles spontaneously over approximately 6 weeks but may take longer.

- Suprascapular nerve entrapment, traction injury or neuritis produces weakness and wasting of the supraspinatus and infraspinatus muscles.
- Long thoracic nerve entrapment, injury or neuritis produces weakness and wasting of the serratus anterior muscle and medial winging of the scapula.
- Spinal accessory nerve entrapment, injury or neuritis produces weakness and wasting of the sternocleidomastoid and trapezius muscles.

The following neuropathies tend to arise from entrapment or injury:

- Dorsal scapular nerve entrapment produces lateral winging of the scapula, best shown on returning the shoulder to neutral from elevation. The nerve is susceptible to entrapment as it passes through the middle scalene.
- Axillary nerve entrapment or injury can be associated with anterior shoulder dislocation, direct trauma or a space-occupying lesion in the quadrilateral space. Pain is poorly localised around the anterolateral shoulder, with possible paraesthesia. There is weakness and wasting of deltoid.

As mentioned, most cases of nerve entrapments respond to conservative management within 6 months (Trojian et al., 2018). Surgical release is not routinely recommended unless pain and/or weakness persists. However, some authors advocate early surgical intervention to avoid permanent nerve impairment (Ganzhorn et al., 1981; Walsworth et al., 2004; Pratt, 2005).

Cervical Myelopathy (Neurological)

Cervical myelopathy is defined as a clinical disease involving loss of fine motor control and coordination, gait dysfunction with long tract signs and imaging evidence of cervical cord compression.

The condition is usually caused by degenerative conditions in the cervical spine. These include spondylosis, disc herniation and facet joint arthropathy as well as ligamentous abnormalities, including calcification, hypertrophy, or ossification of the ligamentum flavum and posterior longitudinal ligament. Metastatic spinal cord compression, usually resulting from the collapse or compression of a vertebral body, can also produce signs and symptoms of cervical myelopathy (Robson, 2014).

The most common symptoms include numb or clumsy hands, impaired gait, neck and leg stiffness, and sensory disturbances in the arms or legs.

Other signs may include:

- Hyper-reflexia.
- Abnormal pathological reflexes (e.g. positive Hoffman, Babinski sign, ankle clonus).
- Increased tone.
- Motor deficits.
- Atrophy of intrinsic hand muscles.
- A broad-based unstable gait.

Cervical myelopathy is diagnosed when a patient presents with signs and symptoms consistent with myelopathy and imaging (usually MRI) evidence of spinal cord compression. A combination of clinical and imaging findings is necessary to confirm the diagnosis of degenerative cervical myelopathy and to rule out other diagnoses. Most patients are first diagnosed in their 50s and it is uncommon before the age of 40.

Although multi-level cervical spondylosis and cervical stenosis are the most common cause of cervical myelopathy, a broad differential diagnosis should be considered, including intracranial pathology, intradural tumour or syrinx, multiple sclerosis and other nerve-related diseases, such as Guillain Barre (Edwards et al., 2003).

Differential diagnosis also includes infectious, inflammatory, and metabolic diseases. In a narrative review, Kim et al. (2013a) identified vitamin B12 deficiency, amyotrophic lateral sclerosis, and peripheral nerve entrapment as the major differential diagnoses of degenerative cervical myelopathy.

In most cases, cervical myelopathy is diagnosed on the basis of the physical examination findings and correlative imaging findings. In cases where a thorough neurological examination reveals inconsistent findings or if imaging is inconsistent with cord compression, a thorough knowledge of other pathologies is paramount for establishing the correct diagnosis.

There are various scales to measure the impact of cervical myelopathy. The modified Japanese Orthopedic Association (mJOA) scale is an investigator-administered cervical myelopathy-specific index that separately addresses motor function of the upper and lower extremities, sensory function of the upper extremities and sphincter function.

Patients presenting with clinical features suggestive of cervical myelopathy should be referred for imaging (preferably MRI). Urgency of imaging is determined by the clinical presentation. When appropriate imaging is available, management depends on the results of imaging and ranges from conservative management to onward referral for surgical opinion.

Inflammatory

Rheumatoid arthritis is an inflammatory polyarthritis, affecting females more than males, with onset usually between the ages of 40 and 50. It tends to follow a relapsing and remitting course.

It is uncommon for rheumatoid arthritis to affect the cervical joints only, without its manifestation elsewhere, and it most commonly affects the smaller peripheral joints bilaterally. However, in patients with rheumatoid arthritis, it may be silent in the cervical joints, and there may be no clinical evidence of cervical spine involvement (Clark, 1994).

The mechanism of the disease in the spinal joints is the same as that seen in peripheral joints, with ligament, cartilage and bone destruction. This loss of the supporting infrastructure of the spine, particularly of the upper cervical segment, is a potential hazard for significant neurological involvement of the brainstem and cervical spinal cord.

Atlantoaxial subluxation is the most common manifestation, but cranial settling (vertical intrusion of the dens) and subaxial subluxation may also occur (Clark, 1994; Zeidman and Ducker, 1994; Mathews, 1995). Rheumatoid arthritis is therefore a contraindication to musculoskeletal medicine techniques.

If there is a suspicion of rheumatoid arthritis but a formal diagnosis has not been made, onward referral is required. Advice, education, and activity modification may be given as appropriate.

Polymyalgia rheumatica (PMR) presents as follows (Dasgupta et al., 2010):

- A history of neck, bilateral shoulder girdle, and/or pelvic girdle stiffness and pain, usually bilateral, occurring in patients aged >50 years (usually women), of >2 weeks' duration.
- Morning stiffness, duration of >45 minutes.
- Evidence of an acute reactive response.

- Patients complain of difficulty rising from seated or prone positions, varying degrees of muscle tenderness, shoulder/hip bursitis, and/or oligoarthritis (arthritis affecting two to four joints during the first six months of disease).
- Rapid improvement is almost invariable within 24 to 48 hours with low-dose prednisolone.

PMR can be diagnosed with normal inflammatory markers if there is a classic clinical picture and response to steroids. These patients should be referred for specialist assessment.

Giant cell arteritis or temporal arteritis is a condition associated with a new-onset unilateral headache (usually temporal), jaw claudication associated with chewing tough foods, diffuse mandibular discomfort, dental discomfort, sinus pain and pressure, and/or tongue pain.

Patients aged greater than 50 years with new-onset headache should be screened for giant cell arteritis or temporal arteritis. About 15% to 20% of patients with PMR have giant cell arteritis and 40% to 60% of giant cell arteritis patients have PMR.

The following may be serious associated features and early diagnosis and management are important:

- Blindness, diplopia or blurry vision, and an abnormally thickened, tender, erythematous or nodular temporal artery may also be found.
- Prominence, beading or diminished pulse on examination of the temporal artery.
- Upper cranial nerve palsies.
- Limb claudication or other evidence of large-vessel involvement.

Vascular Pathologies of the Neck

Vascular pathologies include atherosclerosis, thrombosis, aneurysm, vascular anomalies and dissection. There is a range of potential vascular pathologies of the neck relating to the arterial system which supplies blood to the brain. These pathologies have the potential to present as musculoskeletal pain and dysfunction as 'vascular masqueraders'.

Due to the multiple uses of the acronym 'CAD', the previously used terminology, 'Cervical Artery Dysfunction', has been replaced with 'vascular pathologies of the neck', to avoid confusion (Rushton et al., 2022).

In the early stages of their pathological progression, vascular pathologies of the neck have the potential to mimic musculoskeletal conditions (Murphy, 2010; Taylor and Kerry, 2010), and a patient experiencing symptoms may seek manual therapy for the relief of the associated pain.

Within the cervical spine, vascular pathologies of the neck are rare but important considerations and practitioners should consider them within differential diagnosis. Patient safety is paramount and will be enhanced through an understanding of the risks, pathologies and indications for onward referral.

Vascular pathologies (see Table 8.2) can be recognised if appropriate questions are asked during the patient's history, and the physical examination can be adapted to explore any potential hypothesis of vascular pathologies further.

The history is especially important since there is limited evidence to support the proposed clinical examination tests recommended below. Questioning should explore whether there is any presence or predisposition to vascular pathologies of the neck. The practitioner should use the history to detect subtle symptoms and clues, to be able to make the best judgement on the probability of the presence of either serious pathology or contraindications to treatment (Rushton et al., 2022).

Vascular pathologies may be dissecting or non-dissecting and it is important to be aware that there is a different risk profile for each. That is, dissection events most commonly present with a history of trauma, with cardiovascular factors being less common, whereas non-dissecting events most commonly occur in the presence of cardiovascular factors (Rushton et al., 2022).

Risk factors include:

- Recent trauma (mild-moderate, which may include recent manual therapy).
- Vascular anomaly.
- Current or past smoker.
- Migraine.
- High total cholesterol.
- Recent infection.
- Hypertension.
- Oral contraception.
- Family history of stroke.

As mentioned, the prevalence of vascular pathologies varies between dissection and non-dissection events and between vertebrobasilar and internal carotid artery dissection.

TABLE 8.2	Range of vascular pathologies of the neck	
Structure/site	**Pathology**	**Symptoms/Presentation**
Carotid artery	Atherosclerosis Stenotic Thrombotic Aneurysmal	Carotidynia, neck pain, facial pain, headache, cranial nerve dysfunction, Horner's Syndrome, transient ischaemic attack (TIA), stroke
Carotid artery	Hypoplasia	Commonly silent, rare cerebral ischaemia
Carotid artery	Dissection	Neck pain, facial pain, headache, TIA, cranial nerve palsies, Horner's syndrome
Vertebral artery	Atherosclerosis	Neck pain, occipital headache, possible transient ischaemic attack (TIA), stroke
Vertebral artery	Hypoplasia	Commonly silent, rare cerebral ischaemia
Vertebral artery	Dissection	Neck pain, occipital headache, TIA, cranial nerve palsy
Temporal artery	Giant cell arteritis	Temporal pain (headache), scalp tenderness, jaw and tongue claudication, visual symptoms (diplopia or vision loss – may be permanent)
Cerebral vessels	Reversible cerebral vasoconstriction syndrome (RCVS)	Severe 'thunderclap' headaches
Subarachnoid	Heamorrage	Sudden severe headache, stiff neck, visual disturbance, photophobia, slurred speech, sickness, unilateral weakness,
Jugular vein	Thrombosis	Neck pain, headaches, fever, swelling around neck/angle of jaw
Any cervico-cranial vessel	Vascular anomaly or malformation	Possible headache/neck pain i.e. un-ruptured carotid aneurysm

From Rushton et al., 2022. Reprinted by permission of the Journal of Orthopaedic and Sports Physical Therapy.

It is not possible to identify a definite clinical pattern for each but certain consistent features of the clinical presentation of all vascular pathologies have emerged from case reports, which are supported by observations from systematic studies. These features are presented to allow the practitioner to consider the most likely presentations of different vascular pathologies of the neck and to contribute to diagnosis of the condition (Rushton et al., 2022).

Potential features:
- Dysphasia/dysarthria/aphasia
- Unsteadiness/ataxia
- Weakness (lower limb/upper limb)
- Dysphagia
- Nausea/vomiting
- Facial palsy
- Paraesthesia
- Dizziness/disequilibrium
- Ptosis
- Loss of consciousness
- Confusion
- Drowsiness

If vascular pathology is suspected then referral for medical assessment is required.

Malignancy

Malignant disease is usually extradural with bone metastases produced most commonly from primaries in the bronchus, breast, prostate, ovary, thyroid or kidney. However, a diagnosis of a primary tumour or blood cancer must not be overlooked.

- *Metastatic*
  - Spontaneous but severe, persistent pain, particularly with bony involvement, which does not resolve with initial treatments.
  - Bone invasion is common in known malignancy, but it can often be the initial sign of advanced, undiagnosed malignancy.

- Localised neck pain with a history of primary cancer (breast, lung, prostate, kidney, thyroid), fatigue, history of weight loss; bone pain. Lymphadenopathy and hepatosplenomegaly may be present with more specific findings related to the type of cancer.
- *Primary*
  - Localised neck pain, fatigue, history of weight loss.
  - Localised tenderness with or without neurological compromise.
- *Multiple myeloma*
  - Most common tumour in the spine, along with plasmacytoma. The latter is rare and implies a single lesion with an indolent or slow course clinically. It is seen more commonly in a young person.
  - Multiple myeloma is seen in older patients, is rapidly progressive, and commonly presents with neurological symptoms, due to vertebral body collapse.
  - Patients may also have symptoms associated with hypercalcaemia and renal failure.

If malignancy is suspected, urgent onward referral for further investigation is required, in line with local policy.

Infection

Infection is rare and could include discitis, vertebral osteomyelitis, or spinal epidural abscess. Practitioners should exclude the following symptoms and history:

- Fever.
- Tuberculosis, or recent urinary tract infection.
- Diabetes.
- History of intravenous drug use.
- HIV infection, use of immunosuppressants, or the person is otherwise immunocompromised.
- Fever in a patient with new neck pain.
  - In these patients, neck pain should be assumed to be secondary to an infection until proven otherwise.
  - Patients with an infectious cause may be hypotensive or tachycardic.
  - There may be a history of recent infection (especially skin or urinary tract), or a history of intravenous drug use or immune compromise.
  - Cervical osteomyelitis and cervical epidural abscesses arise from haematogenous spread in most cases. About one-third of cases of cervical epidural abscess arise through spread from adjacent skin.
- Patients with meningitis may also have nuchal rigidity.
- More severe, spontaneous neck pain, often following systemic infection, with marked decreased range of motion, or with progressive neurological changes in upper extremities. It commonly begins as a cervical discitis (i.e. disc space infection) because the disc is highly susceptible to infection. It then spreads to adjacent bone, with severe neck pain. Often this follows some time after the sepsis and the patient may be past the septic episode by the time the actual neck pain begins.

If infection is suspected, emergency onward referral for further investigation is required, in line with local policy.

Other

The pain of *shingles* (herpes zoster) can precede the rash, and cervical pain and headache have been reported prior to the appearance of vesicles in the cervical region.

Thoracic outlet syndrome, *complex regional pain syndrome* and *work-related syndromes* all present with upper limb signs and symptoms that are sometimes difficult to isolate into a simple diagnostic pattern, particularly if symptoms have been present for a long time.

Fibromyalgia usually presents in women as a complex of variable symptoms, including widespread musculoskeletal pain of the neck, shoulders and upper limbs. Fatigue, headache, waking unrefreshed, subjective distal swelling, poor concentration, forgetfulness, depression and gastrointestinal or genitourinary irritability have been described (Doherty, 1995; Kim et al., 2013b). Multiple hyperalgesic tender spots and non-restorative sleep are the main diagnostic features of fibromyalgia.

The condition is difficult to separate from endogenous depression. There are several components to management, including the use of relaxation techniques, exercise, hydrotherapy, physiotherapy and acupuncture. Antidepressants and anticonvulsants such as amitriptyline, duloxetine, gabapentin or pregabalin are commonly prescribed to treat pain and improve sleep, but Kim et al. (2013b) found that these often were not being titrated or taken correctly to achieve the best effects.

The box 'Updated Hierarchical List of Red Flags' presents a weighted list of factors, which, when considered

UPDATED HIERARCHICAL LIST OF RED FLAGS

🏴 🏴 🏴 🏴
- Age >50 years + history of cancer + unexplained weight loss + failure to improve after 1 month of evidence-based conservative therapy

🏴 🏴 🏴
- Age <10 and >51 years
- Medical history (current or past) of:
  - Cancer
  - Tuberculosis
  - Human immunodeficiency virus (HIV)/acquired immune deficiency syndrome (AIDS) or intravenous drug use
  - Osteoporosis
- Weight loss >10% body weight (3–6 months)
- Severe night pain precluding sleep
- Loss of sphincter tone and altered S4 sensation
- Bladder retention or bowel incontinence
- Positive extensor plantar response

🏴 🏴
- Age 11–19
- Weight loss 5%–10% body weight (3–6 months)
- Constant progressive pain
- Band-like pain
- Abdominal pain and changed bowel habits, but with no change of medication
- Inability to lie supine
- Bizarre neurological deficit
- Spasm
- Disturbed gait

🏴
- Loss of mobility, difficulty with stairs, falls, trips
- Legs misbehave, odd feelings in legs, legs feeling heavy
- Weight loss <5% body weight (3–6 months)
- Smoking
- Systemically unwell
- Trauma
- Bilateral pins and needles in hands and/or feet
- Previous failed treatment
- Thoracic pain
- Headache
- Physical appearance
- Marked partial articular restriction of movement

From Greenhalgh and Selfe, 2010. Reprinted by permission of Elsevier Ltd.

together, in the context of the patient's history, signs and symptoms, helps to raise the practitioner's index of suspicion for serious pathology (see Chapter 1).

COMMENTARY ON THE EXAMINATION

Observation

Before proceeding with the history, a general observation of the patient's *face*, *posture* and *gait* is made, noting the posture of the neck and the carriage of the head.

Neck posture will give an immediate indication of the severity and possible irritability of the condition, such as a wry neck associated with acute pain in which the patient has developed an antalgic posture.

History

The 'Updated Hierarchical List of Red Flags' box lists the 'red flags' for the possible presence of serious pathology that should be listened for and identified throughout the history and examination.

In isolation, many of the red flags may have limited significance, but it is for the practitioner to consider the general profile of the patient and to decide whether contraindications to treatment exist and/or whether onward referral is indicated. A combination of the red flags listed should raise the index of suspicion.

The history is particularly important at the spinal joints. Selection of patients for musculoskeletal medicine treatment techniques relies on identifying a musculoskeletal lesion, and certain aspects of the history will assist in this diagnosis as well as highlight patients with contraindications to treatment.

The patient's *age, occupation, sports, hobbies and activities* may give an indication of the nature of onset and its relationship to habitual postural problems associated with a particular lifestyle.

The age of the patient is important, particularly at the cervical spine, since the clinical diagnosis can be related to age. In the young patient, child or adolescent, neck pain may be associated with an acute torticollis. Nonspecific neck pain tends to occur in the working-age group. If there is a posterior or posterolateral disc herniation, there may also be a radiculopathy. Facet joint lesions are also prevalent in this age group.

Arm pain presenting under the age of 35 may be indicative of serious pathology, and this should be excluded. Other degenerative changes in the intervertebral, uncovertebral and facet joints occur in the 'older' neck.

Habitual postures can contribute to postural adjustment, altered biomechanics and muscle imbalance. Examples are provided by the head-forward posture of the computer operator, side-flexed posture of holding the telephone in the crook of the neck to leave the hands free, flexed and rotated posture of the plumber or builder, or head-extended posture allowing the arms to be used above the head in the painter or electrician.

Athletes may assume certain postures or positions related to their sport that may precipitate or contribute to their problem.

The *site and spread* of the symptoms give important clues to diagnosis in the cervical spine and highlight the importance of understanding the mechanisms of referred pain in a segmental or multisegmental pattern. Pain may be localised to the neck or occur in association with symptoms felt in the scapular area, chest, upper limb or head.

Nerve root compression in the cervical spine can only occur at the levels at which the nerve root can be compressed. C1 and C2 nerve roots do not pass through intervertebral foramina, therefore compression of these nerve roots is not the mechanism for upper cervical pain. In the lower cervical segment, the roots are under threat from the intervertebral discs, uncovertebral joints and facet joints that form the boundaries of the intervertebral foramen.

It is important to establish the nature of the *onset and duration* of the symptoms, not just of the current episode of pain, but of all previous episodes. Cervical disc lesions tend to be a progression of the same condition, and establishing a history of increasing and worsening episodes of pain aids diagnosis.

The onset may be sudden or gradual. It may be precipitated by a single incident, such as in WAD due to a road traffic accident, or a sudden unguarded movement, such as missing a footing.

If traumatic in onset, the exact mechanism should be established: was it hyperflexion, hyperextension or excessive rotation? If the condition developed gradually, is it associated with habitual postures, or a change in posture, such as sleeping in a different bed?

The patient with WAD, without serious bony or instability complications, presents with pain felt at the time of the trauma that settles. Twenty-four hours later, pain and stiffness develop due to the ligamentous involvement and muscular strain. The patient who has severe pain persisting from the time of the trauma may have more serious underlying pathology: for example, a fracture and/or dislocation.

Headache of sudden onset, not responding to analgesics, may be an indication of vascular pathology in the cervical spine (Taylor and Kerry, 2005; Kerry and Taylor, 2006).

The duration of the symptoms helps to provide a prognosis of the patient's condition as well as providing an indicator for serious pathology. Generally, the patient who presents with a short duration of symptoms responds better to treatment.

Disc pathology tends to be self-limiting and symptoms will resolve spontaneously. With repeated episodes, however, this tends to take longer and longer. Nerve root compression may follow a mechanism of spontaneous recovery, usually in 6 to 12 months, providing the patient loses the central symptoms.

The *symptoms and behaviour* need to be considered. Recurrent symptoms may indicate a cervical disc lesion or degenerative arthropathy, which both tend to present with periods of exacerbation of symptoms. Inflammatory arthritis may present a similar picture, but it has usually manifested itself in other joints before involving the cervical spine, particularly the hands and feet, where significant morning stiffness is a feature.

The behaviour of the pain can give an indication of the irritability of the condition. Ask about the daily pattern of the pain. If pain is better first thing in the morning and worse as the day goes on, easing again with rest, this could indicate a nerve root compression problem or a postural problem.

If it is uncomfortable and stiff in the morning and painful on certain movements, this could be indicative of an active arthritis. It may be due to an acute episode of degenerative arthropathy, or inflammatory arthritis, such as rheumatoid arthritis or ankylosing spondylitis.

Pain not relieved by rest at all and with unrelenting night pain indicates serious pathology, such as malignancy.

Does the patient complain of other symptoms? Loss of balance, unsteadiness from sitting to standing or numb hands could indicate cervical myelopathy.

Paraesthesia may be related to nerve root compression. Establish the presence of pins and needles and numbness and note exactly where the patient is feeling them. Consider whether the distribution of these symptoms fits with segmental referral or is a sympathetic feature. Sympathetic symptoms such as hot and cold feelings, heaviness, puffiness or circulatory symptoms may be related to nerve root compression or thoracic outlet syndrome, complex regional pain syndrome or peripheral neuropathies.

Other causes of neck pain, which may produce similar symptoms, should be eliminated, such as thoracic outlet syndrome, which may produce similar symptoms to upper cervical syndromes.

From the history, specific questions must be asked to eliminate vascular pathology and problems of instability in the upper cervical joints, which would contraindicate treatment. Ask about headaches, fatigue and stress, or blurred or dull vision. A description of headache as 'unlike any other' should raise concerns of internal carotid dysfunction (Kerry and Taylor, 2006).

Explore any complaint of dizziness, vertigo and disequilibrium. Dizziness is a symptom of cervical vascular pathology, but it is also a symptom associated with cervical dysfunction, cervicogenic headaches, benign positional vertigo and inner ear problems. The vertebrobasilar artery system supplies the vestibular nuclei in the brainstem and in the labyrinth of the inner ear (Grant, 1988). A careful history will aid diagnosis.

It is important to consider any risk factors for vascular disease, specifically atherosclerosis (see page 244), which may help in differential diagnosis to distinguish pain associated with vascular pathologies or to guide treatment selection to minimise the potential risk from cervical techniques.

The list of risk factors for atherosclerosis is extensive and it could be argued that they apply to a large proportion of the population. The advice is to consider the patient's profile but to maintain a wise balance between ensuring patient safety and applying appropriate treatment.

Other joint involvement will give an indication of previous problems that may or may not be related. Listen for evidence of rheumatoid arthritis, usually in the smaller joints, remembering that the disease process may be quiet in the cervical spine. Ankylosing spondylitis usually starts in the sacroiliac joint(s) and lumbar spine or hips. Note the presence of generalised degenerative arthropathy. Shoulder and neck pain can coexist.

Ask about *medical history* and consider any serious illness or operations. It is advisable to ask about previous trauma involving the neck: a history of recent trauma is considered a risk factor in vascular accidents (Kleynhans and Terrett, 1985, Kerry and Taylor, 2006). Explore previous similar episodes of neck pain and any previous treatment.

Practitioners should *screen* routinely for psychosocial factors and consider relevant health co-morbidities and lifestyle factors (see Chapter 1). These factors may contribute to the patient's presenting condition, or form a barrier to recovery and normal function, and should be addressed as an integral part of patient management.

Check the *medications* currently taken by the patient, as anticoagulants and long-term systemic steroid use may present a contraindication to the treatment techniques.

Ask about any pain-relieving drugs to give an indication of how much pain control is required by the patient.

As neuropathic medication may also be prescribed for chronic pain, it can give an indication of the patient's general pain profile. Statins and antihypertensive drugs should also be noted in relation to potential risk factors for diagnosis and treatment selection.

Inspection

The patient should be suitably undressed and in a good light. A general inspection will reveal any *bony deformity*. The general spinal curvatures are assessed, looking for any increased or decreased cervical lordosis, tilt or rotation, abnormalities in the cervicothoracic junction and upper thoracic kyphosis, scoliosis, or the presence of an antalgic posture.

Abnormal fatty tissue sometimes develops over C7, in association with postural deformity at the cervicothoracic junction, and this is known as a 'dowager's hump'. Similar fatty tissue can often be seen in rugby players in the front row of the scrum. The carriage of the head is also noted, looking for excessive protraction or retraction.

Colour changes and swelling would not be expected in the cervical spine unless associated with a history of direct trauma.

A neuritis or nerve entrapment will demonstrate wasting of the muscles supplied by the nerve involved, and the neck, shoulder and scapular area should be inspected for obvious *muscle wasting*. Some unusual nerve pathologies produce bizarre patterns of bilateral asymmetrical wasting, such as brachial neuritis.

In disc pathology with nerve root compression, muscle wasting may not be obvious on inspection but if apparent would indicate long-standing root compression.

State at Rest

Before any movements are performed, the state at rest is established to provide a baseline for subsequent comparison.

Examination by Selective Tension

The suggested sequence for the examination will now be given, followed by a commentary including the reasons for performing the movements and the significance of the possible findings.

A suggested 'star diagram' assessment tool for recording examination of the cervical movements is provided in Section 3.

Articular Signs

- Active cervical extension (Fig. 8.10)
- Active cervical right rotation (Fig. 8.11a)
- Active cervical left rotation (see Fig. 8.11b)
- Active cervical right-side flexion (Fig. 8.12a)
- Active cervical left-side flexion (see Fig. 8.12b)
- Active cervical flexion (Fig. 8.13)
- Passive cervical extension (Fig. 8.14)
- Passive cervical right rotation (Fig. 8.15a)
- Passive cervical left rotation (see Fig. 8.15b)
- Passive cervical right-side flexion (Fig. 8.16a)
- Passive cervical left-side flexion (see Fig. 8.16b)

Resisted tests are not part of the routine examination, but may be applied here

- Resisted cervical extension (Fig. 8.17)
- Resisted cervical rotations (Fig. 8.18)
- Resisted cervical side flexions (Fig. 8.19)
- Resisted cervical flexion (Fig. 8.20)

Elimination of the Shoulder Joint

- Active shoulder elevation (Fig. 8.21)

Resisted tests for objective neurological signs and alternative causes of arm pain; the main nerve roots are indicated in bold

- Shoulder elevation, trapezius (Fig. 8.22): spinal accessory nerve XI C3, 4

- Shoulder abduction, supraspinatus (Fig. 8.23): C4, **5**, 6
- Shoulder adduction, latissimus dorsi, pectoralis major, teres major and minor (Fig. 8.24): C5, 6, **7**, 8, T1
- Shoulder lateral rotation, infraspinatus (Fig. 8.25): C5, **6**
- Shoulder medial rotation, subscapularis (Fig. 8.26), C5, 6
- Elbow flexion, biceps (Fig. 8.27): **C5, 6**
- Elbow extension, triceps (Fig. 8.28): C6, **7**, 8
- Wrist extensors (Fig. 8.29): C6, **7**, 8
- Wrist flexors (Fig. 8.30): C6, 7, **8**, T1
- Thumb adductors, adductor brevis (Fig. 8.31): C8, **T1**
- Finger adductors, palmar interossei (Fig. 8.32): C8, **T1**

Skin Sensation and Reflexes

- Thumb and index finger: C6
- Index, middle and ring fingers: C7
- Middle, ring and little fingers: C8 (Fig. 8.33)
- Biceps (Fig. 8.34): C5, 6
- Brachioradialis (Fig. 8.35): C5, 6, 7
- Triceps (Fig. 8.36): C6, 7, 8
- Skin sensation toes (Fig. 8.37)
- Knee reflex (Fig. 8.38)
- Ankle reflex (Fig. 8.39)
- Plantar response (Fig. 8.40)
- Ankle clonus (Fig. 8.41)

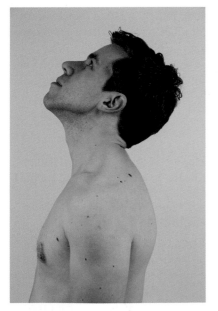

Fig. 8.10 Active extension.

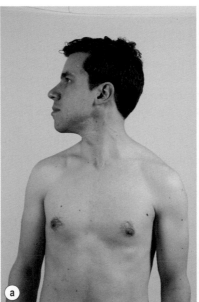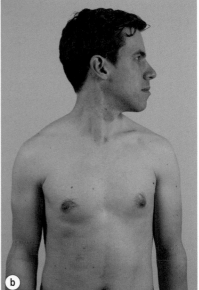

Fig. 8.11 Active rotations.

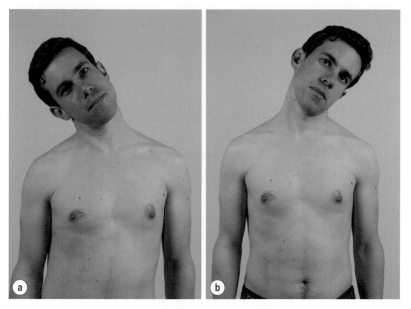

Fig. 8.12 Active side flexions.

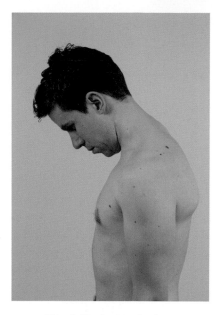

Fig. 8.13 Active flexion.

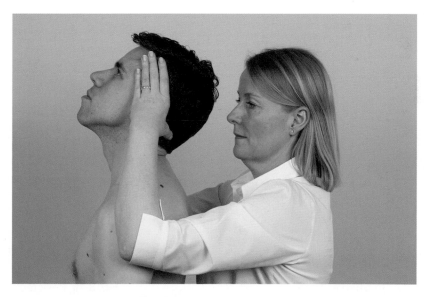

Fig. 8.14 Passive extension.

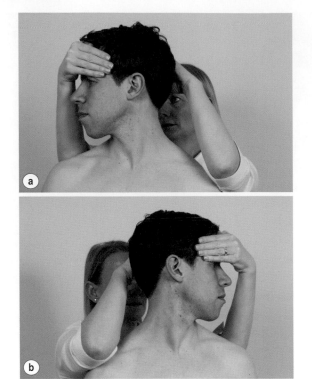

Fig. 8.15 Passive rotations.

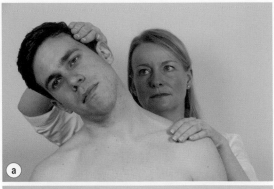
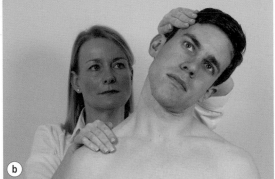

Fig. 8.16 Passive side flexions.

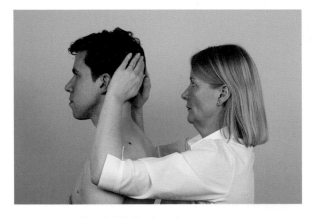

Fig. 8.17 Resisted extension.

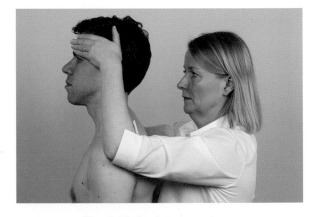

Fig. 8.18 Resisted rotations.

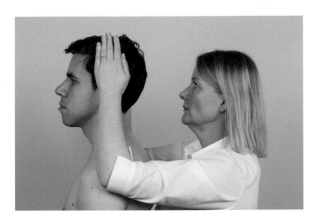

Fig. 8.19 Resisted side flexions.

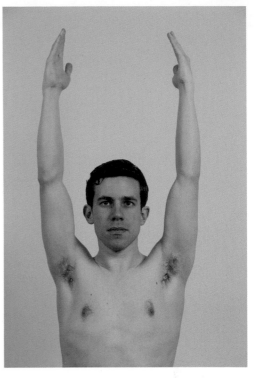

Fig. 8.21 Active shoulder elevation to eliminate the shoulder as a cause of pain.

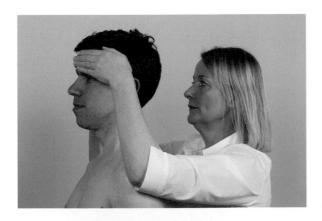

Fig. 8.20 Resisted flexion.

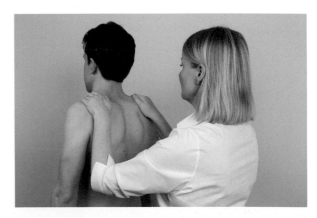

Fig. 8.22 Resisted shoulder elevation.

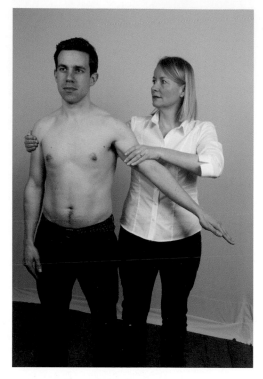

Fig. 8.23 Resisted shoulder abduction.

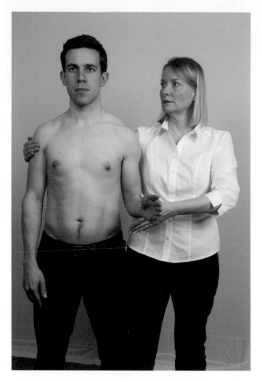

Fig. 8.25 Resisted shoulder lateral rotation.

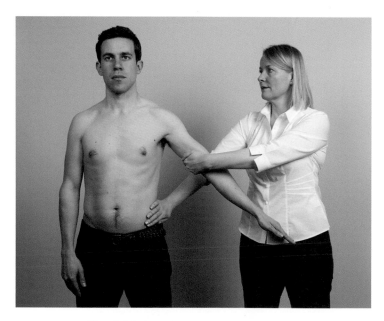

Fig. 8.24 Resisted shoulder adduction.

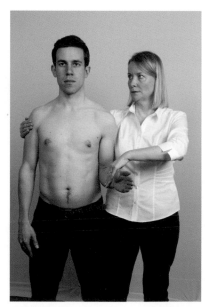

Fig. 8.26 Resisted shoulder medial rotation.

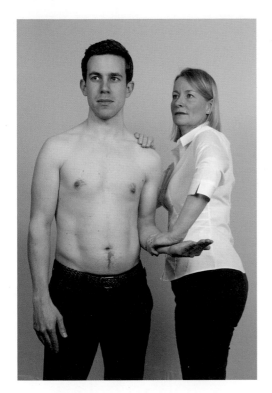

Fig. 8.27 Resisted elbow flexion.

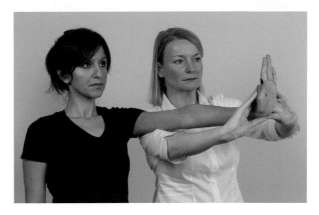

Fig. 8.29 Resisted wrist extension.

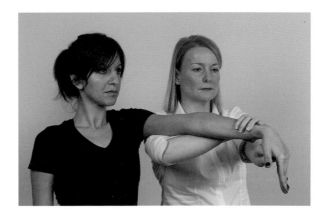

Fig. 8.30 Resisted wrist flexion.

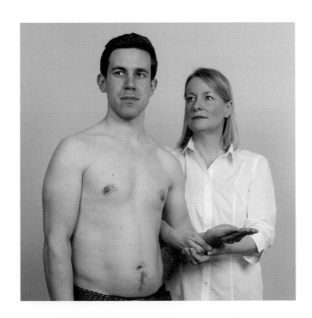

Fig. 8.28 Resisted elbow extension.

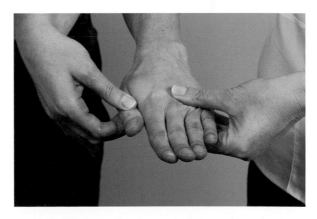

Fig. 8.31 Resisted thumb adduction.

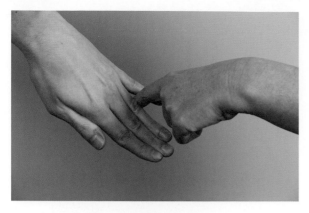

Fig. 8.32 Resisted finger adduction.

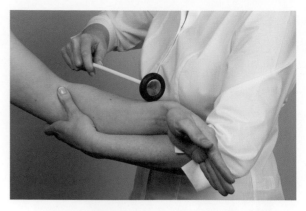

Fig. 8.35 Brachioradialis reflex.

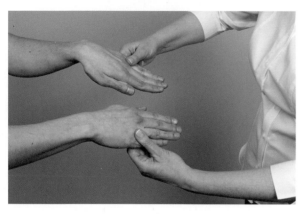

Fig. 8.33 Checking skin sensation.

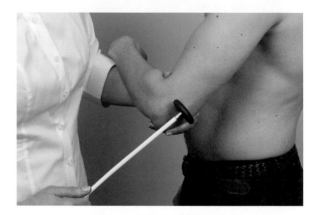

Fig. 8.36 Triceps reflex.

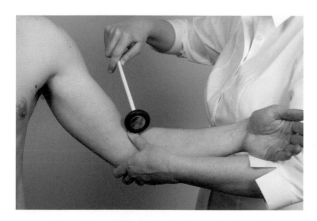

Fig. 8.34 Biceps reflex.

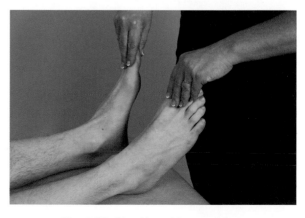

Fig. 8.37 Checking skin sensation.

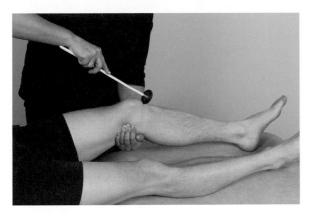

Fig. 8.38 Knee reflex.

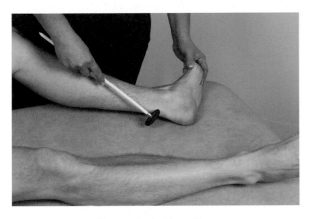

Fig. 8.39 Ankle reflex.

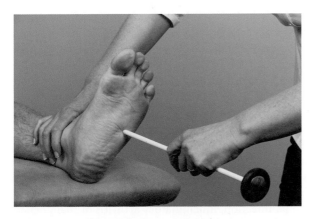

Fig. 8.40 Plantar response.

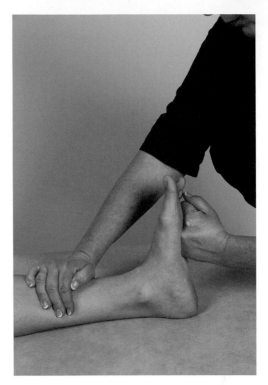

Fig. 8.41 Ankle clonus.

The routine examination of the cervical spine includes active and passive movements and neurological examination. Since the spinal joints are considered to be a potential focus for 'emotional' symptoms, six active movements are conducted assessing willingness to move, range of movement and pain. The capsular or non-capsular pattern may also emerge from these active movements.

In a non-capsular pattern of the cervical spine, some movements are limited and/or painful and others are full and pain-free. Normally, movements at the cervical spine do not occur in isolation, but the examination procedure is conducted simply by assessing the individual movements. It should, however, be remembered that flexion and extension occur with a component of translatory glide, while side flexion and rotation occur as a coupled movement.

The passive movements are assessed to clear a movement and to appreciate the end-feel. Normally, passive extension has a hard end-feel, passive rotations an elastic end-feel and passive side flexions an elastic end-feel due to tissue tension. Passive flexion is not usually assessed because it would tend to aggravate the patient's symptoms.

The resisted cervical movements are not part of the routine examination at the cervical spine but can be applied if felt appropriate: for example, to explore for yellow flags. The wider history should always be considered to signal the presence of serious pathology, such as fracture or malignancy, and whether further investigation or onward referral is required. The resisted cervical movements also assess the C1 and C2 nerve roots.

The shoulder joint is eliminated as a cause of pain by active elevation, which acts as a guide as to whether to proceed with the full shoulder joint examination. If this is full range and pain-free, the shoulder can usually be eliminated from the examination.

Assessment for root signs is conducted by a series of resisted tests for the myotomes, looking for a pattern of muscle weakness that would indicate nerve root compression. Resisted tests also help to establish alternative causes of arm pain, arising from other soft tissues or joints in the upper limb. This explains why the sequence appears to test the same nerve roots several times.

A check of skin sensation to light touch is made looking for differences. Paraesthesia commonly affects the distal end of the dermatomes and these are assessed, followed by the biceps, brachioradialis and triceps reflexes. Additional sensation tests can be conducted if further information is required.

Sensation is also checked on the toes and the knee and ankle reflexes are tested. The plantar response is assessed by stroking up the lateral border of the sole of the foot and across the metatarsal heads. The normal response is flexor. If the response is extensor, or upgoing (Babinski reflex), it is indicative of an upper motor neuron lesion but should be considered in context of other signs and symptoms.

The ankle clonus test/reflex is performed by quickly dorsiflexing the foot and holding it in the dorsiflexed position. A positive sign is rapidly repeated oscillations or 'beats' that can be felt and seen by the practitioner and can be indicative of an upper motor neuron lesion, in the context of other signs and symptoms.

The examination sequence provides a basic assessment framework to glean important information towards the selection of patients appropriate for the treatment techniques used in musculoskeletal medicine.

It also highlights possible contraindications and provides a guide for the specific treatments to be used.

Based on the history and clinical examination, the practitioner should be able to establish the most likely diagnosis, using clinical reasoning and clinical judgement. It is important to recognise potential serious pathology, such as infection, malignancy, vascular pathology, fracture and inflammatory arthritis, and to make any appropriate onward referral in a timely manner. Should additional information be required to aid diagnosis or to add value to management, further investigations can be considered to inform decision making and planning.

The history may lead to the suspicion of vascular pathology and examination should include:
- Blood pressure
- Neurological examination – upper limb, cranial, upper motor neuron testing (as indicated)
- Examination of the carotid artery; palpating for symmetry
- Cranial nerve testing should also be conducted (Table 8.3).

The predictive ability of provocative positional tests to identify at risk individuals is lacking, and there is some evidence against its use (Hutting et al., 2020). Provocative positioning testing is therefore not recommended.

There are no standardised clinical guidelines for medical diagnostic work-up in respect of vertebral and carotid arterial dysfunction, and it is recommended that the practitioner follows local policy in referring for further investigations.

If benign postural vertigo is suspected, diagnosis can be confirmed by performing Hallpike-Dix positional testing, which, if positive, demonstrates a characteristic torsional nystagmus when the head is reclined and turned to the affected side (Lempert et al., 1995; Magaray et al., 2004; Johnson et al., 2008). The test should not be considered in isolation, but in the context of the whole assessment.

The practitioner may consider further investigations such as blood tests, radiological imaging, and other diagnostic procedures as an extension to clinical examination and to aid differential diagnosis. Investigation should be guided by the suspected causes and should be considered with suspected red flags such as fracture, spinal infection, inflammatory arthritis or malignancy, including primary and metastatic tumours.

TABLE 8.3   Cranial Nerve Testing

Nerve		Function/Muscles Controlled	How to Test
I	Olfactory	Sense of smell	With an odorous substance
II	Optic	Vision	Eye test chart
III	Oculomotor	Most eye muscles	Follow the moving finger
IV	Trochlear	Superior oblique muscle	Look down the nose
V	Trigeminal	Facial sensation; muscles of mastication	Touch the face / Clench the teeth
VI	Abducens	Lateral rectus	Look to the side
VII	Facial	Facial expression / Taste	Smile, raise the eyebrows / Sugar or salt
VIII	Vestibulocochlear	Hearing / Balance	Tuning fork / Look for unsteadiness/giddiness
IX	Glossopharyngeal	Pharynx sensation	Gag reflex
X	Vagus	Muscles of larynx and pharynx	Check for hoarseness of speech; open wide and say 'Ahhh'
XI	Accessory	Trapezius and sternocleidomastoid	Shrug shoulders or tilt and turn the head
XII	Hypoglossal	Tongue muscles	Stick out the tongue

Blood tests can be considered if malignancy, inflammatory arthritis or spinal infection is suspected.

Cervical X-rays, and other imaging studies and investigations are not routinely required to assess or diagnose neck pain with radiculopathy. The Royal Australian College of General Practitioners (RACGP, 2013) guidelines suggest that MRI can be considered for confirmation of compressive lesions of the cervical spine in patients who have failed a course of conservative therapy and may be candidates for interventional or surgical treatment, or when cervical radiculopathy has been present for 6 weeks and is not improving.

MRI can also be considered in patients with complex cervical radiculopathy. For example, if there is a high suspicion of myelopathy or abscess, or persistent or progressive objective neurological findings (NICE, 2018a).

Any other assessment procedure may be included throughout the sequence or explored separately afterwards either to elicit extra information for the purposes of the application of other treatment modalities, or to confirm findings necessitating patient referral.

As with other types of spinal pain, there is no gold standard for the diagnosis of cervical radicular pain. Clinical diagnosis is drawn from a combination of the history, clinical examination, and additional tests. The 'Spurling's', 'Arm Squeeze' and 'axial traction' tests can be used to establish the likelihood of cervical radiculopathy and a combined result of four negative neurodynamic tests (upper limb tension tests) and a negative Arm Squeeze test can also be used to rule it out (Thoomes et al., 2018).

TREATMENT OF NECK PAIN

It is recommended that a course in musculoskeletal medicine should be attended before the treatment techniques outlined are applied in clinical practice (see Section 3).

Treatment of cervical lesions depends on the nature of the pain and classification of the symptoms.

If the pain is subacute – with low severity and irritability – a regime of mobilisation can be commenced, progressing to manipulation if necessary. If the pain is acute – with high severity and irritability – a gentler approach to treatment is adopted.

In persistent cervical conditions, a thorough examination may reveal several contributing factors, together with underlying psychological factors such as anxiety and depression. All factors should be considered, and the musculoskeletal medicine approach and treatment techniques should form only part of management. Their use is not intended to be exclusive.

In terms of likely response to manipulation, the ideal patient will fit into the pattern of signs and symptoms that indicate Clinical Model 2: subacute pain/non-irritable.

In this model, there will be a history of sudden or gradual onset of central, short bilateral or unilateral neck and/or scapular pain. On examination, there is a non-capsular pattern of limited movement and no neurological signs.

To be 'ideal' in terms of likely effectiveness of treatment, the symptoms should be of recent onset and have minimal reference of pain. The more peripheral the symptoms, the less successful the techniques described tend to be.

Provided there are no contraindications to treatment, a regime of cervical mobilisation is commenced. Treatment techniques are chosen based on a continuous assessment approach. After every technique the patient's comparable signs are reassessed.

Mobilisation and manipulation techniques are normally used as part of the stepped approach to management. Their pain-relieving effect is often immediate and can be beneficial in the treatment of neck pain. The pain relief achieved improves patients' movement and function and optimises their exercise rehabilitation.

Vernon and Humphreys (2008) reviewed change scores in randomised controlled trials after one session of manual therapy and found moderate- to high-quality evidence that immediate improvements were obtained after one session of manipulation.

The evidence for mobilisation was less substantial, with fewer studies reporting smaller immediate improvements. There was no evidence for a single session of manual traction. Clinical judgement will help to decide when and how to adjust the treatment plan. If the patient is not responding to the treatment approach, other mobilisation and treatment modalities may be introduced as part of the stepped approach.

A CLASSIFICATION SYSTEM OF FOUR CLINICAL MODELS

In the past, treatment in musculoskeletal medicine has been traditionally targeted at the disc, aiming to reduce displacement, relieve pain and restore movement. However, there is a lack of confidence in these traditional pathoanatomical diagnostic labels, since the cause of pain cannot be confidently localised to one specific structure (Peake and Harte, 2005).

Consequently, several authors have established classifications to determine treatment programmes and to predict prognosis (McKenzie, 1981; Riddle, 1998; Laslett and van Wijmen, 1999; Tseng et al., 2006).

The presentation of signs and symptoms of cervical lesions has been classified here into clinical models adapted from Cyriax's original theories. These models are judgement based and contribute to the clinical decision-making process to rationalise appropriate treatment programmes, but they are not intended to be restrictive.

A stepped approach to the management of non-specific neck pain and to the management of cervical radicular pain, with or without radiculopathy, is currently recommended. Less invasive treatments are generally offered first, including education/watchful wait, activity and work modification, simple analgesics and NSAIDs medication, muscle relaxant medication, neuropathic medication if persistent radicular pain and physiotherapy (e.g. exercise, mobilisation).

Consider referral to persistent pain management, occupational health and psychotherapy if appropriate. If symptoms persist, more invasive treatments can be considered, such as cervical epidural injection, transforaminal injection and cervical surgery (NICE, 2018a).

The treatment techniques described in this chapter are by no means a cure-all for every case of neck pain. However, uncomplicated lesions of recent onset may respond well to the mobilisation and manipulative techniques of musculoskeletal medicine. The key is the selection of appropriate patients for treatment.

Clinical Model 1: Acute/Irritable
History
- Adolescent or young adult
- Central or short bilateral or unilateral severe pain with high irritability, often with twinges
- No neurological symptoms
- Patient may wake with severe pain, cause unknown, or may have traumatic onset such as a whiplash mechanism injury
- No red flags or significant yellow flags

Examination
- Antalgic posture
- Non-capsular pattern of pain and limitation of movement
- No neurological signs

Treatment

- Reassurance
- Pain-relieving modalities
- Postural advice
- 'Bridging' technique
- Gentle manual traction
- Grade A mobilisation

The following treatment procedure can be applied to any acute/irritable neck in the absence of contraindications: for example, the acute WAD patient.

Treatment consists of reassurance, and progressive positioning out of the deformity may expedite reduction. Gentle traction may be applied in the form of the 'bridging' technique (see page 264) and progressed to manual traction, depending on irritability. Traction is applied in line with the deformity if the neutral position cannot be assumed. Pain-relieving modalities may be applied: for example, analgesics, soft-tissue massage and gentle mobilisation.

Clinical Model 2: Subacute/Non-Irritable

History

- Central or short bilateral or unilateral, less severe neck or scapular pain
- Sudden or gradual onset
- Patient may or may not recall the exact mode and time of onset
- No red flags or significant yellow flags

Examination

- Non-capsular pattern of pain and limitation of movement
- No neurological signs

Treatment

- If no contraindications, manual traction, mobilisation or manipulation

Treatment of choice is to follow the cervical manual traction and mobilisation routine described providing no contraindications to treatment exist.

Clinical Model 3: Referred Symptoms

History

- Patient usually over 35 but the presentation is most prevalent in the early 50s
- Central or unilateral neck and/or scapular pain, followed by referred arm pain (the central pain usually ceasing or diminishing)

- Sudden or gradual onset
- Often part of a history of increasing, worsening episodes; that is, may be a progression of the aforementioned models
- Patient may or may not recall the exact time and mode of onset
- Patient may complain of root symptoms such as paraesthesia felt in a segmental distribution
- No red flags or significant yellow flags

Examination

- Non-capsular pattern of movements producing neck and/or arm symptoms
- Root signs may be present, such as sensory changes, muscle weakness, absent or reduced reflexes; consistent with the nerve root(s) involved

Treatment

- If pain above the elbow, mild neurological signs and stable
- Subacute level of pain and no contraindications, may try mobilisation/manipulation – often unsuccessful
- Traction – manual or mechanical
- Await spontaneous recovery mechanism

If the nerve root is compressed, there may be neurological signs. Since the nerve roots generally emerge horizontally in the cervical spine, usually only one nerve root should be involved. The quality of the pain helps to distinguish somatic and radicular pain (see Chapter 1).

Treatment is aimed at relieving pain. If neurological signs are present, manipulation is not strictly contraindicated provided the neurological signs are minimal and stable, non-progressive, and no other contraindications exist. However, the more peripheral the signs and symptoms, the less likely manipulation is to succeed, and other modalities, for example, manual or sustained mechanical traction and mobilisation, may be more effective in relieving symptoms.

Clinical Model 4: Persistent

History

- Pain for more than 3 months
- No previous treatment; exacerbation, persistent acute or subacute; or non-responder to mechanical treatment
- 'Aching' central or unilateral neck, scapular and/or arm pain
- Pain worsened by movement

- Often part of a history of increasing, worsening episodes
- Cervical stiffness
- No red flags or significant yellow flags

Examination

- Capsular or non-capsular pattern of movements producing neck and/or arm symptoms

Treatment

- Acute/subacute exacerbation may be treated as the models earlier, as appropriate, provided there are no contraindications
- Pain management
- Multimodal approach

CONTRAINDICATIONS TO CERVICAL MOBILISATION

It is impossible to be absolutely definitive about all contraindications and nothing can substitute for a rigorous assessment of the presenting signs and symptoms and an accurate diagnosis of a musculoskeletal cervical lesion.

'Red flags' are signs and symptoms found in the patient's history and examination that may indicate serious pathology and provide contraindications to cervical manipulation (Sizer et al., 2007; Greenhalgh and Selfe, 2010) (see 'Red flags' box, page 247).

The contraindications are highlighted in the discussion that follows, but there are several cautions that should be considered as well.

It may be useful to use the mnemonic *COINS* (a contraction of '*contra*indications'), as an aide-mémoire to be able to create categories for the contraindications: *C*irculatory, *O*sseous, *I*nflammatory, *N*eurological and suspicious features indicating *S*erious pathology. If the first and last two letters are pushed together as *CONS*, the crucial need for *cons*ent is emphasised.

COINS

- **C**irculatory
- **O**sseous
- **I**nflammatory
- **N**eurological
- **S**erious

The treatment regime discussed in this chapter is absolutely contraindicated in the *absence of informed patient consent* (see Chapter 1).

Patients with a history of *cerebrovascular accident, transient ischaemic attacks* or *other upper motor neuron lesions* would be contraindicated. Upper cervical spine instability is associated with Down's syndrome (Department of Health, 1995) and active cervical rheumatoid arthritic changes and would be a contraindication for these techniques as well. Ligamentous laxity may be a feature of pregnancy, making pregnancy a caution for manipulation.

Ankylosing spondylitis and other spondyloarthropathies may not affect the cervical spine, in which case the cervical mobilisation regime discussed below would not be contraindicated and individual judgements will need to be made for each case.

Rheumatoid arthritis, which usually affects the smaller joints symmetrically, may be progressing subclinically in the cervical spine; therefore, the techniques discussed below would be contraindicated.

The history will screen a patient for symptoms of vascular pathology and, if present, the treatment regime discussed below would be absolutely contraindicated. Consider risk factors and symptoms that could be associated with vascular pathology, including severe headache (Rushton et al., 2022).

Dizziness, a possible symptom of vascular pathology, can also be a symptom of cervical dysfunction. Reid and Rivett (2005) found that there was some evidence, though acknowledged as limited, to support the use of manual therapy in treating cervicogenic dizziness. Therefore, accurate diagnosis is essential, to prevent a large group of patients being denied a worthwhile treatment regime.

Suspicious features indicative of non-musculoskeletal lesions would be contraindications to the musculoskeletal medicine treatment regime. These symptoms should not be considered in isolation but in the general context of the whole examination procedure and may include unexplained weight loss, poor general health, pain unaffected by posture or activity, constant pain (of which night pain is a feature) and double root palsy and cord signs, such as spastic gait and/or an abnormal plantar response.

The patient with a past history of primary tumour is not strictly contraindicated, but diagnosis of a musculoskeletal lesion must be certain before proceeding with the treatment regime since the pain of malignancy may mimic mechanical pain.

A suspicious finding (side flexion away from the painful side as the only positive sign) occurs in Pancoast's tumour (a tumour in the apex of the lung), which may affect the lower trunks of the brachial plexus, resulting in medial arm pain and C8 and/or T1 palsy (Pitz et al., 2004).

Bilateral nerve root involvement at one level is unusual, particularly as the vertebral canal in the cervical region is large and can more readily accommodate a disc prolapse than in the lumbar spine. *Bilateral arm signs and symptoms* would therefore be an unusual presentation of a musculoskeletal lesion. *Cord signs*, which may be associated with cervical myelopathy, are a contraindication to cervical manipulation.

An acute cervical lesion is too irritable for manipulation but may well respond to mobilisation, particularly the bridging or manual traction technique described below. An antalgic posture indicates severity.

In cervical radiculopathy with mild, stable neurological signs, manipulation is not contraindicated but may not be effective. Increasing unstable neurological signs are a contraindication as the herniation could be increased.

A history of *recent trauma* has been identified as a risk factor in vascular pathologies due to damage to the lining of the vertebral artery; therefore, manipulation is contraindicated. Past history of trauma, head injury, fracture and previous surgery are all cautions, and judgements will have to be made on individual cases.

The drug history will identify the contraindication of *anticoagulation therapy* to manipulation due to the risk of intraspinal bleed. The long-term use of *systemic steroid medication* predisposes the patient to osteoporosis; this and *a known diagnosis of osteoporosis* is a contraindication to manipulation. Patients considered susceptible to osteoporosis may provide a relative contraindication, and individual judgements will need to be made.

Caution should be shown with patients who have blood clotting disorders.

Patients with significant psychosocial components, the so-called 'yellow flags', may be unsuitable for manipulation and even the mobilisation regime; again, judgements will need to be made on individual cases.

TREATMENT TECHNIQUES

Before embarking on any cervical technique, the practitioner is recommended to read the previous section on contraindications and cautions, and to follow the guidance for safe practice suggested later, which has been devised to minimise the risk of complications following cervical mobilisation techniques.

Cervical manual traction is used as a technique by itself or in conjunction with mobilisation and manipulation. It is used to unload the cervical joints, protecting the spinal cord from further posterior displacement of a herniated disc during the technique.

Manual traction is recommended as a first technique; it is relatively gentle and can be stopped immediately if adverse effects are noted or reported. It often achieves an increase in range and decrease in pain, making the addition of further techniques unnecessary. Manipulation is only applied when a regime of manual traction and traction with mobilisation has failed to be effective.

Safety recommendations for spinal manipulation techniques are included in Section 3.

There is some evidence that manipulation to the thoracic spine may be useful in the management of patients with neck pain due to the biomechanical link between the cervical and thoracic spines (Cleland et al., 2005, 2007a, b; Huisman et al., 2013).

As the risk of complications is lower with a thoracic spine manipulation, thoracic manipulation might be a suitable, safer alternative to cervical manipulation in some circumstances, provided there are no contraindications. It may also be appropriate to perform thoracic manipulation as well as techniques to the cervical spine for the treatment of neck pain (Massaracchio et al., 2013).

The treatment techniques in this section will be described carefully in a step-by-step fashion to enable their application. However, the professional judgement and existing skill of the practitioner will allow each technique to be adapted.

The order of the techniques as they appear here is to provide a guide towards the development of skills at each stage and it is not necessarily an order of efficacy.

It is important to reassess the patient's comparable signs constantly and to decide on the next step in the light of patient response. In this way, the musculoskeletal medicine approach can be integrated into practice as fresh decisions are made and the underlying hypothesis is modified.

As mentioned previously, it is advised to start each session with manual traction as this technique appears to achieve the greatest response. If progression is required then the other techniques can be applied.

Manipulation is defined as a minimal amplitude, high-velocity thrust at the end of range and it is only carried out if judged to be necessary. The mobilisation procedure suggested is usually sufficient to improve most uncomplicated cervical lesions with no neurological signs or symptoms.

The benefit of this cervical mobilisation procedure outweighs the small risk of vascular complications but that is not to take the risk lightly. The appropriate steps to minimise this risk, suggested in the guidelines provided, should always be taken, but debate continues on the true incidence of complications from cervical manipulation.

The practitioner is recommended to check for the most recent developments before applying the techniques, as safety issues are in a state of change and the most up-to-date guidelines should be adhered to. It is also important to check and follow local policy.

It is not possible to say how many times each technique is to be attempted since the process of reassessment is the basis for each clinical decision, and the circumstances vary in every clinical encounter. Nonetheless, a balance must be found between sidestepping the question and providing a recipe for treatment. Some guidance will be given in terms of expectations, with respect to the different models presenting.

Generally, the more acutely painful lesions require gentle treatment, but education, reassurance and advice on self-management may be more appropriate in the early stages without the application of passive treatment.

For the subacute or less irritable states, if the technique is helping, it is repeated; if no change occurs after a small number of attempts, the next technique is chosen; if the patient's signs and symptoms are abolished, treatment should be stopped. Once improvement plateaus in each session, or if the progress is uncertain, the treatment is either modified to an alternative modality or stopped, with the patient being reassessed at the next session when a new status quo will have emerged.

In general, lesions producing central or short bilateral pain should be treated with central techniques, that is, manual traction, traction with leverage and anteroposterior glide. Lesions producing unilateral pain are treated with manual traction, progressing to rotational mobilisations under traction and manipulation if necessary. The monitoring that takes place during this step-by-step progression of forces is most important for safety.

BRIDGING TECHNIQUE

The indication for use is the patient with an irritable lesion: an acute whiplash mechanism injury or the acute torticollis seen in Clinical Model 1 and an acute presentation of Clinical Models 3 and 4.

'Bridging' is a method of applying gentle traction and should not produce an increase in symptoms. Progression to manual traction may be made as the irritability of the lesion is reduced.

- Position the patient supine on the couch a little way down from the top edge.
- Sit on a chair at the head of the couch and gently adjust the patient's position so that your forearms and elbows are fully supported, with your hands resting under the patient's neck (Fig. 8.42).
- Make a bridge with the fingers and rest them under the occiput.
- Tilt the hands into radial deviation, which tips the head slightly back, and pull, flexing your forearms by pulling yourself towards the patient, to apply minimal traction.
- Hold the pull for a few seconds, according to patient comfort.
- Gently release and repeat as required, gradually applying more traction as the tissues relax.

This technique can be adjusted and applied to different spinal segmental levels. Posterior – anterior and unilateral mobilisations can also be added into the treatment approach in this position.

The following mobilisation procedure is applied to cervical lesions that ideally fall into Clinical Model 2 but manual traction may also be appropriate in Clinical Models 1, 3 and 4. The rotation techniques are not contraindicated for the latter models mentioned but the lesion may be too irritable, and could be made worse, or may not respond to treatment.

The patient who falls into Clinical Model 3 and displays root signs will probably not be helped by manipulation, but again it is not a strict contraindication provided the neurological signs are mild and stable.

MANUAL TRACTION

This is always recommended as the first technique to be performed in each treatment session for the patient with

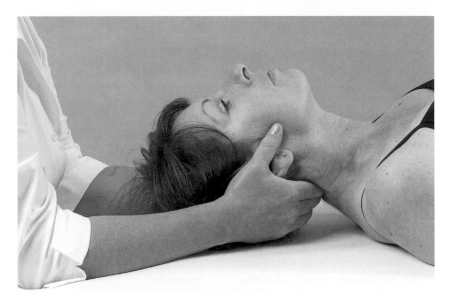

Fig. 8.42 Bridging technique.

less irritable or subacute neck pain. It is generally comfortable and allows both you and the patient to become used to the handling techniques. It is not necessary to progress beyond this stage if positive results are achieved. After each technique, an increase in range and/or decrease in symptoms are expected.

Explain the technique and its aims to the patient. All mobilisation techniques are carefully monitored by the practitioner for a change in symptoms. It is important that patients appreciate that they have control over each technique, and patients are asked to signal if they wish the technique to stop for any reason.

The final overpressure of the Grade C manipulation (see below) is the only exception to this as it is beyond the patient's control – which is why feedback on discomfort should be obtained from the patient right up to the moment of its application.

An assistant is needed to apply counterpressure at the same time as you apply the manual traction, by restraining the movement of the patient's shoulders while adopting a walk-standing position at the side of the couch. If no assistant is available, non-slip matting may be used, or the patient's skin directly against the surface of the plinth should provide enough friction and counterpressure.

Assess the patient's body weight compared with your own. If you are much heavier than the patient, do not apply maximum bodyweight. Less body weight can be achieved by positioning the feet a little further back, but the arms should still be straightened (see below).

- Raise the couch to be approximately level with your hips.
- Position the patient in supine with the shoulders level with the head of the couch and supporting the patient's head in your hands.
- Position one of your hands (it does not matter which for this technique) to cup the occiput or support just below the occiput, allowing the head to tip into slight extension; the cervical spine itself should remain in a neutral position.
- Rest your other hand comfortably around the patient's chin, avoiding the trachea, and let your forearm lie along the side of the face.
- Place both feet directly under the patient's head and bend both your knees; keep them bent throughout the technique.
- Lean out with straight arms to apply the traction using body weight (Fig. 8.43).
- Perform the technique slowly, allowing the traction to establish for several seconds, then pull yourself back to the upright position and release the traction.
- Sit the patient up slowly and reassess.

This technique of manual traction is the first component before applying most of the other techniques and it should be practised to gain confidence and competence.

A patient classified as Clinical Model 3 who experiences a reduction in signs and symptoms after the application of manual traction can be progressed to sustained mechanical traction as described below, since, in the authors' clinical experience, manual traction provides a short temporary effect with this model.

MANUAL TRACTION PLUS ROTATION

(Cyriax, 1984; Cyriax and Cyriax, 1993)

The pain-free, or least painful, rotation is chosen first as this will be more comfortable for the patient. The handholds are similar (Fig. 8.44), but a right rotation requires your right hand to be positioned around the chin (Fig. 8.45), and vice versa for a left rotation.

Three variations of this technique can be applied, and each is a progression of the other.

- Grade A: mid-range rotation (see Fig. 8.44)
- Grade B: to end of available range (see Fig. 8.45)
- Grade C: manipulation, the final high-velocity, minimal amplitude thrust is applied at end of range.

Here, it is so important to understand the nature of end-feel and to be sensitive to any abnormal end-feel such as muscle spasm, which suggests the technique should be abandoned.

- Apply the traction.
- Allow it to establish for a few seconds, then rotate into the least painful rotation by side-flexing your body.
- Return to the mid-position and then release the traction.
- Sit the patient up and reassess.
- Progress through Grade A and Grade B as necessary.
- If these two stages have proved unsuccessful, the procedure is now repeated using the same routine through Grades A and B into the more painful range of rotation. Under traction, this should not produce an increase in symptoms and any increase is an indication to stop.
- Again, progression is only made to the next Grade if necessary.

If this procedure has been followed, but the patient's pain is not resolved, a return can be made to the least painful rotation to apply a Grade C manipulation, and then to the more painful rotation if necessary, provided there are no contraindications to manipulation.

It is important to note that it would be unusual for the full routine to be followed within one treatment session.

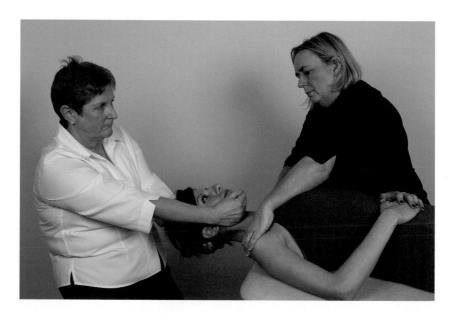

Fig. 8.43 Manual traction.

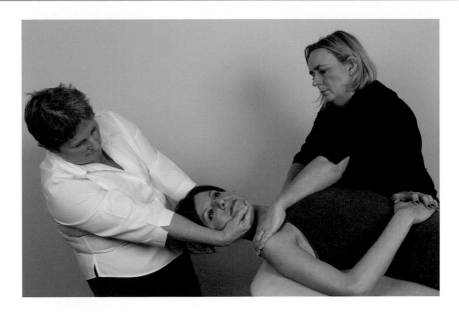

Fig. 8.44 Manual traction plus rotation, Grade A.

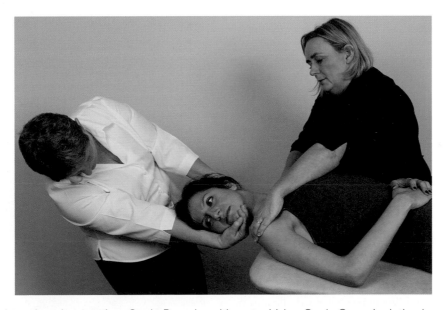

Fig. 8.45 Manual traction plus rotation, Grade B, and position at which a Grade C manipulation is applied.

ANTEROPOSTERIOR GLIDE UNDER TRACTION

(Cyriax, 1984; Cyriax and Cyriax, 1993)

This technique is applied if the symptoms have centralised and the range of movement has increased, but extension remains slightly limited. It aims to improve the range of extension (Cyriax, 1982).

- Place the couch a little lower than hip height.
- Position the patient supine on the couch as before, with an assistant, if available, ready to apply countertraction. Less traction is applied during this technique and it is possible to apply it without an assistant, especially if non-slip matting is used.
- Stand sideways of the patient with both feet parallel, close to the couch and under the patient's head.
- Cup one hand below the occiput and support the weight of the head with your forearm while cradling it against your abdomen.
- The other hand is positioned on the chin to be able to apply both traction and retraction (Fig. 8.46).
- Make a bridge by spreading your index finger and thumb. Apply the web to the chin and curl the remaining fingers so that they tuck around and under the chin (Fig. 8.47).
- Lean out sideways as far as possible to apply traction.
- Once traction is established, bend your knees and apply pressure over the chin, taking the chin into maximum retraction to produce the anteroposterior glide while avoiding pressure from the knuckles against the larynx (Fig. 8.48).
- Allow the chin to return to neutral, avoiding protraction, and release the traction.
- Sit the patient up and reassess.
- If the manoeuvre has helped it can be repeated, this time using several retractions.

LATERAL GLIDE

This manoeuvre is used to relieve post-treatment soreness and to mobilise any residual tightness in the neck. It may be useful in mobilising restricted side flexion in particular.

- The couch is slightly lower than hip height.
- The patient lies supine with the head supported over the end of the couch (Fig. 8.49).

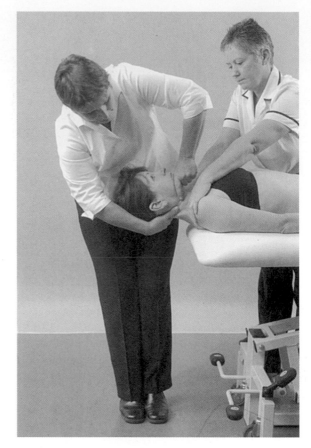

Fig. 8.46 Anteroposterior glide under traction, starting position.

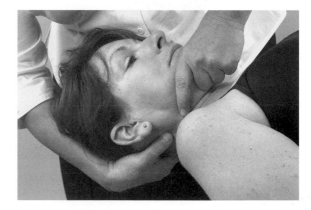

Fig. 8.47 Anteroposterior glide under traction, hand position.

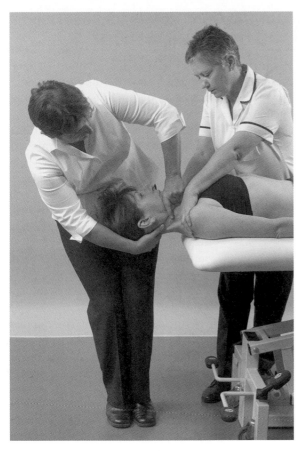

Fig. 8.48 Anteroposterior glide under traction, finishing position.

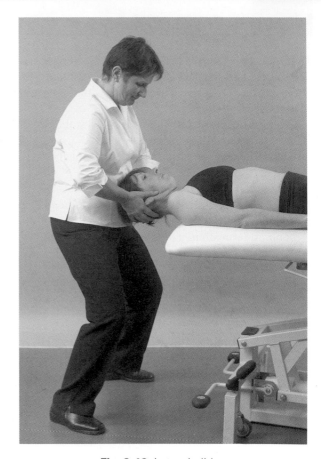

Fig. 8.49 Lateral glide.

- No traction is applied with the lateral glide. An assistant, when available, stands alongside the couch and the patient stays supine but moves closer to the assistant.
- The assistant grasps the patient's opposite arm with both hands and holds the patient close to prevent lateral movement of the thorax.
- Cup the patient's head in both hands with your fingers around the occiput and thumbs parallel with the mandible. Your thenar eminences should support just in front of the ears, resting comfortably over the temporomandibular joint (see Fig. 8.49).
- Bend your knees and position your abdomen against the patient's head but not enough to compress it.

- Apply the lateral glide by rocking from foot to foot, gradually increasing the pressure of your thenar eminences against the patient's head as the patient relaxes and more movement becomes available.
- To ensure that this is a rhythmical lateral gliding movement without side flexion, keep the patient's nose straight and apply gentle pressure to the face as you move towards each side.
- A slight upward movement of the patient's head may occur as your weight moves from each leg.

The following techniques are stronger techniques and it is definitely recommended that they should only be applied after attending a musculoskeletal medicine course.

TRACTION WITH LEVERAGE

(Cyriax, 1984; Cyriax and Cyriax, 1993)

The indication for this technique is that stronger traction is required for central or bilateral symptoms. It is also useful for the larger patient to allow the application of effective manual traction.

- Position the patient in supine lying with the occiput level with the end of the couch.
- Cup the occiput and rest the back of your hand on the couch.
- Apply manual traction as described previously.
- Once the manual traction is in place, bend your knees smartly to apply more traction, using your hand underneath as a pivot (Fig. 8.50).
- Maintain the traction as you straighten your knees, then steadily release the traction.
- Sit the patient up and reassess.

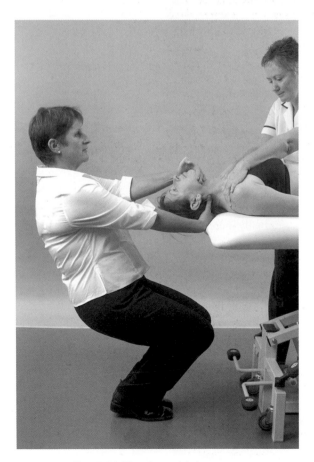

Fig. 8.50 Traction with leverage.

MANUAL TRACTION PLUS ROTATION – ALTERNATIVE HANDHOLD

This is the same technique as the rotation technique described previously, but it applies a different handhold with the neck starting in a small degree of rotation, which gives a stronger rotation overall.

- Start with the patient's head turned into a small degree of rotation before applying the technique in order to secure a good grip.
- Cup your hand, pronate your forearm and place it comfortably on the side of the patient's face with the fingers under the chin, so that they face the direction of the rotation you are aiming towards (Fig. 8.51).
- Stand with your feet rotated a little in that same direction.
- Apply the manual traction and rotation in the progression recommended for the rotation techniques described above, provided there are no contraindications to manipulation.
- Sit the patient up and reassess.

Mechanical Cervical Traction

Cyriax did not advocate the use of cervical traction to the same extent as lumbar and was of the opinion that it was used 'far too often' (Cyriax, 1982). However, there are signs and symptoms that can benefit from the technique and patients in Clinical Model 3, which improve for a short time after manual traction and may benefit from more sustained traction. Similarly, patients with an established capsular pattern associated with degenerative arthropathy and generalised discomfort may also benefit.

Hickling (1972) described the application of sustained cervical traction in either sitting (cervical suspension) or lying. Cervical suspension, the application of vertical traction with the patient sitting, appeared to be the choice of Cyriax, but it may also be applied in supine lying (long traction) or inclined half-lying.

Various studies have looked at the effect of traction at different angles and at different poundages (Judovitch, 1952; Colachis and Strohm, 1965, Deets et al., 1977). The greatest elongation of the posterior portion of the disc was observed with the angle of rope pull at 35 degrees to the horizontal and, unsurprisingly, greater poundages produced great separation throughout the cervical spine.

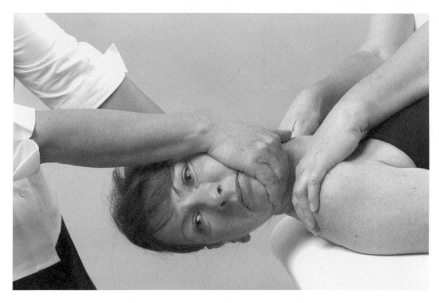

Fig. 8.51 Manual traction plus rotation. The alternative hand position produces stronger rotation (Grade B shown).

Hickling (1972) recounted Cyriax's suggestion that cervical suspension 'should be just sufficient to lift the patient's buttocks from the chair', implying that forces of near body weight were being applied. However, this was for a short duration of 1 to 5 minutes. In lying, average treatments ranged from 15 to 25 lb (7 to 11 kg), according to the size and overall response of the patient. The traction was applied horizontally or in slight flexion with consideration for patient comfort and preference.

The characteristics of the individual patients encountered will form part of the decision-making process in terms of the position adopted.

Some authors propose short applications of traction for just a few seconds. Colachis and Strohm (1965) and Judovitch (1952) suggested that time of application should be decreased as greater forces were applied. Hickling (1972) suggested that traction of 15 to 25 lb (7 to 11 kg) should be continued for between 15 and 25 minutes. This recommendation is based on empirical findings and more work needs to be done to establish the optimum duration of treatment.

Some support for the effect on disc herniation was provided by Chung et al. (2002) who used MRI to evaluate the reducibility of cervical disc herniation under traction on 29 patients and seven healthy volunteers. Using a traction device that essentially consisted of a portable inflatable 'accordion'-shaped neck collar to produce 30 lb of traction force over 10 minutes, an increase in length of the vertebral column was demonstrated in both groups, and 21 patients had complete or partial reduction of the disc herniation.

Contraindications to Mechanical Cervical Traction

These are largely the same as for cervical manipulation (page 262).

Care should be taken in applying traction to the elderly, and they must be thoroughly questioned for the presence of any contraindications.

CERVICAL MANUAL TRACTION TECHNIQUE

Most traction beds and mobile traction equipment of modern design have the facility to apply cervical and lumbar traction. A cervical harness is required to rest under the occiput and chin, with straps or cord passing to a spreader bar above the head.

The straps to the spreader bar should be long enough to give safe clearance above the head. A rope passes from the central point of the spreader bar via a pulley or

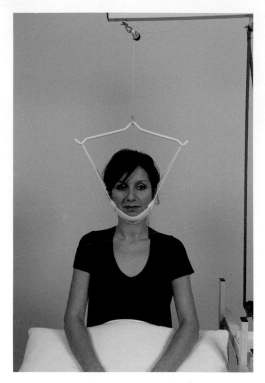

Fig. 8.52 Mechanical cervical traction.

Discuss the treatment time with patients, explaining that the treatment aims to be as 'long and strong' as is comfortable, but they can call a halt to the treatment at any time. In practice, patients are usually comfortable with about 10 to 15 minutes of traction at the first treatment but even on subsequent attendances 20 minutes is usually the maximum required.

Give patients sight of a clock and an alarm bell or buzzer and apply the traction steadily. Keep in close contact with the patient while the traction is being applied, since occasionally patients can become light-headed.

At the end of the treatment time, release the traction slowly and observe the patient's response throughout the release. Let patients sit for a moment or two while they roll their shoulders and relax the tissues, and allow them to get up when they feel ready.

For traction in supine, apply the cervical harness in the same way as for sitting traction. Adjust the angle of pull and select the appropriate setting. Feedback from the patient will ensure that the traction is strong and comfortable. There is a convention that lesser weights are applied in traction in supine than in the sitting position, but for a longer time (Hickling, 1972). On this basis, weights of 5 to 7 kg might be applied on the first treatment for 20 minutes, for example, increasing to 10 kg for 25 to 30 minutes at subsequent attendances.

The traditional advice was for traction to be applied daily, but it would be more realistic to advise as frequently as possible. Patients may not be able to attend daily due to time or financial constraints and the pressures on outpatient departments are also likely to confound this.

Improvement usually occurs after two to four treatments and treatment may be continued over a 2- or 3-week period if necessary. If there is no change in the symptoms after three or four treatments, the position, weight, angle of pull or the time of application may be adjusted, but if there is still no change, the technique should be abandoned and another modality or plan implemented.

pulleys to a fixing cleat in manually applied units, or directly into the housing of the automatic device.

Explain the technique carefully to the patient, mentioning possible after-effects such as stiffness or temporary increase in discomfort, and ask for consent to proceed.

If applying traction in the sitting position, use a firm chair with comfortable back support. Patients often like to have their arms resting on two or three pillows on their lap, both for support and to encourage relaxation (Fig. 8.52). If applying traction in supine, ensure that the patient is comfortable with one or two pillows under the head and knees as desired.

Put the cervical harness in place under the jaw and occiput, providing extra padding if necessary. Place a tissue between the patient and the harness for hygiene purposes or use a disposable harness. Attach the harness to the traction unit and place on the appropriate setting, taking into account the patient's size.

Advice on neck care and posture should be given to patients as part of management and an appropriate exercise programme is normally provided.

REVIEW QUESTIONS

1. Which questions are used to screen for cervical vascular pathology in the history?
2. Discuss the key differences between Clinical Models 1, 2, 3 and 4 in the cervical spine and appropriate treatment protocols for each.
3. How is a spinal nerve formed?
4. Anatomically, how does the cervical disc differ from a lumbar disc?
5. Describe the orientation of the nerve roots in the cervical spine. How many cervical nerve roots are there?

CASE SCENARIOS
Case 1
History
- Madeleine, age 10, woke up with severe neck pain and her head held in a deformity of right rotation and left-side flexion. No precipitating factors, no past history of whiplash-type injuries or congenital deformities. No neurological symptoms. Generally fit and well.

Examination
- An unhappy child not willing to actively move her neck. All neck movement severely limited, resisted tests appear to be negative and no neurological signs.

Task
- Consider differential diagnosis and red flags for a patient this age. What would be the aims of your treatment at this stage?

Case 2
History
- Jasmine, a 37-year-old receptionist, has a 2-month history of pain in the left side of her neck that followed a stressful period at work over Christmas when she was on the phone and typing on her touchscreen computer much more than usual. Pain is intermittent and is worse at the end of the day. She does not have any neurological symptoms, or any risk factors to suspect vascular pathology.

Examination
- No obvious abnormality, painful and limited left cervical rotation, right-side flexion and pain end-range extension. Power, reflexes and sensation normal.

Task
- Which clinical model is this and why? Which treatment techniques could you use and how would you decide on which grade of techniques?

Case 3
History
- Jacob, 21, had a car accident 6 weeks ago and sustained a whiplash injury while driving at 30 mph. He had immediate pain in his neck and had plain X-rays taken at the hospital that were reported as normal. He has constant bilateral neck pain at 5/10 on the visual analogue scale. He has no arm symptoms but does get the occasional headache. He felt dizzy the day after the accident but has been fine since. He is going through motor insurance, as the accident was not his fault. He is currently an out-of-work, qualified stunt man. He is taking ibuprofen and paracetamol.

Examination
- Evidence of muscle spasm in the upper trapezius muscles, very little active neck movements, some pain on resisted testing of the cervical spine but normal power and no other neurological signs.

Task
- Consider a treatment protocol for this patient. Are there any further investigations that may be required if he does not improve? Why would this man not be suitable for manipulation at this stage?

REFERENCES

Aldridge, J.W., Bruno, R.J., Strauch, R.J., et al., 2001. Nerve entrapment in athletes. Clin. Sports Med. 20 (1), 95–122.

Athanassacopoulos, M., Chiverton, N., 2016. Soft tissue problems of the neck. In: Morris, F., Wardrope, J., Hattam, P. (Eds.), ABC of Common Soft Tissue Disorders. Wiley-Blackwell, Edinburgh, pp. 12–18.

Barnsley, L., Lord, S.M., Wallis, B.J., et al., 1995. The prevalence of chronic cervical zygapophyseal joint pain after whiplash. Spine 20, 20–26.

Bogduk, N., Wilson, A.S., Tynan, W., 1982. The human lumbar dorsal rami. J. Anat. 134 (Pt 2), 383–397.

Bogduk, N., 1994. Innervation and pain patterns of the cervical spine. In: Grant, R. (Ed.), Physical Therapy of the Cervical and Thoracic Spine, second ed. Churchill Livingstone, Edinburgh, pp. 65–76.

Bogduk, N., 2023. Clinical and Radiological Anatomy of the Lumbar Spine, sixth ed. Churchill Livingstone, Edinburgh.

Cohen, S.P., 2015. Epidemiology, diagnosis, and treatment of neck pain. Mayo Clinic Proceedings 90 (2), 284–299.

Cohen, S.P., Hooten, W.M., 2017. Advances in the diagnosis and management of neck pain. Br. Med. J. 358, j3221.

Chung, T.-S., Lee, Y.-J., Kang, S.-W., et al., 2002. Reducibility of cervical disk herniation: evaluation at MR imaging during cervical traction with a nonmagnetic traction device. Radiology 225, 895–900.

Clark, C., 1994. Rheumatoid involvement of the cervical spine. Spine 19, 2257–2258.

Cleland, J.A., Childs, J.D., McRae, M., et al., 2005. Immediate effects of thoracic manipulation in patients with neck pain: a randomized clinical trial. Man. Ther. 10, 127–135.

Cleland, J.A., Childs, J.D., Fritz, J.M., et al., 2007a. Development of a clinical predication rule for guiding treatment of a subgroup of patients with neck pain: use of thoracic spine manipulation, exercise and patient education. Phys. Ther. 87 (1), 9–23.

Cleland, J.A., Glynn, P., Whitman, J., et al., 2007b. Short term effects of thrust versus no thrust mobilization/ manipulation directed at the thoracic spine in patients with neck pain: a randomised controlled trial. Phys. Ther. 87 (4), 431–440.

Colachis, S.C., Strohm, B.R., 1965. A study of tractive forces and angle of pull on vertebral interspaces in the cervical spine. Arch. Phys. Med. Rehabil. 46, 820–830.

Cooper, G., Bailey, B., Bogduk, N., 2007. Cervical zygapophyseal joint pain maps. Am. Acad. Pain Med. 8, 344–352.

Croft, P.R., Lewis, M., Papageorgiou, A.C., et al., 2001. Risk factors for neck pain: a longitudinal study in the general population. Pain 93, 17–25.

Cyriax, J., 1982. Textbook of Orthopaedic Medicine, eighth ed. Baillière Tindall, London.

Cyriax, J., 1984. Textbook of Orthopaedic Medicine, eleventh ed. Baillière Tindall, London.

Cyriax, J.H., Cyriax, P.J., 1993. Cyriax's Illustrated Manual of Orthopaedic Medicine. Butterworth Heinemann, Oxford.

Dasgupta, B., Borg, F.A., Hassan, N., et al., 2010. BSR and BHPR guidelines for the management of polymyalgia rheumatica. Rheumatology 49 (1), 186–190.

Deets, D., Hands, K.L., Hopp, S.S., 1977. Cervical traction. Phys. Ther. 57, 255–261.

Department of Health, 1995. Cervical Spine Instability in People with Down Syndrome. Chief Medical Officer's Update, 7. HMSO, London.

Doherty, M., 1995. Fibromyalgia syndrome. In: Lewin, I.G., Seymour, C.A. (Eds.), Collected Reports on the Rheumatic Diseases. Arthritis and Rheumatism Council for Research, London, pp. 83–86.

Duralde, X.A., 2000. Neurologic injuries in the athlete's shoulder. J. Athl. Train. 35 (3), 316–328.

Dwyer, A., Aprill, C., Bogduk, N., 1990. Cervical zygapophyseal joint pain patterns. I: A study in normal volunteers. Spine 15 (6), 453–457.

Edwards 2nd, C.C., Riew, K.D., Anderson, P.A., et al., 2003. Cervical myelopathy. Current diagnostic and treatment strategies. Spine J. 3 (1), 68–81.

Enthoven, P., Skargren, E., Oberg, B., 2004. Clinical course in patients seeking primary care for back or neck pain: a prospective 5-year follow-up of outcome and health care consumption with subgroup analysis. Spine 29 (21), 2458–24565.

Fukui, S., Ohseto, K., Shiotani, M., et al., 1996. Referred pain distribution of the cervical zygapophyseal joints and cervical dorsal rami. Pain 68, 79–83.

Ganzhorn, R.W., Hocker, J.T., Horowitz, M., et al., 1981. Suprascapular-nerve entrapment. J. Bone Joint Surg. Am. 63 (3), 492–494.

Grant, R., 1988. Dizziness testing and manipulation of the cervical spine. In: Grant, R. (Ed.), Physical Therapy of the Cervical and Thoracic Spines. Churchill Livingstone, Edinburgh, pp. 111–124.

Greenhalgh, S., Selfe, J., 2010. Red Flags II. Elsevier, Edinburgh.

Gumina, S., Carbone, S., Albino, P., et al., 2013. Arm Squeeze Test: a new clinical test to distinguish neck from shoulder pain. Eur Spine J. 22 (7), 1558–1563.

Hickling, J., 1972. Spinal traction technique. Physiotherapy 58, 58–63.

Hoving, J.L., de Vet, H.C.W., Twisk, J.W.R., et al., 2004. Prognostic factors for neck pain in general practice. Pain 110, 639–645.

Huisman, P.A., Speksnijder, C.M., de Wijer, A., 2013. The effect of thoracic spine manipulation on pain and disability in patients with non-specific neck pain: a systematic review. Disabil. Rehabil. 35 (20), 1677–1685.

Hussey, A.J., O'Brien, C.P., Regan, P.J., 2007. Parsonage-Turner syndrome – case report and literature review. Hand 2 (4), 218–221.

Hutting, N., Kranenburg, H.A.R., Kerry, R., 2020. Yes, we should abandon pre-treatment positional testing of the cervical spine. Musculoskeletal Sci. Pract. 49, 102181.

Iyer, S., Kim, H.J., 2016. Cervical radiculopathy. Curr. Rev. Musculoskelet Med. 9 (3), 272–280.

Jaumard, N.V., Welch, W.C., Winkelstein, B.A., 2011. Spinal facet joint biomechanics and mechanotransduction in normal, injury and degenerative conditions. J. Biomech. Eng. 133 (7), 1–126.

Johnson, E., Landel, R., Kusunose, R., et al., 2008. Positive patient outcome after manual cervical spine management despite a positive vertebral artery test. Man. Ther. 13, 367–371.

Judovitch, B., 1952. Herniated cervical disc. Am. J. Surg. 84, 646–650.

Kerry, R., Taylor, A., 2006. Cervical arterial dysfunction assessment and manual therapy. Man. Ther. 11, 243–253.

Kim, H.J., Tetreault, L.A., Massicotte, E.M., et al., 2013a. Differential diagnosis for cervical spondylotic myelopathy. Spine 38 (22S), S78–S88.

Kim, S.C., Landon, J.E., Solomon, D.H., 2013b. Clinical characteristics and medication uses among fibromyalgia patients newly prescribed amitriptyline, duloxetine, gabapentin, or pregabalin. Arthritis Care Res. 65 (11), 1813–1819.

Kleynhans, A.M., Terrett, A.G.J., 1985. The prevention of complications from spinal manipulative therapy. In: Glasgow, E.F., Twomey, L.T., Scull, E.R. (Eds.), Aspects of Manipulative Therapy. Churchill Livingstone, Edinburgh, pp. 161–175.

Kristjansson, E., 2005. The cervical spine and proprioception. In: Boyling, J.D., Jull, G.A. (Eds.), Grieve's Modern Manual Therapy. Churchill Livingstone, Edinburgh, pp. 243–256.

Kuijper, B., Tans, J.T.J., de Visser, M., 2009. Cervical collar or physiotherapy versus wait and see policy for recent onset cervical radiculopathy: randomized trial. Br. Med. J. 339, b3883.

Laslett, M., van Wijmen, P., 1999. Low back and referred pain: diagnosis and a proposed new system of classification. NZ J. Physiother. 27 (2), 5–14.

Lempert, T., Gresty, M.A., Bronstein, A.M., 1995. Benign positional vertigo – recognition and treatment. Br. Med. J. 311, 489–491.

Lord, S.M., Barnsley, L., Wallis, B.J., et al., 1996. Chronic cervical zygapophysial joint pain with whiplash: a placebo-controlled prevalence study. Spine 21, 1737–1745.

McKenzie, R.A., 1981. The Lumbar Spine: Mechanical Diagnosis and Therapy. Spinal Publications, Waikanae, New Zealand.

Magaray, M.E., Rebbeck, T., Coughlan, B., et al., 2004. Pre-manipulative testing of the cervical spine review, revision and new guidelines. Man. Ther. 9, 95–108.

Mamula, C.J., Erhard, R.E., Piva, S.R., 2005. Cervical radiculopathy or Parsonage-Turner syndrome: differential diagnosis of a patient with neck and upper extremity symptoms. J. Orthop. Sports Phys. Ther. 35 (10), 659–664.

Manchikanti, L., Singh, V., Pampati, V., et al., 2002a. Is there correlation of facet joint pain in lumbar and cervical spine? Pain Physician 5, 365–371.

Manchikanti, L., Singh, V., Rivera, J., et al., 2002b. Prevalence of cervical facet joint pain in chronic neck pain. Pain Physician 5, 243–249.

Massaracchio, M., Cleland, J.A., Hellman, M., et al., 2013. Short-term combined effects of thoracic spine thrust manipulation and cervical spine nonthrust manipulation in individuals with mechanical neck pain: a randomized clinical trial. J. Orthop. Sports Phys. Ther. 43 (3), 118–127.

Mathews, J.A., 1995. Acute neck pain – differential diagnosis and management. In: Lewin, I.G., Seymour, C.A. (Eds.), Collected Reports on the Rheumatic Diseases. Arthritis and Rheumatism Council for Research, Chesterfield, pp. 142–144.

Mendel, T., Wink, C.S., Zimny, M., 1992. Neural elements in human cervical intervertebral discs. Spine 17, 132–135.

Mercer, S., Bogduk, N., 1999. The ligaments and annulus fibrosus of the human adult cervical intervertebral discs. Spine 24 (7), 619–628.

Mercer, S., Bogduk, N., 2001. Joints of the cervical vertebral column. Phys. Ther. 31 (4), 174–182.

Middleditch, A., Oliver, J., 2005. Functional Anatomy of the Spine, second ed. Butterworth Heinemann, Edinburgh.

Miller, J.D., Pruitt, S., McDonald, T.J., 2000. Acute brachial plexus neuritis: an uncommon cause of shoulder pain. Am. Fam. Physician 62 (9), 2067–2072.

Murphy, D.R., 2010. Current understanding of the relationship between cervical manipulation and stroke: what does it mean for the chiropractic profession? Chiropr. Osteopat. 18 (1), 22.

National Institute for Health and Care Excellence (NICE), 2018a. Neck pain – non-specific. NICE. https://cks.nice.org.uk/topics/neck-pain-non-specific/. Accessed 3 September 2021

National Institute for Health and Care Excellence (NICE), 2018b. Neck pain-whiplash injury. NICE. https://cks.nice.org.uk/topics/neck-pain-whiplash-injury/. Accessed 3 September 2021

National Institute for Health and Care Excellence (NICE), 2018c. Neck pain – acute torticollis. NICE. https://cks.nice.org.uk/topics/neck-pain-acute-torticollis/. Accessed 3 September 2021

Netter, F.H., 1987. Musculoskeletal System, Ciba Collection of Medical Illustrations. Ciba-Giegy, NJ.

Nordin, M., Frankel, V.H., 2001. Basic Biomechanics of the Musculoskeletal System, third ed. Lippincott, Williams & Wilkins, Philadelphia, PA.

Öberg, B., Enthoven, P., Kjellman, G., et al., 2003. Back pain in primary care: a prospective cohort study of clinical outcome and healthcare consumption. Adv. Physiother. 5, 98–108.

Osmotherly, P.G., Rivett, D.A., Mercer, S.R., 2013. Revisiting the clinical anatomy of the alar ligaments. Eur. Spine J. 22, 60–64.

Peake, N., Harte, A., 2005. The effectiveness of cervical traction. Phys. Ther. Rev. 10, 217–229.

Peng, B., DePalma, M.J., 2018. Cervical disc degeneration and neck pain. J. Pain Res. 11, 2853–2857.

Peng, B., Bogduk, N., 2019. Cervical discs as a source of neck pain. An analysis of the evidence. Pain Med. 20 (3), 446–455.

Pitz, C., de la Rivière, A.B., van Swieten, H.A., et al., 2004. Surgical treatment of Pancoast tumours. Eur. J. Cardiothorac. Surg. 26, 202–208.

Pratt, N., 2005. Anatomy of nerve entrapment sites in the upper quarter. J. Hand Ther. 18 (2), 216–219.

Prescher, A., 1998. Anatomy and pathology of the ageing spine. Eur. J. Radiol. 27, 181–195.

Radhakrishnan, K., Litchy, W.J., O'Fallon, W.M., et al., 1994. Epidemiology of cervical radiculopathy. A population-based study from Rochester, Minnesota, 1976 through 1990. Brain 117, 325–335.

Reid, S.A., Rivett, D.A., 2005. Manual therapy treatment of cervicogenic dizziness: a systematic review. Man. Ther. 10, 4–13.

Rhee, J.M., Yoon, T., Riew, K.D., 2007. Cervical radiculopathy. J. Am. Acad. Orthop. Surg. 15 (8), 486–494.

Riddle, D.L., 1998. Classification and low back pain: a review of the literature and critical analysis of selected systems. Phys. Ther. 78 (7), 708–737.

Rivett, D., Sharples, K.J., Milburn, P.D., 1999. Effects of pre-manipulative tests on vertebral artery and internal carotid artery blood flow – a pilot study. J. Manipulative Physiol. Ther. 22 (6), 368–375.

Robson, P., 2014. Metastatic spinal cord compression: a rare but important complication of cancer. Clin. Med. 14 (5), 542–545.

Royal Australian College of General Practitioners (RACGP), 2013. Clinical guidance for MRI referral. https://www.racgp.org.au/getattachment/f8275e83-0489-44a8-893e-461a575ba04a/Clinical-guidance-for-MRI-referral.aspx. Accessed 5 September 2021.

Rushton, A., Carlesso, L., Flynn, T., et al., 2022. Position statement: International framework for examination of the cervical region for potential of vascular pathologies of the neck prior to musculoskeletal intervention: International IFOMPT Cervical Framework. J. Orthop. Sports Phys. Ther. 13 (1), 1–62.

Sizer, P., Brismée, J., Cook, C., 2007. Medical screening for red flags in the diagnosis and management of musculoskeletal spine pain. Pain Pract. 7 (1), 53–71.

Soames, R., Palastanga, N.R., 2018. Anatomy and Human Movement, seventh ed. Elsevier, Oxford.

Standring, S., 2015. Gray's Anatomy: The Anatomical Basis of Clinical Practice, forty-first ed. Churchill Livingstone, Edinburgh.

Sumner, A.J., 2009. Idiopathic brachial neuritis. Neurosurgery 65 (Suppl. 4), A150–A152.

Tanaka, N., Fujimoto, Y., Howard, S., et al., 2000. The anatomic relation among the nerve roots, intervertebral foramina and intervertebral discs of the cervical spine. Spine 25 (3), 286–291.

Taylor, A., Kerry, R., 2005. Neck pain and headache as a result of internal carotid artery dissection: implications for manual therapists. Man. Ther. 10 (1), 73–77.

Taylor, A.J., Kerry, R., 2010. A 'system based' approach to risk assessment of the cervical spine prior to manual therapy. Int. J. Osteopat. Med. 13, 85–93.

Taylor, J.R., Twomey, L.T., 1994. Functional and applied anatomy of the cervical spine. In: Grant, R. (Ed.), Clinics in Physical Therapy of the Cervical and Thoracic Spine, second ed. Churchill Livingstone, Edinburgh, pp. 1–25.

Thoomes, E.J., van Geest, S., van der Windt, D.A., et al., 2018. Value of physical tests in diagnosing cervical radiculopathy: a systematic review. Spine J. 18 (1), 179–189.

Trojian, T.H., Hall, M.L., Aerni, G., 2018. Suprascapular neuropathy treatment and management. Medscape.com. https://emedicine.medscape.com/article/92672-treatment. Accessed 5 September 2021.

Tseng, Y.-L., Wang, W.T.J., Chen, W.-Y., et al., 2006. Predictors for the immediate responders to cervical manipulation in patients with neck pain. Man. Ther. 11, 306–315.

Vernon, H., Humphreys, B.K., 2008. Chronic mechanical neck pain in adults treated by manual therapy: a systematic review of change scores in randomized controlled trials of a single session. J. Man. Manip. Ther. 16 (2), E42.

Walsworth, M.K., Mills, J.T., Michener, L.A., 2004. Diagnosing suprascapular neuropathy in patients with shoulder dysfunction: a report of 5 cases. Phys. Ther. 84 (4), 359–372.

Yoon, S.H., 2011. Cervical radiculopathy. Phys. Med. Rehabil. Clin. N. Am. 22 (3), 439.

Zeidman, S.M., Ducker, T.B., 1994. Rheumatoid arthritis: neuroanatomy, compression, and grading of deficits. Spine 19, 2259–2266.

The Thoracic Spine

CHAPTER CONTENTS

SUMMARY

This chapter outlines the anatomy of the thoracic spine and highlights the structures that are a potential cause of pain. Pain patterns are discussed, and the mechanical and alternative causes of thoracic back pain are presented to aid diagnosis and appropriate management.

Thoracic pain is common and can provide a challenge in diagnosis, since referred pain from visceral problems can mimic pain of somatic origin, and vice versa. The thoracic spine can also be a site for bony metastases that are more commonly found in the thoracic spine than in the cervical or lumbar regions.

Disc lesions are considered by some to be a comparatively rare cause of thoracic pain, probably due to the supportive nature of this relatively stiff area brought about by the sternal and vertebral articulations of the ribs. While this might be so for the mid-thoracic region, lower thoracic disc lesions may be more common than previously thought.

The clinical examination procedure is outlined and interpreted, the contraindications are emphasised, and the treatments used in musculoskeletal medicine are described, with notes on indications for their use.

ANATOMY

The thoracic spine connects with the cervical spine above and the lumbar spine below. It provides attachment for the rib cage and is the longest segment of the spine. The intervertebral, facet and rib joint articulations make it a complex area.

Thoracic Joints

There are 12 thoracic vertebrae, which gradually increase in size from above down, marking a transition between cervical and lumbar vertebrae. A typical thoracic vertebra is easily recognised by its costal facets,

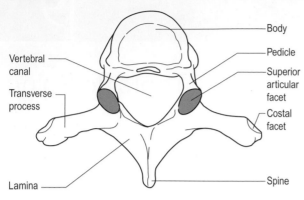

Fig. 9.1 Typical thoracic vertebra. (From Soames and Palastanga, 2018. Reprinted by permission of Elsevier Ltd.)

heart-shaped superior surface and waisted vertebral body (Fig. 9.1).

Short *pedicles* pass almost directly backwards, and thick, broad *laminae* overlap each other from above down. The laminae meet to form the relatively long *spinous process*. The *vertebral canal* in the thoracic region is round and smaller than that found in either the cervical or lumbar spine.

The slope of the long spinous processes gradually increases downwards, with the 5th to 8th spinous processes overlapping each other. The 8th spinous process is the longest, while the 12th is shorter, horizontal and similar to the lumbar spinous processes.

Long, rounded, club-like *transverse processes* are directed posterolaterally and slightly superiorly. Except for the 11th and 12th vertebrae, oval, anterior facets lie at the tips of all transverse processes. These facets articulate with the tubercles of the corresponding ribs.

Flat *articular processes* project superiorly and inferiorly to form the thoracic *facet (zygapophyseal) joints*. The orientation of the plane of the facet joints facilitates the movement of rotation, which is coupled with side flexion, while also permitting a range of flexion and extension. Rotation is a particular feature of the thoracic spine and is facilitated by the direction of the articular facets and rotation of the fibres in the intervertebral discs (Edmondston and Singer, 1997).

The 12th thoracic vertebra is a transitional vertebra with the upper surface being typical of a thoracic vertebra, with the lower surface having lumbar characteristics for articulation with L1.

A dramatic change of direction of the plane of the facet joints occurs over one level at the thoracolumbar junction, permitting rotational stresses between T11 and T12 that are not permitted between T12 and L1. This makes the 12th thoracic vertebra susceptible to fracture (Agur and Dalley, 2009).

The *thoracic intervertebral joints* consist of the vertebral body above and below and the *intervertebral disc*. These joints are supported by anterior and posterior longitudinal ligaments, supraspinous, interspinous and intertransverse ligaments and the ligamentum flavum, which connects adjacent laminae internally. Further support is gained by the costovertebral joints and ligaments.

Movement in the thoracic spine is relatively limited. The thorax comprises the vertebral bodies, ribs, clavicles and sternum and the articulations between them. The bony structure provides support and protection to vital organs but provides little mobility in the sagittal and frontal planes (Heneghan and Rushton, 2016), particularly in the upper segment where the ribs are firmly attached anteriorly and posteriorly (Kapandji, 2019). The largest range of movement is axial rotation (Heneghan and Rushton, 2016).

The restriction of movement may also be due to the thoracic disc height, relative to vertebral body height, which is less than in the cervical or lumbar spines. The shearing movement common to lumbar discs does not occur so readily in the thoracic spine (Kapandji, 2019).

Twelve pairs of ribs attach posteriorly to the thoracic spine. The upper seven pairs are termed true ribs and attach anteriorly to the sternum. The lower five pairs consist of false and floating ribs; the false ribs attach to the costal cartilage above.

A *typical rib* consists of a shaft and anterior and posterior ends. The posterior end of the rib typically has a *head, neck* and *tubercle* and articulates with the thoracic vertebrae, forming the posterior rib joints. The head of the rib is divided into two demifacets by a horizontal ridge that is attached to the disc via an intra-articular ligament. The lower facet articulates with its corresponding vertebra; the upper facet articulates with the vertebra above.

The tubercle of the rib is at the junction of the neck with the shaft and articulates with the transverse process of the corresponding vertebra. Just lateral to the tubercle, the rib turns to run forwards forming the *angle of the rib*.

A cervical rib may be present as an extension of the costal elements of the seventh cervical vertebra. It

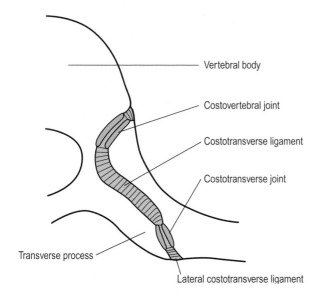

Fig. 9.2 Posterior rib joints. Costovertebral and costotransverse joints, horizontal section. (From Soames and Palastanga, 2018. Reprinted by permission of Elsevier Ltd.)

generally passes forwards and laterally into the posterior triangle of the neck where it is crossed by the lower trunk of the brachial plexus and the subclavian vessels. Compression of these structures may produce motor and sensory signs and symptoms.

Two joints, the costovertebral and costotransverse joints, attach the rib firmly to the vertebral column (Fig. 9.2). These help to stabilise the intervertebral joint while being relatively unstable themselves. Minor subluxations of these joints may be responsible for the mechanical pattern of signs and symptoms associated with thoracic pain.

The *costovertebral joint* is a synovial joint formed between the head of the rib and two adjacent vertebral bodies, except at the 1st, 11th and 12th ribs, where a joint is formed with a single vertebral body. The joint is surrounded by a fibrous capsule that is thickened anteriorly by the radiate ligament. The posterior aspect of the capsule blends with the nearby denticulation of the posterior longitudinal ligament.

The *costotransverse joint* joins the upper 10 ribs to the transverse processes of their corresponding vertebra. It is surrounded by a fibrous capsule and is stabilised by the *lateral costotransverse, costotransverse* and *superior costotransverse ligaments* that join the transverse process

to the neck of the rib. The superior costotransverse ligament also connects the rib to the transverse process of the vertebra above.

Movements occur concurrently at the costovertebral and costotransverse joints and are determined by the shape and direction of the articular facets. This amounts to small rotary and gliding movements that occur with the 'bucket handle' action of the ribs during respiration.

Intervertebral Discs

The thoracic discs are more circular and less wedge-shaped than in the cervical and lumbar regions, and the minimum disc height throughout the whole spine can be found at the T4–T5 level. These differences would appear to be related to the relative immobility in the thoracic region. The tilt of the fibres in the outer annulus is about 70 degrees, which is more than the cervical discs but about the same as in lumbar discs (Pooni et al., 1986).

The bony anatomy, including the primary kyphotic curve and the surrounding ligamentous structures related to the costovertebral joints, may have a stabilising effect on the intervertebral disc, making herniation less likely in this region.

Thoracic Spinal Nerves

The thoracic spine has 12 pairs of spinal nerves (T1 to T12), which are formed from dorsal and ventral nerve roots and emerge through the intervertebral foramina to immediately branch into dorsal and ventral rami. They are named according to the vertebra above.

The dorsal rami pass backwards into the tissues of the back where they innervate the back muscles, ligaments and facet joints and supply cutaneous branches to the skin (Soames and Palastanga, 2018).

The 2nd to 12th ventral rami form intercostal nerves that pass laterally from the intervertebral foramen, under the rib at the same level. The first thoracic ventral ramus forms a small branch from the ventral ramus, which is the first intercostal nerve, but the main ventral ramus passes over the first rib to join into the formation of the brachial plexus (Soames and Palastanga, 2018).

Each intercostal nerve innervates the intercostal muscles and the overlying skin. The lower six intercostal muscles pass onwards onto the abdominal wall, to continue to supply the skin in the same segment and to supply the underlying muscles of the anterior abdominal wall (Soames and Palastanga, 2018).

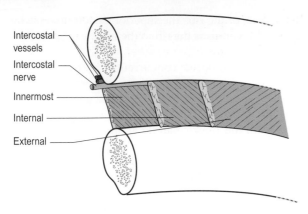

Intercostal vessels

Intercostal nerve

Innermost

Internal

External

Fig. 9.3 Layers of intercostal muscles. (From Soames and Palastanga, 2018. Reprinted by permission of Elsevier Ltd.)

Muscles

The intercostal muscles are relevant to the musculoskeletal medicine approach. Three thin musculotendinous layers occupy the intercostal space between adjacent ribs and may become symptomatic due to strain (Fig. 9.3):

- The *external intercostal muscle* is the most superficial, with fibres running in an oblique direction downwards and forwards.
- The *internal intercostal muscle* lies beneath, with fibres running in the opposite direction.
- The thinnest and deepest layer is formed by the *innermost (intimi) intercostal muscle*, which is thin and may be absent, with fibres running in the same direction as the internal intercostal muscle.

CLINICAL DIAGNOSIS AND MANAGEMENT AT THE THORACIC SPINE

An understanding of the anatomy at the thoracic spine, together with a detailed history and examination of the patient, will help with the selection of patients suitable for manual treatment and will contribute to safe practice.

Musculoskeletal medicine treatment techniques for the thoracic spine are aimed at reducing a musculoskeletal lesion, usually associated with the posterior rib joint or intervertebral disc. The diagnosis is not always certain, however, and there is limited understanding of the aetiology and epidemiology of the range of neuromusculoskeletal conditions that can arise from the thoracic

spine (Heneghan and Rushton, 2016). 'Non-specific thoracic pain' is an appropriate term to describe most of the presentations of thoracic lesions.

The following section is divided into two parts:

- The first part defines non-specific thoracic pain and lists possible causes, incidence, risk factors, diagnosis, management and prognosis. Assessment of the thoracic spine is covered in the next section, 'Commentary on the Examination'.
- The second part looks at other causes of thoracic pain and associated signs and symptoms, diagnosis and management. Most of these conditions have a more specific or identifiable cause. They are generally not appropriate for treatment with manual musculoskeletal medicine treatment techniques and require suitable referral.

Non-specific Thoracic Pain

For many patients presenting with non-specific thoracic pain there is no precise cause. There are several possible musculoskeletal causes, but they usually do not change the management approach, which is the same for most musculoskeletal presentations.

The posterior rib joints can be a common cause of thoracic pain. The articulating surfaces of these joints are relatively shallow and unstable, rendering them susceptible to minor subluxations. The facet joints may also be a cause of signs and symptoms, although they are less susceptible to degenerative change due to the relative immobility of the thoracic spine.

If patients present with a sudden onset of pain, the precipitating event is usually trivial, and they often feel a pop or click. More gradual onset can be associated with working in rotated or flexed postures. The pain presents a typical mechanical picture of pain aggravated by movement and posture and eased by rest. A deep breath or cough often provokes the pain.

On examination, there is a non-capsular pattern of limited movement involving one rotation more than the other.

Management of neck pain and low back pain is led by evidence-based clinical practice guidelines. However, no comparable guidelines exist for the thoracic spine, despite the increasing amount of research on thoracic spine pain and dysfunction (Briggs et al., 2007; Heneghan et al., 2019).

Within a biopsychosocial model of practice, a stepped approach to the management of non-specific thoracic pain is usually applied. Less invasive treatments are generally offered first, including education/watchful wait, activity and work modification, simple analgesics and non-steroidal anti-inflammatory drugs (NSAIDs) medication, physiotherapy (e.g. exercise, manual mobilisation and manipulation), and pain management programmes. If symptoms persist and/or non-musculoskeletal causes of symptoms are suspected, further investigation and onward referral may be required.

Non-specific thoracic pain usually responds rapidly to manipulation and, provided that there are no contraindications present (see page 295), the manipulative techniques described in this chapter can be applied. Postural advice and exercises should also be given to prevent recurrence, which is a typical feature.

Other Causes of Thoracic Pain

Differential diagnosis of thoracic pain is difficult because of the numerous conditions that refer pain to the area and the lesions that mimic mechanical pain. Non-musculoskeletal causes of thoracic pain need to be considered as part of differential diagnosis since treatment may be contraindicated and onward referral required.

Thoracic pain may arise from shoulder, thoracic and cervical spine structures. It may also have a visceral origin and arise from the gastrointestinal, cardiopulmonary and renal systems (Fukui et al., 1997; Fruth, 2006; Briggs et al., 2007).

The thoracic spine is a common site for inflammatory, malignant and infective conditions, which can also contribute to pain and disability (Singer, 2000). The ribs and thoracic vertebrae are common sites for metastases.

The spinal cord is a concern in the thoracic region and thoracic myelopathy should also be considered. Certain signs and symptoms will become evident on examination that require onward referral.

Primary and secondary osteoporosis, particularly associated with vertebral insufficiency fractures (Briggs et al., 2007); hyperkyphosis arising from vertebral bone loss (Kado et al., 2007); ankylosing spondylitis (Sampaio-Barros et al., 2001); degenerative arthropathy (Kramer, 2006) and Scheuermann's disease can all be associated with thoracic pain (Heneghan and Rushton, 2016).

This part of the chapter considers other possible causes of thoracic pain in turn.

Cervical Spine and Shoulder Pathologies

Cervical spine and shoulder pathologies can refer pain to the thoracic spine, particularly into the scapular area.

The cervical spine is excluded with six active movements as part of the routine examination of the thoracic spine, but a full examination of the cervical spine and shoulder joint should be conducted if indicated. Shoulder pathologies referring signs and symptoms to the thoracic spine are discussed in Chapter 5.

Cervical lesions referring pain into the thoracic region are often indicative of dural reference, producing unilateral or bilateral scapular pain. The patient has a typical musculoskeletal presentation, with cervical movements increasing the pain felt in the thoracic region. Pain is not normally reproduced by thoracic movements.

The condition is managed as described in the cervical spine chapter, Chapter 8.

Traumatic

Suspected fractures following major trauma, such as a road traffic accident or a fall from height, will almost always have been dealt with as an emergency.

However, thoracic pain and dysfunction may be associated with whiplash associated disorder (WAD), and there is considerable, but currently low level, evidence to support the association (Heneghan et al., 2018). It primarily involves nerves and muscles and should be considered within differential diagnosis if the patient reports a history of WAD. Having ruled out fracture, it can be managed as for WAD in the cervical spine, as described in Chapter 8.

Spinal fractures associated with osteoporosis may often be encountered in musculoskeletal practice and are more common in the thoracic spine.

Every year, 300,000 insufficiency fractures are sustained from minor injury, and many of them can be prevented by early diagnosis and treatment (Royal Osteoporosis Society, 2021). These are predominantly a risk for older patients, especially women, and practitioners need to be aware of the risk factors and signs and symptoms of spinal fractures and to consider what detailed questions to ask to help with further management.

The incidence of fractures varies greatly by country. However, on average, up to 50% of women over 50 years of age are at risk of fractures (Eastell et al., 2016).

Postmenopausal osteoporosis, resulting from oestrogen deficiency, is the most common type of osteoporosis. Oestrogen deficiency results in an imbalance in bone formation and resorption, which consequently has an effect on trabecular bone (loss of connectivity) and cortical bone (cortical thinning and porosity). Therefore, women have a much higher risk of osteoporotic fracture (Eastell et al., 2016).

From a clinical perspective, it is important to establish when menopause occurred, as fractures commonly start to be a clinical problem 10 to 15 years after menopause (Greenhalgh and Selfe, 2019).

Osteoporotic fractures have a similar distribution to metastases, with 70% in the thoracic region, 20% in the lumbar region, and 10% in the cervical region. Most spinal fractures occur between the T8 and L4 levels (Finucane et al., 2020).

As many as 70% of these fractures are undiagnosed and found during investigation for other health conditions (Finucane et al., 2020). The majority of vertebral compression fractures (50% to 70%) are believed to be asymptomatic (National Institute for Health and Care Excellence [NICE], 2010).

When people seek help, they commonly present with a sudden onset of pain, mostly located in the thoracolumbar region, which may have followed low-impact trauma, such as a slip or trip, or lifting or pushing something while in a flexed position. Pain presentation varies, but it is often severe and well-localised to the area of the fracture. Weight-bearing activities and active movements are restricted and painful, and the person may require strong analgesia, particularly in the early stages.

On examination, the patient may have an increased prominence of the spinous process at the affected level, and/or be hyperkyphotic. There may be marked tenderness to palpation at the affected level, though the absence of tenderness does not exclude fracture. Patients with a suspected fracture should have an X-ray in the first instance to determine whether a fracture is present, and to grade and define its nature (Finucane et al., 2020).

Management is usually conservative, with a focus on alleviating symptoms and providing spinal support, such as pain-relieving medications, bed rest and spinal brace. Patients are advised to stay active within the level of pain tolerance to allow healing to take place (NICE, 2013).

Surgery is rare. Vertebroplasty or balloon kyphoplasty may be considered for patients with severe persistent pain after a recent unhealed vertebral fracture, despite optimal pain management, and in whom the pain has been confirmed to be correlated with the level of fracture observed by physical examination and imaging (NICE, 2013).

Arthropathy

Arthropathy presents with the capsular pattern of limited movement.

CAPSULAR PATTERN OF THE THORACIC SPINE
- Equal limitation of rotations
- Equal limitation of side flexions
- Some limitation of extension
- Usually full flexion

Degenerative arthropathy can affect the spinal joints, causing secondary signs and symptoms. Gross degenerative changes may produce central osteophytes that may cause gradual cord compression. Anterior and lateral lipping of the vertebral body, as well as wedging of mid-thoracic vertebrae, has been associated with degenerative arthropathy of the thoracic spine (Osman et al., 1994).

Thoracic Disc Herniation

Disc herniation is comparatively rare in the thoracic spine. The lordotic shape of the cervical and lumbar spine accommodates the line of gravity that runs through them, and they bear most of the weight of the axial spine, compared to the thoracic and sacral regions. This, with the general restriction of movement in the thoracic spine, may account for why disc herniation occurs more rarely in this region (Fogwe et al., 2020).

Han and Jang (2018) reported the prevalence of thoracic disc herniation at 6.5% (145/2212), being relatively evenly distributed across all age groups, higher in male than female participants and more frequent in patients with lumbar lesions. It was not noted whether the participants with positive findings had thoracic symptoms, however, and Fogwe et al. (2020) suggest that thoracic disc herniations are asymptomatic in most cases. Thoracic disc lesions are usually considered as a condition of working-age, primarily in the third and fourth decades of life (Fogwe et al., 2020).

Mellion and Ladeira (2001) and Han and Jang (2018) suggest that upper thoracic disc herniation is less common and affects the lower thoracic levels more frequently. This is probably because the lower thoracic spine is relatively free of the restriction of the rib cage, making it more mobile. The most common levels reported were T8/9 and T10/11, and 75% of thoracic disc herniations occur below T8. Fogwe et al. (2020) vary slightly in reporting the incidence of the most common level as T11/12.

Radiculopathies that involve T1 share similarities with those occurring at C8, with numbness and weakness in the hand and pain in the arm and medial forearm. Weakness of the intrinsic hand muscles may be involved with T1, but this is an uncommon finding, and the practitioner must exclude non-musculoskeletal causes, such as Pancoast's tumour.

Degenerative change, traumatic incidents, lifting, rotation, falls, exercise, rugby tackles and road traffic accidents can be precipitating factors for thoracic disc herniation (Mellion and Ladeira; 2001; Fogwe et al., 2020). The onset may be sudden and severe or insidious and slowly progressive.

Patients can present with general symptoms such as chest wall pain, epigastric pain, upper limb pain and sometimes a pain in the groin or lower limb pain, leading the practitioner to consider problems that are more common than thoracic disc herniation.

Thoracic pain associated with disc herniation may be constant or intermittent and may be central, localised or diffuse. A posterolateral disc herniation normally produces radicular signs and symptoms, where the pain follows the band-like dermatomal distribution of the nerve root level affected. Segmental referral to the abdomen may occur.

Apart from the confusion with visceral pathologies, other musculoskeletal conditions may be suspected. There is no regular pattern to the history, signs and symptoms, as found at the cervical and lumbar spine. Thoracic disc herniation is often a diagnosis by exclusion but can be confirmed by magnetic resonance imaging (MRI) (Fogwe et al., 2020).

Although thoracic disc herniations are comparatively rare, Ozturk et al. (2006) highlight the potential danger of their being missed, as they could possibly result in progressive myelopathy and paralysis (see below). The thoracic vertebral canal is relatively small to accommodate the spinal cord, and central disc herniation poses the most threat.

In summary, a small uncomplicated thoracic disc herniation may present with sudden or gradual onset of pain that may be felt posteriorly, anteriorly or radiating laterally. Pressure on the dura mater produces multisegmental reference of pain. The pain usually has a typical mechanical behaviour, being aggravated by movement and posture and eased by rest. Dural symptoms of increased pain on a cough, sneeze or deep breath may be present.

On examination, a non-capsular pattern of limited movement will be found, with one rotation being significantly more painful or limited than the other. A dural sign of pain on neck flexion may be present if the dura mater is compromised.

If there are no neurological signs, and signs and symptoms of cord compression are absent, the treatment techniques described in this chapter can be used, provided there are no other contraindications (see page 295). Alternatively, since lower thoracic herniations are more common, they may be treated using the techniques described for the lumbar spine.

Uncomplicated thoracic disc herniations tend to follow a path of recovery similar to that seen in cervical and lumbar disc herniations, responding to physical treatments and eventually stabilising with time (Brown et al., 1992).

Neurological

Central disc herniation can compress the spinal cord, and this can produce the signs and symptoms of *thoracic myelopathy*. Thoracic myelopathy is comparatively uncommon, probably due to the relatively restricted movement, which leads to fewer degenerative changes in the thoracic spine (Ando et al., 2019).

Conditions that can lead to thoracic myelopathy include ossification of the posterior longitudinal ligament, spinal tumour, metastatic spinal cord compression (caused by collapse or compression of a vertebral body [Robson, 2014]), spinal cord tumour, trauma, infection, thoracic disc herniation and calcification or hypertrophy of the ligamentum flavum (Han and Jang, 2018; Ando et al., 2019).

Signs and symptoms can mimic those of cervical or lumbar lesions, and thoracic myelopathy is often overlooked in the initial investigations, leading to delay in diagnosis (Ando et al., 2019).

Ando et al. (2019) reported the principal initial symptoms to be gait disturbance and back pain. Symptoms relating to bladder and bowel are reported later in the development of the condition. Signs may include clonus, hyperreflexia and a positive Babinski sign.

Urgent surgical referral is necessary for patients showing signs of spinal cord compression.

Inflammatory

Inflammatory arthritis can involve the thoracic spine. *Rheumatoid arthritis* commonly affects the costovertebral, costotransverse and facet joints. *Reiter's disease* can affect the spinal joints, although it is more frequently seen in the lower limb joints. *Ankylosing spondylitis*, when it involves the thoracic cage, causes a reduction in chest expansion. Thoracic pain and significant stiffness may be its presenting symptoms.

Visceral Pathology

Visceral pathology can produce local thoracic pain or pain referred to the thoracic region that mimics mechanical pain, making diagnosis difficult. In visceral conditions, the patient is usually unwell, which will aid diagnosis, but this is not always so.

Angina is usually felt in the chest and can be referred into the arms. If mild, it may mimic mechanical pain. The patient experiences increased pain with exertion (e.g., climbing stairs), which may also be felt in the back.

Thoracic aortic aneurysm is a weakened area in the aorta that can 'balloon' under the pressure of the blood passing through it. Dissection of the aortic wall can occur, which can cause life-threatening bleeding or sudden death. As a thoracic aortic aneurysm grows, patients may experience tenderness or pain in the chest, back pain, cough, hoarseness or shortness of breath. Treatment can range from watchful waiting to emergency surgery.

Pulmonary embolism, pleurisy, pneumothorax, etc., all present with chest pain, but other distinguishing features can lead to diagnosis, which is often difficult. A common symptom of pleurisy is a sharp pain in the chest on deep inspiration.

Acute pancreatitis produces abdominal pain localised to the epigastrium or upper abdomen, but pain may be referred to the mid or low thoracic region.

Acute cholecystitis can cause pain in the epigastrium and right hypochondrium, but pain may also be referred to the back and shoulder.

The *testes* may refer pain to the lower thoracic area as they are supplied by nerves derived from the 10th and 11th thoracic spinal segments.

The *lung* (including Pancoast's tumour), *gallbladder* and *pancreas*, as well as *oesophageal, gastrointestinal (ulcer), renal* and *liver pathologies* can all cause referred pain to the interscapular area (Briggs et al., 2009; Knott and Bonsall, 2016)

If any of these conditions is suspected, onward referral is required, and the urgency of the referral depends on the severity of the presenting symptoms

Malignancy

Malignant disease is usually extradural with bone metastases produced most commonly from primaries in the bronchus, breast, prostate, ovary, thyroid or kidney. However, a diagnosis of a primary tumour or blood cancer must not be overlooked.

- *Metastatic*
  - Spontaneous but severe, persistent pain, particularly with bony involvement, which does not resolve with initial treatments.
  - Bone invasion is common in known malignancy, but it can often be the initial sign of advanced, undiagnosed malignancy.
  - Localised thoracic pain with a history of primary cancer (breast, lung, prostate, kidney, thyroid), fatigue, history of weight loss; bone pain. Lymphadenopathy and hepatosplenomegaly may be present with more specific findings related to the type of cancer. Tumours in the bronchus, breast, kidney, prostate and thyroid commonly metastasise to bone, and the thoracic spine is the most common site (70%), followed by lumbar spine (20%) and cervical spine (10%) (Klimo and Schmidt, 2004). Although uncommon, radiotherapy to the thorax can cause damage to the bony structure of the thoracic cage, manifested as rib fractures and providing a source of pain (Whitfield et al., 1963; Iyer and Jhingran, 2006).
- *Primary*
  - Localised thoracic pain, fatigue, history of weight loss
  - Localised tenderness with or without neurological compromise
  - Bronchial carcinoma accounts for 95% of all primary tumours of the lung and may present with a cough and chest pain (Feather et al., 2020).
- *Multiple myeloma*
  - This is the most common tumour in the spine, along with plasmacytoma. The latter is rare and implies a single lesion with an indolent or slow course clinically. It is seen more commonly in a young person.
  - Multiple myeloma is seen in older patients, is rapidly progressive, and commonly presents with

neurological symptoms, due to vertebral body collapse.

- Patients may also have symptoms associated with hypercalcaemia and renal failure.

If malignancy is suspected, urgent onward referral for further investigation is required, in line with local policy.

Infection

Infection is rare and could include *discitis, vertebral osteomyelitis, or spinal epidural abscess.* Practitioners should exclude the following symptoms and history:

- Fever.
- Tuberculosis, or recent urinary tract infection.
- Diabetes.
- History of intravenous drug use.
- HIV infection, use of immunosuppressants, or the person is otherwise immunocompromised.
- Fever in a patient with new thoracic pain:
  - In these patients, thoracic pain should be assumed to be secondary to an infection until proven otherwise.
  - Patients with an infectious cause may be hypotensive or tachycardic.
  - There may be a history of recent infection (especially skin or urinary tract), or a history of intravenous drug use or immune compromise.
  - Osteomyelitis and epidural abscesses arise from haematogenous spread in most cases.
- More severe, spontaneous thoracic pain, often following systemic infection, with marked decreased range of motion, or with progressive neurological changes in upper extremities.

If infection is suspected, emergency onward referral for further investigation is required, in line with local policy.

Other

Scheuermann's disease is vertebral osteochondritis, most commonly seen in males 12 to 18 years old. It usually involves the lower thoracic vertebrae, often T9. The disc may move forwards between the cartilage endplate and the anterior longitudinal ligament, producing wedging. It may produce minor thoracic backache, and a local dorsal kyphosis may be evident on spinal flexion (Corrigan and Maitland, 1989).

Scheuermann's disease has been associated with Schmorl's nodes and degenerative lumbar disc disease in relatively young patients (Heithoff et al., 1994). Management can range from a conservative approach, including analgesics, NSAIDs and bracing, to surgery for those with deformities that produce neurological signs or respiratory compromise.

Schmorl's nodes are protrusions of the intervertebral disc into the cancellous bone of the vertebral body. This may produce an anterior prolapse, causing separation of a small fragment of bone, seen on X-ray as a limbus vertebra (Taylor and Twomey, 1985). Management can range from a conservative approach, including analgesics, anti-inflammatories, advice and exercise, to vertebroplasty for those with persisting symptoms.

Shingles (herpes zoster) is related to a chickenpox virus infection and affects one posterior nerve root. The patient presents with a dermatomal reference of pain that may be present for some days before the typical rash appears. The rash consists of vesicles following a segmental course related to the affected nerve root. Shingles can be recurrent and may provide a persistent cycle of thoracic pain.

Family history, older age, trauma, female sex, immunosuppression, HIV/AIDS, and the presence of comorbid conditions (such as diabetes, rheumatoid arthritis, cardiovascular disease, renal disease, systemic lupus erythematosus and irritable bowel disease), are all factors that increase the risk of herpes zoster (Marra et al., 2020).

Soft tissue conditions can produce thoracic pain. Muscle lesions are relatively common in the thoracic region; therefore, resisted tests are included in the routine examination. Commonly, the *intercostal muscles* are affected, particularly if there is a history of a fractured rib. Palpation determines the site of the lesion.

Tietze's syndrome is a condition affecting the costochondral or chondrosternal joints. It is usually unilateral, affecting one, two or three joints that are tender to palpation. The cause is not known, but the condition may follow a respiratory condition that involves prolonged coughing. The condition is self-limiting and may be treated with physiotherapeutic pain-relieving modalities, NSAIDs or injection with corticosteroid and local anaesthetic (Feather et al., 2020).

Epidemic myalgia (Bornholm's disease) is due to infection by the Coxsackie B virus. The features are an upper respiratory tract illness and fever followed by pleuritic and abdominal pain and muscular tenderness. It may occur in young adults in the late summer and autumn, but resolves spontaneously within a week (Feather et al., 2020).

The box 'Updated Hierarchical List of Red Flags' presents a weighted list of factors, which, when considered together, in the context of the patient's history, signs and

symptoms, help to raise the practitioner's index of suspicion for serious pathology (see Chapter 1).

COMMENTARY ON THE EXAMINATION

Observation

A general observation of the patient is made, assessing the *face, posture and gait*. Serious pathology shows in the face, with the patient appearing tired and drawn.

An assessment of the gait is important; the presentation of a disc lesion at the thoracic spine may present a serious threat to the spinal cord, and signs of myelopathy may show disturbances and/or balance problems in the gait pattern.

History

The box 'Updated Hierarchical List of Red Flags' lists the 'red flags' for the possible presence of serious pathology that should be listened for and identified throughout the history and examination.

In isolation, many of the red flags may have limited significance, but it is for the practitioner to consider the general profile of the patient and to decide whether contraindications to treatment exist and/or whether onward referral is indicated. A combination of the red flags listed should raise the index of suspicion (see Chapter 1).

The patient's *age, occupation, sports, hobbies and activities* will indicate possible lesions and any contributing factors to the condition that may need to be addressed to prevent recurrence.

Thoracic pain has been found to be more prevalent in the working-age population, with concurrent musculoskeletal conditions, psychosocial factors and increased biomechanical loading. In children or adolescents, thoracic pain has been found to be more prevalent in females and may be caused by postural changes, such as backpack use (Briggs et al., 2009).

Musculoskeletal lesions tend to be found in the working age group. Osteoporosis can affect postmenopausal women. Postmenopausal loss of bone mass can be as high as 5% per year due to oestrogen deficiency (Eastell et al., 2016) and osteoporotic fractures commonly start to be a clinical problem 10 to 15 years post menopause (Greenhalgh and Selfe, 2019). Serious conditions may present in both the very young and the elderly, and caution is required if these particular age groups present with symptoms mimicking a mechanical lesion.

UPDATED HIERARCHICAL LIST OF RED FLAGS

- Age >50 years + history of cancer + unexplained weight loss + failure to improve after 1 month of evidence-based conservative therapy

- Age <10 and >51 years
- Medical history (current or past) of:
  - Cancer
  - Tuberculosis
  - Human immunodeficiency virus (HIV)/acquired immune deficiency syndrome (AIDS) or intravenous drug use
  - Osteoporosis
- Weight loss >10% body weight (3–6 months)
- Severe night pain precluding sleep
- Loss of sphincter tone and altered S4 sensation
- Bladder retention or bowel incontinence
- Positive extensor plantar response

- Age 11–19
- Weight loss 5%–10% body weight (3–6 months)
- Constant progressive pain
- Band-like pain
- Abdominal pain and changed bowel habits, but with no change of medication
- Inability to lie supine
- Bizarre neurological deficit
- Spasm
- Disturbed gait

- Loss of mobility, difficulty with stairs, falls, trips
- Legs misbehave, odd feelings in legs, legs feeling heavy
- Weight loss <5% body weight (3–6 months)
- Smoking
- Systemically unwell
- Trauma
- Bilateral pins and needles in hands and/or feet
- Previous failed treatment
- Thoracic pain
- Headache
- Physical appearance
- Marked partial articular restriction of movement

From Greenhalgh and Selfe., 2010. Reprinted by permission of Elsevier Ltd.

Habitual postures may have relevance to the symptoms, as could the patient's sports, hobbies or general activities.

The *site and spread* of symptoms can indicate the site of the lesion. The initial site of the symptoms may be different to the current site, and it can be helpful to know this.

Thoracic lesions can produce central pain, anterior pain or both. Pain may radiate around the chest wall, and this may be indicative of nerve root involvement. If pain is constant, severe and progressive, without any relief from bed rest or postural modification, then it should be considered to be suspicious.

Progressively increasing and radiating pain is usually sinister. Symptoms may spread in a multisegmental distribution, indicating dural involvement, or separate satellite areas of pain may be related to visceral causes.

Cardiac pain characteristically radiates from the chest into one or both arms. Mechanical lesions of the posterior rib joints produce relatively local pain, but movement may provoke sharp, shooting or twinging pain.

The nature of the *onset and duration* of the symptoms will help to differentiate mechanical lesions from more serious pathology.

If the onset is sudden, it is hypothesised that it could be a minor mechanical lesion of the posterior rib joint, with the patient recalling the exact moment the pain came on. The mode of onset is usually trivial and is often associated with a popping or cracking sound. The duration of the pain is generally short, but the patients seek help early as they 'felt it go.' Minor lesions may also have a gradual onset following the adoption of an awkward posture for some time.

A disc herniation may have a gradual or sudden onset. A history of trauma could indicate possible fracture. More serious pathology generally starts insidiously for no apparent reason, and the duration of the symptoms may be many weeks or months. Recurrent episodes may be indicative of mechanical instability or inflammatory arthritis.

The *behaviour* of the pain is important since mechanical lesions produce a recognisable pattern of behaviour. The pain is better during rest and worse during activity. Providing the mechanical lesion does not wake the patient on turning, night pain is not usually a feature, and the patient can sleep. The provoking activities are consistent, and every time the patient repeats a particular aggravating movement, the pain is produced.

The 24-hour pain pattern gives an indication of severity and irritability of the condition. Inflammatory symptoms are worse at night. Pain at night, especially in the second half of the night (Poddubnyy, 2020), with significant early morning stiffness of an hour or more would generally indicate inflammatory arthritis

If night pain is a feature, particularly if it is unremitting and prevents the patient from lying in supine or getting to sleep, the patient will look tired, and this can indicate serious pathology.

Other *symptoms* may indicate a mechanical lesion. A deep breath and cough may aggravate the pain, and this needs to be distinguished from such conditions as pleurisy and pulmonary embolism, for example. These conditions can also produce pain on a deep breath, but the subsequent findings on assessment will confirm whether the lesion is mechanical.

Although movements are small at the posterior rib joints, the length of the ribs produces a greater proportion of movement at the anterior ends. This movement may also be painful in an intercostal muscle strain. A cough or sneeze increasing the pain could be indicative of minor subluxation or, more commonly, dural irritation, and symptoms are generally increased with activity and relieved by rest.

As the vertebral canal in the thoracic spine is small, disc displacement can threaten the spinal cord and produce symptoms of myelopathy. These must be ruled out. The patient is asked about the presence of paraesthesia in the feet, weakness in the legs and difficulty in walking. Specific questioning must be asked about bladder and bowel function, to rule out myelopathy (Oppenheim et al., 1993). If any impairment is suspected, the patient should be referred for neurosurgical opinion.

Other joint involvement may give an indication of rheumatoid arthritis, ankylosing spondylitis and systemic lupus erythematosus. All can cause pain in the thoracic region.

Medical history will give information concerning conditions that may be relevant to the patient's current complaint or reveal possible alternative diagnoses and contraindications to treatment. An indication of the patient's general health will indicate any systemic illness. It may be pertinent to take the patient's temperature. The patient should be asked about any recent unexplained weight loss.

As well as past medical history, establish any ongoing conditions and treatment. Explore other previous or current musculoskeletal problems including previous episodes of the current complaint, any treatment given and the outcome of treatment.

Practitioners should *screen* routinely for psychosocial factors and consider relevant health co-morbidities and lifestyle factors (see Chapter 1). These factors may contribute to the patient's presenting condition, or form a barrier to recovery and normal function, and should be addressed as an integral part of patient management.

On considering *medications*, the patient should be asked specifically about anticoagulants, long-term oral steroids, antidepressant medication and the current intake of analgesics, as an objective measure of pain control requirement.

Inspection

The patient should be suitably undressed, and an inspection carried out in a good light. A general inspection of the posture is made, assessing *bony deformity*. Note the position of the head and neck, cervical, thoracic and lumbar curves. Is there any evidence of cervical protraction or 'dowager's hump' (a localised soft-tissue 'bump' at the base of the neck usually associated with neck protraction), excessive or local thoracic kyphosis? Note the position of the scapulae and any evidence of scoliosis.

Colour changes or *swelling* would not be expected unless associated with a history of recent trauma. The typical appearance of shingles may be seen, or the mottled reddening produced after prolonged application of excessive heat (erythema ab igne), giving an indication of the severity of the pain.

Muscle wasting may be seen in the scapular area associated with neuritis.

State at Rest

Before any movements are performed, the state at rest is established to provide a baseline for comparison.

Examination by Selective Tension

The suggested sequence for the examination will now be given, followed by a commentary that includes the reason for performing the movements and the significance of the possible findings.

A suggested 'star diagram' assessment tool for recording examination of the cervical movements is provided in Section 3.

The cervical spine is a possible source of pain felt in the thoracic region and it must first be eliminated. If cervical flexion is the only movement to reproduce the thoracic pain, it is considered to be a dural sign for the thoracic spine since neck flexion draws the dura upwards (see Fig. 9.4f).

The routine examination of the thoracic spine includes active, passive and neurological examination. Since the spinal joints are considered to be a potential focus for 'emotional' symptoms, six active movements

---

Eliminate the Cervical Spine

- Active cervical extension (Fig. 9.4a)
- Active right cervical rotation (Fig. 9.4b)
- Active left cervical rotation (Fig. 9.4c)
- Active right cervical side flexion (Fig. 9.4d)
- Active left cervical side flexion (Fig. 9.4e)
- Active cervical flexion (a dural sign due to the upward migration of the dura mater in this area during cervical flexion) (Fig. 9.4f)

Articular and Muscle Signs

Standing

- Active thoracic extension (Fig. 9.5)
- Active right thoracic side flexion (Fig. 9.6a)
- Active left thoracic side flexion (Fig. 9.6b)
- Active thoracic flexion (Fig. 9.7)
- Resisted thoracic side flexions (Fig. 9.8a and b)

Sitting

- Active thoracic right rotation (Fig. 9.9a)
- Active thoracic left rotation (Fig. 9.9b)
- Passive thoracic right rotation (Fig. 9.10a)
- Passive thoracic left rotation (Fig. 9.10b)
- Resisted thoracic right rotation (Fig. 9.11a)
- Resisted thoracic left rotation (Fig. 9.11b)
- Resisted thoracic flexion (Fig. 9.12)

Supine Lying

- Checking skin sensation (Fig. 9.13)
- Knee reflex (Fig. 9.14)
- Ankle reflex (Fig. 9.15)
- Plantar response (Fig. 9.16)
- Ankle clonus (Fig. 9.17)

Prone Lying

- Resisted thoracic extension (Fig. 9.18)

Palpation

- Spinous processes for pain, range and end-feel (Fig. 9.19)

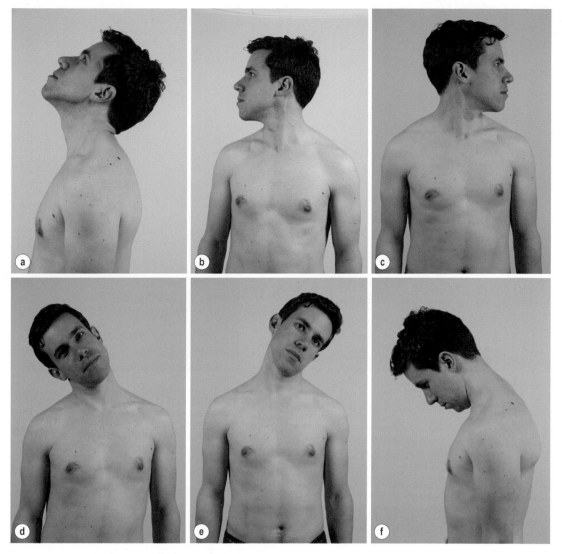

Fig. 9.4 Six active cervical movements to eliminate the cervical spine as a cause of pain. (a) Extension; (b, c) rotations; (d, e) side flexions; (f) flexion.

are conducted (four in standing and two while seated), assessing willingness to move, range of movement and pain. A capsular or non-capsular pattern will become evident through these movements.

Resisted side flexion is assessed to look for evidence of a muscle lesion. Resisted tests can be applied if a muscle lesion or significant yellow flags are suspected.

The patient sits to fix the pelvis while the rotations are assessed for willingness, pain, range of movement, end-feel and the capsular pattern. End-feel, which is normally elastic, is particularly pertinent to the rotations

since these movements may show minimal limitation and pain in minor subluxations of the posterior rib joints. Passive overpressure can be applied to any of the other movements, if appropriate. Resisted flexion may also be assessed in this position.

The non-capsular pattern involves pain and/or limitation of at least one of the rotations.

The patient is positioned in supine lying to test for skin sensation and the knee and ankle reflexes. The plantar response, is assessed by stroking up the lateral border of the sole of the foot and across the metatarsal

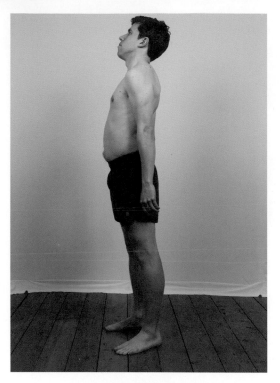

Fig. 9.5 Active extension.

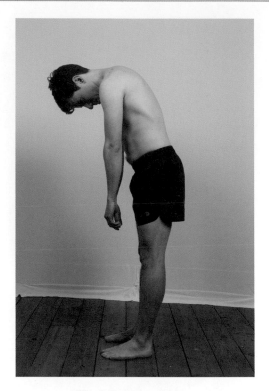

Fig. 9.7 Active flexion.

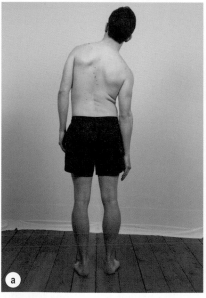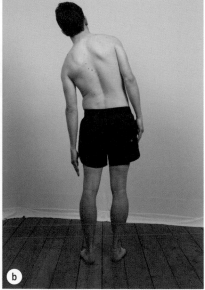

Fig. 9.6 (a, b) Active side flexions.

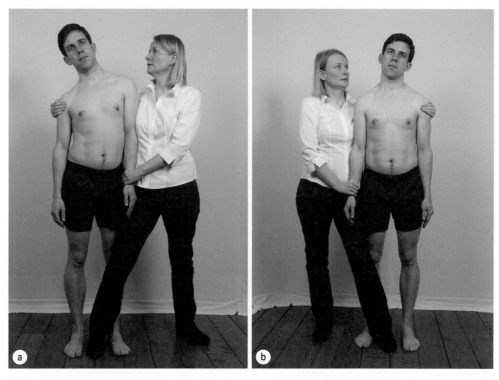

Fig. 9.8 (a, b) Resisted side flexions.

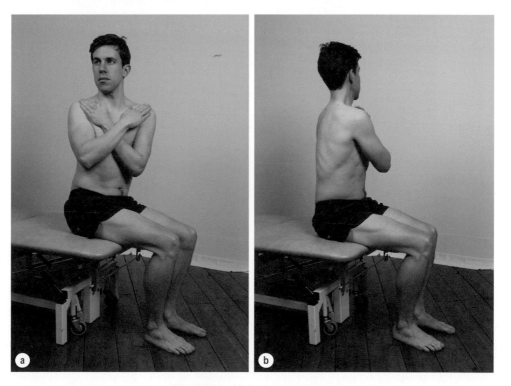

Fig. 9.9 (a, b) Active rotations.

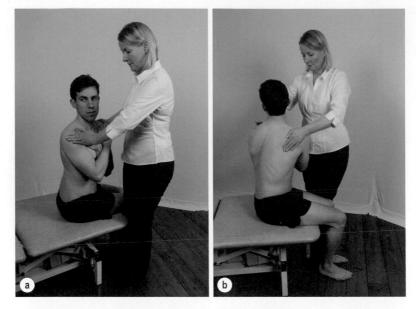

Fig. 9.10 (a, b) Passive rotations.

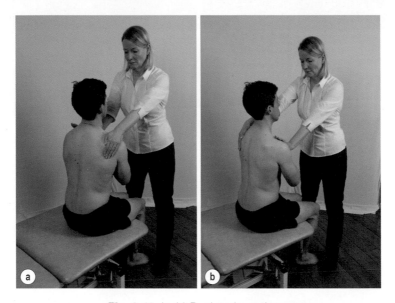

Fig. 9.11 (a, b) Resisted rotations.

heads. If the response is extensor, or upgoing (Babinski reflex), it is indicative of an upper motor neuron lesion; the normal response is flexor.

The ankle clonus test/reflex is performed by rapidly dorsiflexing the foot and holding it in the dorsiflexed position. A positive sign is rapidly repeated oscillations or 'beats' that can be felt and seen by the practitioner and can be indicative of an upper motor neuron lesion, in the context of other signs and symptoms.

The patient is positioned in prone lying to complete the examination. Resisted extension is applied, and the spinous processes are palpated, assessing

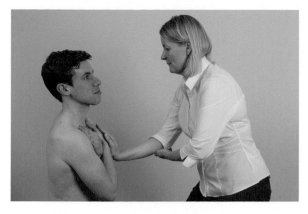

Fig. 9.12 Resisted flexion.

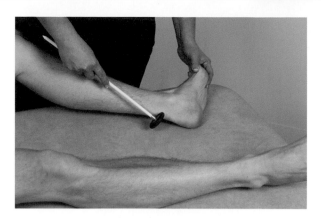

Fig. 9.15 Ankle reflex.

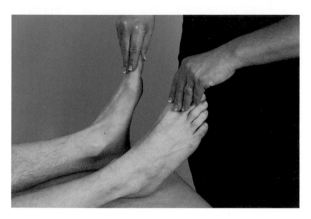

Fig. 9.13 Checking skin sensation.

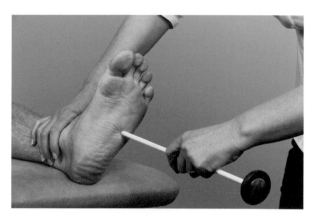

Fig. 9.16 Plantar response.

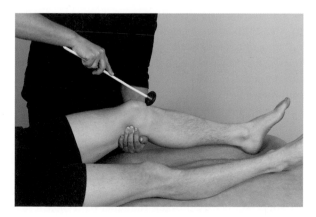

Fig. 9.14 Knee reflex.

pain, range of movement and end-feel at each segmental level.

Based on the history and clinical examination, the practitioner should be able to establish the most likely diagnosis, using clinical reasoning and clinical judgement.

It is important to recognise potential serious pathology, such as infection, malignancy, fracture and inflammatory arthritis, and to make any appropriate onward referral in a timely manner. Should additional information be required to aid diagnosis or to add value to management, further investigations can be considered to inform decision making and planning.

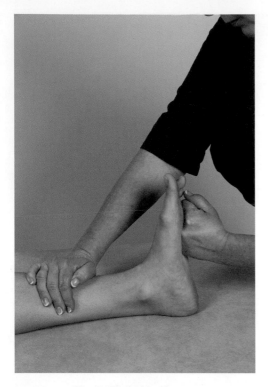

Fig. 9.17 Ankle clonus.

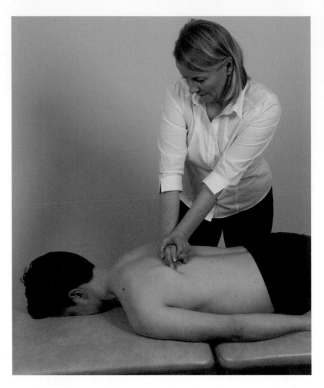

Fig. 9.19 Palpation.

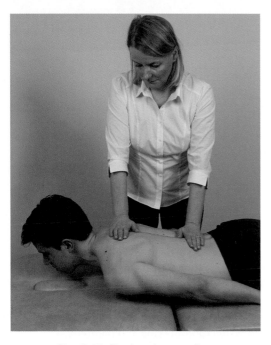

Fig. 9.18 Resisted extension.

Any other tests can be added to this basic routine examination of the thoracic spine, including repeated, combined and accessory movements and neural tension testing, as appropriate. Determination of the Cobb angle for scoliosis and kyphosis, from X-rays, may be appropriate.

If indicated, the practitioner may consider further investigations such as blood tests, radiological imaging, and other diagnostic procedures (see Chapter 1). Investigation should be guided by suspected causes and differential diagnosis, as an extension to the clinical examination process.

Investigation should be considered with suspected red flags, such as spinal fracture due to trauma or osteoporotic collapse, spinal infection, inflammatory arthritis, including ankylosing spondylitis, or suspected malignancy, including primary or metastatic tumours and multiple myeloma. MRI can be considered if the patient presents with thoracic radicular pain since it may be an early sign of impending cord compression. Basic blood tests and a blood test to screen for rheumatoid factor and HLA-B27 can be considered if inflammatory arthritis is suspected.

TREATMENT OF THORACIC PAIN

Manipulation is the treatment of choice for thoracic mechanical lesions.

Indications for Thoracic Manipulation
- Mechanical thoracic lesion – minor subluxation or disc herniation
- A sudden or gradual onset of pain
- Central, unilateral, local or referred pain
- Non-capsular pattern, usually limitation and/or pain of at least one thoracic rotation, or one more than the other
- No neurological signs
- No contraindications

CONTRAINDICATIONS TO THORACIC MANIPULATION

It is impossible to be definitive about all contraindications to thoracic manipulation, and nothing can substitute for a rigorous assessment of the presenting signs and symptoms and an accurate diagnosis.

'Red flags' are signs and symptoms reported in the history and observed in the examination that may indicate serious pathology and provide contraindications to thoracic manipulation (Sizer et al., 2007; Greenhalgh and Selfe, 2010). In isolation, many of the flags may have limited significance, but it is for the practitioner to consider the general profile of the patient and to decide whether contraindications to treatment exist and/or whether onward referral is indicated. A combination of the flags listed should raise the index of suspicion (see Red Flags on page 286).

The contraindications are highlighted in the following discussion, but there are several cautions that should be considered as well. It may be useful to use the mnemonic COINS (a contraction of 'contraindications'), as an aide-mémoire to be able to create categories for the contraindications: Circulatory, Osseous, Inflammatory, Neurological and suspicious features indicating Serious pathology. If the first and last two letters are pushed together as CONS, the crucial need for consent is emphasised.

> **COINS**
> - **C**irculatory
> - **O**sseous
> - **I**nflammatory
> - **N**eurological
> - **S**erious

The treatment regime discussed here is absolutely contraindicated in the absence of informed patient consent (see Chapter 1).

Signs and symptoms of *spinal cord compression* require urgent neurosurgical referral, especially if symptoms are progressing rapidly. *Inflammatory arthritis* affecting the thoracic synovial joints is a contraindication to manipulation, and if suspected, but undiagnosed, appropriate onward referral is required.

Suspicious features indicative of non-mechanical lesions would be a contraindication to the musculoskeletal medicine treatment regimen. These symptoms should not be considered in isolation but in the general context of the whole examination procedure. They may include unexplained weight loss, poor general health, pain unaffected by posture or activity, constant pain, of which night pain is a feature, and cord signs, such as abnormal gait and/or abnormal plantar response.

Secondary tumour needs to be eliminated as a cause of pain in patients with a past history of primary tumour, but a past history of primary tumour is not a contraindication in itself.

It is important to explore any past history of irradiation of the thorax, however, with respect to possible rib fractures. Diagnosis of a mechanical lesion must be certain before proceeding with the treatment regime since, as mentioned previously, bony metastases can form in the thoracic cage and may mimic mechanical pain.

The ill patient should be investigated for the cause of the systemic illness. As mentioned previously, *Horner's syndrome* is a contraindication to manipulation or mobilisation of the thoracic joints until the cause of the symptoms has been determined, due to its association with more serious pathology.

Anticoagulation therapy and *blood clotting disorders* are contraindications unless medical advice is sought. Known *osteoporosis* with *prolonged corticosteroid therapy* is a contraindication to manipulation. Pathological fracture must be excluded.

Safety recommendations for spinal manipulation techniques are included in Section 3.

TREATMENT TECHNIQUES

It is recommended that a course in musculoskeletal medicine is attended before the treatment techniques described are applied in clinical practice (see Section 3 [Appendix 3]).

The treatment techniques in this section will be described carefully in a step-by-step fashion to enable their application. However, the professional judgement and existing skill of the practitioner will allow each technique to be adapted.

The techniques presented have been adapted from those originally described by Cyriax (1984) and Cyriax and Cyriax (1993).

As with all manipulations and mobilisations, the comparable signs are reassessed after each technique and a decision made about the next. If the first techniques described below do not produce a reduction in signs and symptoms, the techniques following are applied under traction and may be more effective (Cyriax, 1984; Cyriax and Cyriax, 1993).

The following extension thrust techniques are best conducted with the bed as low as possible.

EXTENSION WITH A ROTATIONAL COMPONENT

- Position the patient comfortably in prone, preferably with the cervical spine in neutral, with the face positioned in the face hole and the arms resting over the edge of the couch or down at the patient's side.
- Locate the most tender spinous process by palpation.
- The technique can be applied in one of two ways, but it may be necessary to do both if, on reassessment, the first technique is unsuccessful.
- Position your hands as follows on either side of the spinous processes over the paraspinal muscle bulk, approximately over the underlying transverse processes.

Technique 1

- Take the pisiform of your hand which is nearest to the patient's head and place it adjacent to the spinous

process and on the side nearest to yourself at the painful level (fingers pointing caudally). The pisiform will now be resting over the transverse process (Figs 9.20–9.22).
- Place the first carpometacarpal joint of your other hand adjacent to the spinous process on the level

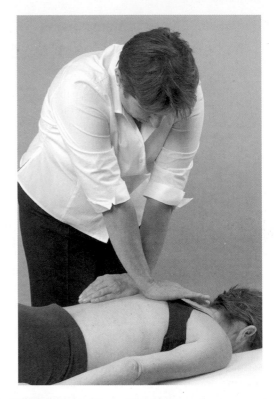

Fig. 9.20 Extension with a rotational component.

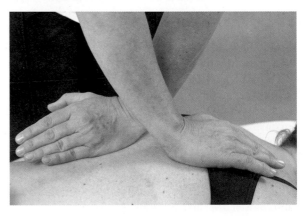

Fig. 9.21 Extension with a rotational component showing hand position.

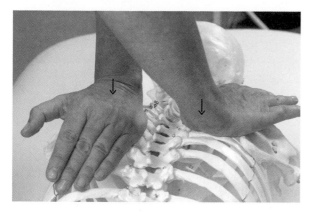

Fig. 9.22 Extension with a rotational component: hand position demonstrated on spine.

above, resting on the transverse process on the opposite side.
- With the patient relaxed, apply downward pressure to test the end of range of the tissues.
- Remove all pressure and ask the patient to take in a small breath.
- Follow the movement down as the patient breathes out; the position of your hands will automatically apply the rotation/extension movement and rotation of the hands is unnecessary.
- Apply a minimal-amplitude, high-velocity thrust through straight arms once all of the slack is taken up.
- Reassess.

Technique 2

This technique is the reverse of that described earlier, or a similar effect will be achieved by performing Technique 1, but from the other side of the bed.
- Take the first carpometacarpal joint of your hand which is nearest to the patient's head and place it adjacent to the spinous process at the painful level (fingers pointing caudally). The first carpometacarpal joint will now be resting over the transverse process on the side opposite to yourself (Figs 9.23–9.25).
- Place the pisiform of your other hand on the level above, over the transverse process on the side nearest to yourself.
- With the patient relaxed, apply downward pressure to test the end of range of the tissues.
- Remove all pressure and ask the patient to take in a small breath.
- Follow the movement down as the patient breathes out; the position of your hands will automatically

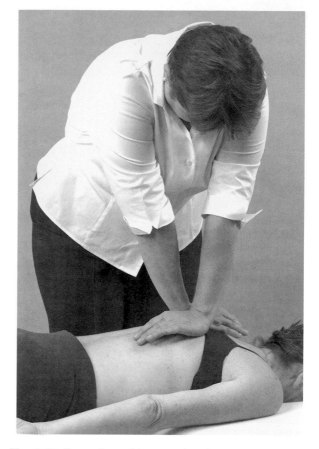

Fig. 9.23 Extension with a rotational component: alternative position.

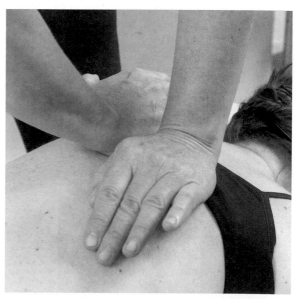

Fig. 9.24 Extension with a rotational component showing alternative hand position.

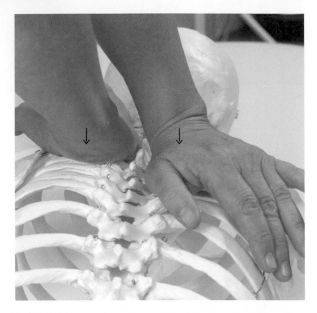

Fig. 9.25 Extension with a rotational component: alternative hand position demonstrated on spine.

apply the rotation/extension movement and rotation of the hands is unnecessary.

- Apply a minimal-amplitude, high-velocity thrust through straight arms once all of the slack is taken up.
- Reassess.

It is common to find one, two or even three tender levels and this technique, and the following 'Straight Extension Thrust', may have to be applied at one or two levels. The most tender level to palpation is chosen first.

STRAIGHT EXTENSION THRUST

This technique can be uncomfortable for the patient, and the previous 'Extension with a Rotational Component' is more comfortable, as the thrust is not applied directly to the tender spinous process.

- Position the patient comfortably in prone, as for the previous technique.
- Palpate for the tender thoracic level.
- Apply the ulnar border of your hand, reinforced with the other hand, to the most tender spinous process, which will indicate the level of the lesion (Fig. 9.26).
- With the patient relaxed, apply downward pressure to test the end of range of the tissues. At the mid and upper thoracic levels, angle your pressure slightly in

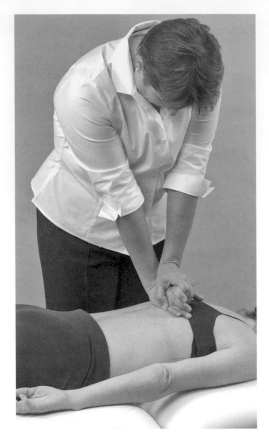

Fig. 9.26 Straight extension thrust.

a cephalad direction to accommodate the direction of the spinous processes and the planes of the facet joints.

- Remove all pressure and ask the patient to take in a small breath.
- Follow the breath out and apply pressure downwards with straight arms, angled slightly towards the head if appropriate.
- Apply a minimal amplitude, high-velocity thrust once all the slack is taken up.
- Reassess.

SITTING ROTATION

Rotate the patient into the least painful rotation first. If that fails to improve symptoms, the technique can be repeated in the opposite direction.

- Position the patient astride the end of a narrow couch to fix the pelvis, with the patient's back towards you and the patient's arms folded across the chest.

- Stand close to the patient and bend your knees.
- Hug the patient so that your shoulder sits below the patient's shoulder (Fig. 9.27).
- Keep the patient as close as possible, while the heel of your other hand rests adjacent to the spinous process just above the painful level (Fig. 9.28).
- Ask the patient to rotate actively as far as possible.
- Rotate the spine a little further passively, then straighten your knees to apply some traction to the patient's upper trunk (Fig. 9.29).
- Rotate a little further until all of the slack is taken up.

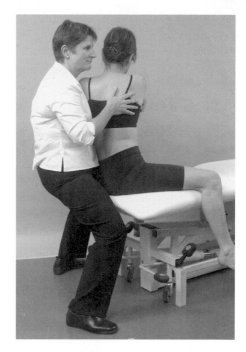

Fig. 9.28 Sitting rotation, showing hand position just above painful level.

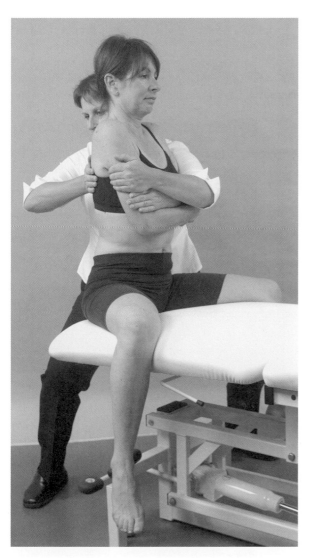

Fig. 9.27 Sitting rotation, starting position.

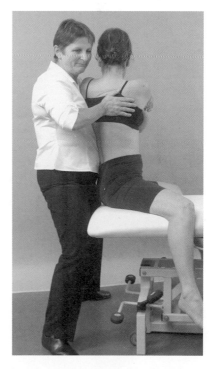

Fig. 9.29 Sitting rotation: traction applied by straightening knees, before application of the Grade C manipulation.

- Apply a minimal-amplitude, high-velocity thrust towards rotation, by smartly rotating your body and pushing through the heel of your hand.
- Support the patient as you return back towards the starting position.
- Reassess.

SITTING EXTENSION THRUST WITH A DEGREE OF TRACTION

This technique is useful if the patient is large and the practitioner small, as body weight can be used more effectively to apply the traction.

- Position the patient sitting on the end of the couch with the patient's hands overlapping each other, behind his or her head.

- Stand on the couch behind the patient and place one knee at the painful level, with a pillow or padding placed between your knee and the patient's back.
- Wrap your hands over and below the patient's upper arms, with your thumbs on the side chest wall and your fingers resting over the patient's scapulae (Fig. 9.30).
- Apply traction by moving your body weight upwards and backwards onto your other leg (Fig. 9.31). Keep your back straight by moving your weight backwards as you apply the traction. Be careful not to bend the patient backwards over the fulcrum of your knee, as this is very uncomfortable for the patient.
- Once the patient has relaxed, smartly extend the thoracic spine by applying a small-amplitude, high-velocity upward jerk of your knee against the spine.
- Reassess.

This technique may be applied without the thrust as a means of applying strong traction to the thoracic spine.

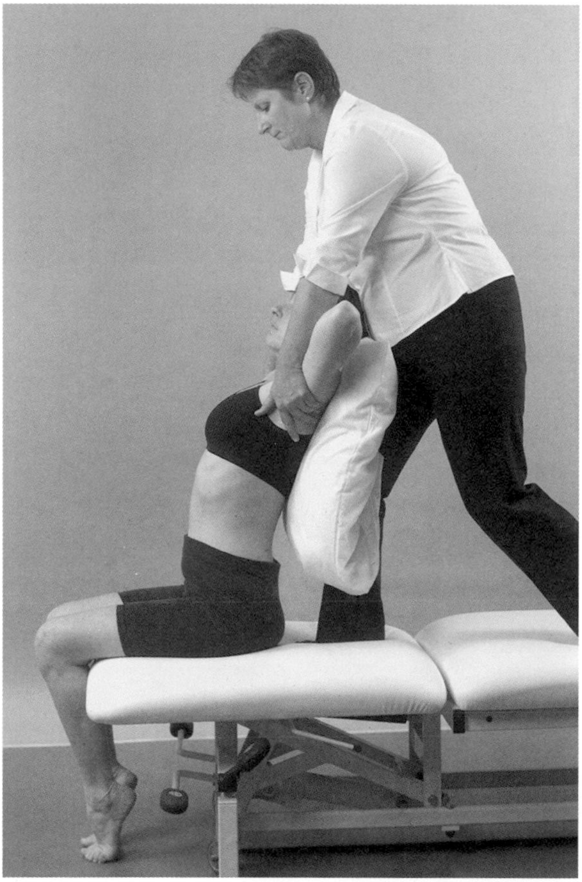

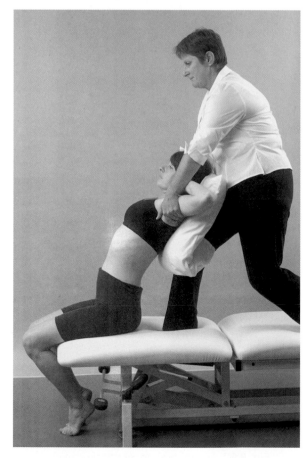

Fig. 9.30 Sitting extension thrust, starting position.

Fig. 9.31 Sitting extension thrust with a degree of traction.

The aim will be to hold the traction for as long as possible, provided it can be tolerated by both the patient and the practitioner.

INTERCOSTAL MUSCLE STRAIN

(Cyriax, 1984)

Generally, muscle lesions at the spinal joints are rare. However, it is not uncommon to find a lesion in the intercostal muscles.

The onset of pain may follow a chest infection with prolonged coughing, overexertion, or as the result of a fractured rib. Pain is felt locally and reproduced on resisted testing. Palpation reveals an area of tenderness, usually in one intercostal space.

The lesion responds well to transverse frictions. Position the patient in side lying (Fig. 9.32), or half-lying if respiratory distress is present or the patient is uncomfortable. Locate the tender area. Using an index or middle reinforced finger, direct the pressure up or down against the affected rib and apply transverse frictions parallel to the rib, according to the general principles.

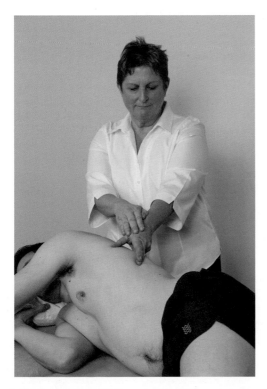

Fig. 9.32 Transverse frictions to the intercostal muscles.

REVIEW QUESTIONS

1. Which viscera can refer pain to the thoracic region?
2. What are the contraindications to thoracic manipulation?
3. How many articulations are associated with one thoracic vertebra?
4. What is the capsular pattern of the thoracic spine?
5. Which positive examination findings would lead you to the diagnosis of mechanical thoracic back pain?

CASE SCENARIOS

Case 1

History

- Kerry, a 42-year-old housewife, had a sudden onset of thoracic pain when twisting to pull her suitcase down from the overhead storage on a plane 3 days ago. The pain is intermittent but sharp and is causing her to catch her breath. She has no neurological symptoms and no previous episodes of pain. Her GP has given her co-codamol for the pain.

Examination

- Pain end-range cervical extension, limited right thoracic rotation, tender on palpation of T6/T7 centrally. Resisted thoracic movements pain-free. No neurological signs.

Task

- What are the contraindications to thoracic manipulation? Which manipulation techniques would be suitable for this patient?

Case 2

History

- Retired politician Trevor, 66, had a sudden onset of thoracic left-sided pain when he awoke one morning last week. Pain is constant and it is keeping him awake at night. The pain is travelling round his ribs on the left. He is generally feeling a bit under the weather. Paracetamol and ibuprofen are not helping the pain. No suspicious past medical history.

Examination

- Increased thoracic kyphosis, thoracic movements do not alter his pain and are not restricted. Neurological examination normal. Extremely tender on palpation around the mid-thoracic region spinous processes and to the left.

Task

- Is this a normal thoracic mechanical presentation? What are the potential pathologies for differential diagnosis? What approach will you take with this patient?

Case 3

History

- Finlay, a 36-year-old croupier, has a 3-week history of right-side thoracic pain that developed following an extended shift of overtime on the roulette tables. His pain is intermittent and aggravated by twisting and reaching. It is getting better but slowly. He had a previous whiplash injury 8 years ago, but all symptoms resolved at the time.

Examination

- No obvious abnormality, full cervical range of movement. Limited thoracic rotations with right rotation more restricted. All resisted tests pain-free. No neurology.

Task

- Describe mechanical thoracic pain as if explaining to the patient. Which treatments are suitable for this patient and consider any advice to give to the patient to prevent recurrence?

REFERENCES

Agur, A.M.R., Dalley, A.F., 2009. Grant's Atlas of Anatomy, twelfth ed Lippincott Williams & Wilkins, Philadelphia.

Ando, K., Imagama, S., Kobayashi, K., et al., 2019. Clinical features f thoracic myelopathy: A single-center study. J. Am. Acad. Orthop. Surg. Glob. Res. Rev. 3 (11), e10.5435.

Briggs, A.M., Greig, A.M., Wark, J.D., 2007. The vertebral fracture cascade in osteoporosis. A review of aetiopathogenesis. Osteoporos. Int. 18 (5), 575–584.

Briggs, A.M., Smith, A.J., Straker, L.M., et al., 2009. Thoracic spine pain in the general population: prevalence, incidence and associated factors in children, adolescents and adults. A systematic review. BMC Musculoskelet. Disord. 10 (77), 1–12.

Brown, C.W., Deffer, P.A., Akmakjian, J., et al., 1992. The natural history of thoracic disc herniation. Spine 17, S97–S102.

Corrigan, B., Maitland, G.D., 1989. Practical Orthopaedic Medicine. Butterworths, London.

Cyriax, J., 1984. Textbook of Orthopaedic Medicine, eleventh ed. Baillière Tindall, London.

Cyriax, J., Cyriax, P., 1993. Cyriax's Illustrated Manual of Orthopaedic Medicine. Butterworth Heinemann, Oxford.

Eastell, R., O'Neill, T.W., Hofbauer, L.C., et al., 2016. Postmenopausal osteoporosis. Nat. Rev. Dis. Primers 2, 16069.

Edmondston, S.J., Singer, K.P., 1997. Thoracic spine: anatomical and biomechanical considerations for manual therapy. Man. Ther. 2 (3), 132–143.

Feather, A., Randall, D., Waterhouse, M., 2020. Kumar and Clark's Clinical Medicine, tenth ed. Elsevier, London.

Finucane, L.M., Downie, A., Mercer, C., et al., 2020. International Framework for Red Flags for Potential Serious Spinal Pathologies. J. Orthop. Sports Phys. Ther. 50 (7), 350–372.

Fogwe, D.T., Petrone, B., Mesfinfin, F.B., 2020. Thoracic discogenic syndrome. StatPearls Publishing. https://www.ncbi.nlm.nih.gov/books/NBK470388/. Accessed 5 September 2021

Fruth, S.J., 2006. Differential diagnosis and treatment in a patient with posterior upper thoracic pain. Phys. Ther. 86, 254–268.

Fukui, S., Ohseto, K., Shiotani, M., 1997. Patterns of pain induced by distending the thoracic zygapophyseal joints. Reg. Anesth. 22 332–236

Greenhalgh, S., Selfe, J., 2010. Red Flags II: A guide to solving serious pathology of the spine. Elsevier, Edinburgh.

Greenhalgh, S., Selfe, J., 2019. E-Book-Red Flags: Managing Serious Pathology of the Spine. Elsevier Health Sciences.

Han, S., Jang, I.T., 2018. Prevalence and distribution of incidental thoracic disc herniation, and thoracic hypertrophied ligamentum flavum in patients with back or leg pain: a magnetic resonance imaging-based cross-sectional study. World Neurosurg. 120, e517–e524.

Heithoff, K.B., Gundry, C.R., Burton, C.V., et al., 1994. Juvenile discogenic disease. Spine 19, 335–340.

Heneghan, N., Rushton, A., 2016. Understanding why the thoracic region is the 'Cinderella' region of the spine. Man. Ther. 21, 274–276.

Heneghan, N.R., Gormley, S., Hallam, C., et al., 2019. Management of thoracic spine pain and dysfunction: A survey of clinical practice in the UK. Musculoskelet. Sci. Pract. 39, 58–66.

Heneghan, N.R., Smith, R., Tyros, I., et al., 2018. Thoracic dysfunction in whiplash associated disorders: A systematic review. PLoS One 13 (3), e0194235.

Iyer, R., Jhingran, A., 2006. Radiation injury: imaging findings in the chest, abdomen and pelvis after therapeutic radiation. Cancer Imaging 6, S131–S139.

Kado, D.M., Prenovost, K., Crandall, C., 2007. Narrative review: Hyperkyphosis in older persons. Ann. Int. Med. 147, 330–338.

Kapandji, I.A., 2019. The Physiology of the Joints: The Spinal Column, Pelvic Girdle and Head, seventh ed. Handspring Publishing, London.

Klimo Jr., P., Schmidt, M.H., 2004. Surgical management of spinal metastases. Oncologist 9, 188–196.

Knott, L., Bonsall, A., 2016. Thoracic Back Pain. Patient. https://patient.info/doctor/thoracic-back-pain. Accessed 5 September 2021.

Kramer, P.A., 2006. Prevalence and distribution of spinal osteoarthritis in women. Spine 31, 2843–2848.

Marra, F., Parhar, K., Huang, B., et al., 2020. Risk factors for Herpes Zoster infection: a meta-analysis. Opem Forum Infect. Dis. 7 (1), ofaa005.

Mellion, L.R., Ladeira, C., 2001. The herniated thoracic disc: a review of the literature. J. Man. Manip. Ther. 9 (3), 154–163.

National Institute for Health and Care Excellence (NICE), 2010. Vertebroplasty and kyphoplasty for the treatment of osteoporotic vertebral fractures. Draft scope (Pre-referral). NICE. https://www.nice.org.uk/guidance/ta279/documents/vertebral-fractures-vertebroplasty-and-kyphoplasty-draft-scope-for-consultation-prereferral-november-20102. Accessed 5 September 2021.

National Institute for Health and Care Excellence (NICE), 2013. Percutaneous vertebroplasty and percutaneous balloon kyphoplasty for treating osteoporotic vertebral compression fractures. NICE. https://www.nice.org.uk/guidance/ta279. Accessed 5 September 2021.

Oppenheim, J.S., Rothman, A.S., Sachdev, V.P., 1993. Thoracic herniated discs – review of the literature and 12 cases. Mt. Sinai J. Med. 60 (4), 321–326.

Osman, A.A., Bassiouni, H., Koutri, R., et al., 1994. Aging of the thoracic spine: distinction between wedging on osteoarthritis and fracture in osteoporosis – a cross-sectional and longitudinal study. Bone 15 (4), 437–442.

Ozturk, C., Tezer, M., Sirvanci, M., et al., 2006. Far lateral thoracic disc herniation presenting with flank pain. Spine J. 6, 201–213.

Poddubnyy, D., 2020. Classification vs diagnostic criteria: the challenge of diagnosing axial spondyloarthritis. Rheumatology 59, iv6–iv17.

Pooni, J.S., Hukins, D.W.L., Harris, P.F., et al., 1986. Comparison of the structure of human intervertebral discs in the cervical, thoracic and lumbar regions of the spine. Surg. Radiol. Anat. 8, 175–182.

Robson, P., 2014. Metastatic spinal cord compression: a rare but important complication of cancer. Clin. Med. 14 (5), 542–545.

Royal Osteoporosis Society, 2021. Vertebral fractures. ROS. https://theros.org.uk/healthcare-professionals/vertebral-fractures/. Accessed 5 September 2021.

Sampaio-Barros, P.D., Bertolo, M.B., Kraemer, M.H.S., et al., 2001. Primary ankylosing spondylitis: Patterns of disease in a Brazilian population of 147 patients. J. Rheum. 28, 560–565.

Singer, K.P., 2000. Pathology of the thoracic spine. In: Giles, L.G.F., Singer, K.P. (Eds.), Clinical Anatomy and Management of Thoracic Spine Pain. The Clinical Anatomy and Management of Back Pain Series. Oxford, Butterworth Heinmann.

Sizer, P., Brismée, J., Cook, C., 2007. Medical screening for red flags in the diagnosis and management of musculoskeletal spine pain. Pain Pract. 7 (1), 53–71.

Soames, R., Palastanga, N. 2018. Anatomy and Human Movement, seventh ed. Elsevier, Oxford.

Taylor, J.R., Twomey, L.T., 1985. Vertebral column development and its relation to adult pathology. Aust. J. Physiother. 31, 83–88.

Whitfield, A.G.W., Bond, W.H., Kunkler, P.B., 1963. Radiation damage to thoracic tissues. Thorax 18, 371–380.

The Hip

CHAPTER CONTENTS

SUMMARY

Differential diagnosis at the hip can be challenging. Pain in the hip region can be incorrectly attributed to the lumbar spine and/or sacroiliac joint, while the bursae in the area may be overlooked and can evade diagnosis. Pathology in the hip region may refer pain predominantly to the knee, which can also be misleading.

Degenerative arthropathy of the hip, even before the development of X-ray changes, is frequently overlooked as a treatable condition, when symptomatic relief can often be obtained by applying the mobilisation techniques described in musculoskeletal medicine or injection, normally under image guidance.

Groin strain and hamstring injury are familiar to the practitioner and are included to enhance effective treatment.

This chapter describes the anatomy relevant to common lesions in the hip region. A commentary follows, highlighting the relevant points of the history and suggesting a methodical sequence for examination. Lesions are then discussed with treatment alternatives and overall management.

ANATOMY

The *hip joint* is a synovial joint formed between the head of the femur and the acetabulum of the innominate bone of the pelvis (Fig. 10.1)

Inert Structures

Each *innominate* bone is made up of the *ilium* above, the *pubis* in front and the *ischium* behind. The *acetabulum* is the cup-shaped hollow on its outer surface at the junction of the three component bones. The *acetabulum* is deepened by a fibrocartilaginous *acetabular labrum.*

The *head of the femur* is slightly more than half a sphere and faces anteriorly, superiorly and medially to articulate with the acetabulum, forming a ball-and-socket joint. This articulation offers great stability and provides sufficient mobility for gait. All articular surfaces are covered by articular cartilage.

The *fibrous capsule*, lined with synovium, surrounds most of the neck of the femur, attaching above to the acetabular rim, below and anteriorly to the intertrochanteric line and 1 cm above the intertrochanteric crest posteriorly. Both the joint capsule and the articular cartilage tend to be thicker anterosuperiorly, which is the region of most stress in weight-bearing.

The close packed position of the hip joint is full extension, with a degree of abduction and medial rotation (Hartley, 1995; Standring, 2015).

Synovial plicae (folds or reflections of the synovial membrane) are found mainly on the external surface of the lower medial part of the acetabular labrum (labral plicae) but also at the base of the ligament of the head of the femur and on the base of the femoral neck (Fu et al., 1997; Bencardino et al., 2011). The labral plicae may potentially be a source of pain if torn or thickened.

Three ligaments reinforce the articular capsule and control movement. All three are taut in extension and relaxed in flexion:

- The *iliofemoral ligament* has strong medial and lateral bands that form a Y-shape, passing from the anterior inferior iliac spine to the intertrochanteric line.
- The *pubofemoral ligament* passes from the superior pubic ramus to blend distally with the capsule and the medial border of the iliofemoral ligament.
- The *ischiofemoral ligament* passes from the ischium and winds superiorly and laterally to the upper part

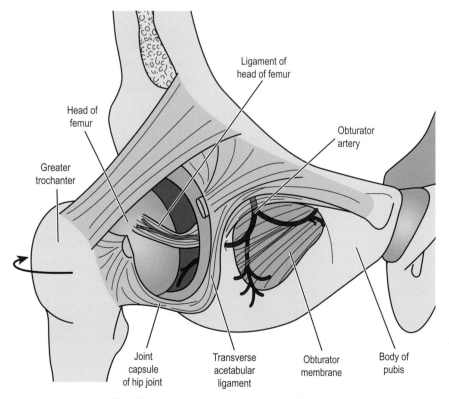

Fig. 10.1 Anterolateral view of the hip joint.

of the femoral neck, blending with the capsule of the hip joint and supporting it posteriorly.

The *psoas bursa* (also referred to as the iliopsoas or iliopectineal bursa) (L2–L3; Cyriax, 1982) is 5 to 7 cm long and 2 to 4 cm wide in its normal collapsed state (Underwood et al., 1988; Toohey et al., 1990; Flanagan et al., 1995; Zimmermann et al., 1995) (Fig. 10.2). In 15% of cadaveric specimens, the psoas bursa was seen to communicate with the hip joint via an aperture between the iliofemoral and pubofemoral ligaments (Flanagan et al., 1995). It may be a simple bursa or multiloculated with well-defined thin walls (Meaney et al., 1992).

The psoas bursa lies beneath the musculotendinous junction of the iliopsoas muscle and the front of the capsule of the hip joint, where it cushions the iliopsoas tendon as it winds around the front of the hip joint to its insertion onto the lesser trochanter. It is related anteromedially to the femoral artery and anteriorly to the femoral nerve (Canoso, 1981). Its point of location is just distal to the midpoint of the inguinal ligament, deep to the femoral artery.

The *gluteal bursa* (L4–L5; Cyriax and Cyriax, 1993) is not a single entity, but the term is often used clinically to describe the general area. At least four separate bursae lie between the different planes of the gluteal muscles as they attach to or pass over the greater trochanter, collectively forming the gluteal bursa:

- Two bursae are associated with gluteus maximus: a large *trochanteric bursa* (Figs 10.2 and 10.3), separating it from the lateral aspect of the greater trochanter, and a gluteofemoral bursa, lying between it and vastus lateralis (Standring, 2015).
- The trochanteric bursa of gluteus medius lies between its tendon and the anterosuperior aspect of the greater trochanter (Figs 10.2 and Fig. 10.3).

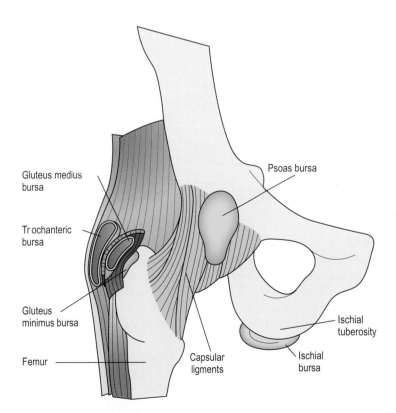

Fig. 10.2 Bursae around the hip.

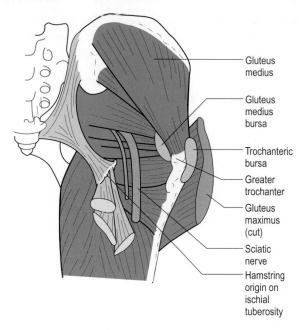

Gluteus medius

Gluteus medius bursa

Trochanteric bursa

Greater trochanter

Gluteus maximus (cut)

Sciatic nerve

Hamstring origin on ischial tuberosity

Fig. 10.3 Position of trochanteric bursa and adjacent structures.

- The trochanteric bursa of gluteus minimus separates its insertion from the medial part of the greater trochanter (Standring, 2015) (Fig. 10.2).
- One further bursa may be present, the ischial bursa, lying between the ischial tuberosity and the lower part of gluteus maximus (Fig. 10.2).

The hip joint is innervated by the femoral, obturator and superior gluteal nerves (L2–S1).

Contractile Structures

The *anterior muscles* are flexors of the hip, although they may also assist other hip movements. Some pass over the knee where they also have an effect.

Psoas major (ventral rami L1–L3) has its origin from the lumbar spine. It descends to pass under the centre of the inguinal ligament, receiving the fibres of iliacus on its lateral side. The iliopsoas tendon crosses the front of the hip joint where it is cushioned by the underlying psoas bursa. The combined tendon winds backwards to insert into the posteromedial lesser trochanter of the femur.

Sartorius (femoral nerve L2–L3) passes from the anterior superior iliac spine to cross the thigh medially,

inserting into the upper medial aspect of the tibia. It marks the lateral border of the femoral triangle. Sartorius flexes and laterally rotates the hip and flexes the knee.

Rectus femoris (femoral nerve L2–L4) is part of the quadriceps mechanism and has its main effect at the knee. However, its origin above the hip makes it a two-joint muscle, and it also acts as a powerful hip flexor, being most efficient when the knee is flexed (Kapandji, 2019). It has two heads of origin: a straight head from the anterior inferior iliac spine and a reflected head from just above the acetabular rim. It joins the rest of the quadriceps to insert into the patellar tendon. Resisted flexion of the hip mainly tests psoas major, but with the knee flexed it is also testing rectus femoris.

The *posterior muscles* are extensors of the hip.

Gluteus maximus (inferior gluteal nerve L5, S1–S2) is the largest and most superficial of the gluteal muscles. It passes from behind the posterior gluteal line on the blade of the ilium to the *iliotibial band (or tract)* (ITB) and upper femur. The large trochanteric bursa separates the insertion of gluteus maximus from the lateral aspect of the greater trochanter. Gluteus maximus acts principally as a hip extensor.

Biceps femoris (sciatic nerve L5, S1–S2) is the lateral hamstring with two heads of origin. A long head arises from an inferomedial facet on the ischial tuberosity (which it shares with semitendinosus) and a short head from the lateral lip of the linea aspera. Its fibres converge into a fusiform muscle belly, and its tendon of insertion attaches to the head of the fibula.

The *medial hamstrings* comprise semitendinosus and semimembranosus.

Semitendinosus (sciatic nerve L5, S1–S2) takes origin from the inferomedial facet on the ischial tuberosity. Its muscle belly ends in the middle of the thigh, and its long tendon of insertion lies on semimembranosus before winding around to the medial aspect of the upper tibia.

Semimembranosus (sciatic nerve L5, S1–S2) takes origin from the superolateral facet on the ischial tuberosity and has its main insertion onto the posterior aspect of the medial tibial condyle into the tuberculum tendinis.

The hamstrings assist hip extension, but their main effect is in flexing the knee. Because the hamstring muscles run over two joints, their efficiency in extending the hip increases if the knee is locked into extension (Kapandji, 2019).

Functionally, the small, *deep muscles* of the hip are responsible for lateral rotation.

Piriformis (L5, S1–S2) originates in the pelvis, exiting through the greater sciatic foramen to attach to the upper border of the greater trochanter.

Obturator externus (posterior branch of the obturator nerve L3–L4) and *obturator internus* (nerve to obturator internus L5, S1) pass posteriorly to the hip joint and insert into the medial surface of the greater trochanter and trochanteric fossa.

Gemelli (L5, S1) pass from the ischial spine and ischial tuberosity to the medial aspect of the greater trochanter.

Quadratus femoris (nerve to quadratus femoris L5, S1) passes from the ischial tuberosity to the quadrate tubercle in the middle of the trochanteric crest.

The *lateral muscles* are abductors and lateral rotators:

Gluteus medius (superior gluteal nerve L5, S1) is partially overlapped by maximus and lies in a slightly deeper plane. It originates from the blade of the ilium between posterior and anterior gluteal lines and inserts into the lateral aspect of the greater trochanter.

Gluteus minimus (superior gluteal nerve L5, S1) is the deepest gluteal muscle and arises between the anterior and inferior gluteal lines, inserting into the medial part of the anterior trochanteric surface.

Tensor fascia lata (superior gluteal nerve L4–L5) arises from the anterior 5 cm of the outer lip of the iliac crest and the anterior superior iliac spine. It passes downwards and laterally to insert into the anterior border of the ITB.

Gluteus medius is the main hip abductor, while medius and minimus together are responsible for maintaining the position of the opposite side of the pelvis in single-leg stance. Weakness of the hip abductors produces a positive Trendelenburg sign.

Tensor fascia lata and the anterior fibres of gluteus medius and minimus also produce medial rotation and flexion because they lie anteriorly to the frontal plane of the hip joint. Lying posteriorly, some fibres of gluteus medius and minimus are responsible for lateral rotation and extension (Kapandji, 2019).

Functionally, the *medial muscles* are responsible for adduction of the hip. The adductor muscles originate in the pelvis and pass to the medial aspect of the high.

Gracilis (obturator nerve L2–L3) is the most medial hip adductor. It passes from the lower half of the body of the pubis, the inferior pubic ramus and the adjacent ischial ramus, to run vertically downwards to just below the medial tibial condyle.

Pectineus (femoral nerve L2–L3) passes from the pecten pubis running posterolaterally to a line joining the lesser trochanter to the linea aspera.

Adductor longus (obturator nerve L2–L4) is the most superficial adductor. It passes from the body of the pubis, in the angle between the crest and the symphysis pubis, to descend posterolaterally to the middle third of the linea aspera.

Adductor brevis (obturator nerve L3) lies deep to adductor longus, passing from the lower aspect of the body of the pubis and the inferior pubic ramus to its attachment on the femur, between the lesser trochanter and the linea aspera.

Adductor magnus (upper fibres, obturator nerve; lower fibres, tibial branch of the sciatic nerve, L2–L4) is the largest and deepest adductor muscle. It is considered to have two separate portions, one an adductor portion and the other a hamstring portion, each with its own separate nerve supply. It takes origin from the inferior pubic ramus, the adjacent ischial ramus and the inferolateral aspect of the ischial tuberosity.

Its upper fibres pass mainly horizontally to the linea aspera of the femur and form the adductor part of the muscle. Its lower fibres pass more vertically to the adductor tubercle on the medial femoral condyle and form the hamstring part.

A GUIDE TO SURFACE MARKING AT THE HIP

Pelvis Region

With the model in standing, palpate the *iliac crest*, which should be obvious in most people as no muscles attach to its superior border. The highest point of the crest lies just behind the midpoint and gives an approximate indication of the level of the spinous process of L4.

Palpate the *anterior superior iliac spine*, which is subcutaneous and located at the anterior end of the iliac crest. It marks the lateral attachment of the inguinal ligament and the origin of the sartorius muscle.

Palpate the *posterior superior iliac spine*, which is situated at the posterior end of the iliac crest. It is not as readily palpable as the anterior spine, but lies under a dimple in the upper buttock, approximately 4 cm lateral to the spinous process of S2. It gives attachment to the sacrotuberous ligament.

Imagine a line drawn from the posterior superior iliac spine to the spinous process of S2; this line crosses the centre of the *sacroiliac joint* and gives an indication of the joint's position.

Consider the position of the *anterior and posterior inferior iliac spines*, which lie below the superior spines and are not as readily palpable. The anterior inferior spine gives origin superiorly to the long head of rectus femoris and inferiorly to part of the iliofemoral ligament.

Locate the position of the *pubic tubercle* at the medial end of the inguinal crease, lying at the same level as the top of the greater trochanter. It marks the medial attachment of the inguinal ligament.

Palpate the bony *ischial tuberosity*, which lies in the buttock approximately 5 cm lateral to the midline just above the gluteal fold. In the sitting position, body weight is supported by the ischial tuberosities. Each tuberosity is most easily palpated with the patient in side-lying with the uppermost hip placed in flexion, to bring the ischial tuberosity out from under the bulk of gluteus maximus.

Lateral Aspect of the Thigh

With the model in side-lying, palpate the *greater trochanter*, which is a large quadrangular bony prominence situated at the upper lateral shaft of the femur, approximately one hand's width below the iliac crest.

Grasp the greater trochanter with your thumb, index and middle fingers (Fig. 10.4), lifting the leg passively into abduction to relax the ITB. The greater trochanter will be a useful bony landmark for some injection techniques around the hip.

Anterior Aspect of the Thigh

With the model in supine-lying, consider the position of the *femoral triangle* on the anterior thigh (Fig. 10.5).

Place the leg into the FABER position – a combination of *F*lexion, *AB*duction and *E*xternal (lateral) *R*otation of the hip – to give you an indication of the borders of the femoral triangle. The inguinal ligament forms the base of the triangle, sartorius its lateral border and adductor longus its medial border. Iliopsoas and pectineus lie in the floor of the femoral triangle.

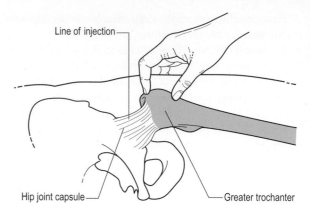

Fig. 10.4 Grasping the greater trochanter to locate the hip joint line.

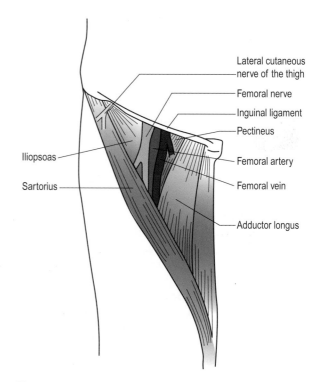

Fig. 10.5 Femoral triangle, also showing emerging lateral cutaneous nerve of thigh.

Consider the position of the *lateral femoral cutaneous nerve* of the thigh (L2–L3) as it passes under or through the inguinal ligament, just medial to the anterior superior iliac spine.

Palpate for the *femoral artery*, which passes down through the middle of the triangle with the femoral vein situated medially and the femoral nerve laterally. You will locate a strong pulse just distal to the midpoint of the inguinal ligament.

Locating the femoral pulse will prove a useful landmark for the structures passing deep to it. From superficial to deep, this is the iliopsoas tendon, which is en route to its insertion into the lesser trochanter, the psoas bursa and the hip joint.

Medial Aspect of the Thigh

With the model still in supine-lying, place the leg into the FABER position (see earlier) to identify the thick, cordlike tendon of *adductor longus*. Palpate this tendon to appreciate its width and depth.

Posterior Aspect of Buttock and Thigh

With the model in prone-lying, consider the position of the *sciatic nerve* in the buttock (Fig. 10.6). You can locate its approximate position by marking a point midway between the posterior apex of the sacrum and the top of greater trochanter, which

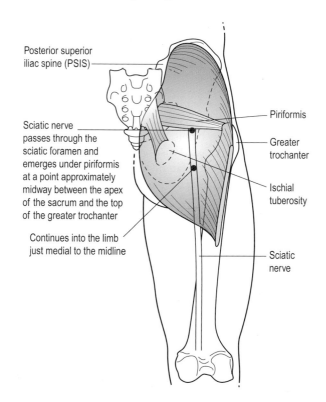

Fig. 10.6 Approximate course of the sciatic nerve in the buttock and thigh.

Posterior superior iliac spine (PSIS)

Sciatic nerve passes through the sciatic foramen and emerges under piriformis at a point approximately midway between the apex of the sacrum and the top of the greater trochanter

Continues into the limb just medial to the midline

Piriformis

Greater trochanter

Ischial tuberosity

Sciatic nerve

identifies the position of the nerve as it leaves the pelvis via the greater sciatic foramen and emerges under piriformis.

Join this to another mark at a point just medial to the midpoint between the greater trochanter and the ischial tuberosity. This indicates the position of the nerve as it continues to exit the buttock under the lower border of gluteus maximus (Standring, 2015).

COMMENTARY ON THE EXAMINATION

Observation

A general observation is made of the patient's *face and overall posture*, but particular attention is paid to the *gait*. Since the function of the hip joint is to support body weight, lesions involving the joint mechanics tend to cause alterations in the gait pattern.

An uneven stride will indicate restricted movement, as found in arthropathy, or may be due to pain on weight-bearing. Excessive lateral rotation on walking may indicate a slipped epiphysis in the young or may be present with pain or advanced capsular contracture in the elderly, indicating an arthropathy with a marked capsular pattern. A Trendelenburg gait will indicate weak abductor muscles and there can be various causes of this.

History

The patient's *age, occupation, sports, hobbies and activities* may alert the examiner to the possible cause of the lesion.

The age of the patient is relevant to conditions at the hip (Table 10.1). Degenerative arthropathy typically presents in the working-age to older age group, although it is not uncommon to find it in younger athletes, especially road runners. Muscle lesions and bursitis affect the working-age group, while loose bodies can present as a complication of degenerative arthropathy in the older age group, or as osteochondritis dissecans in adolescents.

Children can develop hip problems, which if misdiagnosed can be potentially serious, and an orthopaedic opinion should always be sought:

- Hip dysplasia.
- 'Irritable hip' is a non-specific diagnosis for groin pain, limited movement and a limp.
- Perthes' disease affects boys aged 3 to 10 and is an osteochondritis of the femoral epiphysis.

TABLE 10.1   **Lesions Suspected at Different Ages**

Lesions	Young	Middle	Old
Degeneration in hip joint	‡	**	***
Dislocation/instability	*	‡	‡
Perthes' disease	***	‡	‡
Slipped epiphysis	***	‡	‡
Labral injuries	***	*	‡
Bursitis	*	***	*
Tendinopathy	‡	***	‡
Tendon apophysitis	***	‡	‡
Fracture	**	*	***
Malignancy	**	**	**

Key: ***common, **less common, *rare, ‡highly unlikely.

- Slipped epiphysis is either a sudden or gradual slipping of the superior epiphyseal plate, which may produce a lateral rotation deformity. It tends to occur in overweight adolescents (ages 10 to 16) and is more common in boys, who present with pain on exercise.
- Transient synovitis is of unknown aetiology and affects children under 10 years old with an acute onset (Gough-Palmer and McHugh, 2007).
- Juvenile chronic arthritis usually begins in other joints, but it can also affect the hip joints.

It is well known that the hip can refer pain to the knee in children (Emms et al., 2002). Groin pain or pain referred to the knee in a child or adolescent, without obvious cause, must be considered as suspicious and a specialist opinion sought for the possibility of the conditions mentioned earlier.

Excessive muscle contraction, as involved in explosive sports changing rapidly from running to jumping (hurdling, etc.), can lead to avulsion fractures and chronic apophysitis in adolescents. These occur most commonly at the attachment of the hamstring muscles at the ischial tuberosity and the long head of rectus femoris at the anterior inferior iliac spine (Brukner et al., 2017).

Occupation, sports, hobbies and activities will indicate the aggravating factors of the condition and allow the practitioner to formulate a programme of treatment and advice that is tailored to the patient's individual needs.

Specific sports-related conditions should be considered. Stress fracture of the femoral neck may be encountered in young adults who are involved in endurance and high-intensity sports. Initially, anterior hip pain comes on later in the sporting activity, but it then progresses to limit activity, becoming present during any weight-bearing episode and even at rest.

It should also be suspected in women with the female athletic triad of amenorrhoea, eating disorder and osteoporosis. Diagnosis is essential to prevent progression to avascular necrosis of the femoral head (O'Kane, 1999; Adkins and Figler, 2000).

Hip fractures are regarded as the most severe, and second most common, osteoporotic fracture (Johnell and Kanis, 2005). Osteoporotic fracture (also known as insufficiency or fragility fracture) should be considered in all women aged 50 to 64 years and all men aged 50 to 74 years who have risk factors (National Institute for Health and Care Excellence NICE, 2021).

Osteitis pubis, a pathological condition involving the pubic bone and symphysis pubis, presents with groin pain that may be bilateral. The symptoms may be aggravated by exercise, twisting, turning and kicking. Pain is provoked by bilateral resisted adduction (the 'squeeze test'), which is usually accompanied by weakness, and there is tenderness to palpation over the pubic tubercles and symphysis pubis (Brukner et al., 2017).

'Sports hernias' should also be considered as a cause of anterior hip pain. These are thought to be responsible for activity-related hip pain, particularly in football, rugby and ice hockey players (O'Kane, 1999). Inguinal hernia presents as a lump in the groin that goes away when the patient lies down. The lump reappears or increases on coughing and is not usually painful (Jenkins and O'Dwyer, 2008). 'Gilmore's groin' (see page 332) is not a hernia but should be considered in the differential diagnosis of groin pain, particularly in the sporting male.

Low levels of activity, as well as overuse or repetitive movements, may also be a cause of conditions at the hip, particularly tendinopathies or bursitis.

The *site and spread* of pain may be local, indicating a superficial or less irritable lesion, such as a muscle strain, or diffuse, indicating a larger lesion or gross inflammation.

Pain originating from hip pathology is most commonly located in the groin (88%) (Luthra et al., 2019). It may also occur anywhere around the hip, thigh or be referred to the knee via the obturator nerve (Fig. 10.7).

Patients with possible intra-articular hip pathologies tend to cup the trochanter, making a 'C-sign', indicating where they feel the pain by spreading their finger and thumb widely against the side of the hip joint, to point to both the anterior and posterior aspects of the joint.

Trochanteric pain may be a result of gluteal tendinopathy, greater trochanteric pain syndrome (GTPS) or ITB friction syndrome. Adductor pathologies usually result in medial thigh pain. Pain in the hip joint region may originate in the lumbar spine, particularly if the pain is predominantly in the buttock, and there may also be associated referred leg pain.

The sensory nerve supply to the hip joint is mainly through the femoral nerve L2–L3. Part of the L2 and L3 dermatomes also cover the upper buttock, and a hip lesion may present as low back pain only. The hip joint itself can refer pain further into these dermatomes,

depending on the size of the lesion. A detailed history will help to differentiate lesions in the area.

As well as in children, hip pathology can masquerade as knee pain in adult patients (Emms et al., 2002). There is apparently a Spanish saying that translates as 'the hip cries through the knee', which may help to remember this common clinical finding.

The *onset* of the symptoms may be gradual or sudden.

In degenerative arthropathy, the pain has a gradual onset, initially during weight-bearing activities but progressing to hip pain without weight-bearing, and being present at rest (Cailliet, 1990). A history of previous trauma such as fracture, which can alter joint biomechanics, can predispose the joint to degenerative changes.

Relatively minor trauma can fracture the pubic ramus in the elderly, producing severe local and groin pain of sudden onset.

Loose bodies present suddenly, as do traumatic muscular lesions. Muscles around the hip joint can be strained easily, since several are two-joint muscles, and a sudden explosive contraction, such as that seen in sprinting, may produce overstretching (Hartley, 1995).

A severe pain that gradually increases in intensity and remains so, coupled with other findings in the

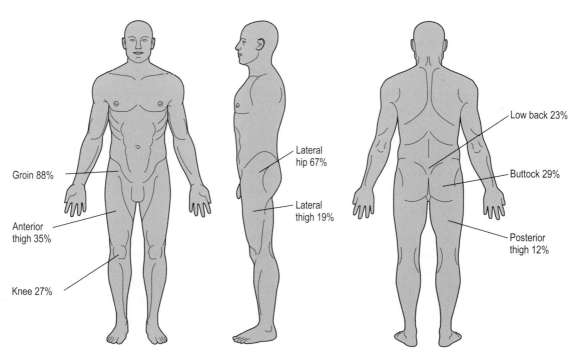

Fig. 10.7 Possible sites of pain associated with hip pathology in young adults. (From Luthra et al., 2019.).

history, suggests a serious lesion. The 'sign of the buttock' (see page 321) may also be produced.

The *duration* of symptoms can help with differential diagnosis and indicate the stage of the lesion in the healing process.

Degenerative arthropathy usually presents with a typical history of gradually worsening episodes of pain. Bursitis tends to give a gradual onset of aching pain and is often present for many months before the patient seeks treatment.

The *symptoms and behaviour* need to be considered. Symptoms described by the patient may give essential clues to diagnosis. Loose bodies tend to produce twinging pain and a sensation of giving way on weight-bearing. Similar symptoms may be associated with labral tears or anterior acetabular chondral defects where clicking or locking may also be present (Neumann et al., 2007).

Unrelenting pain should be considered serious, especially if the patient is feeling systemically unwell with a fever, night sweats and chills.

To determine if the pain is being referred from the lumbar spine, the patient is questioned about the presence of paraesthesia and pain produced by a cough or sneeze. Also consider peripheral nerve compression as a cause of paraesthesia.

Compression of the lateral cutaneous nerve (L2–L3) of the thigh can cause a condition called meralgia paraesthetica, which produces paraesthesia and pain in the nerve's distribution on the anterolateral side of the thigh. Impaired or altered sensation may also be experienced in the same area, but there is no motor weakness or wasting, and the knee reflex is preserved, helping to differentiate it from lumbar radiculopathy (Pearce, 2006).

The behaviour of the pain gives an indication of the nature of the lesion. For example, degenerative arthropathy at the hip joint or inflamed bursae may be aggravated by activity and weight-bearing, and muscle strains are worse with use and eased by rest. Bursae produce pain on activities that squeeze or compress them, such as lying on the side or sitting.

Inflammatory arthritis tends to produce morning pain and significant early stiffness (usually lasts more than an hour) due to accumulation of intracapsular swelling overnight (Hartley, 1995). Degenerative arthropathy also often produces night pain.

An indication of *medical history, other joint involvement* and *medications* may give a clue to diagnosis and will establish whether contraindications to treatment techniques exist. Patients should be asked red flag screening questions, such as unexpected recent weight loss and unrelenting night pain, which are indicative of more serious lesions (Paice, 1995).

In addition to past medical history, establish any ongoing conditions and treatment. Explore other previous or current musculoskeletal problems with previous episodes of the current complaint, any treatment given and the outcome of treatment. For example, previous osteoporotic fragility fracture, frequent use of oral corticosteroids, history of falls, low body mass index (less than 18.5kg/m^2), smoking, or excessive drinking.

Differential diagnosis should also consider the exclusion of hip pain associated with pathology of the abdominal and pelvic organs, as well as femoral or inguinal hernias.

Practitioners should routinely screen for psychosocial factors and consider relevant health co-morbidities and lifestyle factors (see Chapter 1). These factors may contribute to patients' presenting condition or form a barrier to their recovery and normal function, which should be addressed as an integral part of patient management.

Inspection

An inspection of the general posture in weight-bearing will reveal any *bony deformity*. Look for general postural asymmetry that may be relevant, the position of the buttock creases, posterior superior iliac spines, anterior superior iliac spines, level of the iliac crests, any leg length discrepancy and the position of the feet.

Colour changes and *swelling* are not expected at the hip because it is such a deep joint, but they may be associated with trauma, bruising and abrasions. If redness and swelling are present in the buttock area, without a history of trauma, the 'sign of the buttock' (see page 321) may be suspected.

Muscle wasting may be seen in the glutei, associated with a lumbar lesion, or in the quadriceps, associated with degenerative arthropathy of the hip or a lumbar lesion.

State at Rest

Before any movements are performed, the state at rest is established to provide a baseline for subsequent comparison.

Examination by Selective Tension

The suggested sequence for the examination will now be given, followed by a commentary that includes the reason for performing the movements and the significance of the possible findings. Comparison should always be made with the other side.

The routine examination of the hip is conducted in the order given, as it allows the tests to be completed in each of the positions of standing, supine and prone lying and prevents frequent changes of position.

Eliminate the Lumbar Spine
- Active lumbar extension (Fig. 10.8)
- Extension repeated with foot on stool if indicated (Fig. 10.9)
- Active lumbar right-side flexion (Fig. 10.10)
- Active lumbar left-side flexion (Fig. 10.11)
- Active lumbar flexion (Fig. 10.12)
- Passive straight leg raise (Fig. 10.13)

Supine Lying
- Passive hip flexion (Fig. 10.14)
- Passive hip medial rotation for end-feel (Fig. 10.15)
- Passive hip lateral rotation (Fig. 10.16)
- Passive hip abduction (Fig. 10.17)
- Passive hip adduction (Fig. 10.18)
- Resisted hip flexion (Fig. 10.19)
- Resisted hip abduction (Fig. 10.20)
- Resisted hip adduction (Fig. 10.21)
- Resisted hip extension (Fig. 10.22)

Prone Lying
- Passive femoral stretch test (Fig. 10.23)
- Passive hip extension (Fig. 10.24)
- Passive hip medial rotation for range (Fig. 10.25)
- Resisted hip medial rotation (Fig. 10.26)
- Resisted hip lateral rotation (Fig. 10.27)
- Resisted knee flexion (Fig. 10.28)
- Resisted knee extension (Fig. 10.29)

Accessory Test for the Psoas Bursa
- Passive hip flexion and adduction (Fig. 10.30)

Accessory test for the 'sign of the buttock'
- Passive straight leg raise (Fig. 10.31a and b)

Palpation
- Once a diagnosis has been made, the structure at fault is palpated for the exact site of the lesion

---

The lumbar spine is first assessed by the four active movements. If active lumbar extension reproduces the pain, it should be repeated with the hip joint eliminated by placing it into flexion with the foot up on a stool. If extension is still painful, the lesion is more likely to be in the lumbar spine and a more thorough lumbar examination is necessary.

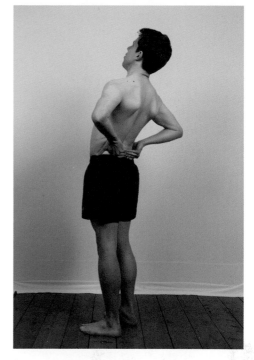

Fig. 10.8 Active extension.

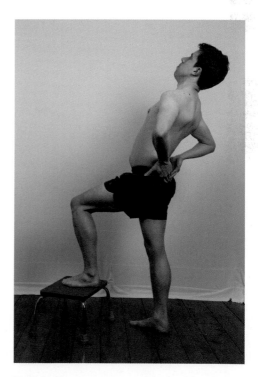

Fig. 10.9 Active extension with hip flexed to differentiate between hip and lumbar spine as the cause of pain.

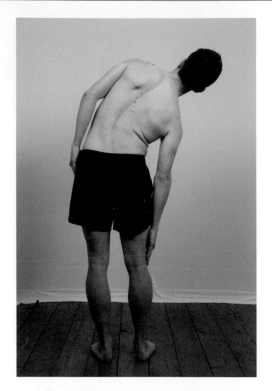

Fig. 10.10 Active right-side flexion.

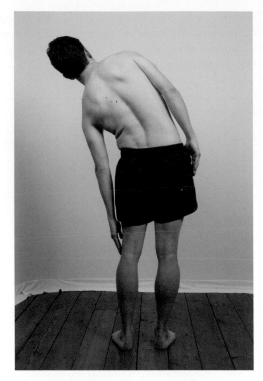

Fig. 10.11 Active left-side flexion.

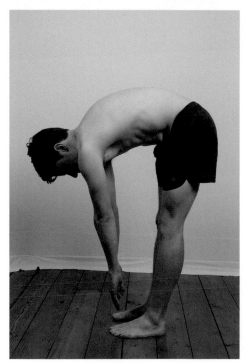

Fig. 10.12 Active flexion.

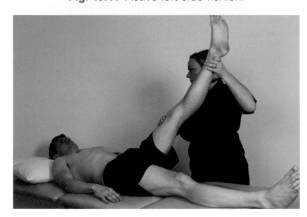

Fig. 10.13 Passive straight leg raise.

The straight leg raise and femoral stretch tests are applied passively within the examination sequence to test for neural involvement. This needs to be considered within clinical reasoning.

Tests for sacroiliac joint involvement may also be included at this stage, as indicated by the history, and are described in Chapter 14.

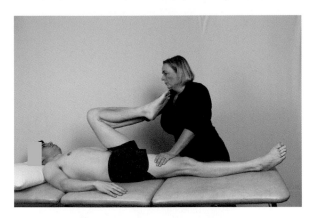

Fig. 10.14 Passive flexion.

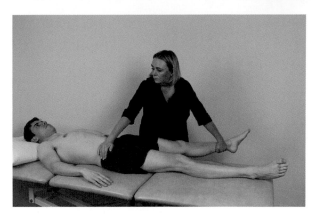

Fig. 10.17 Passive abduction.

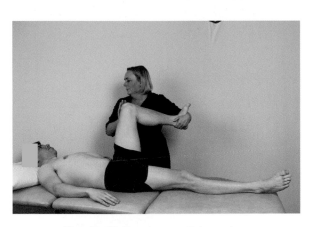

Fig. 10.15 Passive medial rotation.

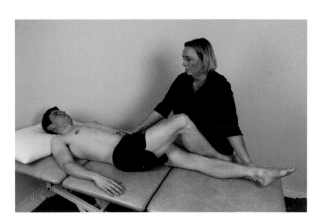

Fig. 10.18 Passive adduction.

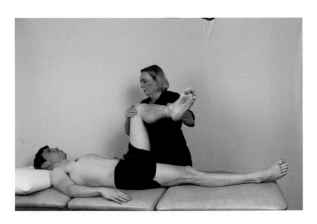

Fig. 10.16 Passive lateral rotation.

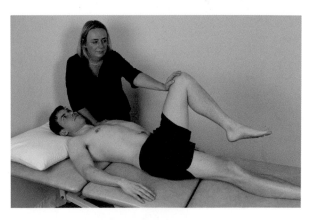

Fig. 10.19 Resisted flexion.

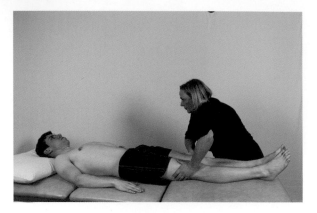

Fig. 10.20 Resisted abduction.

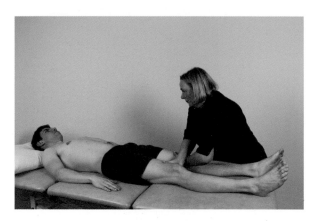

Fig. 10.21 Resisted adduction.

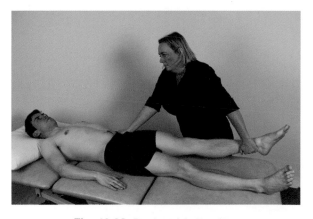

Fig. 10.22 Resisted extension.

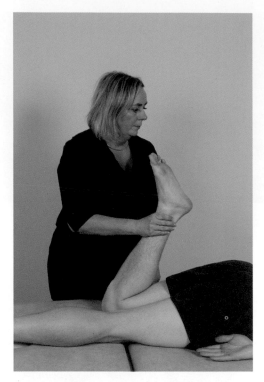

Fig. 10.23 Passive femoral stretch test.

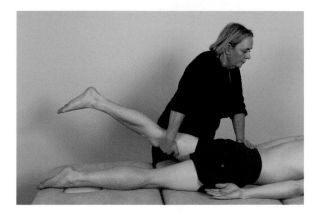

Fig. 10.24 Passive extension.

The passive hip movements test the inert structures for pain, range of movement and end-feel. Limited movement may be typical of the capsular pattern of limitation due to arthritis. Normally, passive flexion has a 'soft' end-feel while passive medial rotation, lateral rotation and extension have an 'elastic' end-feel.

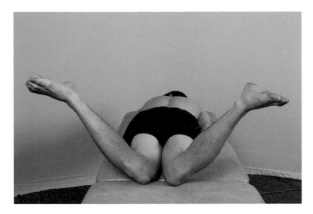

Fig. 10.25 Passive medial rotation.

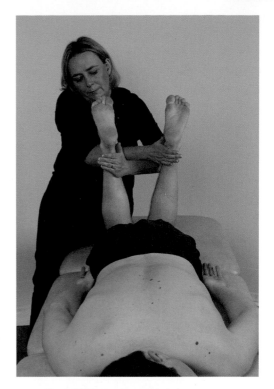

Fig. 10.27 Resisted lateral rotation.

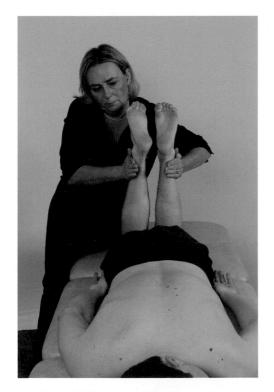

Fig. 10.26 Resisted medial rotation.

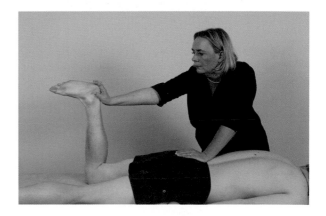

Fig. 10.28 Resisted knee flexion.

It is not possible to appreciate the end-feel of the capsule on passive abduction and adduction, as the tension in the overlying soft tissue structures provides the end of range of these movements before the capsule can be stressed. Abduction may still be limited as part of the capsular pattern, nonetheless.

A bursitis or a loose body in the joint produces a non-capsular pattern of movement.

The resisted movements test the contractile structures for pain and power. At the hip, muscle lesions are commonly found in the adductors, quadriceps and hamstrings, but positive resisted tests may also be an accessory sign in bursitis.

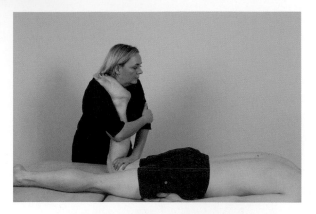

Fig. 10.29 Resisted knee extension.

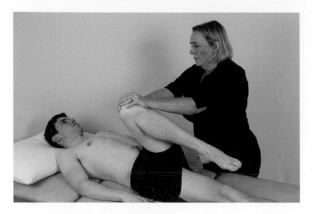

Fig. 10.30 Combined flexion and adduction to compress the psoas bursa.

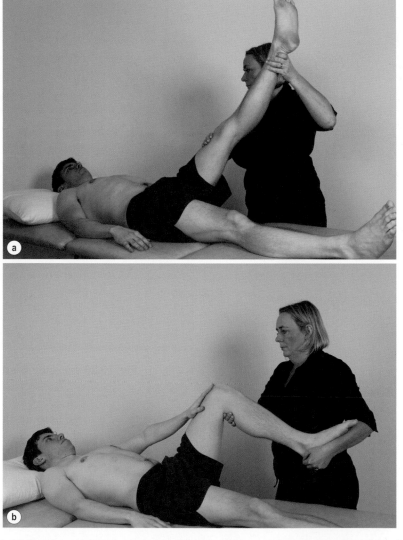

Fig. 10.31 (a) Passive straight leg raise and (b) hip flexion, accessory test for 'sign of the buttock'.

Movement	Main Muscles	'Assistors'
Flexion	Psoas	Iliacus, rectus femoris
Extension	Gluteus maximus	Adductor magnus, hamstrings
Lateral rotation	Externus and internus obturators, piriformis, superior and inferior gemelli, quadratus femoris	Gluteus maximus, adductor magnus
Medial rotation	Gluteus medius, gluteus minimus, tensor fasciae latae	Adductor brevis, adductor longus, adductor magnus
Abduction	Gluteus medius, gluteus minimus, tensor fasciae latae	
Adduction	Adductor brevis, adductor longus, adductor magnus, pectineus, gracilis	

Accessory tests can be applied if indicated by the history and are described with the relevant pathologies following in the chapter. The straight leg raise can also be an accessory test to look for serious pathology in the hip or pelvis (see 'sign of the buttock').

Based on the history and clinical examination, the practitioner should be able to establish the most likely diagnosis, using clinical reasoning and clinical judgement.

It is important to recognise potential serious pathology, such as infection, malignancy, fracture and inflammatory arthritis, and to make any appropriate onward referral in a timely manner. Should additional information be required to aid diagnosis or to add value to management, further investigations can be considered to inform decision making and planning.

Investigations should be guided by suspected causes as an extension to the clinical examination. If necessary, the practitioner may consider further investigations such as blood tests, radiological imaging, and other diagnostic procedures. They should be considered with suspected red flags such as fracture, infection, inflammatory arthritis or malignancy.

If severe degenerative arthropathy, avascular neurosis of the femoral head, or hip impingement syndrome are suspected, X-ray or magnetic resonance imaging (MRI) (with or without contrast) may be appropriate.

Blood tests can be considered if malignancy, polymyalgia rheumatica, inflammatory arthritis or infection are suspected.

The differential diagnosis of hip pain is extensive. It includes intra-articular pathology and extra-articular pathology of the hip joint, as well as pathologies within the lumbar spine and sacroiliac joint.

The causes of intra-articular hip pain include degenerative arthropathy, femoroacetabular impingement, synovitis, labral tears, loose bodies, capsular laxity, tears of the ligamentum teres, and chondral damage.

Extra-articular hip pain can be associated with greater trochanteric pain syndrome (GTPS), ITB syndrome, iliopsoas tendonitis, 'internal' snapping hip, 'external' snapping hip, greater trochanteric bursitis, gluteal tendinopathy, femoral neck stress fracture, adductor strain, 'sports hernia', or 'Gilmore's groin'.

Sign of the Buttock

The sign of the buttock is pain produced on straight leg raise that increases on flexing the knee and hip (Cyriax and Cyriax, 1993). An empty end-feel is experienced as more range of movement is available, but any attempt to produce more hip flexion is prevented by voluntary muscle spasm, and the patient puts out a hand to stop the movement due to pain.

A positive sign indicates a major lesion in the buttock or hip region. The history may reveal a patient in severe pain or an unwell patient who looks ill and may have a fever with night sweats and chills. The pain may be unrelenting in the buttock, hip or leg. It is not eased by rest and therefore night pain is a feature.

On examination, a non-capsular pattern of movement at the hip, and often the lumbar spine, is discovered. Pain may be increased by lumbar flexion and resisted tests at the hip, but the cardinal feature is the positive sign of the buttock.

Possible causes of the sign of the buttock are malignancy in the upper femur or ilium, fracture, ischiorectal abscess, sepsis, either septic bursitis or arthritis, or osteomyelitis of the upper femur (Cyriax and Cyriax,

1993). Urgent medical attention and further investigation are required.

CAPSULAR LESIONS

The movements limited in the capsular pattern have a characteristically 'hard' end-feel. The capsular pattern of the hip is most limitation of medial rotation, less limitation of flexion and abduction and least limitation of extension.

> **CAPSULAR PATTERN OF THE HIP JOINT**
> - Most limitation of medial rotation
> - Less limitation of flexion and abduction
> - Least limitation of extension

Klässbo et al. (2003) supported medial rotation, flexion and abduction as the three most limited movements but found it difficult to identify the exact proportions lost to be able to establish an ordering or pattern of limitation. However, the capsular patterns at all the joints are intended as a clinical guide, and it may not be appropriate to expose them to rigorous investigation.

The limitation of medial rotation is clinically the most useful component of the pattern. If, on examination, the capsular pattern exists at the hip joint, then an arthropathy is present. At the hip this could be degenerative arthropathy, traumatic arthritis, rheumatoid arthritis and any of the spondyloarthropathies.

Arthropathy at the hip is commonly degenerative arthropathy, usually occurring over the age of 60 but frequently younger (Feather et al., 2020). Prevalence varies between communities and ranges from 10% to 12% across local authorities in England (Arthritis Research UK and Public Health England, 2012).

Men and women are generally equally affected (Dieppe, 1995; Sims, 1999), with possibly a slightly higher prevalence in women (Quintana et al., 2008), and the female femoral and pelvic shape may predispose women to degenerative arthropathy (Kersnic et al., 1997), especially in association with increased body weight. Obesity increases the load on the weight-bearing surfaces, progressing the degenerative process more rapidly (Dieppe, 1995).

Intrinsic factors such as physical inactivity, altered biomechanics, or extrinsic factors such as hardness of the floor, and the influence of sporting and leisure activities, may also contribute to degenerative change (Sims, 1999).

Abnormal loading may also occur as a result of alteration in the centre of gravity, for example, associated with an antalgic gait pattern. Although this reduces the compressive forces of the abductor muscles as the centre of gravity shifts towards the stance limb, the load is transferred to the superior aspect of the femoral head where it becomes concentrated, leading to cartilage degradation (Sims, 1999).

An abnormal gait pattern may be the result of pathology anywhere in the lower limb kinetic chain, from the lumbar spine to the foot, and need not be confined to the hip.

The articular surfaces of the hip are slightly incongruent such that the apex of the acetabulum is a non-contact area allowing lubrication of the articular cartilage. The joint becomes more congruent during the ageing process, reducing lubrication and possibly contributing further to degenerative change.

Neumann et al. (2007) looked at the prevalence of labral tears and cartilage loss in patients with mechanical symptoms of the hip using magnetic resonance arthrography (MRA). They concluded that cartilage loss, labral tears and bone marrow oedema appear to be interrelated and may represent important risk factors for the development and progression of degenerative arthropathy in the hip joint.

The pain of degenerative arthropathy usually has a gradual onset and may be felt in the upper buttock, groin and anterior thigh, down to or beyond the knee. Pain is associated with activity in the early stages, but as the condition advances, pain is also present at rest, including at night. Joint stiffness and loss of movement, such as difficulty in reaching to put on shoes and socks, are also presenting factors.

X-ray changes are not a good indicator of symptoms, as the pain tends to be worse before changes become apparent and can often ease as the changes become more significant (C. Speed, Society of Musculoskeletal Medicine Conference, March 2014).

Differential diagnosis of hip arthropathy includes malignancy, fracture, inflammatory arthritis, septic arthritis, avascular neurosis of femoral head, acetabular protrusion, slipped epiphysis, Perthes disease, GTPS, meralgia paraesthetica, spinal stenosis, and ITB syndrome (NICE, 2018; Tibor and Sekiya, 2008).

A stepped approach to the management of degenerative arthropathy of the hip is currently recommended (NICE, 2020). Less invasive treatments are generally offered first, including education/watchful wait, activity and work modification, weight management, suitable footwear, simple analgesics and non-steroidal anti-inflammatory drugs (NSAIDs) medication, physiotherapy (e.g. exercise, mobilisation) and then injection therapy (e.g. corticosteroid, local anaesthetic, hyaluronic acid). If symptoms persist, more invasive treatments can be considered, such as arthroplasty.

After diagnosis, degenerative arthropathy may stabilise and the prognosis can be good, but it usually progresses with periods of exacerbation and remission (Dieppe, 1995).

Research continues for evidence to support that some foodstuffs or dietary compounds can actually change the progressive nature of the disease. Following a Mediterranean diet may help (Arthritis Foundation, 2021) and the overweight patient should be encouraged to lose weight. Sticks and other walking support may be appropriate to aid daily living.

Treatment in the musculoskeletal approach aims to provide pain relief and increase mobility. It depends on the stage and activity of the disease, as indicated by the severity/irritability of the lesion, and can be divided into mild, moderate and severe stages to guide the application of appropriate treatment.

Mild Degenerative Arthropathy of the Hip

This is usually the initial phase of diagnosis of the condition. At this stage, the key findings are as follows:

- The patient complains of buttock or groin pain associated with weight-bearing activities and the pain sometimes disturbs sleep.
- On examination, the patient has a mild capsular pattern of limited medial rotation, flexion and perhaps abduction, with extension not yet affected.
- The limited movements have an abnormal 'hard' end-feel due to muscle spasm, but some elasticity remains.

The principle of treatment, applied during this mild stage, is to mobilise the restricted hip movements, using a Grade B capsular stretching technique in conjunction with heat applied to the joint. The aim of treatment is to relieve pain and to allow a greater range of pain-free movement to be established.

GRADE B MOBILISATION FOR MILD DEGENERATIVE ARTHROPATHY

(Saunders, 2000)

The movements limited in the capsular pattern are stretched using peripheral Grade B mobilisation. However, functional benefit is often gained by stretching flexion alone.

To stretch flexion:

- Position the patient in supine lying with counter-pressure on the other leg to stabilise it and to ensure that maximum stretch is applied to the affected hip joint capsule (Fig. 10.32).
- Place one hand under the patient's lower thigh, to avoid involving the knee and to give a little distraction, which makes the technique more comfortable.
- Place the patient's foot against your shoulder to help with stretching and to guide the movement.
- Hold the stretch at the end of the available range for as long as the patient can tolerate.
- Ease off the end of the range to allow the patient to rest and then repeat several times.
- Observe the patient's reaction throughout and gradually increase the range with each stretch.
- After stretching flexion, slide the patient's leg over your shoulder and return the leg steadily to the bed under some distraction to reduce discomfort (Fig. 10.33).

To stretch extension:

- Reverse the position described for stretching flexion, with pressure applied to stretch extension of the affected leg (Fig. 10.34).

To stretch abduction:

- Fix the good leg over the edge of the couch and position the affected leg in as much abduction as possible (Fig. 10.35).
- Increase this range of movement periodically as creep occurs and the range of movement increases.
- After stretching, allow the patient to return the legs from the stretch position at their own pace, to avoid discomfort.

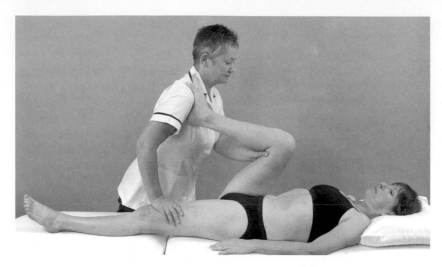

Fig. 10.32 Grade B mobilisation, stretching flexion.

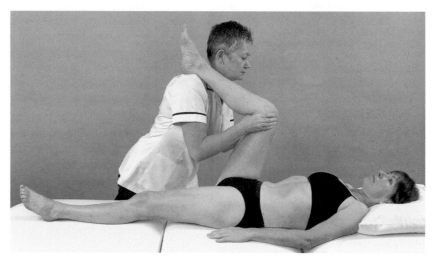

Fig. 10.33 Grade B mobilisation, returning leg under some distraction.

To stretch medial rotation:
- Position the patient in prone-lying with the knee flexed to 90 degrees.
- Fix the opposite buttock and apply the pressure carefully to the medial aspect of the knee.
- Stretch and repeat, gradually increasing range and checking carefully with the patient during each technique.

- Take care with this stretch, as it can apply a strong torsion force to the neck of the femur and may also affect the knee (Fig. 10.36).

The stretching techniques, as applied previously, are used as an adjunct to the core treatment, and self-stretches are an important part of the overall exercise programme to maintain and improve range.

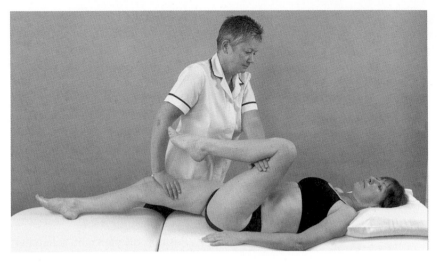

Fig. 10.34 Grade B mobilisation, stretching extension.

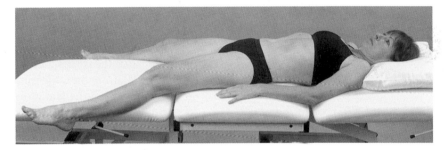

Fig. 10.35 Grade B mobilisation, stretching abduction.

Clinical judgement should be used to guide how long each session of stretching should last. The pain may be aggravated afterwards for 2 to 4 hours and this should be explained to the patient. If the patient reports that the pain lasted much longer than the 2 to 4 hours, then reduce the intensity and number of stretches at the next session, or consider increasing the stretches if there is little after-treatment soreness.

Initially, the patient is seen regularly to assess the effect of the capsular stretching and to teach the patient self-management. Treatment continues until either a plateau is reached or patients are confident to continue with their own stretching exercises and management.

Moderate Degenerative Arthropathy of the Hip

Here, the patient's symptoms and signs indicate a progression of the disease. Pain may be present at rest as well as exacerbated by weight-bearing activities. On examination, a moderate to severe capsular pattern is found and the limited movements have a 'hard' end-feel.

Capsular stretching may no longer provide benefit. Injection may be considered to provide short term pain relief, but practitioners should check with local policy prior to injecting the hip, since most are now conducted under image guidance in a sterile theatre. Current practice appears to be to avoid injecting into the hip within 3 to 6 months of planned surgery.

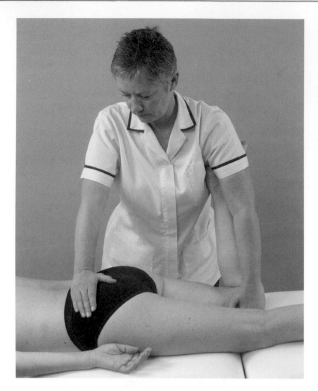

Fig. 10.36 Grade B mobilisation, stretching medial rotation.

Kaspar and de Van de Beer (2005) conducted a retrospective study of 40 patients who had injections prior to hip arthroplasty and 40 who had not. The hip injections had all been given under sterile theatre conditions with the same dosages of corticosteroid and local anaesthetic, but the study found a significantly increased rate of postoperative infection in those hips that had had previous injection.

In contrast to this finding, a similar study to establish the influence of corticosteroid injections on the incidence of infection following total knee arthroplasty found no link between previous injection and subsequent postoperative infection (Horne et al., 2008; see Chapter 11). A review by Wang et al. (2014) also identified no increased risk of infection among patients who had received injections prior to surgery in either the hip or knee joints.

Controversy also exists concerning repeated steroid injections into weight-bearing joints and the risk of steroid arthropathy (Cameron, 1995). Therefore, as a general precaution, repeated corticosteroid injections into the hip joint are not advised.

A minimum dose of 40 mg triamcinolone acetonide is recommended, but support for a larger dose of 80 mg is provided by a study conducted by Robinson et al. (2007), who found significant and longer lasting improvements in pain, stiffness and disability with the higher dose.

INJECTION OF THE HIP JOINT (CYRIAX, 1984 CYRIAX AND CYRIAX, 1993)

Suggested needle size: 20 G × 3½ in. (0.9 × 90 mm) spinal needle

Dose: 40–80 mg triamcinolone acetonide in a total volume of 5–6 mL

- Position the patient in side-lying with the painful leg uppermost and supported in a neutral position on a pillow.
- Locate the greater trochanter by grasping it between thumb, index and middle fingers; the index finger should be resting on the top of the trochanter.
- To test you are in the correct position, move the leg passively into some abduction (Fig. 10.37), to relax the ITB, and you should feel your index finger sink in over the top of the trochanter.
- The capsule of the hip joint almost completely surrounds the neck of the femur. Insert the needle just above the index finger, i.e. above the greater trochanter, and aim vertically downward towards the neck of the femur (Fig. 10.38).
- You will feel a resistance as the needle pierces first the fascia lata, then the capsule, before gently 'caressing' bone (Fig. 10.39); the needle should now be intracapsular.
- Withdraw away from the bone a little and deliver the injection as a bolus.

The patient should minimise or modify activities for 2 weeks following injection.

Severe Degenerative Arthropathy of the Hip

Conservative management no longer controls the patient's pain, and functional disability may now be serious. Surgery is probably indicated, but there are no agreed criteria or guidelines for electing to perform hip surgery (Dieppe, 1995). Pain, age and disability, as well as the patient's general health, potential for rehabilitation, social factors and psychological factors, should all be taken into consideration by the patient and surgeon.

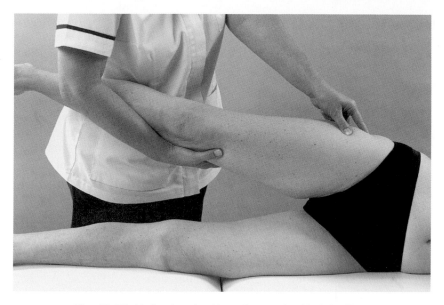

Fig. 10.37 Abducting the hip to locate the hip joint line.

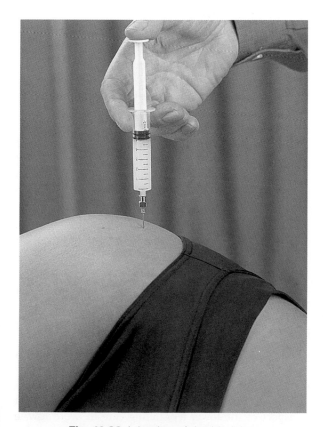

Fig. 10.38 Injection of the hip joint.

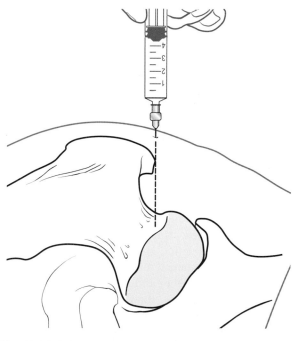

Fig. 10.39 Injection of the hip joint, showing direction of approach and needle position.

Injection for this stage may be given for diagnostic or therapeutic purposes, especially if the patient is young and/or not eligible for surgery.

Rheumatoid Arthritis

This may affect the hip joint, and symptomatic relief may be gained from intra-articular injection, as described previously.

NON-CAPSULAR LESIONS

Loose Body

A loose body in the hip joint may be associated with the rare condition osteochondritis dissecans in adolescents, but most commonly occurs secondary to the onset of degenerative arthropathy (Cyriax and Cyriax, 1993; Saotome et al., 2006; Tibor and Sekiya, 2008).

Loose bodies associated with degenerative arthropathy can be chondral, osteochondral or osseous. They can increase in size and progressively worsen the damage to the joint surfaces as well as the clinical symptoms (Bianchi and Martinoli, 1999). To avoid this, they should be removed arthroscopically (Tibor and Sekiya, 2008).

A loose body in the hip joint can cause twinges of pain felt in the groin or radiating down the front of the leg. These twinges may be associated with a momentary sensation of locking or giving way and an inability to bear weight. This history suggests a loose body in the joint that periodically becomes impacted between the joint surfaces.

A short stance phase in gait may be evident, or a Trendelenburg gait. Pain is usually felt in the groin with clicking, locking and/or giving way (O'Kane, 1999; Hickman and Peters, 2001; Neumann et al., 2007).

Signs of a loose body consist of a non-capsular pattern, commonly with pain at the end of range of full passive hip flexion and lateral rotation. If the range of movement demonstrates limitation, a springy end-feel may be appreciated. Impingement tests, combining forced flexion, adduction and medial rotation, or flexion, abduction with lateral rotation, may reproduce pain (Martin et al., 2008; Tibor and Sekiya, 2008).

Differential diagnosis should exclude labral tears, which are found in the young adult. Labral pathology is often associated with traumatic incidents that may be minor twisting, repetitive flexion or hyperextension injuries, especially in athletes. There may also be predisposing congenital factors where the onset of pain is more likely to be gradual. MRI, and more specifically MRA, can be used to confirm a labral tear (Bharam, 2006).

Other conditions to consider in differential diagnosis for a loose body at the hip include osteochondritis dissecans, femoroacetabular impingement, tears of the ligamentum teres, chondral damage, iliopsoas tendinopathy, 'internal' snapping hip, 'external' snapping hip, ITB and GTPS (Tibor and Sekiya, 2008).

The principle of treatment is to reduce the loose body using strong traction together with Grade A mobilisation. If successful, the loose body will be moved to a position within the joint where symptoms are more manageable. A surgical opinion should be sought in the young, or for those with persistent symptoms of pain, locking and instability, which have a significant impact on function.

LOOSE BODY MOBILISATION TECHNIQUE

(Cyriax, 1984; Cyriax and Cyriax, 1993)

Position the patient in supine on the couch with an assistant applying counter-pressure at the anterior superior iliac spines; padding may make it more comfortable for the patient (see Fig. 10.41). The assistant must start by applying pressure in an anterior–posterior direction and be prepared to change to apply cephalad pressure towards the end of the technique.

The choice of technique, with either lateral or medial rotation, will depend on the physical findings during examination, and the least painful rotation is attempted first; this is usually medial rotation.

Local health and safety requirements or an unsuitable treatment couch may make it difficult to perform the technique as described here. The technique can also be performed with the operator standing on the floor, although it is harder to apply and maintain the traction throughout the technique in this position (Fig. 10.44a and b).

Mobilisation A: With Medial Rotation

- Stand on the end of the couch, at its lowest height, with your feet close together and parallel to the edge.
- Face the direction of medial rotation and apply a butterfly grip with the thumbs parallel on the lateral aspect of the lower leg, taking care to avoid undue pressure around the malleoli (Fig. 10.40).

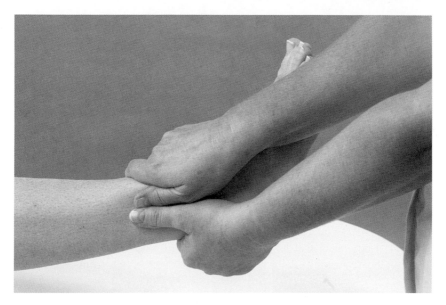

Fig. 10.40 Loose-body mobilisation A for the hip, showing hand position for mobilisation into medial rotation.

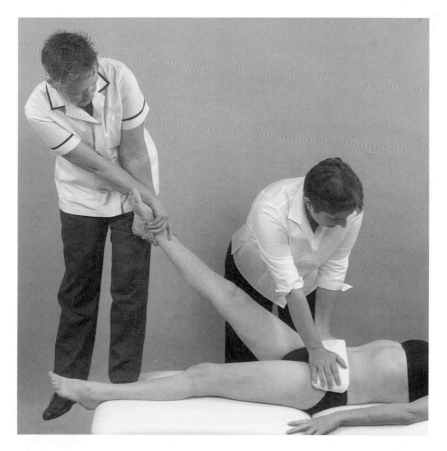

Fig. 10.41 Loose-body mobilisation A for the hip, showing body positioning and assistant's counter-pressure.

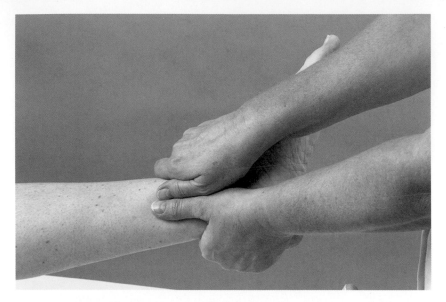

Fig. 10.42 Loose-body mobilisation B for the hip, showing hand position for mobilisation into lateral rotation.

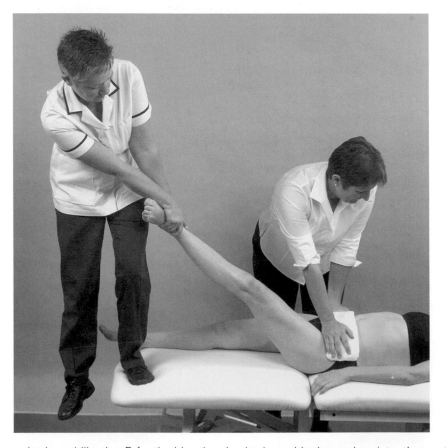

Fig. 10.43 Loose-body mobilisation B for the hip, showing body positioning and assistant's counter-pressure.

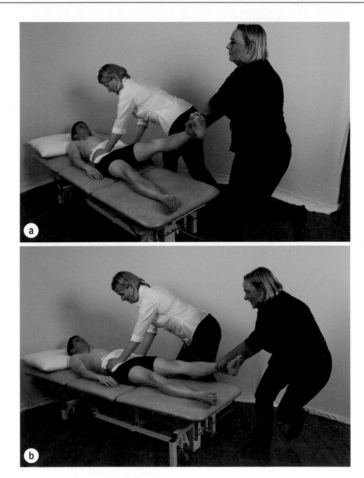

Fig. 10.44 Alternative position for loose-body mobilisation, standing on the floor: (a) starting position and (b) ending the technique.

- Wrap the hands comfortably around the talus and calcaneus to provide anchorage points and pull the ankle into a degree of dorsiflexion to prevent undue movement at the ankle joint. The forearm rests against the lateral border of the patient's foot, helping to direct the movement towards medial rotation.
- Take your distal leg off the couch and lean out to apply traction with your elbows straight (Fig. 10.41).
- Maintain the traction throughout the rest of the technique, which is to rotate the patient's leg smartly back and forth towards medial rotation while simultaneously stepping down off the couch. This automatically takes the hip from flexion, towards extension.
- Reassess.

Mobilisation B: With Lateral Rotation

This technique is exactly the same as that described earlier, but in the opposite direction.
- Face the movement of lateral rotation
- Rotate the patient's leg under strong traction, back and forth towards lateral rotation (Figs 10.42 and 10.43).

If a comparable sign was identified on clinical examination, then this can guide whether to continue with one technique or to change to the other. It may be a diagnosis reached on the history alone, however, and in both cases, a judgment will need to be made on when to stop applying the technique and to adopt a 'watchful wait' approach to see if the symptoms have improved.

Bursitis

Bursitis may be a cause of pain at the hip although this condition is difficult to diagnose definitively and may be overlooked. Because of the close anatomical relationship of bursae to tendons, bursitis may coexist with tendinopathy.

Bursitis may be managed by addressing the causative factors and by injection, which is normally performed under image-guidance and requires onward referral. Notwithstanding, it is helpful to be aware of the signs and symptoms of bursitis at the hip to help with differential diagnosis.

Trochanteric, psoas, gluteal or occasionally ischial bursitis may be a cause of pain at the hip. Trochanteric bursitis is the most common but is generally considered within GTPS, which is discussed below.

In general terms, patients with bursitis commonly present with a gradual onset of pain, often with no obvious cause. Although it is possible to induce a bursitis by direct trauma, it is usually the result of a change in use or repetitive activity, with the pain increased by activity and made better with rest.

Diabetes, degenerative arthropathy, thyroid problems and rheumatoid arthritis can be associated with bursitis.

On examination, a muddled clinical picture emerges of a non-capsular pattern with some resisted tests and some passive tests reproducing the pain, leading to confusion in diagnosis.

Tendinopathy usually produces a predictable clinical picture of pain on the appropriate resisted test and pain on passive stretching in the opposite direction. In contrast, a bursitis may produce pain when passively squeezed under a contracted muscle or tendon and thus the muddled presentation emerges.

'Gilmore's groin' is also a condition to consider within differential diagnosis since it can present with similar signs and symptoms to bursitis.

Psoas Bursitis

Psoas bursitis produces local groin pain but can also cause referred pain in the L3 dermatome. It has a gradual onset of pain, with the patient usually unable to recall the precipitating factors.

It may be associated with a change in use or repetitive movements and is exacerbated by hip flexion movements. For example, bending to put on shoes and socks, rising from sitting with hips flexed, walking upstairs or

hills, brisk walking, jogging or kicking (Broadhurst, 1995a). The pain may produce a shortened gait stride and, through underuse, a secondary capsulitis.

On examination, there is a non-capsular pattern, and a combination of passive hip flexion and adduction squeezes the bursa and can produce pain. The test is not specific to the bursa, however, and may also be positive with a labral tear and sacroiliac joint pathology. Other signs could include pain on passive lateral rotation, passive extension and resisted flexion of the hip.

Pain on resisted flexion can also indicate iliopsoas tendinopathy, which can coexist with psoas bursitis or be present as a separate condition. Treatment with progressive loading is appropriate for the tendinopathy.

As well as considering iliopsoas tendinopathy, differential diagnosis should exclude lumbar spine and sacroiliac joint involvement and other pelvic and hip joint pathology, such as stress and avulsion fractures and labral tears, as well as 'Gilmore's groin'.

Gilmore's groin (inguinal disruption or sportsmen's groin) describes a disruption of the external oblique aponeurosis causing dilatation of the superficial inguinal ring, torn conjoined tendon and dehiscence between the inguinal ligament and the torn conjoined tendon. Males are more commonly affected. It is common in athletes, particularly footballers.

Inguinal disruption presents as pain, of either an insidious or acute onset, felt predominantly in the groin area, near the pubic tubercle (Sheen et al., 2014), and over the lateral edge of the rectus abdominis muscle, with or without radiation to the testis or adductor longus origin. It is increased by sporting activity, on getting out of bed (especially the day after a game), and on sudden movement, such as sprinting or coughing.

On examination, The British Hernia Society (Sheen et al., 2014) recommends that a diagnosis of inguinal disruption can be made if at least three of the following five clinical signs are positive:

- Pinpoint tenderness over the pubic tubercle at the point of insertion of the conjoint tendon
- Palpable tenderness over the deep inguinal ring
- Pain and/or dilation of the external ring with no obvious evidence of hernia
- Pain at the origin of the adductor longus tendon
- Dull, diffuse pain in the groin, often radiating to the perineum and inner thigh or across the midline.

Tenderness at or just above the pubic crest on the affected side may be aggravated by a resisted sit-up. Resisted hip adduction may be painful, and the adductor 'squeeze test' is usually positive in supine and/or 90-degree hip flexed positions (Garvey et al., 2010).

Diagnosis may be confirmed by the practitioner inverting the patient's scrotum and examining the superficial inguinal ring. On the symptomatic side, the ring is dilated and tender and there may be a cough impulse. Imaging, such as ultrasound or MRI, is recommended for all patients with inguinal disruption because it is important to exclude other conditions that may cause chronic groin pain.

A stepped approach, beginning with a tailored physiotherapy regime and rehabilitation back to sport is recommended. A progressive programme to improve core and gluteal stability often forms the basis of rehabilitation. Surgery with post-operative rehabilitation can be considered when conservative management has failed (Sheen et al., 2014).

Ischial Bursitis

Ischial bursitis (weaver's bottom) involves the ischial bursa of gluteus maximus. It produces pain on prolonged sitting, especially on hard surfaces, and the pain is relieved by standing. Pain may be reproduced near the end of range of the straight leg raise (Broadhurst, 1995b).

It is a rare cause of buttock pain but the principles of treatment of bursitis can be applied.

Complicated Bursitis

Septic bursitis at the hip has been described, but this occurs more commonly in the olecranon and prepatellar bursae (Hoppmann, 1993; Zimmermann et al., 1995). A case of tuberculosis of the trochanteric bursa has been described (Rehm-Graves et al., 1983).

Bursitis has been reported as a cause of hip pain associated with rheumatoid arthritis (Raman and Haslock, 1982), and occasionally bursitis may be complicated by calcification, making it resistant to normal conservative management (Gerber and Herrin, 1994).

Pain referred from the lumbar spine and sacroiliac joint may produce a similar pattern of signs and symptoms, and this has been described as pseudotrochanteric bursitis (Traycoff 1991).

CONTRACTILE LESIONS

The mode of onset of contractile lesions around the hip may be sudden through strain, gradual through overuse or traumatic through direct injury, causing muscle contusion. Lesions commonly affect the gluteal tendons, hamstrings, quadriceps and adductor longus muscles. Less common lesions of the psoas and sartorius are not described, although the principles of diagnosis and treatment would apply to any muscle lesion in the region.

Differential diagnosis between contractile lesions and their associated bursae can be difficult. They can often coexist and can present as syndromes with a group of symptoms appearing together.

Greater Trochanteric Pain Syndrome

GTPS is a common regional pain syndrome with patients experiencing buttock, lateral hip or groin pain. It has traditionally been referred to as 'trochanteric bursitis', but tendinopathy can also be a cause of pain, and the two conditions can exist together.

GTPS is often due to gluteus medius and minimus tendinopathy, rather than trochanteric bursitis alone. Histopathological findings have shown tendinopathy and bursal pathology coexisting in GTPS (Fearon et al., 2013). Bursal swelling is an inconsistent feature of lateral hip pain, and typically the bursa is not inflamed and is not the primary cause of symptoms (Silva et al., 2008).

Differential diagnosis of pain around the greater trochanter is extensive, and includes hip degenerative arthropathy, referred pain from lumbar spine, lumbar radiculopathy, ITB syndrome, avascular necrosis, greater trochanteric bursitis, gluteal tendinopathy, stress fracture of the femoral neck, sacroiliac joint pain and polymyalgia rheumatica (Tibor and Sekiya, 2008; Klauser et al., 2013).

Myofascial pain and piriformis syndrome should also be considered. Piriformis syndrome presents with pain in a similar distribution and is associated with tenderness to palpation at the sciatic notch and greater trochanter (Tibor and Sekiya, 2008; Brukner et al., 2017).

The cause of GTPS is occasionally trauma, through direct injury, but it is more commonly due to a change in use through occupational or sporting activities, where degenerative change may also be a factor.

GTPS is common in obese, middle-aged women (Rasmussen and Fano, 1985; Allwright et al., 1988; Gerber and Herrin, 1994), especially those with poor core stability. It may also be secondary to degenerative arthropathy of the hip joint, and it is not uncommon to find the bursa and associated tissues tender after total hip replacement (Dennison and Beverland, 2002).

The angle of insertion of the glutei is greater in females than males, which could lead to increased compression forces and the greater prevalence of the condition in women. Both gluteal tendinopathy and trochanteric bursitis may be associated with a tight ITB, where the tendons and bursa may be irritated by direct friction. It can also be a consequence of altered biomechanics of gait, leg length discrepancy, low back pain or sacroiliac dysfunction (Haller et al., 1989; Collée et al., 1991; Caruso and Toney, 1994, Norris, 2004).

Fearon et al. (2013) set out to differentiate GTPS from hip degenerative arthropathy. They concluded that patients with lateral hip pain were more likely to have GTPS than degenerative arthropathy if they had no difficulty putting on shoes and socks, if they had tenderness on palpation of the greater trochanter and the FABER test reproduced their lateral hip pain (see below).

GTPS is a clinical diagnosis. There is no one specific test to confirm GTPS. However, diagnostic accuracy can be improved when a combination of tests is used (Speers and Bhogal, 2017):

- Single leg stance for 30 seconds. Positive when pain is produced within 30 seconds of standing on the painful side
- Resisted hip medial rotation, lateral rotation and abduction can also be used to assess for GTPS. Resisted lateral rotation has the highest sensitivity (88%) and specificity (97.3%) when compared to resisted medial rotation and abduction (Grimaldi and Fearon, 2015)
- The FABER (flexion, abduction and external rotation), FADER (flexion, adduction and external rotation) and Ober tests aim to increase the tensile load on the gluteal tendon
- Direct palpation of greater trochanter, which has a positive predictive value of 83% (Speers and Bhogal, 2017)
- The Trendelenburg sign is present in patients with GTPS and when used to assess for a gluteus medius tear. It has a sensitivity of 73% and a specificity of 77% (Lin and Fredericson, 2015).

Gluteal Tendinopathy

Gluteal tendinopathy mostly affects the anterior portion of the gluteus medius tendon, but it can also involve gluteus minimus and occasionally gluteus maximus. The anterior and posterior tendons of gluteus medius and the tendon of gluteus minimus can be involved alone or together (Connell et al., 2003). The cause is uncertain, but as with trochanteric bursitis, tension in the ITB may result in frictional trauma.

A stepped approach to the management of GTPS is currently recommended. Less invasive treatments are generally offered first, including education/watchful wait, activity and work modification, weight management, suitable footwear, simple analgesics and NSAIDs medication, physiotherapy (e.g. exercise, mobilisation, extracorporeal shortwave therapy) and then injection therapy (e.g. corticosteroid, local anaesthetic, hyaluronic acid, platelet-rich plasma [PRP]). If symptoms persist, more invasive treatments can be considered, such as ITB release, ITB bursectomy and lateral synovial recess resection.

In the musculoskeletal medicine approach, transverse frictions can be applied to the area of tenderness, particularly in the degenerative phase.

TRANSVERSE FRICTIONS TO GLUTEAL TENDONS

- Lower the couch to approximately the level of your knees.
- Position the patient comfortably in side-lying, painful side uppermost, with the hips and knees flexed to approximately 80 degrees.
- Palpate for the area of tenderness over the superolateral aspect of the greater trochanter.
- Stand in front of the patient, level with the patient's waist, facing diagonally across the couch (Fig. 10.45).
- Apply the frictions transversely across the fibres using the fingers of one hand reinforced with the other hand to maintain pressure down against the tendons, while rocking forwards and backwards with straight arms.
- Maintain the technique for an appropriate time, according to the irritability of the lesion and stage of healing, to achieve analgesia and to mobilise the tissues.

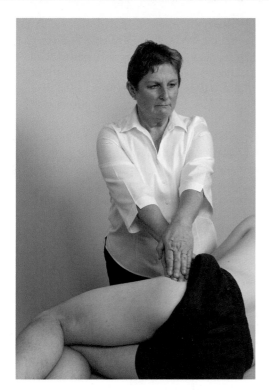

Fig. 10.45 Transverse frictions to gluteal tendons.

Relative rest is advised where functional movements and a progressive optimal loading exercise programme may continue, but no overuse or stretching until pain-free on resisted testing.

Biomechanical or postural problems with muscle tightness will need to be addressed, and stability exercises are an important part of rehabilitation (Brukner et al., 2017).

An alternative position may be used if the symptoms are bilateral and the patient is uncomfortable in side-lying.

- Place the patient in prone-lying and stand on the side to be treated, just below the patient's hip and facing towards the patient's head.
- Place the fingers of one hand reinforced with the other onto the painful area, pointing downwards, and apply the frictions across the tendons by moving downwards and upwards with straight arms.
- Maintain the technique for an appropriate time, according to the irritability of the lesion and stage of healing, to achieve analgesia and to mobilise the tissues.

Iliotibial band syndrome has been described as a separate condition, but tightness of the ITB may also be considered as one of the contributing factors to GTPS.

ITB syndrome presents with a similar pattern of lateral hip and/or knee pain, but is painful on provocative testing using Ober's test as follows:

- Place the patient in side-lying (painful side uppermost), the hip neutral and the upper knee flexed.
- Extend the hip and adduct the femur.
- ITB tightness and/or lateral hip pain will be demonstrated as the knee will extend when the femur is adducted (Adkins and Figler, 2000; Brukner et al., 2017; Hattam and Smeatham, 2020).

As mentioned previously, 'trochanteric bursitis' was the most common clinical diagnosis for pain in the region of the greater trochanter before other structures were recognised as a possible cause of pain.

Long et al. (2013) performed a retrospective review of 877 musculoskeletal sonographic examinations over a 6-year period for GTPS to assess the prevalence of trochanteric bursitis, gluteal tendon and ITB or a combination of findings. Only 20.2% of patients had observable trochanteric bursitis, with 49.9% having gluteal tendinosis, 0.5% gluteal tendon tears and 28.5% a thickened ITB.

From these findings, now that scanning techniques have become more readily available, 'trochanteric bursitis' may be diagnosed less often.

Imaging may be considered if other pathologies are suspected to be the cause of patients' symptoms. The choice of investigation should be guided by suspected cause and as an extension to the clinical examination process.

Once a diagnosis of GTPS is established, an option for treatment is an injection of low-dose, large-volume local anaesthetic with an appropriate amount of corticosteroid.

INJECTION FOR GREATER TROCHANTERIC PAIN SYNDROME

Suggested needle size: 21 G × 1½ in. (0.8 × 40 mm) or 21 G × 2 in. (0.8 × 50 mm) green needle
Dose: 20 mg triamcinolone acetonide in a total volume of 3–5 mL

- Position the patient comfortably in side-lying, painful side uppermost.

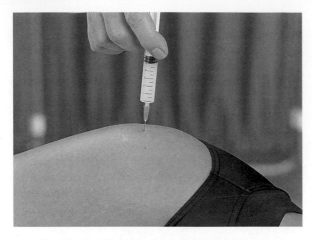

Fig. 10.46 Injection of the trochanteric bursa.

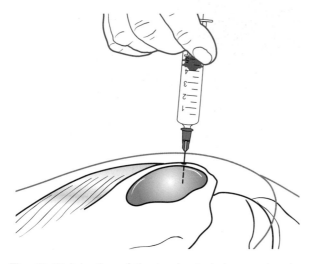

Fig. 10.47 Injection of the trochanteric bursa, showing direction of approach and needle position.

- Palpate for the area of tenderness over the superolateral aspect of the greater trochanter where gluteus maximus inserts into the ITB (Fig. 10.46).
- Deliver the injection by a bolus technique if no resistance is felt; or
- If this is not possible due to synovial folds and adhesions within the bursa, redirect the needle and use a series of smaller injections to infiltrate the area of tenderness (Fig. 10.47).

The patient should minimise or modify activities for 2 weeks following injection.

Hamstrings

The hamstrings act to extend the hip and flex the knee, and hamstring injury is common, perhaps due to the muscles' relative weakness in comparison to the quadriceps (Sutton, 1984). As two-joint muscles, they are susceptible to injury because there is a greater potential for overuse.

Injury can occur at the tendinous origin at the ischial tuberosity, within the muscle belly, or at the musculotendinous junction. Predominant risk factors include age and previous injury (Hunter and Speed, 2007).

The onset is usually sudden (e.g. on a sudden stretch or a rapid contraction against resistance, such as the ballistic action of sprinting), which produces acute pain, further increased by activity, and swelling and bruising. The vulnerable phase in the running cycle appears to be at the end of the swing phase, where peak muscle lengths occur, and the beginning of the stance phase. Biceps femoris is more susceptible, as its peak length exceeds that of the medial hamstrings (Hunter and Speed, 2007).

Symptoms may include stiffness, muscle cramps and spasms in the posterior aspect of the distal thigh or weak knee flexion. Patients with a complete distal hamstring tear may also report a sensation of instability at the knee, and diagnostic imaging may be required as an adjunct to clinical examination to aid decision-making in the management of more severe lesions (Lempainen et al., 2007).

On examination, the patient has pain on resisted knee flexion and pain on passive straight leg raising. In most clinical situations, testing for hamstring strain is conducted statically in a non-weight-bearing position. In reality, the hamstrings function, and are most often injured, in dynamic weight-bearing situations. This is an important point to remember for full rehabilitation of any muscle lesion in the region.

Many pathologies may cause buttock and thigh pain. To add further complexity to both diagnosis and management, isolated hamstring pathology may coexist with other pathologies that may also cause buttock and thigh pain. Therefore, other conditions should be considered in differential diagnosis, particularly when the patient's presentation does not follow the typical behavior of hamstrings tendinopathy.

For example, more diffuse symptoms may indicate lumbar, hip, or sacroiliac joint somatic referral and lumbar radiculopathy. Sciatic nerve irritation at the piriformis muscle or near the ischial tuberosity can be a possible pathology because of its proximity to the hamstring origin.

Other pathologies include ischiofemoral impingement; unfused ischial growth plate in a postadolescent athlete; apophysitis or avulsion among adolescents; deep gluteal muscle tear; posterior pubic or ischial ramus stress fracture; and partial or complete rupture of the proximal hamstring tendon (Goom et al., 2016). Differential diagnosis can be assisted by screening with imaging, palpation and provocative tests.

Treatment options depend on the severity of the injury and extent of retraction. Partial tears with avulsion and full tears involving all three tendons, and retraction greater than 2 cm, improve with surgical repair and are less likely to respond to conservative treatment.

Partial tears involving one or two tendons, albeit with retraction greater than 2 cm, should generally be treated non-operatively with activity modification, physiotherapy, stretching, non-steroidal anti-inflammatory medication, extracorporeal shockwave therapy, or local injection with either corticosteroid or PRP (Bowman et al., 2013).

Tendinopathy at the origin from the ischial tuberosity may come on gradually if associated with prolonged over- or underuse, or more quickly if associated with sudden trauma or unaccustomed activity. It can be treated by transverse frictions or injection. Palpation reveals the site of the lesion.

TRANSVERSE FRICTIONS TO THE ORIGIN OF THE HAMSTRINGS

- Position the patient into side-lying on the unaffected side with the hips and knees flexed to 90 degrees to expose the ischial tuberosity from under the lower border of gluteus maximus (Fig. 10.48).
- Stand behind the patient's waist, facing across the couch.
- Frictions can then be applied transversely across the fibres using the fingers of one hand reinforced with the other hand to maintain pressure back against the origin, and rocking body weight downwards and upwards through straight arms.
- Maintain the technique for an appropriate time, according to the irritability of the lesion and stage of healing, to achieve analgesia and to mobilise the tissues.

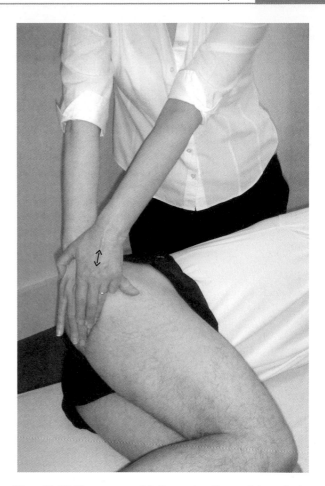

Fig. 10.48 Transverse frictions to the origin of the hamstrings.

Relative rest is advised where functional movements may continue with progressive loading, but no overuse or stretching until resisted testing is pain-free.

INJECTION OF THE ORIGIN OF THE HAMSTRINGS
Suggested needle size: 23 G × 1¼ in. (0.6 × 25 mm) blue needle (or as appropriate for the patient)
Dose: 20 mg triamcinolone acetonide in a total volume of 1.5 mL

Injection of the origin of the hamstrings is usually conducted under image guidance as the tendon is weight-bearing. It is important to check local policy.

- Place the patient in the position described for transverse frictions of the hamstrings' origin.
- Locate the area of tenderness over the ischial tuberosity
- Insert the needle perpendicular the tender area (Fig. 10.49).
- Deliver the injection by a peppering technique into the teno-osseous junction (Fig. 10.50).

The patient should minimise or modify activities for 2 weeks following injection.

Hamstring injuries may also occur in the muscle bellies, commonly deep in the mid-thigh region. Palpation reveals the site of the lesion, and the treatment for acute and chronic muscle belly lesions will now be described.

The principles of treatment for acute soft tissue lesions (see Chapter 4) should be applied as soon as possible after the onset and for 2 to 3 days following injury to promote conditions favourable for healing.

Treatment is ideally conducted on a daily basis and transverse frictions are initially applied gently, followed by Grade A mobilisation to maintain the muscle belly function.

TRANSVERSE FRICTIONS FOR ACUTE MUSCLE BELLY

- Position the patient in prone-lying with the knee flexed to place the muscle belly in the shortened position; this allows the muscle fibres to be moved transversely by the frictions (Fig. 10.51).
- Maintain the technique for an appropriate time, according to the irritability of the lesion and stage of healing, to achieve analgesia and to mobilise the tissues.

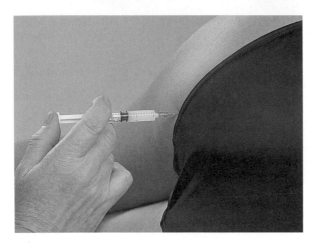

Fig. 10.49 Injection of the origin of the hamstrings.

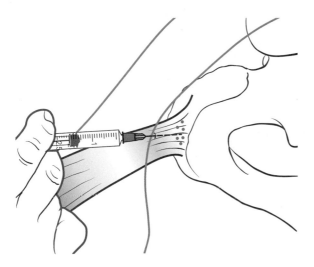

Fig. 10.50 Injection of the origin of the hamstrings, showing direction of approach and needle position.

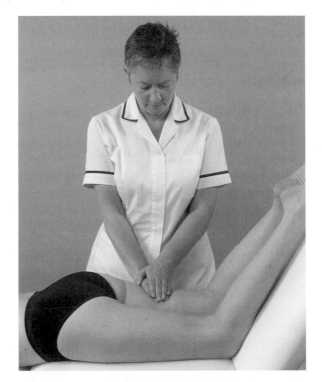

Fig. 10.51 Transverse frictions to the hamstring muscle bellies.

- Follow this immediately with Grade A mobilisation, encouraging an active muscle contraction within the pain-free range to broaden the fibres.
- Teach the patient to use a normal heel–toe gait, with the aid of crutches if necessary.

After approximately 5 days (depending upon irritability), the depth of transverse frictions and Grade A mobilisations can be increased progressively until a full range of pain-free movement is achieved. Treating an acute muscle belly lesion in this way should avoid shortening of the muscle fibres and the need to apply stretching techniques.

Home exercises can be given to support this approach, taking care to avoid overstressing the healing fibres by avoiding pain.

TRANSVERSE FRICTIONS FOR CHRONIC MUSCLE BELLY

- Place the patient in prone lying with the knee flexed, as described earlier.
- Apply the transverse frictions with the knee flexed to place the muscle belly in a relaxed position and apply transverse frictions, either using one hand reinforced with the other, or the flat (not the point) of the elbow guided by the other hand on the forearm (Figs 10.51 and 10.52).
- Maintain the technique for an appropriate time, according to the irritability of the lesion and stage of healing, to achieve analgesia and to mobilise the tissues.
- Follow this with vigorous Grade A exercises to maintain the gained mobility.

It is important that the hamstrings are not undertreated and, to prevent recurrence of symptoms, transverse frictions should be continued for approximately 1 week after cessation of symptoms. If the muscle is tight, traditional stretches can be applied once the resisted tests are pain-free but the stretches themselves should never go further than nudging into pain.

Rehabilitation Following Hamstring Lesions

In either the acute or the chronic situation, once the pain has been eased by transverse frictions and Grade A mobilisations, a full rehabilitation programme can be implemented, with a focus on strengthening and including stretching to lengthen the muscle, if appropriate.

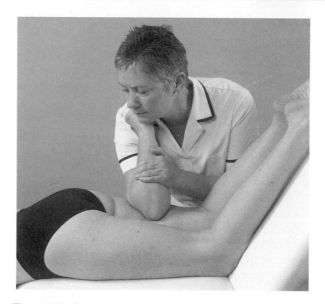

Fig. 10.52 Transverse frictions to the hamstring muscle bellies, alternative technique (chronic).

Mason et al. (2008) support the use of graded stretching exercises within the pain-free range and also advise that consideration should be given to the lumbar spine, sacroiliac and pelvic alignment and postural control mechanisms in the rehabilitation of hamstring injuries.

Attention should be paid to the dynamic rather than the static function of the hamstrings and weight-bearing sport-specific activities and rehabilitation under speed are important considerations (Coole and Gieck, 1987).

Strengthening is essential for rehabilitation and prevention of hamstring injuries. Training programmes should include eccentric muscle contractions and extensive lengthening (Brukner et al., 2017).

Hunter and Speed (2007) summarise that the aim of rehabilitation is to cause adaptation in the muscle tendon unit of the hamstrings and the adjacent supporting tissues to allow the entire system to absorb sufficient energy and to facilitate a full return to functional activity.

Quadriceps

The mechanism of injury of the quadriceps is similar to that of the hamstrings and the principles of treatment and rehabilitation can be applied in much the same way.

The patient presents with anterior thigh pain, pain on resisted knee extension and pain on resisted hip flexion (if rectus femoris is involved). As a two-joint muscle, rectus femoris is the most susceptible to injury. Rupture, particularly relating to the traumatic onset, and the development of myositis ossificans should be considered within the assessment. Both should be referred for specialist opinion.

Palpation reveals the site of the lesion, which may be within the tendon of rectus femoris from the anterior inferior iliac spine, or in the belly of the muscle, usually mid-thigh (see Chapter 11).

TRANSVERSE FRICTIONS TO THE ORIGIN OF RECTUS FEMORIS

(Cyriax, 1984; Cyriax and Cyriax, 1993)

- Position the patient in half-lying to allow the hip flexors to relax.
- Locate the origin of rectus femoris and apply two fingers to the tendon (Fig. 10.53).
- Push down onto the tendon and apply transverse frictions across the fibres.
- Maintain the technique for an appropriate time, according to the irritability of the lesion and stage of healing, to achieve analgesia and to mobilise the tissues.

Relative rest is advised where functional movements may continue with progressive loading, but no overuse or stretching until the muscle is pain-free on resisted testing.

Management of quadriceps muscle belly injuries is discussed in Chapter 11.

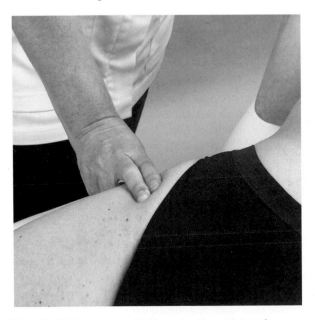

Fig. 10.53 Transverse frictions to the origin of rectus femoris.

Adductor Longus

Adductor longus is the most common adductor to be strained at the hip. It is sometimes known as a 'rider's strain' due to overuse of adductor longus in working a horse while riding.

The patient has groin or medial thigh pain, often presenting as a dull ache, with pain on resisted adduction and passive abduction (Tibor and Sekiya, 2008).

The lesion is at one of two sites: either the origin from the pubis (teno-osseous site) or the musculotendinous junction.

Treatment of the teno-osseous site is by either transverse frictions or anatomically- or image-guided injection. The musculotendinous junction usually responds well to transverse frictions and injection is not usually necessary. It is important to check local policy before injecting.

TRANSVERSE FRICTIONS TO ADDUCTOR LONGUS

Teno-osseous Site

- Position the patient in supine with the leg in a degree of abduction and lateral rotation, supported on a pillow.
- With an index finger reinforced by the middle finger, locate the area of tenderness at the teno-osseous junction (Fig. 10.54).
- Apply the frictions first in a direction down onto the bone, then transversely across the fibres, until analgesia has been achieved.
- Maintain the technique for an appropriate time, according to the irritability of the lesion and stage of healing, to achieve analgesia and to mobilise the tissues.

Musculotendinous

- Position the patient as described and locate the area of tenderness at the musculotendinous junction.
- With consideration of the shape of the tendon and patient comfort, the transverse frictions may be imparted by a pinching technique (Fig. 10.55) (Cyriax, 1984; Cyriax and Cyriax, 1993), or by pressure directed first down against the tendon and then transversely across the fibres (Fig. 10.56).
- Maintain the technique for an appropriate time, according to the irritability of the lesion and stage of healing, to achieve analgesia and to mobilise the tissues.

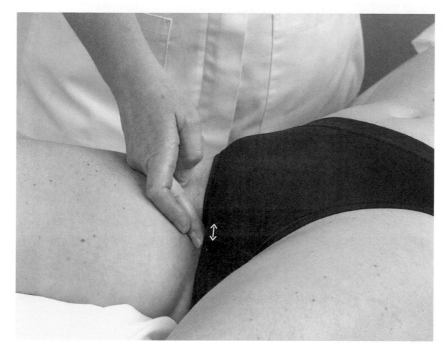

Fig. 10.54 Transverse frictions to the origin of adductor longus.

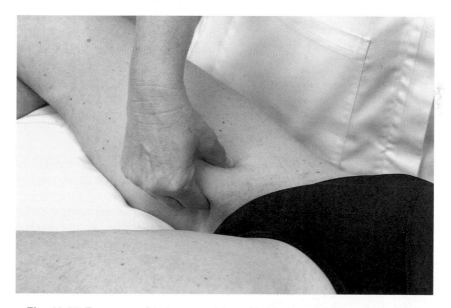

Fig. 10.55 Transverse frictions to adductor longus, musculotendinous site.

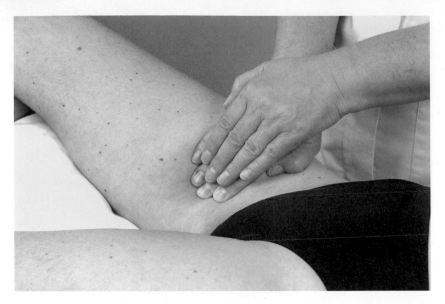

Fig. 10.56 Transverse frictions to adductor longus, musculotendinous site, alternative hand position.

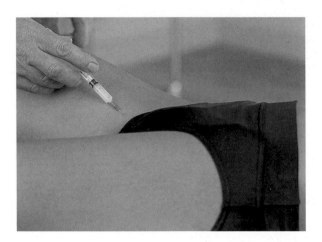

Fig. 10.57 Injection of the origin of adductor longus.

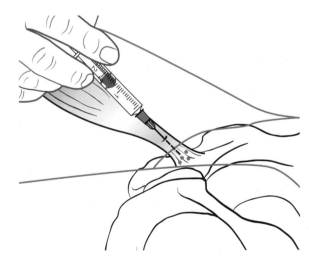

Fig. 10.58 Injection of the origin of adductor longus, showing direction of approach and needle position.

Relative rest is advised where functional movements and progressive loading should continue, but no overuse or stretching until resisted testing is pain-free.

INJECTION OF THE ORIGIN OF ADDUCTOR LONGUS (CYRIAX AND CYRIAX, 1993)

Suggested needle size: 23 G × 1¼ in. (0.6 × 30 mm) blue needle

Dose: 20 mg triamcinolone acetonide in a total volume of 1.5 mL

- Position the patient as for the transverse frictions.
- Insert the needle into the origin of adductor longus, which is situated in the angle between the symphysis and the obturator crest (Fig. 10.57).
- Once in the teno-osseous junction and in contact with bone, deliver the injection by the peppering technique (Fig. 10.58).

The patient should minimise or modify activities for 2 weeks following injection.

REVIEW QUESTIONS

1. Discuss the differential diagnosis of groin pain.
2. What are the key principles of a Grade B mobilisation at the hip?
3. How could you treat gluteal tendinopathy?
4. What would be the positive findings and potential sites for a lesion in the adductor longus tendon?
5. Describe the origins and insertions of the hamstring muscles.

CASE SCENARIOS

Case 1
History
- A retired footballer named Jamie, aged 38, has noticed increasing stiffness in his left hip since he finished being a full-time player (2 years ago). Pain is in his groin and occasionally in his buttock. The stiffness is worse first thing on the morning and eases with walking. He is training for a marathon by road running, which he commenced 6 weeks ago. This aggravates his symptoms. Anti-inflammatories help. Past medical history of a sports hernia operation on the right side 8 years ago.

Examination
- Lumbar movements clear. Pain end-range hip flexion, a loss of 20 degrees medial rotation, with a hard/elastic end-feel. Resisted tests all pain-free and full power.

Task
- Are any further investigations required at this stage? Discuss patient management. What are the principles of treatment and advice regarding his training for a marathon?

Case 2
History
- Ellie is a 26-year-old national hockey player and part-time receptionist. She trains 6 days a week and plays in goal. She has a 2-week history of pain in her right hamstring following an over reach for a ball during training. She felt something 'go' and has been unable to run since because she has had fairly constant pain. Ice and compression were applied immediately and have been continued. She is concerned about her recovery as she has an important tournament coming up in 4 weeks.

Examination
- There is some bruising tracking down the hamstring to the knee. She has pain on full lumbar flexion and straight leg raising limited by 20 degrees by muscle pain. She has pain on resisted knee flexion with full power. There is tenderness on deep palpation muscle bulk of biceps femoris.

Task
- What would the treatment protocol be? Consider how you may advise her to progress the Grade A mobilisations throughout her rehabilitation. What is the likelihood she will be ready for the tournament?

Case 3
History
- Georgina is a 62-year-old retired housewife who regularly hill-walks with her family. She has a 4-month history of pain in her right buttock and lateral hip region that came on following an overnight walking challenge. She cannot remember slipping or any injury, but the pain has gradually got worse. It is painful to lie on that side in bed, and she has stopped her walking. Medical history includes osteopenia and a deep vein thrombosis 10 years ago.

Examination
- Slim woman with no obvious bony deformities. Lumbar movements clear. Pain on passive hip lateral rotation and adduction with normal end-feel. Pain on resisted abduction and extension with normal power. Tender on palpation over the upper outer section of the right greater trochanter.

Task
- What is your primary diagnosis? Which structures can be involved? Discuss the treatment options for this case and the rehabilitation exercises you could prescribe.

REFERENCES

Adkins, S.B., Figler, R.A., 2000. Hip pain in athletes. Am. Fam. Phys. 61 (7), 2109–2118.
Allwright, S.J., Cooper, R.A., Nash, P., 1988. Trochanteric bursitis: bone scan appearance. Clin. Nucl. Med. 13, 561–564.
Arthritis Foundation, 2021. Mediterranean diet for osteoarthritis. Arthritis Foundation. https://www.arthritis.org/health-wellness/healthy-living/nutrition/

healthy-eating/mediterranean-diet-for-osteoarthritis. Accessed 5 September 2021.

Arthritis Research UK, Public Health England, 2012. Prevalence of osteoarthritis in England and local authorities: Birmingham. https://www.versusarthritis.org/media/13374/birmingham-oa-1.pdf. Accessed 5 September 2021.

Bencardino, J.T., Kassarjian, A., Vieira, R.L., et al., 2011. Synovial plicae of the hip: evaluation using MR arthrography in patients with hip pain. Skelet. Radiol. 40 (4), 415–421.

Bharam, S., 2006. Labral tears, extra-articular injuries and hip arthroscopy in the athlete. Clin. Sports Med. 25, 279–292.

Bianchi, S., Martinoli, C., 1999. Detection of loose bodies in joints. Radiol. Clin. N. Am. 37 (4), 679–690.

Bowman, K.F., Cohen, S.B., Bradley, J.P., 2013. Operative management of partial-thickness tears of the proximal hamstring muscles in athletes. Am. J. Sports Med. 41, 1363–1371.

Broadhurst, N., 1995a. Iliopsoas tendinopathy and bursitis. Aust. Fam. Phys. 24, 1303.

Broadhurst, N., 1995b. Ischial bursitis. Aust. Fam. Phys. 24, 1121.

Brukner, P., Clarson, B., Cook, J., et al., 2017. Clinical Sports Medicine, Volume 1: Injuries, fifth ed. McGraw-Hill, Sydney.

Cailliet, R., 1990. Soft Tissue Pain and Disability, second ed. F.A. Davis, Philadelphia.

Cameron, G., 1995. Steroid arthropathy – myth or reality? J. Orthop. Med. 17, 51–55.

Canoso, J.J., 1981. Bursae, tendons and ligaments. Clin. Rheum. Dis. 7, 189–221.

Caruso, F.A., Toney, M.A.O., 1994. Trochanteric bursitis – a case report of plain film, scintigraphic and MRI correlation. Clin. Nucl. Med. 19, 393–395.

Collée, G., Dijkmans, B.A.C., Vandenbroucke, J.P., et al., 1991. Greater trochanteric pain syndrome trochanteric bursitis in low back pain. Scand. J. Rheumatol. 20, 262–266.

Connell, D.A., Bass, C., Sykes, C.A., et al., 2003. Sonographic evaluation of gluteus medius and minimus tendinopathy. Eur. Radiol. 13 (6), 1339–1347.

Coole, W., Gieck, J.H., 1987. An analysis of hamstring strains and their rehabilitation. J. Orthop. Sports Phys. Ther. 9, 77–85.

Cyriax, J., 1982. Textbook of Orthopaedic Medicine, eighth ed. Baillière Tindall, London.

Cyriax, J., 1984. Textbook of Orthopaedic Medicine, eleventh ed. Baillière Tindall, London.

Cyriax, J., Cyriax, P., 1993. Cyriax's Illustrated Manual of Orthopaedic Medicine. Butterworth Heinemann, Oxford.

Dennison, J., Beverland, D.E., 2002. An audit of trochanteric bursitis in total hip arthroplasty and recommendations for treatment. J. Orthop. Nurs. 6 (1), 5–8.

Dieppe, P., 1995. Management of hip osteoarthritis. Br. Med. J. 311 (7009), 853–857.

Emms, N.W., O'Connor, M., Montgomery, S.C., 2002. Hip pain can masquerade as knee pain in adults. Age Ageing 31, 67–69.

Fearon, A.M., Scarvell, J.M., Neeman, T., et al., 2013. Greater trochanteric pain syndrome: defining the clinical syndrome. Br. J. Sports Med. 47, 649–653.

Feather, A., Randall, D., Waterhouse, M., 2020. Kumar and Clark's Clinical Medicine, tenth ed. Elsevier, London.

Flanagan, F.L., Sant, S., Coughlan, R.J., et al., 1995. Symptomatic enlarged iliopsoas bursae in the presence of a normal plain hip radiograph. Br. J. Rheumatol. 34, 365–369.

Fu, Z., Peng, M., Peng, Q., 1997. Anatomical study of the synovial plicae of the hip joint. Clin. Anat. 10 (4), 235–238.

Garvey, J.F.W., Read, J.W., Turner, A., 2010. Sportsman hernia: what can we do? Hernia 14, 17–25.

Gerber, J.M., Herrin, S.O., 1994. Conservative management of calcific trochanteric bursitis. J. Manip. Physiol. Ther. 17, 250–252.

Goom, T.S., Malliaras, P., Reiman, M.P., et al., 2016. Proximal hamstring tendinopathy: clinical aspects of assessment and management. J. Orthop. Sports Phys. Ther. 46 (6), 483–493.

Gough-Palmer, A., McHugh, K., 2007. Investigating hip pain. a well child. Br. Med. J. 334, 1216–1217.

Grimaldi, A, Fearon, A., 2015. Gluteal tendinopathy: Integrating pathomechanics and clinical features in its management. J. Orthop. Sports Phys. Ther. 45(11), 910–922.

Haller, C.C., Coleman, P.A., Estes, N.C., et al., 1989. Traumatic trochanteric bursitis. Kans. Med. 90, 17–22.

Hartley, A., 1995. Practical Joint Assessment – Lower Quadrant, second ed. Mosby, London.

Hattam, P., Smeatham, A., 2020. Handbook of Special Tests in Musculoskeletal Examination, second ed. Elsevier, Oxford.

Hickman, J.M., Peters, C.L., 2001. Hip pain in the young adult. Am. J. Orthop. 30 (6), 459–467.

Hoppmann, R.A., 1993. Diagnosis and management of common tendinopathy and bursitis syndromes. J. S. C. Med. Assoc. 89, 531–535.

Horne, G., Devane, P., Davidson, A., et al., 2008. The influence of steroid injections on the incidence of infection following total knee arthroplasty. N. Z. Med. J. 121 (1268), 1–11.

Hunter, D.G., Speed, C.A., 2007. The assessment and management of chronic hamstring/posterior thigh pain. Best. Pract. Res. Clin. Rheumatol. 21 (2), 261–277.

Jenkins, J.T., O'Dwyer, P.J., 2008. Inguinal hernias. Br. Med. J. 336, 269–272.

Johnell, O., Kanis, J., 2005. Epidemiology of osteoporotic fractures. Osteoporos. Int. 16 (Suppl. 2), S3–S7.

Kapandji, I.A., 2019. The Physiology of the Joints: Lower Limb, seventh ed. Handspring Publishing.

Kaspar, S., de Van de Beer, J., 2005. Infection in hip arthroplasty after previous injection of steroid. J. Bone Jt. Surg. 87-B, 454–457.

Kersnic, B., Iglic, A., Kralj-Iglic, V., et al., 1997. Increased incidence of arthrosis in women could be related to femoral and pelvic shape. Arch. Orthop. Trauma. Surg. 116 (6–7), 345–347.

Klässbo, M., Harms-Ringdahl, K., Larrson, G., 2003. Examination of passive ROM and capsular patterns in the hip. Physiother. Res. Int. 8 (1), 1–12.

Klauser, A.S., Martinoli, C., Tagliafico, A., et al., 2013. Greater trochanteric pain syndrome. Semin. Musculoskelet. Radiol. 17 (1), 43–48.

Lempainen, L., Sarimo, J., Mattila, K., et al., 2007. Distal tears of the hamstring muscles: review of the literature and our results of surgical treatment. Br. J. Sports Med. 41 (2), 80–83.

Lin, C.Y., Fredericson, M., 2015. Greater trochanteric pain syndrome: An update on diagnosis and management. Curr. Phys. Med. Rehabil. Rep. 3 (1), 60–66.

Long, S.S., Surrey, D.E., Nazarian, L.N., 2013. Sonography of greater trochanteric pain syndrome and the rarity of primary bursitis. Am. J. Roentgen. 201, 1083–1086.

Luthra, J.S., Salim, A.H., Suwailim, A.G., et al., 2019. Understanding painful hip in young adults: a review article. Hip Pelvis 31 (3), 129–135.

Martin, R.L., Irrgang, J.J., Sekiya, J.K., 2008. The diagnostic accuracy of clinical examination in determining intra-articular hip pain for potential hip arthroscopy candidates. J. Arthrosc. Relat. Surg. 24 (9), 1013–1018.

Mason, D.L., Dickens, V., Vail, A., 2008. Rehabilitation for hamstring injuries. Cochrane Database Syst. Rev. 1, CP004575.

Meaney, J.F., Cassar-Pullicino, V.N., Ethrington, R., et al., 1992. Ilio-psoas bursa enlargement. Clin. Radiol. 45, 161–168.

National Institute for Health and Care Excellence (NICE), 2018. Osteoarthritis: What else might it be? NICE. https://cks.nice.org.uk/topics/osteoarthritis/diagnosis/differential-diagnosis/. Accessed 5 September 2021.

National Institute for Health and Care Excellence (NICE), 2020. Osteoarthritis: care and management. NICE. https://www.nice.org.uk/guidance/cg177. Accessed 5 September 2021.

National Institute for Health and Care Excellence (NICE), 2021. Osteoporosis – prevention of fragility fractures. NICE https://cks.nice.org.uk/topics/osteoporosis-prevention-of-fragility-fractures/. Accessed 5 September 2021.

Neumann, G., Mendicuti, A.D., Zou, K.H., et al., 2007. Prevalence of labral tears and cartilage loss in patients with mechanical symptoms of the hip: evaluation using MR arthrography. Osteoarthr. Cartil. 15, 909–1017.

Norris, C.M., 2004. Sports Injuries: Diagnosis and Management for Physiotherapists, Third ed. Butterworth Heinemann, Oxford.

O'Kane, J.W., 1999. Anterior hip pain. Am. Fam. Phys. 60 (6), 1687–1696.

Paice, E., 1995. Pain in the hip and knee. Br. Med. J. 310, 319–322.

Pearce, J.M.S., 2006. Meralgia paraesthetica (Bernhardt-Roth syndrome). J. Neurol. Neurosurg. Psychiatry 77 (1), 84.

Quintana, J.M., Arostegui, I., Escobar, A., et al., 2008. Prevalence of knee and hip osteoarthritis and the appropriateness of joint replacement in an older population. Arch. Intern. Med. 168 (14), 1576–1584.

Raman, D., Haslock, I., 1982. Trochanteric bursitis – a frequent cause of 'hip' pain in rheumatoid arthritis. Ann. Rheum. Dis. 41, 602–613.

Rasmussen, K.-J.E., Fano, N., 1985. Trochanteric bursitis: treatment by corticosteroid injection. Scand. J. Rheumatol. 14, 417–420.

Rehm-Graves, S., Weinstein, A.J., Calabrese, L.H., et al., 1983. Tuberculosis of the greater trochanter bursa. Arthritis Rheum. 26, 77–81.

Robinson, P., Keenan, A.-M., Conaghan, P.G., 2007. Clinical effectiveness and dose of image-guided intra-articular corticosteroid injection for hip osteoarthritis. Rheumatology 46 (2), 285291.

Saotome, K., Tamai, K., Osada, D., et al., 2006. Histologic classification of loose bodies in osteoarthrosis. J. Orthop. Sci. 11 (6), 607–613.

Saunders, S., 2000. Orthopaedic Medicine Course Manual. Saunders, London.

Sheen, A.J., Stephenson, B.M., Lloyd, D.M., et al., 2014. 'Treatment of the Sportsman's groin': British Hernia Society's 2014 position statement based on the Manchester Consensus Conference. Br. J. Sports Med. 48 (14), 1079–1087.

Silva, F., Adams, T., Feinstein, J., et al., 2008. Trochanteric bursitis: refuting the myth of inflammation. J. Clin. Rheumatol. 14 (2), 82–86.

Sims, K., 1999. The development of hip osteoarthritis: implications for conservative management. Man. Ther. 4 (3), 127–135.

Speers, C.J., Bhogal, G.S., 2017. Greater trochanteric pain syndrome: a review of diagnosis and management in general practice. Br. J. Gen. Pract. 67 (663), 479–480.

Standring, S., 2015. Gray's Anatomy: The Anatomical Basis of Clinical Practice, forty-first ed. Churchill Livingstone, Edinburgh.

Sutton, G., 1984. Hamstrung by hamstring strains: a review of the literature. J. Orthop. Sports Phys. Ther. 5, 184–195.

Tibor, L.M., Sekiya, J.K., 2008. Differential diagnosis of pain around the hip joint. Arthroscopy 24 (12), 1407–1421.

Toohey, A.K., LaSalle, T.L., Martinez, S., et al., 1990. Iliopsoas bursitis: clinical features, radiographic findings, and disease associations. Semin. Arthritis Rheum. 20, 41–47.

Traycoff, R.B., 1991. 'Pseudotrochanteric bursitis': the differential diagnosis of lateral hip pain. J. Rheumatol. 18, 1810–1812.

Underwood, P.L., McLeod, R.A., Ginsburg, W.W., 1988. The varied clinical manifestations of iliopsoas bursitis. J. Rheumatol. 15, 1683–1685.

Wang, Q., Jiang, X., Tian, W., 2014. Does previous intra-articular steroid injection increase the risk of joint infection following total hip arthroplasty or total knee arthroplasty? A meta-analysis. Med. Sci. Monit. 20, 1878–1883.

Zimmermann, B., Mikolich, D.J., Ho, G., 1995. Septic Bursitis. Semin. Arthritis Rheum. 24, 391–410.

The Knee

CHAPTER CONTENTS

SUMMARY

This chapter presents the anatomy of the knee relating to commonly encountered lesions. The commentary that follows explores the relevant points of history, aiding diagnosis, and the suggested method of examination adheres to the principles of selective tension. The lesions, their treatment and management are then discussed.

Degenerative arthropathy of the knee is a common condition in musculoskeletal practice along with knee injuries, which are largely in the province of sport. Initial diagnosis is crucial to appropriate management, particularly of the ligamentous and contractile lesions. Scanning techniques have done much to facilitate diagnosis and aid appropriate onward management. Pain referred from the lumbar spine, sacroiliac joint or hip can be wrongly ascribed to the knee.

ANATOMY

The knee joint is the largest joint in the body. It is a synovial bicondylar hinge joint between the femur and tibia with the patella placed anteriorly.

Inert Structures

The lower end of the *femur* consists of two large femoral condyles that articulate with, and transfer weight to, corresponding surfaces on the tibial condyles at the tibiofemoral joint. The two femoral condyles are separated posteriorly and inferiorly by the intercondylar notch or fossa. The anterior aspect of the femur bears an articular surface for the patella to form the patellofemoral joint.

The lateral femoral epicondyle gives attachment to the proximal end of the *lateral (fibular) collateral ligament*. Below this lies a smooth groove that contains the tendon of popliteus in full flexion of the knee.

The medial femoral condyle displays a prominent *adductor tubercle* on the medial supracondylar line and, just below this, the medial epicondyle gives origin to the *medial (tibial) collateral ligament*.

The *tibia* has an expanded upper end that overhangs the shaft posteriorly. The upper weight-bearing surface bears two shallow tibial condyles divided by the intercondylar area. Below the posterolateral tibial condyle lies an oval facet for articulation with the head of the fibula.

The prominent *tibial tuberosity* lies anteriorly and marks the insertion of the infrapatellar tendon (ligamentum patellae). *The iliotibial band (or tract)* (ITB) inserts into *Gerdy's tubercle* which lies anterolaterally (Burks, 1990; Kapandji, 2019).

The upper end of the *fibula* is expanded to form the head, which articulates with the tibia on its superomedial side, at the *superior tibiofibular joint*. The apex of the head of the fibula gives attachment to the lateral collateral ligament and the biceps femoris tendon. The common peroneal nerve winds around the neck of the fibula.

The *patella*, the largest sesamoid bone in the body, lies within the quadriceps tendon and articulates with the lower end of the femur at the *patellofemoral joint*. It is a flat triangular-shaped bone with its base uppermost and apex pointing inferiorly (Fig. 11.1).

The patella has anterior and posterior surfaces and upper, medial and lateral borders. Its anterior surface shows vertical ridges produced by the fibres of the quadriceps that pass over it. The posterior articulating surface of the patella is covered with thick articular cartilage, which is divided by a vertical ridge into medial and lateral articular facets for articulation with the femur, with an 'odd' facet on the medial side.

The tibiofemoral and patellofemoral joints share the same fibrous capsule, but each has a separate function.

The *tibiofemoral joint* is involved in weight-bearing activities. It is a synovial hinge joint between the convex

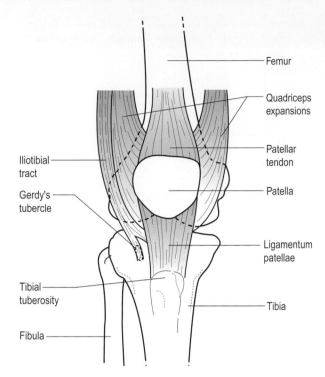

Fig. 11.1 Anterior aspect of the knee.

condyles of the femur and the slightly concave articular surfaces of the tibia. Mobility is not normally compatible with stability in a joint, but the incongruent joint surfaces of the knee make it a mobile joint, while the shape of the articular surfaces and the interaction of muscles, tendons and strong ligaments all contribute to stability.

The *patellofemoral joint* is the joint of the extensor mechanism of the knee. It is formed between the posterior aspect of the patella and the anterior surface of the femur.

As the joint of the extensor mechanism of the knee, it gives rise to symptoms on antigravity activities. The patella performs two important biomechanical functions at the knee (Nordin and Frankel, 2020):

- It produces anterior displacement of the quadriceps tendon throughout movement, assisting knee extension by increasing the lever arm of the quadriceps muscle force
- It increases the area of contact between the patellar tendon and the femur, distributing compressive forces over a wider area

As the knee moves from full extension to full flexion, the patella rotates and glides caudally approximately 7 cm. In full knee flexion, the patella sinks into the intercondylar groove (Nordin and Frankel, 2020).

There is a tendency for the patella to slip laterally, particularly as the knee moves towards full extension, and this is counteracted by the high lateral border of the patellar groove on the femur; the active muscle pull of the oblique fibres of vastus medialis and the medial quadriceps expansion.

The *superior tibiofibular joint* is a synovial plane joint between the lateral tibial condyle and the head of the fibula; it communicates with the knee joint in 10% of adults (Bozkurt et al., 2003). The joint capsule is reinforced by anterior and posterior tibiofibular ligaments.

The superior tibiofibular joint is linked mechanically to the inferior tibiofibular joint and is influenced by movements at the ankle joint. Small accessory movements are possible that dissipate torsional stresses applied to the ankle (Bozkurt et al., 2003).

The main function of the knee joint as a whole is to bear weight and consequently, symptoms are usually produced on weight-bearing activities. During the gait cycle, the forces across the tibiofemoral joint amount to two to five times body weight according to position and activity. However, the forces may increase to 24 times body weight during activities such as jumping (Soames and Palastanga, 2018).

The range of movement at the knee joint is greatest in the sagittal plane, with an active range from 0 degree extension to 140 degrees of flexion. Approximately 5 to 10 degrees of passive extension is usually available and up to 160 degrees of passive flexion, which is halted when the calf and hamstring muscles approximate and the heel reaches the buttock.

Active and passive axial rotation occur with the knee joint in flexion and the range is greatest at 90 degrees of flexion. Active lateral rotation amounts to approximately 45 degrees and medial rotation to 35 degrees, with a little more movement in each direction available passively.

A few degrees of automatic rotation occur to achieve the locked or unlocked positions of the knee. During the last 20 degrees or so of knee extension, lateral rotation of the tibia on the femur occurs to produce the terminal 'screw-home' or 'locking' phase of the knee. This achieves the close packed position of the knee joint, where it is most stable.

Rotation and accessory movements are impossible to perform on the normal extended knee. The ligaments around the knee contribute to stability in extension when most fibres are under tension. The knee is unlocked by the action of popliteus medially rotating the tibia on the femur.

Two semilunar cartilages, the *menisci*, deepen the tibial articulating surface and contribute to the congruency of the joint. The menisci facilitate load transmission, shock absorption, lubrication and stability (Bessette, 1992; Bikkina et al., 2005).

The menisci are composed of collagen fibres and the orientation of the fibres facilitates dispersion of compressive loads and resistance to longitudinal stresses. The fibre orientation at the surface of the meniscus is a random meshwork, thought to be important for distributing shear stress (Greis et al., 2002).

There is some vascularity within the outer 10% to 15% or 'red' zone of the meniscus but not in the inner 'white' zone, and the location and severity of meniscal tears can be used to guide the choice between conservative and surgical management (Hauger et al., 2000).

The *medial meniscus* is the larger of the two and is almost semicircular in shape. Its periphery attaches to the deep part of the medial collateral ligament, which forms part of the fibrous capsule of the knee joint.

The *lateral meniscus* is almost circular and is separated from the capsule of the knee joint at its periphery by the tendon of popliteus, to which it is attached. Posteriorly, the lateral meniscus contributes a ligamentous slip to the posterior cruciate ligament, known as the *posterior meniscofemoral ligament.*

The peripheral rim of each meniscus is attached to deep fibres of the capsule, which secure it to the edge of the tibial condyles and attach several millimetres below the articular cartilage (Bikkina et al., 2005). These deep capsular fibres are known as the *coronary ligaments* or meniscotibial ligaments (Fig. 11.2). They are strong, but lax enough to allow axial rotation to occur at the meniscotibial surface. The lateral coronary ligaments are longer than the medial and allow for greater excursion of the lateral meniscus (Burks, 1990).

The *fibrous capsule* of the knee joint is strengthened by ligamentous thickenings and independent ligamentous reinforcements, as well as by expansions from the tendons that cross the joint.

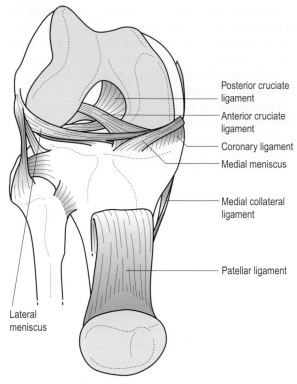

Fig. 11.2 Anterior view of the knee with patella reflected to show cruciate and coronary ligaments.

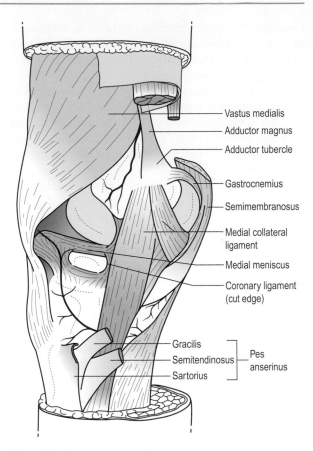

Fig. 11.3 Medial aspect of the knee.

The ligaments of the knee provide a dynamic guide during movement and act as a passive restraint to abnormal translation (Barrack and Skinner, 1990). Each ligament is oriented in a direction to produce stability (Woo et al., 1990).

The *medial collateral ligament* is a strong, broad, flat band lying posteriorly over the medial joint line (Fig. 11.3). Approximately 8 to 10 cm long, it arises from the medial femoral epicondyle, just distal to the adductor tubercle. It descends vertically across the joint line, running forwards to its attachment on the medial condyle and shaft of the upper tibia, approximately 5 cm below the joint line.

As the ligament crosses over the knee joint its anterior fibres blend with fibres of the medial patellar expansion (El-Dieb et al., 2002). It is the primary stabiliser of the medial aspect of the knee joint and is assisted by the quadriceps expansions and the tendons of sartorius,

gracilis and semitendinosus, which cross over its lower part. It is separated from the tendons by the pes anserine bursa.

The medial collateral ligament is composed of superficial and deep layers. The fibres of the superficial part pass directly from the femur to the tibia (Staron et al., 1994; Schweitzer et al., 1995). These fibres are relatively strong and provide 80% of the resistance to valgus force (Schenck and Heckman, 1993). Beneath the superficial fibres, the capsule is thickened to form the weaker, deep part, which is firmly anchored to the medial meniscus (Pope and Winston-Salem, 1996).

The primary stabilising role of the medial collateral ligament is to support the medial aspect of the knee joint, preventing excessive valgus movement. Its secondary stabilising role is to prevent lateral rotation of the tibia, anterior translation of the tibia on the femur and hyperextension of the knee. Most of the ligament is taut in full extension, preventing hyperextension (Pope and Winston-Salem, 1996).

The *lateral collateral ligament* is a shorter, cord-like ligament separated from the capsule of the knee joint by the tendon of popliteus. It is approximately 5 cm long and roughly the size of half a pencil (Evans, 1986; Soames and Palastanga, 2018; Fig. 11.4). It runs from the lateral femoral epicondyle to the head of the fibula where it blends with the insertion of biceps femoris to form a conjoined tendon, which is an important lateral stabiliser.

The primary stabilising role of the lateral collateral ligament is to restrain varus movement, supporting the lateral aspect of the knee (Burks, 1990), with a secondary stabilising role in controlling posterior drawer and lateral rotation of the tibia.

The lateral collateral ligament is closely related to the overlying *ITB*, which is similar in width and direction to the medial collateral ligament and may also provide dynamic stability to the lateral aspect of the knee joint.

The *cruciate ligaments* cross in the intercondylar fossa and are strong intracapsular, but extrasynovial, ligaments about as thick as a pencil (Evans, 1986; Bowditch,

2001). Their primary stabilising role is to resist anterior and posterior translation of the tibia under the femur. Their secondary stabilising function is to act as internal collateral ligaments controlling varus, valgus and rotation (Schenck and Heckman, 1993). They are named anterior or posterior by their tibial attachments (Figs 11.2 and 11.5).

The *anterior cruciate ligament* passes from the anterior tibial intercondylar area upwards, posteriorly and laterally, twisting as it goes, to attach to the posteromedial aspect of the lateral femoral condyle. Functionally, the ligament has a stabilising effect throughout the range of movement (Katz and Fingeroth, 1986; Perko et al., 1992).

The anterior cruciate ligament's primary stabilising role is to resist anterior translation and medial rotation of the tibia on the femur. It has a secondary stabilising role, working with the collateral ligaments, to resist valgus, varus and hyperextension stresses (Evans, 1986). The most common mechanism of injury to the anterior cruciate ligament is lateral rotation combined with a valgus force applied to the fixed tibia.

Complete ruptures of the anterior cruciate ligament most commonly result in disruption of all fibres and synovial coverings, leading to a haemarthrosis. With

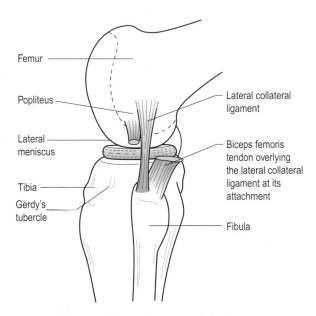

Fig. 11.4 Lateral aspect of the knee.

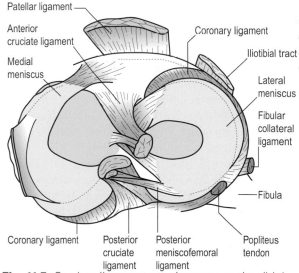

Fig. 11.5 Cruciate ligament attachments on the tibial plateau.

partial tears the synovial envelope may not be disrupted, leading to a contained haematoma without a haemarthrosis (Bowditch, 2001).

The *posterior cruciate ligament* passes upwards, anteriorly and medially from the posterior intercondylar area, to attach to the anterolateral aspect of the medial femoral condyle. The ligament is said to be twice as strong and less oblique than the anterior cruciate ligament, and its close relationship to the centre of rotation of the knee joint makes it a principal stabiliser (Soames and Palastanga, 2018).

The posterior cruciate ligament controls posterior translation of the tibia on the femur as well as restraining rotation of the tibia, since posterior translation occurs with concomitant lateral rotation of the tibia. It is less commonly injured than the anterior cruciate ligament.

Forced posterior translation of the tibia on the flexed knee, the typical 'dashboard' injury, is the most common mechanism of injury, but it may also be injured in forced hyperextension (El-Dieb et al., 2002).

Several fat pads are interposed between the knee joint capsule and synovial lining. The *infrapatellar fat pad of Hoffa* lies between the infrapatellar tendon and the knee joint and may be subjected to trauma or impingement (Jacobson et al., 1997).

Plicae (folds of synovium that protrude inwards) exist in the knee joint and may be responsible for symptoms. Three are usually recognised: the superior, inferior and medial plicae (Boles and Martin, 2001).

Numerous bursae are associated with the knee, facilitating the function of the tendons that exert a lengthwise pull across the joint (Soames and Palastanga, 2018).

A subcutaneous *superficial infrapatellar bursa* lies between the infrapatellar tendon and the skin; a *deep infrapatellar bursa* lies deep to the distal portion of the infrapatellar tendon and the underlying tibia.

The cylindrical knee joint capsule is invaginated posteriorly and lined with synovial membrane. The synovium is reflected upwards anteriorly under the quadriceps, approximately three fingers' breadth, to form the *suprapatellar bursa*.

The anterior surface of the patella is separated from the skin by a synovial-lined potential space, the subcutaneous *prepatellar bursa*. It contains minimal fluid and is only obvious when inflamed (Pope and Winston-Salem, 1996).

Anteromedially, the *pes anserine bursa* sits between the distal medial collateral ligament and the tendons of sartorius, gracilis and semitendinosus in front, known collectively as the *pes anserinus* (goose's foot) *tendon complex*. A variable number of small bursae lie deep to the medial collateral ligament.

Posteriorly, a bursa sits under each head of origin of gastrocnemius. A *semimembranosus bursa* sits medially between the tendon of semimembranosus and the medial tibial condyle of the tibia. Laterally, bursae lie on either side of the lateral collateral ligament, providing cushions between the ligament and biceps femoris and popliteus. There is also a bursa between popliteus and the lateral femoral condyle.

The knee joint is innervated by the femoral nerve (L2, 3, 4).

Contractile Structures

The contractile structures at the knee consist of muscles that originate from the hip region and insert at the knee, or originate at the knee and insert below the ankle. The muscles will be described in relationship to the knee in this chapter and are referred to in relation to the hip and ankle in Chapters 10 and 12 respectively.

Quadriceps femoris (femoral nerve L2–L4) is composed of four muscles: rectus femoris, vastus lateralis, vastus medialis and vastus intermedius, uniting around the patella to form the *infrapatellar tendon*, which passes from the apex of the patella to insert into the tibial tuberosity.

Rectus femoris originates above the hip joint and inserts into the base of the patella (upper border) with fibres continued over and on each side of the patella to contribute to the infrapatellar tendon.

Vastus lateralis passes down from the upper anterolateral femur to form a broad tendon that eventually tapers as it inserts into the lateral border of the patella as the lateral quadriceps expansion. Vastus lateralis contributes to the main quadriceps tendon, passing over the patella, as well as blending with fibres of the ITB to support the anterolateral joint capsule.

Vastus medialis passes from the upper anteromedial femur downwards to join the common quadriceps tendon and the medial border of the patella as the medial quadriceps expansion. The medial quadriceps expansion is a strong sheet of fibres on the anteromedial aspect of the knee with fibres continuing to run inferiorly and posteriorly to insert onto the tibia beside the fibres of the medial collateral ligament (Greenhill, 1967).

The lower fibres of the muscle run more horizontally and have their origin from adductor magnus, with which they share a nerve supply. These fibres are commonly known as the *vastus medialis obliquus* (VMO) muscle. The VMO traditionally has a role in the 'screwing home' of the tibia in the final locking stage of knee extension (Greenhill, 1967).

Vastus intermedius is the deepest part of the quadriceps and inserts with rectus femoris into the base of the patella as the *suprapatellar tendon*. The roughened posterior aspect of the apex gives attachment to the proximal end of the *infrapatellar tendon (ligamentum patellae)*.

As mentioned previously, the vastus lateralis and medialis muscles send tendinous insertions to the lateral and medial borders of the patella in the form of *quadriceps expansions* (or the *patellar retinacula*) (see Fig. 11.1). The *lateral expansion* receives an extension from the ITB. The *medial expansion* blends with the anterior fibres of the medial collateral ligament. The quadriceps expansions together are responsible for transverse stability of the patella.

Quadriceps femoris is the main extensor muscle of the knee joint. Vastus medialis is believed to be particularly active during the later stages of knee extension, when it exerts a stabilising force on the patella to prevent it slipping laterally. Although quiet in standing, the quadriceps femoris muscle contracts strongly in activities such as climbing.

The *hamstrings* (sciatic nerve L5, S1–S2), comprising biceps femoris, semimembranosus and semitendinosus, produce flexion of the knee and medial and lateral rotation of the knee when in the mid-flexed position.

Biceps femoris inserts into the head of the fibula (Fig. 11.6), splitting around the lateral collateral ligament, with which it forms a conjoined tendon.

Semimembranosus has its main attachment into the posterior aspect of the medial tibial condyle, but slips onwards to blend with other structures to support the posteromedial capsule.

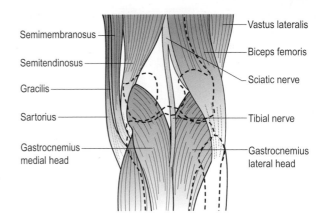

Fig. 11.6 Posterior aspect of the knee.

Semitendinosus curves around the medial tibial condyle to the upper surface of the medial tibia and together with sartorius and gracilis forms the pes anserine tendon complex. These tendons blend with and support the medial capsule.

The *pes anserine tendon complex* is responsible for flexion of the knee and medial rotation of the tibia on the femur (Valley and Shermer, 2000).

The ITB inserts into Gerdy's tubercle on the anterolateral aspect of the upper tibia and blends with the lateral capsule and the lateral quadriceps expansion. Functionally, it is related to the lateral collateral ligament. Tensor fascia lata, acting with gluteus maximus, tightens the tract and assists extension of the knee.

Popliteus (tibial nerve L4–L5, S1) originates within the capsule of the knee joint as a tendon arising from the groove on the lateral aspect of the lateral femoral condyle. It separates the lateral collateral ligament from the fibrous capsule of the knee joint and, as it passes downwards and medially, it sends tendinous fibres to the posterior horn of the lateral meniscus. It forms a fleshy, triangular muscle belly and attaches to the posterior aspect of the tibia above the soleal line.

Popliteus is the primary medial rotator of the knee, medially rotating the tibia on the femur and unlocking the knee joint from the close packed position. Through its attachment to the lateral meniscus, it can pull the meniscus backwards during rotatory movements, possibly preventing it from being trapped (Safran and Fu, 1995). The muscle also plays a role in dynamic stability,

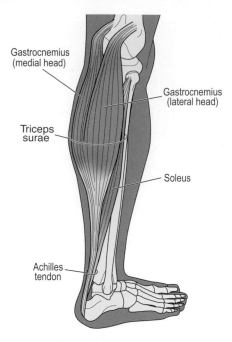

Fig. 11.7 Triceps surae.

particularly in preventing forward displacement of the femur on the tibia (Burks, 1990; Safran and Fu, 1995; El-Dieb et al., 2002).

Gastrocnemius (tibial nerve S1–S2) arises by two heads from the posterior aspect of the medial and lateral femoral condyles and together with soleus and plantaris (not shown) forms the triceps surae (Fig. 11.7). As well as its action at the ankle, gastrocnemius is a strong flexor at the knee, but is unable to act strongly at both joints simultaneously.

A GUIDE TO SURFACE MARKING AND PALPATION

Anterior Aspect

Locate the *patella* at the front of the knee and identify its base (upper border), apex (lower border), medial and lateral borders (Fig. 11.1). With the knee extended and relaxed, you should be able to move the patella from side to side to palpate the insertion of the *quadriceps expansions* under the edge of each border. Tilt the base and apex to locate the *suprapatellar* and *infrapatellar tendons*, respectively.

Follow the *infrapatellar tendon* down to its insertion onto the tibial tuberosity, which lies approximately 5 cm below the apex of the patella in the flexed knee.

Palpate and mark in the *knee joint line* with the knee in flexion. The anterior articular surface of each femoral condyle and the anterior articular margins of the tibia should be palpable at either side of the patella. Both can be followed round onto the medial and lateral aspects, but it is not possible to palpate the joint line posteriorly since it is covered by many musculotendinous structures.

With the knee joint flexed, the apex of the patella marks the approximate position of the joint line. In extension, the apex of the patella lies approximately one finger's breadth above the joint line. This information may provide a useful guide if the joint is very swollen, making it difficult to palpate the joint line.

The *quadriceps muscle* forms the major anterior muscle bulk. On static contraction of this muscle, locate rectus femoris, which forms the central part of the muscle bulk. Vastus lateralis forms an obvious lateral muscle bulk, and vastus medialis terminates in oblique fibres (VMO) that blend into the medial quadriceps expansion.

Lateral Aspect

On the anterolateral surface of the tibia, approximately two-thirds of the way forward from the head of the fibula to the tibial tuberosity, palpate for *Gerdy's tubercle* (see Figs 11.1 and 11.4), which gives attachment to the ITB. The ITB should be obvious as the quadriceps contracts.

Palpate the *head of the fibula* just below the posterior part of the lateral condyle of the tibia where it forms the proximal tibiofibular joint (Fig. 11.4). The common peroneal nerve can be rolled over the neck of the fibula.

Place the leg into the FABER position of hip *f*lexion, *ab*duction and *e*xternal (lateral) *r*otation, palpate the lateral aspect of the knee and find the head of the fibula again. Move your fingers slightly proximally and you should be able to roll over the cord-like *lateral collateral ligament*.

Medial Aspect

Palpate the medial condyle of the femur and locate the prominent *adductor tubercle* on the upper part of the condyle (Fig. 11.3). Deep palpation is necessary, and the tubercle will feel tender to palpation.

Move directly distally from the adductor tubercle until you are over the joint line and see if you can identify, by palpation, the anterior edge of the *medial collateral ligament*. This ligament is approximately 8 to 10 cm long (Soames and Palastanga, 2018) and two and a half fingers wide as it broadens to cross the joint line. Its anterior border may be palpated in most people, and it is usually in line with or just behind the central axis of the joint.

Visualise the position of the *sartorius, gracilis and semitendinosus* tendons (the pes anserine complex) as they cross the lower part of the medial collateral ligament to their insertion on the upper part of the medial tibia.

Posterior Aspect

Resist knee flexion and palpate the *hamstrings*, which form the muscle bulk of the posterior thigh (Fig. 11.6). The point at which the medial and lateral hamstrings separate can be identified, with semitendinosus lying on semimembranosus to form the medial wall of the popliteal fossa and biceps femoris forming the lateral wall.

Palpate the medial side of the popliteal fossa, where *semitendinosus* can be felt as an obvious tendon. Medial to it is *gracilis*, made more prominent by adding resisted medial rotation. Deeper to this is *semimembranosus*, remaining more muscular as it blends into its aponeurotic attachment.

Biceps femoris can be followed down to its insertion onto the head of the fibula.

Posteriorly, locate the two heads of *gastrocnemius* as they originate above the knee joint from the medial and lateral femoral condyles.

COMMENTARY ON THE EXAMINATION

Observation

A general observation is made of the patient's *face and overall posture*, but as the knee is a weight-bearing joint, particular attention is paid to the *gait* pattern.

Note if an antalgic posture or gait has been adopted; a limp will be evident during gait if the patient has an abnormal stride length or is not weight-bearing evenly. 'Toeing' in or out, together with abnormalities of foot posture, should also be noted.

History

The anatomy at the knee makes the structures susceptible to direct and indirect trauma. The menisci and ligaments are often the sites of acute lesions, while the contractile structures are susceptible to change in use, as well as acute trauma.

The superior tibiofibular joint is linked mechanically to its inferior counterpart and influenced by mechanisms of injury at the foot and ankle.

A detailed history is required at the knee since it gives important diagnostic clues, including typical injury patterns, which may be confirmed by clinical examination. It also assists in the identification of lesions that may be better suited for specialist referral.

The patient's *age, occupation, sports, hobbies and activities* are particularly relevant.

Some conditions affect certain age groups. Knee pain in children is commonly referred from the hip, and it is necessary to carry out a thorough examination of both joints. Slipped upper femoral epiphysis, Perthes' disease, osteochondritis dissecans and tumour can all refer pain to the knee and require urgent referral (Brukner et al., 2017). Meniscal lesions are unusual in children and increase in incidence from adolescence onwards.

Juvenile idiopathic arthritis (JIA), formerly juvenile rheumatoid arthritis, is an autoimmune disorder that occurs before the age of 16. JIA causes multiple joint pain, swelling and significant stiffness and commonly affects knees, hands and feet (National Institute of Arthritis and Musculoskeletal and Skin Diseases, 2021).

The young adult, particularly male, may present with a traumatic meniscal lesion associated with rotational injury during sporting activities (Greis et al., 2002). Females, more than males, tend to present with instability, subluxation or episodes of dislocation of the patella.

Rheumatoid arthritis may affect the knee, and onset usually occurs between the ages of 30 and 40. Degenerative arthropathy affects the older age group but may occur earlier if predisposed by previous injury or surgery. It is important to remember that degenerative arthropathy can affect both the patellofemoral and tibiofemoral joints.

Degenerative meniscal lesions occur more commonly in males in the fourth to sixth decades and can develop in association with degenerative joint disease (Greis et al., 2002).

The patients' activities will reflect whether occupational or recreational activities are a contributing factor to their condition. Sport in particular may be responsible for traumatic incidents to the relatively unstable knee, especially in positions of flexion. Progressive microtrauma may be the result of incorrect training or overtraining, muscle imbalances or poor joint biomechanics.

The *site* of the pain indicates whether it is local or referred.

Superficial structures tend to give local pain and point tenderness and lesions of the medial collateral ligament, coronary ligaments or the tendinous insertions of the muscles around the knee give reasonably accurate localization of pain.

Acutely inflamed lesions or deep lesions, such as of the tibiofemoral joint, menisci or cruciate ligaments, produce a vague, more widely felt, deep pain, with the patient unable to localise the lesion accurately.

The *spread* of pain generally indicates the severity of the lesion. While pain is expected to refer distally to the site of the lesion, the knee as a central limb joint may also produce some proximal pain in the thigh. Pain referred from the hip or lumbar spine can be felt at the knee and both may need to be eliminated as a cause of pain.

Anterior knee pain is a description of where the symptoms are felt by the patient, although the term is often misused as a diagnosis. It usually indicates patellofemoral joint involvement. Degenerative arthropathy of the patellofemoral joint can be a cause of anterior knee pain. Chondromalacia patellae is a softening of the articular cartilage of the patella that can be explored with magnetic resonance imaging (MRI) to establish the nature of the lesion. Stress fracture of the patella is a rare cause of anterior knee pain.

Patellar tendinopathy is a common cause of anterior knee pain with prepatellar and infrapatellar bursitis, fat pad impingement or synovial plicae being less common causes (Brukner et al., 2017).

The *onset* of the pain is highly relevant to lesions at the knee. Recalling the exact onset of the injury, the direction of forces involved and the position of the leg at the time of injury will give an idea of the likely anatomical structures involved in the lesion.

Trauma is a common precipitating cause and the sudden nature of the injury makes it easily recalled by the patient. A direct injury can cause muscular contusion and commonly involves the quadriceps.

A direct blow to the patella, such as a fall on the flexed knee, may result in fracture, may cause contusion of the periosteum or involvement of the prepatellar bursa. A direct blow to the anterior aspect of the upper tibia or,

again, a fall on the flexed knee can injure the posterior cruciate ligament.

In contact sports such as rugby and football the lateral side of the knee is vulnerable to impact, which may result in excessive valgus strain affecting the medial collateral ligament or medial meniscus. Injury may be produced by excessive forces applied to the flexed knee while the foot is fixed, such as skiing injuries which may affect the medial collateral ligament, anterior cruciate ligament and medial meniscus.

The coronary ligaments may also be involved in rotational injuries. Major ligamentous rupture, particularly of the anterior cruciate ligament, is usually accompanied by a 'pop' or tearing sound as the patient feels the ligament 'go' (Edwards and Villar, 1993).

Hyperextension injuries can affect any of the ligaments, since all are taut in extension, but the anterior cruciate ligament and medial collateral ligament are most commonly affected.

Muscle injuries are common around the knee, as the major muscle groups span two joints and may affect the origin, insertion or mid-belly. Strain results from sudden eccentric contraction (attempting to contract when the muscle is on the stretch) when the muscle is unable to overcome the resistance.

Explosive sprinting action affects the hamstrings and the quadriceps, and rectus femoris particularly may be affected by kicking against strong resistance. A direct blow to the quadriceps may cause a severe haematoma. Patellar instability with subluxation or dislocation affects the medial quadriceps expansions, vastus medialis or the medial capsule.

Repetitive minor injury results in microtrauma, making the onset of the lesion difficult to recall, and the examiner will have to be aware of contributing factors such as overtraining, training errors, foot posture and biomechanics.

Lateral knee pain due to ITB friction syndrome is common in long-distance runners, with a more gradual onset. Patellar tendinopathy is common in activities associated with repetitive jumping, and the bursae can become symptomatic as a result of a change in use.

A gradual onset of anterior knee pain in adolescents may be related to patellofemoral joint syndromes or Osgood–Schlatter's disease, an osteochondritis at the growth plate of the tibial tuberosity, which presents as localised tenderness over the tibial tuberosity and is associated with pain on repeated strong knee extension as in basketball, football or gymnastics (Brukner et al., 2017).

The *duration* of the symptoms will indicate the stage reached in the healing process, or the persistent or recurrent nature of the condition. Different treatment approaches depend on the acute, subacute or chronic nature of a ligamentous or muscle belly injury. Lesions due to a change in use around the knee tend to be chronic in nature and can be present for some considerable time before the patient seeks treatment.

Recurrent episodes of pain and swelling may be due to instability and derangement of the joint. Patellar subluxation, meniscal lesions or partial ligamentous tears may produce pain and joint effusion after use. Degenerative arthropathy may be symptom-free until unaccustomed use and/or overuse triggers a synovitis with increased pain and swelling.

The *symptoms and behaviour* need to be considered. The behaviour of the pain and the symptoms described by the patient are relevant to diagnosis at the knee. The ability to continue with the sport or activity after the onset of pain is often indicative of minor ligamentous injury, whereas major ligament disruption and muscle tears, meniscal lesions or cruciate rupture often result in the patient being totally incapacitated.

Total rupture of a ligament may produce severe pain at the time of injury but, following the initial injury, pain may not be a particular feature since the structure is totally disrupted. Partial ligamentous rupture continues to produce pain on movement.

Aggravating factors can be activity, which can indicate a mechanical or muscular lesion, or rest, which can indicate a ligamentous lesion with an inflammatory component.

Postures such as prolonged sitting may affect the patellofemoral joint in particular. A pseudo-locking effect often occurs when the patient first gets up to bear weight. This is not the same as true locking of the knee joint, but is a stiffness experienced by the patient that usually resolves after a few steps.

Walking, squatting and using stairs all aggravate patellofemoral conditions, particularly going downstairs, when the forces acting on this joint are increased to approximately three times body weight.

The tibiofemoral joint, as the weight-bearing joint, usually produces symptoms on weight-bearing activities, such as the stance phase of walking or running or going upstairs and prolonged standing. There can also be pain when the joint is off-loaded, especially at night. Pain produced on deep knee bends, rising from kneeling and rotational strains may indicate a meniscal lesion.

The other symptoms described by the patient give important clues to diagnosis. Swelling may be a symptom and it is important to know if it is constant, intermittent/recurrent or provoked by activity.

Swelling that usually occurs quickly, within 2 to 6 hours of injury, is indicative of a haemarthrosis or disruption in the joint but these cannot be excluded if the swelling takes longer to develop. The joint may feel warm to touch and the swelling may be tense. Structures responsible for a haemarthrosis are those with a good blood supply. The anterior cruciate ligament associated with torn synovium is the most common cause of a haemarthrosis (Shaerf and Banerjee, 2008).

Amiel et al. (1990) quoted a study by Noyes in which more than 70% of patients presenting with acute haemarthrosis of the knee had a tear of the anterior cruciate ligament. In children, however, haemarthrosis is more likely to be indicative of an osteochondral fracture than an anterior cruciate ligament injury (Baker, 1992).

The forces required for rupture of the posterior cruciate ligament are great, and therefore the posterior capsule usually tears as well, with blood escaping into the calf, where swelling and bruising are reported by the patient.

Swelling that develops more slowly, over 6 to 24 hours, is usually synovial in origin due to traumatic arthritis. Structures with a relatively poor blood supply tend to produce this traumatic arthritis, such as meniscal lesions; the deep part of the medial collateral ligament involving the capsule of the knee joint; and subluxation or dislocation of the patella.

Activity may provoke swelling in conditions such as degenerative arthropathy, chronic instability or internal derangement. This may be confirmed after the examination, which may provoke the swelling as well as pain.

Localised swelling may indicate bursitis, synovial effusion into the gastrocnemius or semimembranosus bursa due to effusion in the knee joint, or meniscal cysts which more commonly affect the lateral meniscus.

A swollen hot knee, in an unwell patient, that is, pyrexial with night sweats or with constant unremitting pain, should be investigated urgently to rule out red flags, such as a joint infection.

The presence of an effusion may affect the gait pattern and limit full extension. Reflex inhibition of the quadriceps muscle and an inability to lock the knee gives a feeling of insecurity on weight-bearing with the patient complaining of a sensation of 'giving way'. Giving way on weight-bearing may also be due to a loose body or meniscal lesion; it is momentary and occurs together with a twinge of pain.

Muscle imbalances, particularly involving the VMO, may produce a feeling of apprehension as the knee feels as if it will give way. This may occur when bearing weight after sitting for prolonged periods or walking downstairs.

True locking of the knee is indicative of a meniscal lesion and usually occurs in conjunction with a rotary component to the injury. Locking usually occurs at 10 to 40 degrees short of full extension (Hartley, 1995). The locking may resolve spontaneously over several hours or days or a truly locked knee should be referred for urgent surgical opinion.

Meniscal lesions can present with acute pain and swelling and the patient may report giving way, catching or locking. Degenerative meniscal lesions occur in older patients who present with an atraumatic history, mild swelling, joint line pain and mechanical symptoms (Greis et al., 2002). A ruptured anterior cruciate ligament can cause locking as the ligamentous flap catches between the joint surfaces. True locking must be distinguished from the pseudo-locking associated with the patellofemoral joint after prolonged sitting.

Provocation of pain on the stairs is important. The patellofemoral joint characteristically produces more pain on coming downstairs, due to the greater joint reaction force. The tibiofemoral joint may be more painful when going upstairs.

Clicking, snapping or catching may be due to internal derangement. Patients often describe a 'popping' sensation on injury that can indicate cruciate ligament rupture. Grating and pain associated with crepitation are usually indicative of degenerative changes of the tibiofemoral joint, patellofemoral joint or both.

To exclude symptoms arising from the lumbar spine and peripheral neuropathies, the patient should be questioned about paraesthesia and weakness.

Other joint involvement should be explored to establish the possibility of inflammatory joint disease. Have there been any previous knee problems or knee surgery?

Medical history should exclude serious pathology, and questions about *medications* will highlight any contraindications to treatment.

Practitioners should routinely *screen* for psychosocial factors and consider relevant health comorbidities and lifestyle factors (see Chapter 1). These factors may contribute to patients' presenting condition or form a barrier to their recovery and normal function, which should be addressed as an integral part of patient management.

If degenerative arthropathy is considered a factor in the diagnosis, the patient can be questioned about substantial weight gain, since obesity has a significant impact on degenerative arthropathy. Weight loss can impart clinically significant improvements in pain and delay progression of structural joint damage (King et al., 2013).

As well as past medical history, establish any ongoing conditions and treatment. Explore other previous or current musculoskeletal problems with previous episodes of the current complaint, any treatment given and the outcome of treatment.

Inspection

The knee should be fully extended in standing. If not, some compromise of the terminal screw home or locking mechanism exists, or an effusion with limited extension is present as part of the capsular pattern.

The knee should be inspected in both the weight-bearing and non-weight-bearing positions. In standing, the normal slight valgus tibiofemoral angle should be obvious.

The whole lower limb is inspected for leg length discrepancy and obvious *bony deformity* such as genu valgum, varum, recurvatum or 'wind-swept' knees (one varus, one valgus). The posture of the feet is important.

Overpronation or a tight Achilles tendon may be related to the knee symptoms and a detailed biomechanical assessment is then required. Position of the pelvis and obvious spinal deformities may be important to note if relevant to symptoms.

The position, shape and size of the patellae are also noted if relevant to the presenting symptoms. Patellar alignment is measured by the Q-angle – the angle between the line of the quadriceps muscle (anterior superior iliac spine to the midpoint of the patella) and the patellar tendon (midpoint of the patella to the tibial tuberosity). An angle of between 15 and 20 degrees is considered normal for patellar alignment and tracking, and less or more than this can be considered to be a malalignment (Norris, 2004).

Congenital malformation of the patella – small or absent – may lead to instability and recurrent subluxation of the patella as a rare cause of knee pain (Bongers et al., 2005).

Colour changes may be present, especially if the condition is acute, when the joint looks red due to inflammatory activity. Direct trauma may produce bruising and acute muscle lesions may show bruising, particularly in the quadriceps and hamstring muscles. Distal colour changes may be indicative of circulatory problems.

In standing, all muscle groups are inspected for *wasting*. The quadriceps wastes rapidly due to reflex inhibition if pain, swelling or degenerative change is present. In patellofemoral problems wasting of the VMO may be obvious.

Loss of the dimple on the medial aspect of the knee will indicate the presence of *swelling*. Minor swelling may not be obvious, however, and may only be apparent on testing by palpation in the supine position.

State at Rest

Before any movements are performed, the state at rest is established to provide a baseline for subsequent comparison.

Examination by Selective Tension

The suggested sequence for the examination will now be given, followed by a commentary that includes the reasoning in performing the movements and the significance of the possible findings. Comparison should always be made with the other side.

Supine Lying
- Palpation for heat (Fig. 11.8), swelling (Fig. 11.9) and synovial thickening (Fig. 11.10)
  Eliminate the hip
- Passive hip flexion (Fig. 11.11)
- Passive hip medial rotation (Fig. 11.12)
- Passive hip lateral rotation (Fig. 11.13)
- Passive knee flexion (Fig. 11.14)
- Passive knee extension, once for range (Fig. 11.15a), once for end-feel (see Fig. 11.15b)
- Passive valgus stress (Fig. 11.16)
- Passive varus stress (Fig. 11.17)
- Passive lateral rotation (Fig. 11.18a)
- Passive medial rotation (see Fig. 11.18b)
- Posterior drawer test (Figs 11.19–11.21)
- Anterior drawer test (Fig. 11.22)
- Lachman test (Fig. 11.23)

Provocation Tests for the Menisci (Saunders, 2000)
- Flexion, lateral rotation and valgus (Fig. 11.24)
- Flexion, lateral rotation and varus (Fig. 11.25)
- Flexion, medial rotation and valgus (Fig. 11.26)
- Flexion, medial rotation and varus (Fig. 11.27)

Prone Lying
- Resisted knee flexion (Fig. 11.28)
- Resisted knee extension (Fig. 11.29)

Palpation
- Once a diagnosis has been made, the structure at fault is palpated for the exact site of the lesion

The combined history and examination are important at the knee. The symptoms described by the patient result from functional weight-bearing activities. Additional functional tests may be required following the initial examination of the knee in the non-weight-bearing position.

Lesions vary from simple contusions, muscle strains and ligament injuries to arthropathy and major ligamentous rupture and instability. It is clinically important to be able to diagnose lesions at the knee, but also to appreciate the limits of clinical examination and determine when further investigation or onward referral for a specialist opinion is necessary.

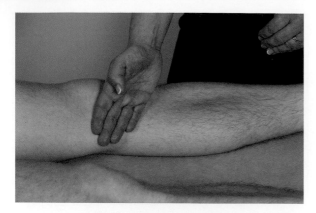

Fig. 11.8 Palpation for heat.

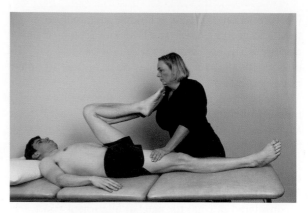

Fig. 11.11 Passive hip flexion.

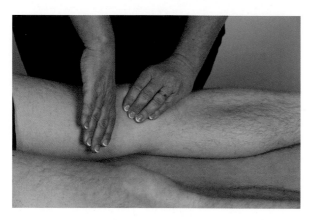

Fig. 11.9 Palpation for swelling.

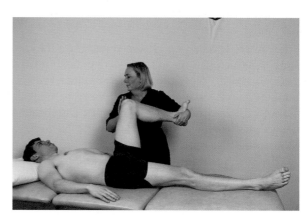

Fig. 11.12 Passive hip medial rotation.

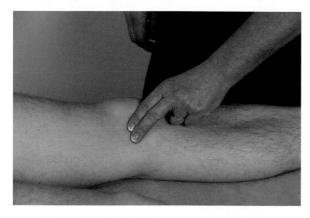

Fig. 11.10 Palpation for synovial thickening.

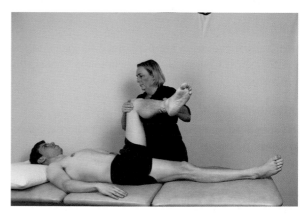

Fig. 11.13 Passive hip lateral rotation.

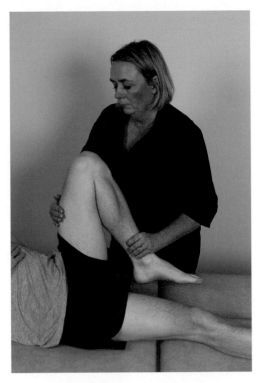

Fig. 11.14 Passive knee flexion.

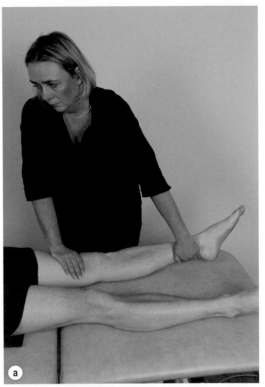

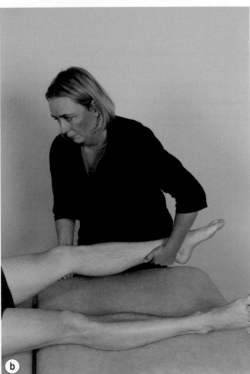

Fig. 11.15 Passive knee extension: (a) for range and (b) for end-feel.

With chronic knee problems and in children, the hip and lumbar spine should be cleared first to eliminate more proximal causes of pain referring to the knee.

The acute knee should be examined as soon as possible after injury: for instance, on the side of the pitch, before effusion causes pain, apprehension and limited movement. Effusion makes it difficult to test accurately for ligamentous instability and to apply provocative meniscal tests.

Palpation tests are conducted for signs of activity within the joint. Temperature changes are assessed using the dorsal aspect of the same hand and comparing like with like. Inflammatory conditions and infection will show an increase in *heat* compared with the other side. It may be necessary to repeat this test at the end of the examination to assess whether an inflammatory response has been triggered by the examination, giving an indication of the irritability of the lesion.

Several tests exist for *swelling* and the choice is left to the practitioner on the basis of personal opinion on effectiveness and preference. A sensitive test for minor swelling involves placing the finger and thumb of one hand on

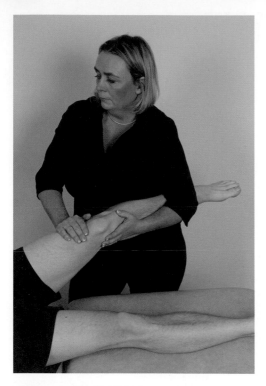

Fig. 11.16 Valgus stress.

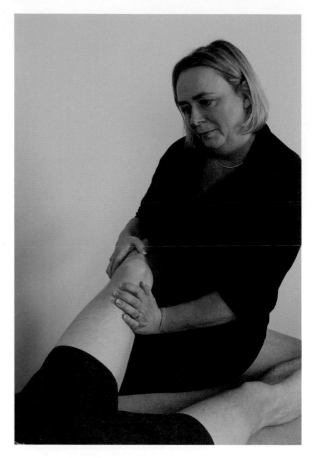

Fig. 11.17 Varus stress.

either side of the patella just below the bony periphery. The web between the index finger and thumb of the other hand applies compression to the suprapatellar bursa, which squeezes fluid out into the joint cavity and, if positive, is felt to part the finger and thumb of the other hand.

Other tests involve wiping the fluid from one side of the joint to the other; compression of the suprapatellar bursa; compression at the front of the joint just below the patella to assess fluctuation of fluid; or pressing down on the patella to assess for the presence of a patellar 'tap'.

Synovial thickening is assessed by palpation of the medial and lateral femoral condyles.

Thickening of the synovium is normal here because of the presence of synovial plicae and the medial plica is more obvious to palpation. Assessment for excessive thickening of the synovium is confirmed if the tissue feels 'boggy' to the touch. Hill et al. (2001) regard synovial thickening as a contributor to pain in the degenerative arthropathic knee and an indication of the severity of the disease.

The position of the patella should be assessed for size and to see if it is shifted, tilted or rotated with respect to the other side.

After excluding the hip, the primary passive movements of flexion and extension are performed to assess the tibiofemoral joint. Pain, range of movement and end-feel are noted, which will indicate the presence of the capsular or non-capsular pattern. Passive flexion normally has a soft end-feel and passive extension a hard end-feel. The thigh is fixed above the knee and the foot is lifted to assess the range of hyperextension present, normally 5 to 10 degrees.

A further test is conducted for the end-feel of extension whereby the leg is lifted into approximately 10 degrees of flexion and dropped into extension to assess for the normal, bony hard end-feel. This is sometimes known as the 'bounce home' test and an

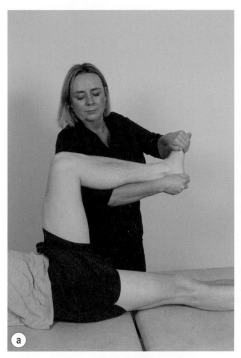
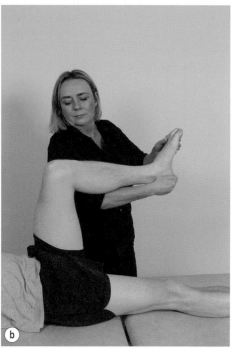

Fig. 11.18 Passive (a) lateral and (b) medial rotation.

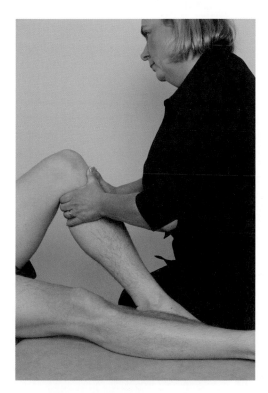

Fig. 11.19 Posterior drawer test.

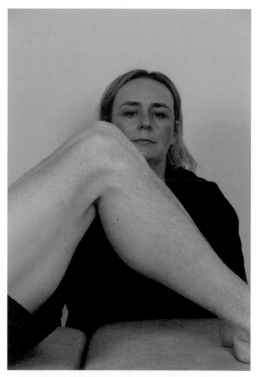

Fig. 11.20 Assessment of laxity of the posterior cruciate ligament.

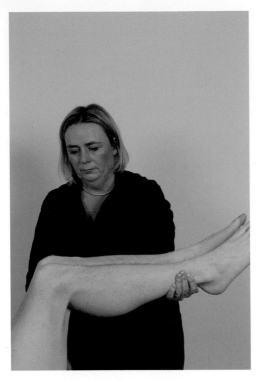

Fig. 11.21 Assessment of laxity of the posterior cruciate ligament, alternative position.

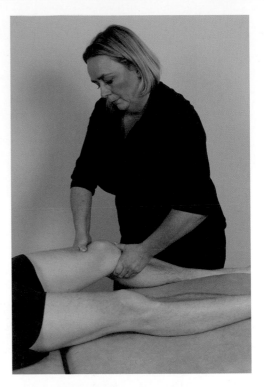

Fig. 11.23 Lachman test.

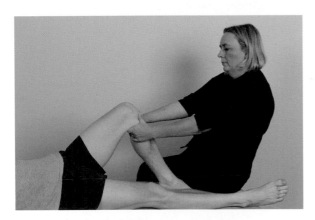

Fig. 11.22 Anterior drawer test.

abnormally 'soft' or 'springy' end-feel indicates the end of range has not been reached due to a meniscal lesion, loose body or joint effusion. This test is not suitable for the very irritable and painful knee.

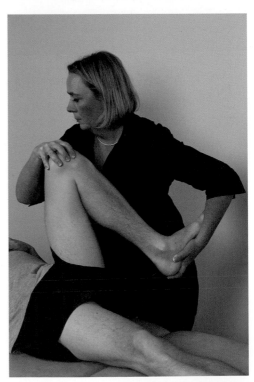

Fig. 11.24 Flexion, lateral rotation and valgus.

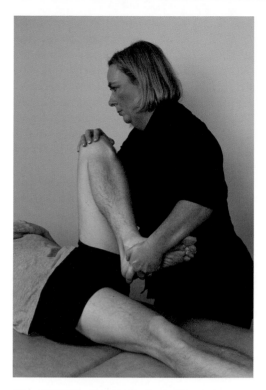

Fig. 11.25 Flexion, lateral rotation and varus.

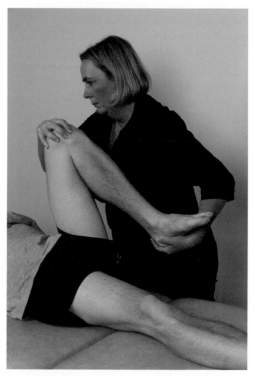

Fig. 11.26 Flexion, medial rotation and valgus.

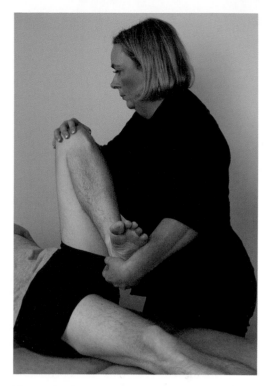

Fig. 11.27 Flexion, medial rotation and varus.

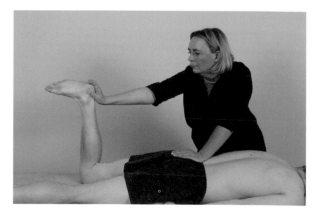

Fig. 11.28 Resisted knee flexion.

The presence of the non-capsular pattern indicates a ligamentous lesion, a loose body in the joint or possibly a meniscal problem.

The secondary passive movements at the knee are applied to assess the ligaments. It is important to compare the two limbs since, although joint motion varies

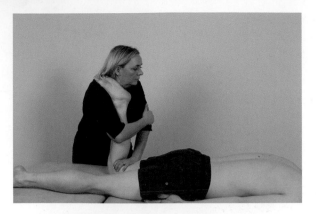

Fig. 11.29 Resisted knee extension.

considerably within the population, there is little variation between right and left in a normal subject (Daniel, 1990).

The tests depend on the muscles being relaxed and the eye, feel and experience of the practitioner, who is looking for an excessive range of movement compared with the asymptomatic knee and an abnormal soft endfeel with no definite endpoint if laxity is present.

Secondary passive movements are applied to the knee in a loose packed position of 20 to 30 degrees of flexion since no passive or accessory movement should be possible with the knee in full extension. If movement can be detected in the close packed position, serious ligamentous disruption is present, with accompanying damage to capsular components.

Musculoskeletal medicine treatment techniques will be directed at simple ligamentous injuries, but it is important to recognise more serious ligament disruption or intra-articular derangement due to a meniscal lesion, in order to conduct the appropriate investigations or refer for specialist opinion.

The suggested testing positions for the ligaments are provided in the figures within the clinical examination procedure. They are not described in detail here, but the interested practitioner is referred to fuller descriptions of these and other methods to be found in textbooks devoted to musculoskeletal examination (see Hattam and Smeatham, 2020), the knee and sports injuries.

Valgus and varus stresses are applied to the knee in approximately 20 to 30 degrees of flexion and assess the primary stabilising function of the medial and lateral

collateral ligaments, respectively. The range of movement available and any pain reproduced are noted and compared with the asymptomatic knee. The end-feel is assessed, which is normally firm elastic.

Axial rotation should be tested at 90 degrees of knee flexion as the range of movement is greatest in this position. Passive lateral rotation is usually 45 degrees and assesses the medial coronary ligaments, and passive medial rotation is usually 35 degrees and tests the lateral coronary ligaments.

The posterior and anterior drawer tests are both performed with the knee at 90 degrees of flexion. The neutral position of the injured knee must be established and compared with the other knee. A lax or ruptured posterior cruciate ligament will allow the tibial tuberosity to drop backwards with respect to the other knee.

For this reason, the posterior drawer test is applied first for the posterior cruciate ligament since a deficient posterior cruciate ligament could give a false positive to anterior translation. As the tibia is pushed posteriorly, the thumbs rest over the anterior joint line to assess the 'sag-back' or step created anteriorly by the excessive posterior drawer.

Isolated rupture of the posterior cruciate ligament is a rare lesion, but the posterior drawer test is a sensitive and specific test for the posterior cruciate ligament as part of a complete assessment and if accompanied by other relevant tests (Malanga et al., 2003; Soames and Palastanga, 2018; Hattam and Smeatham, 2020).

The anterior drawer test assesses the anterior cruciate ligament, although it is considered an insensitive and poor diagnostic indicator of acute lesions of this ligament (Wagemakers et al., 2010; van Eck et al., 2013; Huang et al., 2016; Decary et al., 2017). Haemarthrosis and traumatic arthritis 'splint' the knee and may make it difficult to place the knee in 90 degrees of flexion. Pain can also produce protective spasm in the hamstrings, preventing anterior tibial translation. In a chronic knee, the secondary stabilising role of an intact medial collateral ligament may prevent anterior translation at 90 degrees of knee flexion.

The Lachman test is a clinical test with excellent diagnostic accuracy to determine anterior cruciate laxity (Nickinson et al., 2010; van Eck et al., 2013; Huang et al., 2016; Decary et al., 2017). The Lachman test may be difficult to perform, especially if the limb is large or the patient unable to relax sufficiently. Several modifications have been made to the Lachman test since it was first described by Torg et al. (1974), including a 'drop leg' Lachman test described by Adler et al. (1995) and a reversed Lachman test described by Hattam and Smeatham (2020). It is important to check the range with the unaffected knee as this varies considerably in the normal population.

An intact anterior cruciate ligament should provide a normal hard end-feel or 'stop' to the drawer movement applied. The end-feel with a ruptured anterior cruciate ligament will feel 'soft' or absent when compared to the other knee (Bowditch, 2001; Shaerf and Banerjee, 2008). Haemarthrosis and the presence of a positive Lachman test indicate the need for onward referral for orthopaedic opinion.

With a more chronic injury the reliability of both the anterior drawer test and the Lachman test is good at 95% to 99% (Nickinson et al., 2010; van Eck et al., 2013; Huang et al., 2016; Decary et al., 2017). Bowditch (2001) was less convinced, believing that a positive drawer test at 90 degrees in the chronic knee may be due to laxity of the secondary constraints: for example, the medial collateral ligament.

The pivot-shift test is a dynamic test to determine the degree of instability related to anterior cruciate ligament injury and has a low false-negative rate (Shaerf and Banerjee, 2008; Hattam and Smeatham, 2020). However, it may also be difficult to apply in the acute knee due to pain and swelling.

Four provocation tests are applied if the history indicates a meniscal lesion. Each meniscus is put under compression and stress during combined movements of flexion, valgus, varus and both rotations.

Other traditional tests for a meniscal lesion include the 'bounce home' test of passive knee extension for end-feel; the McMurray's test, which takes the leg from a position of flexion towards extension, with medial or lateral rotation of the tibia; Apley's grind or compression test; and Thessaly's (weight-bearing rotation) test (see Hattam and Smeatham, 2020). There is mixed support for the various meniscal tests in the literature.

Mohan and Gosal (2007) used the McMurray test and joint line tenderness along with the history to examine their own reliability in clinical diagnosis of meniscal tears. They recorded their accuracy as 88% for medial meniscal lesions and 92% for lateral, being as reliable, and in some cases more reliable, than MRI. Ryzewicz et al. (2007) also supported that an experienced practitioner can generally identify patients with a meniscal tear as accurately as MRI but emphasised that the tests applied should always be interpreted in the context of the patient's history.

Notwithstanding Mohan and Gosal's and Ryzewicz's et al.'s claim for the accuracy of clinical diagnosis, MRI is still proposed as the 'gold standard' in non-invasive investigation of knee pain, having a high negative predictive value and helping to avoid unnecessary knee arthroscopy. It has greater than 89% accuracy and 90% sensitivity for detection of medial meniscal tears (Curtin et al., 1992; Skinner, 2012; Hattam and Smeatham, 2020).

Negative clinical testing is not conclusive evidence that a meniscal lesion does not exist. If the history is indicative, or the patient is experiencing progressive, recurrent episodes of locking and/or giving way, referral should be considered for MRI and specialist opinion.

The resisted tests are applied, looking for pain and power. Resisted knee extension tests the quadriceps and resisted knee flexion tests the hamstrings. Having established that there is no pain on testing the muscles in the mid-position, accessory provocation tests may be included to provoke minor contractile lesions.

Movement	Main Muscles	'Assistors'
Flexion	Hamstrings	Gracilis, sartorius
Extension	Quadriceps	
Medial rotation	Popliteus	Semimembranosus, semitendinosus, gracilis, sartorius
Lateral rotationss	Biceps femoris	Popliteus

The quadriceps and hamstrings can be tested in varying degrees of knee flexion and extension, and isotonically. The hamstring muscles can be tested in conjunction with medial or lateral rotation to isolate the lesion to the medial or lateral hamstrings. Popliteus is assessed by testing resisted knee flexion in conjunction with resisted medial rotation of the tibia.

At this stage, palpation of the structure determined to be at fault may be made to identify the exact site of the lesion. Interestingly, as mentioned, joint line tenderness is considered to be highly sensitive in meniscal lesions and palpation is therefore a good adjunct to the highly specific McMurray test (Hegedus et al., 2007; Meserve et al., 2008; Speziali et al., 2016; Decary et al., 2017).

Based on the history and clinical examination, the practitioner should be able to establish the most likely diagnosis, using clinical reasoning and clinical judgment.

It is important to recognise potential serious pathology, such as infection, malignancy, fracture and inflammatory arthritis, and to make any appropriate onward referral in a timely manner. Should additional information be required to aid diagnosis or to add value to management, further investigations can be considered to inform decision making and planning.

Investigations should be guided by suspected causes as an extension to the clinical examination. If necessary, the practitioner may consider further investigations such as blood tests, radiological imaging, and other diagnostic procedures (see Chapter 1). They should be considered with suspected red flags such as fracture, infection, inflammatory arthritis or malignancy. If severe degenerative arthropathy is suspected, X-ray or MRI (with or without contrast) may be appropriate. Blood tests can be considered if malignancy, polymyalgia rheumatica, inflammatory arthritis or infection are suspected.

CAPSULAR LESIONS

CAPSULAR PATTERN AT THE KNEE JOINT
- More limitation of flexion than extension.

The movements limited in the capsular pattern have a characteristically 'hard' end-feel. The capsular pattern at the knee is more limitation of flexion than extension. The history indicates the cause of the arthropathy which could be degenerative arthropathy, inflammatory arthritis, such as rheumatoid arthritis, or traumatic arthritis.

Traumatic arthritis is usually a secondary response to a ligamentous lesion at the knee. As a capsular ligament, damage to the medial collateral ligament can produce a secondary traumatic arthritis; a ruptured cruciate ligament may also produce a haemarthrosis.

A number of differential diagnoses should also be considered. These include patellofemoral pain, fracture, malignancy, pes anserine bursitis, ITB syndrome or degenerative meniscal tear (NICE, 2020).

A stepped approach to the management of degenerative arthropathy is recommended (McAlindon et al., 2014; NICE, 2020). Less invasive treatments are generally offered first including weight management, suitable footwear, simple analgesics and non-steroidal anti-inflammatory drugs (NSAIDs) medication, physiotherapy (e.g. exercise, manual therapy, gait re-education) and then injection therapy (e.g. corticosteroid, local anaesthetic, hyaluronic acid, platelet-rich plasma (PRP)). If symptoms persist, more invasive treatments can be considered, such as arthroplasty.

Considerations for knee arthroplasty should be personalised to include patients' symptoms, age, medical/drugs history, weight and evidence of symptoms correlating to imaging such as moderate or severe degenerative changes and joint space narrowing. General indications for knee replacement are persistent severe symptoms (e.g. pain and significant impact on function), and when good quality non-surgical intervention has failed (NICE, 2020).

Symptomatic degenerative arthropathy and inflammatory arthritis may benefit from an intra-articular injection of corticosteroid with some evidence for relief of moderate to severe pain (Conaghan et al., 2008; Ringdahl and Pandit, 2011; Bannuru, et al., 2015). Treatment for traumatic arthritis should be directed to the cause of the lesion, or the ligamentous injury.

INJECTION OF THE KNEE JOINT (CYRIAX, 1984; CYRIAX AND CYRIAX, 1993)
Suggested needle size: 21 G × 1½ in. (0.8 × 40 mm) green needle.
Dose: 30–60 mg triamcinolone acetonide in a total volume of 4 mL.

- Position the patient comfortably in supine lying with the knee supported in extension.
- Tilt the patella by pressing down on the lateral edge to lift the medial border (Fig. 11.30).
- Insert the needle halfway along the medial border of the patella, aiming laterally and slightly posteriorly, parallel with the articular surface of the patella (Fig. 11.31).
- Once the needle is intra-articular, deliver the injection as a bolus.

The patient should minimise or modify activities for 2 weeks following injection.

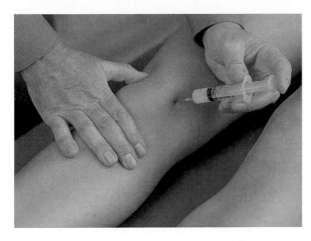

Fig. 11.30 Injection of the knee joint.

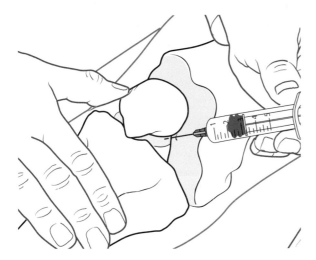

Fig. 11.31 Injection of the knee joint, showing direction of approach and needle position.

NON-CAPSULAR LESIONS

Loose Body

From the history, symptoms of momentary giving way on weight-bearing accompanied by twinges of pain indicate a possible loose body in the knee joint. The loose body may be a fragment of cartilage or bone, or both (osteochondral), and can be associated with degenerative arthropathy in the older adult (Saotome et al., 2006), or a flap of meniscus that may momentarily give way or lock on weight-bearing.

Although its ability to act as a loose body is unclear, a 'floating' meniscus may be visible on MRI where the coronary ligaments are disrupted or stretched, rather than the meniscus itself, and the meniscus commonly stays intact (Bikkina et al., 2005). An anterior cruciate ligament tear can present as a loose body, and a tear should be considered if the symptoms arose after trauma.

Loose bodies can be stable, fixed in a synovial recess or bursa, or attached to synovial membrane, where they tend not to be displaced. Unstable loose bodies can move freely in the joint to become trapped at irregular intervals between the articular bone ends, causing intermittent symptoms and internal joint derangement (Bianchi and Martinoli, 1999).

Osteochondritis dissecans may affect the knee in adolescents, usually between the ages of 15 and 20 years. A small fragment of bone becomes separated from a condyle and forms a loose body. The symptoms are usually pain, swelling, locking and giving way. On examination, a non-capsular pattern is present with a small limitation of flexion or extension, but not both. The end-feel is characteristically springy.

If the joint should lock, it is usually temporary and unlocks spontaneously. A truly locked knee should be referred for urgent surgical opinion.

A loose body may become impinged between the joint surfaces in degenerative arthropathy. If the loose fragment impinges on the medial side of the joint, the patient presents with signs of an intrinsic medial collateral injury in the absence of trauma. The capsular pattern of degenerative arthropathy is present with a non-capsular pattern superimposed upon it; the patient complains of increased pain on a valgus stress. The primary lesion of the loose body should be treated and the secondary ligamentous injury should then subside.

The treatment of choice to reduce a loose body is strong traction together with Grade A mobilisation, theoretically, aiming to move the loose body to another part of the joint and to restore full, pain-free movement. This technique can also be used as a distraction/mobilisation technique for non-irritable knee degenerative arthropathy or mild meniscal irritation, where joint stiffness is the main complaint.

Strong traction is applied to the joint, and a medial or lateral movement is applied simultaneously with a movement from flexion towards extension.

LOOSE BODY MOBILISATION TECHNIQUE

(Saunders, 2000)

This technique can only be applied to a relatively fit patient, but it enables the technique to be applied single-handedly.

- Position the patient in supine lying with the legs hanging over the end of the couch and the thighs supported.

- Arrange the couch so that it is as high as it will go and elevate the head end of the couch.
- Run your hand down the posterior aspect of the ankle, grasping the calcaneus and pulling the ankle into dorsiflexion.
- Place the other hand on top of the talus in order to rotate the leg into either medial or lateral rotation (Figs 11.32 and 11.33) (position your hands such that the hand on top of the foot will be pulling, not pushing, into rotation).

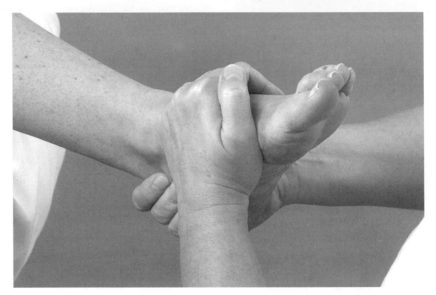

Fig. 11.32 Loose-body mobilisation for the knee; hand position for mobilisation into medial rotation.

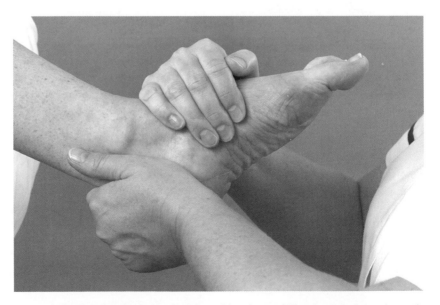

Fig. 11.33 Loose-body mobilisation for the knee; hand position for mobilisation into lateral rotation.

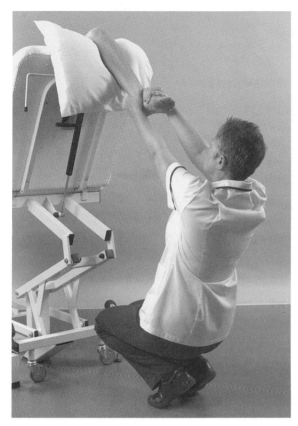

Fig. 11.34 Loose-body mobilisation for the knee; starting position applying traction.

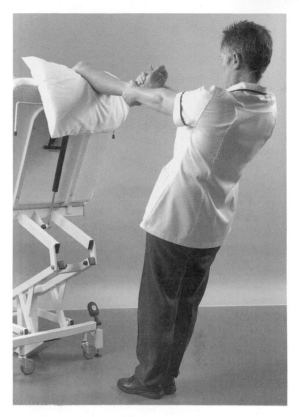

Fig. 11.35 Loose-body mobilisation for the knee; ending the manoeuvre, avoiding full extension of the patient's knee.

- Bend your knees and straighten your arms to apply traction (Fig. 11.34).
- Once traction is established, straighten your knees to extend the patient's knee, leaning backwards to maintain the traction as you stand, smartly rotating the leg at the same time (Fig. 11.35).
- Reassess.

If the technique has helped, it can be repeated; if not, change your hand position to perform the opposite rotation.

As mentioned, the basis of this technique is traction, rotation and a movement towards extension of the knee. It can be modified to suit the patient or operator and you are encouraged to be inventive with the technique. It can be applied with the patient sitting sideways on the couch and the technique is described below.

LOOSE BODY TECHNIQUE– ALTERNATIVE POSITION

- Sit the patient sideways on the couch with the legs hanging over the side and leaning backwards a little to hold onto the edge of the couch behind.
- Make sure that the bend of the knee is at the edge of the couch, for comfort.
- Raise the couch to an appropriate height, depending on the length of the patient's leg, and sit on the floor in front of the patient, resting your feet against the bar underneath the couch (Fig. 11.36a).
- Grasp the ankle using the same handhold as described above, according to which way the leg will be rotated.
- Pull down through the line of the tibia and allow a moment for the traction to establish.

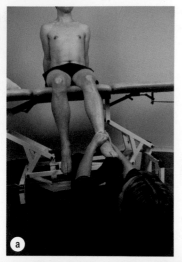

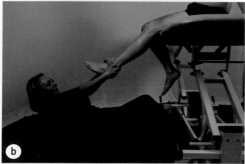

Fig. 11.36 Alternative position, loose-body mobilisation of the knee, sitting on floor: (a) starting position applying traction; (b) ending the manoeuvre, avoiding full extension of the patient's knee.

- Lean backwards while rotating the leg smartly towards either medial or lateral rotation, whilst extending the knee (see Fig. 11.36b).
- Reassess.

If the technique has helped, it can be repeated; if not, change your hand position to effect the opposite rotation.

A 'seat belt' may be used to help to maintain the traction while the technique is being performed.

If a comparable sign was identified on clinical examination, then this can guide whether to continue with one technique or to change to the other.

The diagnosis may have been reached on the history alone, however, and in both cases, a judgment will need to be made on when to stop applying the technique and to adopt a 'watchful wait' approach to see if the symptoms have improved.

Should the patient fail to improve or continue to experience symptoms, differential diagnosis such as osteochondritis dissecans, meniscal tear, tibial plateau fracture, degenerative, traumatic or inflammatory arthritis should be considered.

Medial Collateral Ligament Injury

The medial collateral ligament is the ligament most vulnerable to injury at the knee, but the following principles of treatment may also be applied to the lateral collateral ligament if it is the site of the lesion. As the lateral collateral ligament is not associated with the joint capsule, the acute effusion common to medial collateral injury is likely to be absent.

The collateral and cruciate ligaments function together to control and stabilise the knee. The medial collateral ligament is anatomically related to the medial meniscus and functionally related to the anterior cruciate ligament.

The mechanism of injury can be through a valgus strain, due to direct impact to the lateral aspect of the knee, or it commonly includes a rotation stress to the knee which may result in 'O'Donoghue's unhappy triad', affecting all three structures (Evans, 1986; Staron et al., 1994).

If tears of the medial meniscus and anterior cruciate ligament are confirmed by MRI or arthroscopy, subtle signs of medial collateral ligament injury should be sought, since the three conditions usually coexist (Staron et al., 1994).

Rupture of the cruciate ligaments or a meniscal lesion produces an acute effusion that can be managed conservatively as for the acute phase of medial collateral ligament injury. Once the acute phase has settled, a full assessment of the knee can be carried out, including assessment for ligamentous laxity and the provocative meniscal tests. A decision may then be taken concerning onward referral for specialist opinion.

Ligament injuries are graded I–III according to the amount of laxity and the end-feel (Hartley, 1995; Nakamura and Shino, 2005; Azar, 2006). The following grading is applied to the medial collateral ligament, but it should be noted that assessment for laxity on the acute knee may not be possible due to the effusion and painful muscle spasm. Brotzman and Wilk (2003) have proposed ranges of valgus movement that are likely to be associated with the grades of injury as a guide:

Grade I

In a Grade I injury, there is stretching and microfailure of some fibres of the ligament, pain, tenderness and swelling at the site of the injury, possibly a mild capsular pattern as the medial collateral ligament is an integral part of the capsule, no notable elongation or clinical instability, and a firm elastic end-feel. Normal valgus laxity 0 to 5 mm in 20 to 30 degrees flexion.

Grade II

Grade II injury is associated with moderate-major tearing of the ligament fibres, some exceeding their elastic limit, pain and tenderness at the site of injury, moderate to severe swelling, movement limited in the capsular pattern, a minor degree of ligamentous laxity noted clinically, and a relatively firm elastic end-feel with a definite endpoint. Valgus stress test applied at 20 degrees flexion 5 to 10 mm.

Grade III

Grade III injury is diagnosed when there is macrofailure, or complete rupture of the ligament, swelling, possibly haemarthrosis and a capsular pattern of limited movement, severe pain at the time of injury, but relatively little since, definite ligamentous laxity noted, and the joint may click as it returns to the neutral position. There is a soft end-feel with no definite endpoint. Valgus stress test at 30 degrees flexion greater than 10 mm.

Not all major ligamentous ruptures require surgical reconstruction, and decisions are based on the lifestyle of the patient or the site of the injury.

Azar (2006) explored the consensus for treatment of Grade III injuries and found that there was a tendency towards non-operative management if the injury was at the femoral attachment of the ligament, with surgical repair for lesions at the tibial insertion. A good functional recovery from ligamentous laxity may be achieved by strengthening the dynamic stabilisers of the knee, the hamstrings and quadriceps muscles, while maintaining control with appropriate braces.

A stepped approach to the management of medial collateral ligament injury is currently recommended. Less invasive treatments are generally offered first, including education/watchful wait, knee bracing, activity and work modification, simple analgesics and NSAIDs medication, physiotherapy (e.g. exercise, mobilisation). If symptoms persist despite good non-surgical management or the patient has a Grade III ligament injury (i.e. ligament rupture), more invasive treatments can be considered, such as surgical repair (Tandogan and Kayaalp, 2016).

Acute Medial Collateral Ligament Injury

Initially, the lesion can be accompanied by a secondary traumatic arthritis that presents with a capsular pattern of limited movement. It may be difficult to apply provocative stress tests to either the ligament or menisci to assess associated damage.

Differential diagnosis of acute medial collateral ligament injury includes an acute flare of medial compartment knee degenerative arthropathy, fracture, infection and acute inflammatory arthritis. However, the history of the mechanism of the injury, the position of the leg and the direction of the forces applied will aid the diagnosis of medial collateral ligament injury. The valgus test will produce pain to confirm diagnosis, but the grade of injury will be difficult to ascertain initially, since the reflex muscle spasm and effusion effectively splint the knee.

The presence of haemarthrosis indicates possible anterior cruciate ligament damage and the Lachman test at least can usually be applied to the acute knee.

The acute situation is managed conservatively with daily treatment initially (preferably), following the guidelines for management of soft tissue lesions (see Chapter 4).

Transverse frictions are started as early as possible, to gain some movement of the ligament over the underlying bone. This is followed by Grade A mobilisation to maintain the function of the ligament.

The patient is encouraged to maintain a normal gait pattern with the aid of crutches if necessary.

Once it is judged that the tensile strength of the healing ligament has improved, the depth of transverse frictions is gradually increased, and the range of active pain-free movement becomes greater, aiming to apply a directional stress to encourage alignment of fibres.

The regime continues until a full range of pain-free movement is restored, always guided by reassessment for a reduction or exacerbation of symptoms.

Other exercises are incorporated as appropriate, aiming towards full rehabilitation of the patient.

TRANSVERSE FRICTIONS FOR ACUTE INJURY OF THE MEDIAL COLLATERAL LIGAMENT

(Cyriax, 1984; Cyriax and Cyriax, 1993)

- Position the patient in half-lying with enough pillows to support the knee in the maximum amount of extension that can be achieved without causing pain.

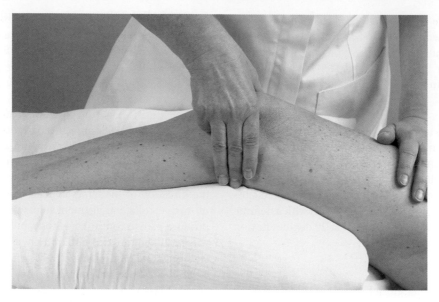

Fig. 11.37 Transverse frictions for acute medial collateral ligament injury, in extension.

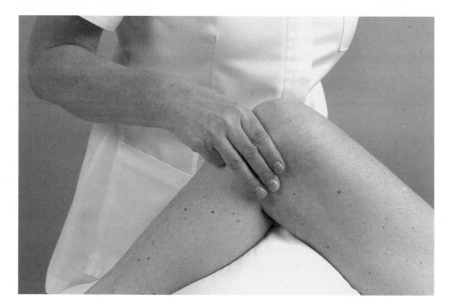

Fig. 11.38 Transverse frictions for acute medial collateral ligament injury, in flexion.

- Palpate for the site of the lesion, which may be difficult to locate due to the swelling. However, the most common site of injury is at the joint line, and this can be located by following the advice given in the surface marking and palpation section earlier in the chapter.

- Place two or three fingers across the site of the lesion and gently apply transverse frictions to achieve an analgesic effect (Fig. 11.37).
- Maintain the technique for an appropriate time, according to the irritability of the lesion and stage of healing, to achieve analgesia and to mobilise the tissues.

- Follow this immediately with Grade A active mobilisation towards extension.
- Next, support the knee in the maximum amount of flexion that can be achieved without pain, and repeat the friction technique as above (Fig. 11.38).
- Follow this immediately with Grade A active exercises towards flexion.

The pain and swelling usually reduce steadily over a few days and the range of movement increases. The knee should not be pushed towards extension as the medial collateral ligament is taut in extension and may become overstretched.

The usual exercises for maintenance of muscle strength should be included together with gait re-education and, eventually, full rehabilitation according to the patient's needs. Treating the ligament in this way maintains its mobility, length and function and should avoid the need to stretch. Active movement of the knee joint is continued.

An uncommon complication of medial collateral ligament injury is Stieda–Pellegrini's syndrome (also known as Pellegrini–Stieda syndrome or Pellegrini–Stieda disease) and this should be considered if the range of movement at the knee fails to improve as expected (Cyriax, 1982). It is believed that, following trauma to the medial collateral ligament, calcium is deposited within the ligament, usually near the superior medial femoral condyle (Wang and Shapiro, 1995).

Chronic Medial Collateral Ligament Injury

The patient has a past history of injury to the ligament that may have largely settled without treatment. However, activity still causes pain and transient swelling around the ligament. On examination, the patient may have end-range pain or limitation of movement of passive flexion, extension or both.

The valgus stress test produces the pain, as may hyperextension and passive lateral rotation – movements that tighten the ligament. Assessment should be made for instability and any associated structural damage of the cruciate ligaments and/or menisci.

Should patients fail to improve, differential diagnosis should be considered, such as medial compartment degenerative arthropathy, inflammatory arthritis, meniscal tear or pes anserine bursitis. Poor foot posture may need to be addressed.

The principle of treatment is to mobilise the ligament with a Grade C manipulation once the ligament has been numbed by transverse frictions. Following manipulation, the patient is instructed to mobilise vigorously in order to maintain the movement gained.

GRADE C MANIPULATION FOR CHRONIC INJURY OF THE MEDIAL COLLATERAL LIGAMENT

(Cyriax, 1984; Cyriax and Cyriax, 1993)

The ligament is prepared for the manipulation with transverse frictions to achieve the analgesic effect. If passive extension is limited, position the patient in half-lying with the knee in maximum extension and locate the site of the lesion by palpation, commonly at the joint line.

- Apply the transverse frictions with the index finger reinforced by the middle finger and the thumb placed on the opposite side of the knee for counterpressure (Fig. 11.39).
- Direct the pressure back against the ligament and sweep transversely across the fibres, keeping the finger parallel to the upper border of the tibia.
- Treatment is applied until analgesia is achieved.

The Grade C manipulation follows immediately after achieving the analgesia.

- Place one hand just above the knee to maintain the thigh on the couch.
- Wrap the other hand around the posterior aspect of the heel.
- Lean on the thigh, lifting the lower leg.
- Once end-range extension is achieved, apply the overpressure by a minimal amplitude, high-velocity thrust applied by side-flexing your body (Fig. 11.40).

If flexion is limited, next place the knee in maximum flexion. The direction of the transverse frictions will have to be adjusted to run parallel to the upper tibia, remembering that the ligament moves backwards a little in flexion (Fig. 11.41).

The Grade C manipulation follows immediately after achieving the analgesic effect by applying an overpressure towards flexion with the knee placed into lateral

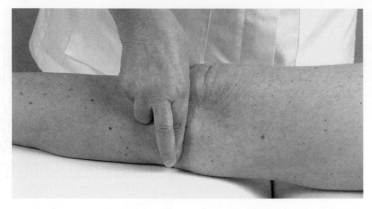

Fig. 11.39 Transverse frictions for chronic medial collateral ligament injury, in extension.

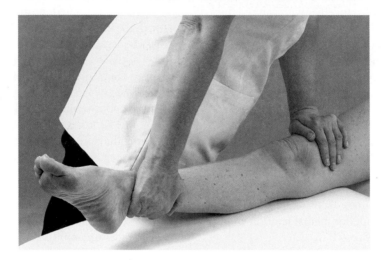

Fig. 11.40 Grade C manipulation into extension.

rotation, to achieve full range, since the insertion of the medial collateral ligament sweeps forward.

- Place the hip and knee into maximum flexion.
- Cup the heel into your hand and place the leg into lateral rotation by resting your forearm along the medial border of the foot (Fig. 11.42a).
- Maintain the lateral rotation and take the leg into maximum passive flexion.
- A minimal amplitude, high-velocity thrust is applied into flexion (see Fig. 11.42b).

The technique can be modified to apply the thrust in the direction of the lateral rotation, or to add a valgus stress if assessment of the patient shows movement to be limited in these directions.

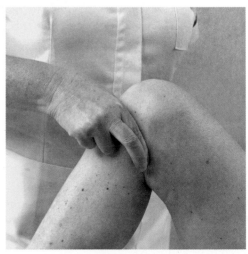

Fig. 11.41 Transverse frictions for chronic medial ligament injury, in flexion.

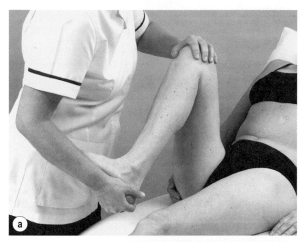

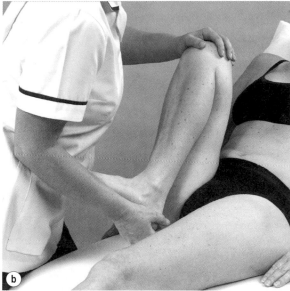

Fig. 11.42 Grade C manipulation into flexion: (a) starting position; (b) completion of the manoeuvre.

CLINICAL TIP

When performing a Grade C peripheral manipulation for appropriate chronic lesions, the transverse frictions are ONLY applied to gain some analgesia.

Treatment of chronic collateral ligament injury is expected to be successful in two or three treatment sessions. It is important that the patient exercises the knee vigorously to maintain the mobility of the ligament.

Coronary Ligaments

The patient presents with a history of rotational strain and on examination there is pain on the appropriate passive rotation.

The coronary ligaments may be involved in a hyperextension injury since the menisci move forwards during extension of the tibiofemoral joint. Ligament injury can coexist with meniscal injury, or the ligaments can be disrupted or stretched rather than the adjacent meniscus itself, which stays intact. This may appear as a floating meniscus on MRI (Bikkina et al., 2005).

The longer lateral coronary ligaments are less vulnerable to trauma than the shorter medial coronary ligaments, and the attachment of the medial meniscus to the deep part of the medial collateral ligament makes the medial aspect of the joint more susceptible to injury.

Injury of the medial coronary ligaments will be discussed, but if the lesion lies in the lateral coronary ligaments, the same principles apply.

An effusion may be present, depending on the severity of the lesion, but this is not usually as obvious as that associated with injury to the collateral or cruciate ligaments.

Injury of the medial coronary ligaments produces pain on passive lateral rotation of the tibia with the tibiofemoral joint at 90 degrees of flexion. Pain may also be provoked by passive extension as the menisci move forwards on the tibia.

Palpation confirms the site of the lesion, which is usually on the superior surface of the anteromedial aspect of the medial meniscus where the coronary ligaments attach the meniscus to the tibial plateau. It is essential that full palpation is conducted, to determine the extent of the lesion.

The treatment of choice is transverse frictions.

TRANSVERSE FRICTIONS TO THE CORONARY LIGAMENTS

- Position the patient comfortably, half-lying with the knee in flexion and lateral rotation to expose the medial tibial condyle.
- Place an index finger reinforced by the middle finger on top of the edge of the medial meniscus at the site of the lesion within the medial coronary ligaments.

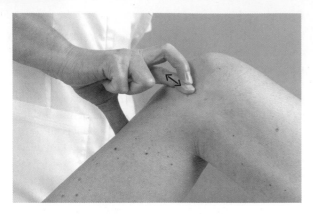

Fig. 11.43 Transverse frictions to the medial coronary ligaments.

- Consider the position of the coronary ligaments that act as oblique 'staples' between the medial meniscus and the edge of the tibial plateau.
- Direct the pressure down onto the ligaments and sweep transversely across the fibres (Fig. 11.43).
- Maintain the technique for an appropriate time, according to the irritability of the lesion and stage of healing, to achieve analgesia and to mobilise the tissues.

Bursitis

Unaccustomed use or overuse can affect any of the bursae around the knee. The patient presents with pain localised to the site of the lesion and there may be local swelling.

The prepatellar and infrapatellar bursae are commonly involved. Bursitis may respond to an injection of corticosteroid, which is normally performed under image guidance, into the bursa. Before injecting, it is important to be sure that no infection is present, since septic bursitis is possible in the superficial bursae.

Pes anserinus syndrome may involve the bursa and/or tendons and the condition can mimic medial collateral ligament injury. Pain and tenderness occur 5 to 6 cm below the medial joint line. This is aggravated by activity and there may be slight swelling and crepitus over the bursal area. General principles of treatment for bursitis and/or tendinopathy may be applied (see Chapter 3).

Excessive friction may cause ITB syndrome, which is a non-traumatic overuse injury involving the ITB and the underlying bursa. It occurs particularly in long-distance runners and cyclists and is often associated with tightness of the ITB (Safran and Fu, 1995; van der Worp et al., 2012; Aderem and Louw, 2015).

Several other aetiologies have been proposed for ITB syndrome, including friction of the ITB against the lateral femoral epicondyle, compression of the fat and connective tissue deep to the ITB, and chronic inflammation of the ITB bursa (Strauss et al., 2011).

Pain is felt laterally, 2 to 3 cm proximal to the knee joint. Aggravating factors are downhill running and climbing stairs. Treatment is mainly nonsurgical and topical anti-inflammatory preparations may be applied.

Other conservative management, including physiotherapy, exercise rehabilitation, education, pacing, ice/heat application, activity modification, myofascial release, deep tissue massage and orthotics can be considered. General treatment principles may be applied (see Chapter 3). In persistent or chronic cases, surgical management can be considered.

CONTRACTILE LESIONS

Quadriceps

Strains of the quadriceps muscle are common and usually happen during jumping, sprinting and kicking, especially if suddenly kicking the ground while playing football, for example.

Complete ruptures of rectus femoris are uncommon but can be suspected if the patient reports a deep tearing sensation at the time of injury and subsequent weakness, out of proportion to the pain experienced. A gap may be palpable initially and an orthopaedic opinion should be sought.

Direct trauma to the quadriceps muscle belly causes swelling and superficial bruising that eventually tracks down the leg. Known in sporting circles as 'cork thigh', it has the potential to develop myositis ossificans traumatica, particularly if the contusion is accompanied by persistent gross limitation of knee flexion (Norris, 2004).

With a quadriceps muscle injury, pain is produced on resisted knee extension and palpation reveals the site of the lesion.

A stepped approach to the management of contractile lesions is currently recommended. Less invasive treatments are generally offered first, including education/watchful wait, activity and work modification, simple analgesics and NSAIDs medication and physiotherapy (e.g. exercise, mobilisation). If symptoms persist, further investigation or onward referral may be required.

Principles of the early management of soft tissue lesions should be applied. Within the musculoskeletal approach, treatment is by transverse frictions.

TRANSVERSE FRICTIONS TO THE QUADRICEPS MUSCLE BELLY

- Position the patient in long-sitting with the knee straight to place the muscle belly in a shortened position.
- Locate the site of the lesion and, using the fingers, apply transverse frictions across the extent of the lesion (Fig. 11.44).
- Maintain the technique for an appropriate time, according to the irritability of the lesion and stage of healing, to achieve analgesia and to mobilise the tissues.
- Follow with Grade A exercises.

Tendinopathy of the Medial and Lateral Quadriceps Expansions

The patient usually presents with a gradual onset of pain felt locally at the front of the knee, normally associated with a change in use. On examination, there is pain on resisted knee extension and tenderness located at the medial, lateral or both borders of the patella. Often the lesion lies at the 'corners' of the patella.

TRANSVERSE FRICTIONS TO THE QUADRICEPS EXPANSIONS

(Cyriax, 1984; Cyriax and Cyriax, 1993)

Having established the site of the lesion, transverse frictions are applied, with consideration for the direction of the fibres.

- Position the patient comfortably with the knee supported and relaxed in extension.
- Push and hold the patella to one side.
- Use the middle finger, reinforced by the index finger, and rotate the forearm to direct the pressure up and under the edge of the patella (Figs 11.45 and 11.46).
- Sweep transversely across the fibres in a superior–inferior direction.

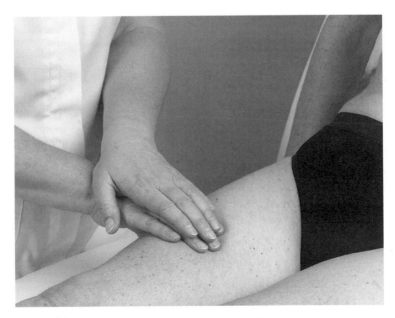

Fig. 11.44 Transverse frictions to the quadriceps muscle belly.

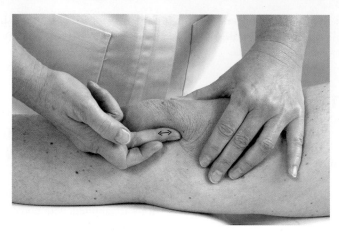

Fig. 11.45 Transverse frictions to the quadriceps expansions, medial.

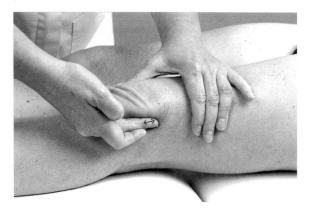

Fig. 11.46 Transverse frictions to the quadriceps expansions, lateral.

- Maintain the technique for an appropriate time, according to the irritability of the lesion and stage of healing, to achieve analgesia and to mobilise the tissues.

It may be necessary to treat several areas around the patella.

Relative rest is advised where functional movements may continue, but no stretching until the structure is pain free on resisted testing.

Lesions of the quadriceps expansions may be secondary to malalignment or abnormal tracking of the patella.

Treatment may be incorporated into a regime of corrective taping and re-education of the oblique portion of vastus medialis, gluteal muscles, etc.

Patellar Tendinopathy

Patellar tendinopathy or jumper's knee is a clinical diagnosis of pain and dysfunction in the patellar tendon. It is distinguished by activity-related anterior knee pain associated with focal patellar tendon tenderness and intra-tendinous imaging changes (Warden and Brukner, 2003).

Normally the patellar tendon is pain free and has the capacity to withstand load, being able to adapt to functional tasks such as jumping and running. However, if excessive load is placed on the tendon, with insufficient rest, pathology may develop. The continuum of tendinopathy suggests that there are three stages of tendinopathy: reactive tendinopathy, tendon disrepair and degenerative tendinopathy (Cook and Purdam, 2009; Leong et al., 2018) See Chapter 3.

For example, reactive tendinopathy can occur with a sudden increase in training, or on returning to normal training after an injury or holiday. If the tendon continues to be excessively loaded, the tendon will progress toward tendon disrepair, which, if overloading continues and the tendon is not allowed to settle, will progress to the final stage of tendon pathology, i.e. degenerative tendinopathy.

Management of patellar tendinopathy relies on understanding the pathophysiology of patellar tendinopathy. A detailed history and assessment are essential to differentiate it from other potential diagnoses of anterior knee pain.

Clinically, the differential diagnosis of patellar tendinopathy is broad, including patellofemoral degenerative arthropathy, meniscal tear, osteochondral lesion, plica syndrome, calcification of the tendon and chondromalacia. Infrapatellar fat pad inflammation (Hoffa's disease) produces symptoms that mimic infrapatellar tendinopathy, but pain is produced by gentle squeezing of the fat pad at either side of the apex of the patella (Curwin and Stanish, 1984; Brukner et al., 2017).

There are two sites for patellar tendinopathy:
- At the apex of the patella (infrapatellar tendon)
- At the base of the patella (suprapatellar tendon)

The most common is infrapatellar tendinopathy and it may be associated with repetitive jumping actions (jumper's knee).

The signs and symptoms are similar to those described for tendinopathy of the quadriceps expansions, but the site of the lesion will be located to either of the infrapatellar or suprapatellar tendons.

In the musculoskeletal medicine approach, treatment of patellar tendinopathy is by transverse frictions followed by progressive loading.

TRANSVERSE FRICTIONS TO THE INFRAPATELLAR AND SUPRAPATELLAR TENDONS; TENO-OSSEOUS JUNCTIONS

(Cyriax, 1984; Cyriax and Cyriax, 1993)

- Position the patient comfortably with the knee relaxed and supported in extension.
- Apply the web space between your index finger and thumb of one hand to the base of the patella, tilting the apex.
- Using the middle finger of the other hand reinforced by the index, supinate the forearm to direct the pressure up under the apex of the patella and sweep transversely across the fibres of the infrapatellar tendon (Fig. 11.47).
- The lesion may be found slightly to either side of the apex. If so, after tilting the patella, angle the finger to friction in line with the edge of the patella.
- Start gently and maintain the technique for an appropriate time, according to the irritability of the lesion and stage of healing, to achieve analgesia and to mobilise the tissues.

Relative rest is advised where functional movements may continue with progressive loading, but no overuse or stretching until the structure is pain free on resisted testing.

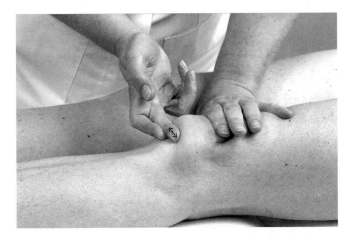

Fig. 11.47 Transverse frictions to the infrapatellar tendon, teno-osseous junction.

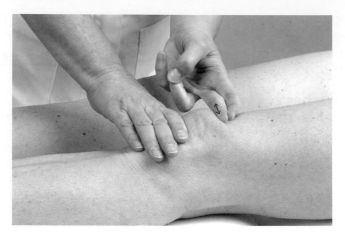

Fig. 11.48 Transverse frictions to the suprapatellar tendon, teno-osseous junction.

For treatment of suprapatellar tendinopathy, the above principles are applied with the base of the patella tilted upwards (Fig. 11.48).

As well as activity modification and biomechanical correction, Brukner et al. (2017) propose that gym-based isometric exercises can provide pain relief and that strengthening strategies should involve the entire kinetic chain, paying attention to the calf and gluteal muscles as well as improving quadriceps strength on the unaffected side.

A review conducted by Rodriguez-Merchan (2013) concluded that physical training, particularly including eccentric exercises, appears to be the treatment of choice for patellar tendinopathy. However, Rudavsky and Cook (2014) warn that adding eccentric exercise as part of rehabilitation for athletes in a high-load environment (e.g. jumping sports such as volleyball or basketball) can be detrimental to the tendon. Decline squat exercises may provoke pain and they can be detrimental when used during a playing season (Brukner et al., 2017).

Other modalities such as ice, taping extracorporeal shock wave therapy, image-guided corticosteroid injections and PRP injections can be used for pain relief. NSAIDs may be useful in the reactive stage of tendinopathy.

The emphasis continues to be on progressive loading in the rehabilitation of tendinopathy. A progressive strengthening programme is appropriate, with the next stage being approached when the previous workload is managed easily, the pain remains under control and the improvement in function is satisfactory (Cook and Purdam, 2009).

Tendinopathy of the Insertions of the Hamstrings

The patient presents with pain localised to the posterior aspect of the knee following a history of overuse. Pain is reproduced by resisted knee flexion and the site of tenderness is located medially or laterally according to the tendons involved.

Principles of treatment can be applied using transverse frictions. Relative rest is advised where functional movements may continue but no stretching until the structure is pain free on resisted testing. An appropriate progressive loading rehabilitation programme should be applied.

Lesions of the hamstrings muscle belly and the tendon of origin are discussed in Chapter 10. Lesions of gastrocnemius are discussed in Chapter 12.

REVIEW QUESTIONS

1. The presence of a haemarthrosis in a knee suggests what?
2. What could synovial thickening mean if found on palpation of the medial joint line? What would be appropriate treatment on this finding?
3. Describe the anatomy of the medial collateral ligament.
4. Giving way can be a symptom of knee pathology. Discuss differential diagnosis.
5. Why is it important to screen the hip joint in a patient presenting with knee pain?

CASE SCENARIOS

Case 1

History

- A 23-year-old ski instructor, Adrian, fell whilst on a night out après ski 5 days ago. He slipped on black ice and twisted his left knee. Pain is over the medial aspect and he was initially unable to bear weight. The knee swelled immediately. Pain and stiffness are worst first thing in the morning and after periods of inactivity. He is taking anti-inflammatories and paracetamol. He is keen to get back to work and is seeking a second opinion on diagnosis as the medical team wants to put his knee in a backslab for 6 weeks.

Examination

- Adrian is walking with crutches; his knee is swollen and slightly warm to touch. He has lost 15 degrees of extension and 30 degrees of flexion. Valgus testing is painful with slight laxity. All other ligament testing normal, unable to test menisci fully at this stage. There is tenderness on palpation over the medial joint line.

Task

- What is the likely primary diagnosis? Review the grading of ligament injury. What is occurring at this stage of the healing process? Discuss the principles of treatment at this stage and home advice?

Case 2

History

- 47-year-old Craig is a fireman and club runner who has a 3-month history of pain in his left infrapatellar tendon following an increase in his mileage. Pain is worse descending stairs, first thing in the morning and running downhill. He has a past history of Osgood–Schlatter's bilaterally.

Examination

- Pain on resisted knee extension and palpation of the inferior pole of the patella.

Task

- Review current thinking on tendon pathology. What advice can you give Craig? Does he need to completely rest the tendon? What are the treatment options? Would you ever consider injecting this?

Case 3

History

- 72-year-old John is a retired head teacher with a 2-week history of pain and 'giving way' in his right knee. A previous X-ray highlighted some degeneration of the medial joint space. There is no pattern to the 'giving way', but he is concerned it happens whilst descending the stairs. He is on medication for high blood pressure and hypercholesterolaemia.

Examination

- Full hip range of movement. A loss of 15 degrees knee flexion with a springy end-feel, full extension with a hard end-feel. All ligament tests are negative and meniscal test ineffective due to the loss of flexion.

Task

- Consider the likelihood of this being a meniscal lesion or loose body. Are there factors that would differentiate between those diagnoses? What would be your treatment protocol for this gentleman?

REFERENCES

Aderem, J., Louw, Q.A., 2015. Biomechanical risk factors associated with iliotibial band syndrome in runners: a systematic review. BMC Musculoskelet. Disord. 16 (1), 1–16.

Adler, G.G., Hoekman, R.A., Beach, D.M., 1995. Drop leg Lachman test. Am. J. Sports Med. 23, 320–323.

Amiel, D., Kuiper, S., Akeson, W.H., 1990. Cruciate ligaments. In: Daniel, D., Akeson, W.H., O'Connor, J.J. (Eds.), Knee Ligaments: Structure, Function, Injury and Repair. Lippincott, Williams & Wilkins, Philadelphia, pp. 365–376.

Azar, F., 2006. Evaluation and treatment of chronic medial collateral ligament injuries of the knee. Sports Med. Arthrosc. Rev. 14 (2), 84–90.

Baker, C.L., 1992. Acute haemarthrosis of the knee. J. Med. Assoc. Ga. 81 (6), 301–305.

Bannuru, R.R., Schmid, C.H., Kent, D.M., et al., 2015. Comparative effectiveness of pharmacologic interventions for knee osteoarthritis: a systematic review and network meta-analysis. Ann. Intern. Med. 162 (1), 46–54.

Barrack, R.L., Skinner, H.B., 1990. The sensory function of knee ligaments. In: Daniel, D., Akeson, W.H., Akeson, W.H. (Eds.), Knee Ligaments: Structure, Function, Injury and Repair. Lippincott, Williams & Wilkins, Philadelphia, pp. 95–112.

Bessette, G.C., 1992. The meniscus. Orthopaedics 15, 35–42.

Bianchi, S., Martinoli, C., 1999. Detection of loose bodies in joints. Radiol. Clin. N. Am. 37 (4), 679–690.

Bikkina, R., Tujo, C., Schraner, A., et al., 2005. The 'floating' meniscus: MRI in knee trauma and implications for surgery. Am. J. Roentgenol. 184, 200–204.

Boles, C.A., Martin, D.F., 2001. Synovial plicae in the knee. Am. J. Roentgenol. 177, 221–227.

Bongers, E., van Kampen, A., van Bokhoven, H., et al., 2005. Human syndromes with congenital anomalies and the underlying defects. Clin. Genet. 68 (4), 302–319.

Bowditch, M., 2001. Anterior cruciate ligament rupture and management. Trauma 3 (4), 246–261.

Bozkurt, M., Yilmaz, E., Atlihan, D., et al., 2003. The proximal tibiofibular joint. Clin. Orthop. Relat. Res. 406, 136–140.

Brotzman, S.B., Wilk, K.E., 2003. Clinical Orthopaedic Rehabilitation, second ed. Mosby, Edinburgh.

Brukner, P., Clarson, B., Cook, J., et al., 2017. Clinical Sports Medicine. In: Injuries, vol. 1, fifth ed. McGraw-Hill, Sydney.

Burks, R.T., 1990. Gross anatomy. In: Daniel, D., Akeson, W.H., O'Connor, J.J. (Eds.), Knee Ligaments: Structure, Function, Injury and Repair. Lippincott, Williams & Wilkins, Philadelphia, pp. 59–75.

Conaghan, P.G., Dickson, J., Grant, R.L., Guideline Development Group. 2008. Care and management of osteoarthritis in adults: summary of NICE guidance. Br. Med. J. 336, 502–503.

Cook, J.L., Purdam, C.R., 2009. Is tendon pathology a continuum? A pathology model to explain the clinical presentation of load-induced tendinopathy. Br. J. Sports Med. 43, 409–416.

Curtin, W., O'Farrell, D., McGoldrick, F., et al., 1992. The correlation between clinical diagnosis of knee pathology and findings in arthroscopy. Irish J. Med. Sci. 161, 135136.

Curwin, S., Stanish, W.D., 1984. Jumper's Knee, Tendinitis – Its Etiology and Treatment. Collamore Press, Massachusetts.

Cyriax, J., 1982. Textbook of Orthopaedic Medicine, eighth ed. Baillière Tindall, London.

Cyriax, J., 1984. Textbook of Orthopaedic Medicine, eleventh ed. Baillière Tindall, London.

Cyriax, J., Cyriax, P., 1993. Cyriax's Illustrated Manual of Orthopaedic Medicine. Butterworth Heinemann, Oxford.

Daniel, D.M., 1990. Diagnosis of a ligament injury. In: Daniel, D., Akeson, W.H., O'Connor, J.J. (Eds.), Knee Ligaments: Structure, Function, Injury and Repair. Lippincott, Williams & Wilkins, Philadelphia, pp. 3–10.

Decary, S., Ouellet, P., Vendittoli, P.A., et al., 2017. Diagnostic validity of physical examination tests for common knee disorders: An overview of systematic reviews and meta-analysis. Phys. Ther. Sport 23, 143–155.

Edwards, D., Villar, R., 1993. Anterior cruciate ligament injury. Practitioner 237, 113–117.

El-Dieb, A., Yu, J.S., Huang, G.-S., et al., 2002. Pathologic conditions of the ligaments and tendons of the knee. Radiol. Clin. N. Am. 40, 1061–1079.

Evans, P., 1986. The Knee Joint. Churchill Livingstone, Edinburgh.

Greenhill, B.J., 1967. The importance of the medial quadriceps expansion in medial ligament injury. Can. J. Surg. 10 (3), 312–317.

Greis, P.E., Bardana, D.D., Holmstrom, M.C., et al., 2002. Meniscal injury, I. Basic science and evaluation. J. Am. Acad. Orthop. Surg. 10 (3), 168–176.

Hartley, A., 1995. Practical Joint Assessment – Lower Quadrant, second ed. Mosby, London.

Hattam, P., Smeatham, A., 2020. Handbook of Special Tests in Musculoskeletal Examination, second ed. Elsevier, Oxford.

Hauger, O., Frank, L.R., Boutin, R.D., et al., 2000. Characterization of the 'red zone' of knee meniscus; MR imaging and histologic correlation. Radiology 217, 193–200.

Hegedus, E.J., Cook, C., Hasselbad, V., et al., 2007. Physical examination tests for assessing a torn meniscus in the knee: a systematic review with meta-analysis. J Orthop. Sports Phys. Ther. 37 (9), 541–550.

Hill, C.L., Gale, D.G., Chaisson, C.R., et al., 2001. Knee effusions, popliteal cysts and synovial thickening: Association with knee pain. J. Rheumatol. 28 (6), 1330–1337.

Huang, W., Zhang, Y., Yao, Z., et al., 2016. Clinical examination of anterior cruciate ligament rupture: a systematic review and meta-analysis. Acta Orthop. Traumatol. Turc. 50 (1), 22–31.

Jacobson, J.A., Lenchik, L., Ruhoy, M.K., et al., 1997. MR imaging of the infrapatellar fat pad of Hoffa. Radiographics 17 (3), 675–691.

Kapandji, I.A., 2019. The Physiology of the Joints: Lower Limb, seventh ed. Churchill Livingstone, Edinburgh.

Katz, J.W., Fingeroth, R.J., 1986. The diagnostic accuracy of ruptures of the anterior cruciate ligament comparing the Lachman test, the anterior drawer sign, and the pivot shift test in acute and chronic knee injuries. Am. J. Sports Med. 14, 88–91.

King, L.K., March, L., Anandacoomarasamy, A., 2013. Obesity & osteoarthritis. Indian J. Med. Res. 138 (2), 185–193.

Leong, H.T., Cook, J., Docking, S., et al., 2018. Physiotherapy management of patellar tendinopathy in tennis players. In: Tennis Medicine. Springer, Cham, pp. 401–413.

McAlindon, T.E., Bannuru, R.R., Sullivan, M.C., et al., 2014. OARSI guidelines for the non-surgical management of knee osteoarthritis. Osteoarthr. Cartil. 22 (3), 363–368.

Malanga, G.A., Andrus, S., Nadler, S.F., et al., 2003. Physical examination of the knee: a review of the original test description and scientific validity of common orthopaedic tests. Arch. Phys. Med. Rehabil. 84, 592–603.

Meserve, B.B., Cleland, J.A., Boucher, T.R., 2008. A meta-analysis examining clinical test utilities for assessing meniscal injury. Clin. Rehabil. 22 (2), 143–161.

Mohan, B., Gosal, H., 2007. Reliability of clinical diagnosis in meniscal tears. Int. Orthop. 31, 57–60.

Nakamura, N., Shino, K., 2005. The clinical problems of ligament healing of the knee. Sports Med. Arthrosc. Rev. 13 (3), 118–126.

National Institute of Arthritis and Musculoskeletal and Skin Diseases, 2021. Health Information: Juvenile Arthritis. http://www.niams.nih.gov/Health_Info/Juv_Arthritis/default.asp. Accessed 18 August 2021.

National Institute for Health and Care Excellence (NICE), 2020. Osteoarthritis: Care and Management. NICE. https://www.nice.org.uk/guidance/cg177. Accessed 5 September 2021.

Nickinson, R., Darrah, C., Donell, S., 2010. Accuracy of clinical diagnosis in patients undergoing knee arthroscopy. Int. Orthop. 34 (1), 39–44.

Nordin, M., Frankel, V.H., 2020. Basic Biomechanics of the Musculoskeletal System, fifth ed. Wolters Kluwer, Philadelphia.

Norris, C.M., 2004. Sports Injuries: Diagnosis and Management for Physiotherapists, third ed. Butterworth Heinemann, Oxford.

Perko, M.M.J., Cross, M.J., Ruske, D., et al., 1992. Anterior cruciate ligament injuries, clues for diagnosis. Med. J. Aust. 157, 467–470.

Pope, T.L., Winston-Salem, N.C., 1996. MR imaging of the knee ligaments. J. South. Orthop. Assoc. 5 (1), 46–62.

Ringdahl, E.N., Pandit, S., 2011. Treatment of knee osteoarthritis. Am. Fam. Physician 83 (11), 1287–1292.

Rodriguez-Merchan, E.C., 2013. The treatment of patellar tendinopathy. J. Orthopaed. Traumatol. 14, 77–81.

Rudavsky, A., Cook, J., 2014. Physiotherapy management of patellar tendinopathy (jumper's knee). J. Physiother. 60, 122–129.

Ryzewicz, M., Peterson, B., Siparsky, P.N., et al., 2007. The diagnosis of meniscus tears: the role of MRI and clinical examination. Clin. Orthop. Relat. Res. 455, 123–133.

Safran, M.R., Fu, F.H., 1995. Uncommon causes of knee pain in the athlete. Orthop. Clin. N. Am. 26 547–259

Saotome, K., Tamai, K., Osada, D., et al., 2006. Histologic classification of loose bodies in osteoarthrosis. J. Orthop. Sci. 11 (6), 607–613.

Saunders, S., 2000. Orthopaedic Medicine Course Manual. Saunders, London.

Schenck, R.C., Heckman, J.D., 1993. Injuries of the knee. Clin. Symp. 45, 2–32.

Schweitzer, M.E., Tran, D., Deely, D.M., et al., 1995. Medial collateral ligament injuries: evaluation of multiple signs, prevalence and location of associated bone bruises, and assessment with MR imaging. Radiology 194 (3), 825–829.

Shaerf, D., Banerjee, A., 2008. Assessment and management of posttraumatic haemarthrosis of the knee. Br. J. Hosp. Med. 69 (8), 459–460. 462–463

Skinner, S., 2012. MRI of the knee. Aust. Fam. Physician 41 (11), 867–869.

Soames, R., Palastanga, N., R., 2018. Anatomy and Human Movement, seventh ed. Elsevier, Oxford.

Speziali, A., Placella, G., Tei, M.M., et al., 2016. Diagnostic value of the clinical investigation in acute meniscal tears combined with anterior cruciate ligament injury using arthroscopic findings as golden standard. Musculoskelet. Surg. 100 (1), 31–35.

Staron, R.B., Haramati, N., Feldman, F., et al., 1994. O'Donaghue's triad: magnetic resonance imaging evidence. Skeletol. Radiol. 23, 633–636.

Strauss, E.J., Kim, S., Calcei, J.G., et al., 2011. Iliotibial band syndrome: evaluation and management. J. Am. Acad. Orthop. Surg. 19 (12), 728–736.

Tandogan, N.R., Kayaalp, A., 2016. Surgical treatment of medial knee ligament injuries: current indications and techniques. EFORT Open Rev. 1 (2), 27–33.

Torg, J.S., Conrad, W., Kalen, V., 1974. Clinical diagnosis of anterior cruciate ligament instability in the athlete. Am. J. Sports Med. 4, 84–93.

Valley, V.T., Shermer, C.D., 2000. Use of musculoskeletal ultrasonography in the diagnosis of pes anserine tendinopathy: a case report. J. Emerg. Med. 20 (1), 43–45.

van der Worp, M.P., van der Horst, N., de Wijer, A., et al., 2012. Iliotibial band syndrome in runners. Sports Med. 42 (11), 969–992.

van Eck, C.F., van den Bekerom, M.P., Fu, F.H., et al., 2013. Methods to diagnose acute anterior cruciate ligament rupture: a meta-analysis of physical examinations with and without anaesthesia. Knee Surg. Sports Traumatol. Arthrosc. 21 (8), 1895–1903.

Wagemakers, H.P., Luijsterburg, P.A., Boks, S.S., et al., 2010. Diagnostic accuracy of history taking and physical examination for assessing anterior cruciate ligament lesions of the knee in primary care. Arch. Phys. Med. Rehabil. 91 (9), 1452–1459.

Wang, J.C., Shapiro, M.S., 1995. Pellegrini–Steida syndrome. Am. J. Orthop. 24 (6), 493–497.

Warden, S.J., Brukner, P., 2003. Patellar tendinopathy. Clin. Sports Med. 22, 743–759.

Woo, S.L.-Y., Wang, C., Newton, P.O., et al., 1990. The response of ligaments to stress deprivation and stress enhancement. In: Daniel, D., Akeson, W.H., O'Connor, J.J. (Eds.), Knee Ligaments: Structure, Function, Injury and Repair. Lippincott, Williams & Wilkins, Philadelphia, pp. 337–350.

The Ankle and Foot

CHAPTER CONTENTS

SUMMARY

This chapter confines itself to common lesions in the ankle and foot arising from arthropathy, trauma or a change in use and begins with a presentation of the relevant anatomy and palpation techniques. Points from the history are considered, and a logical sequence of examination is given, followed by a presentation of lesions and suggestions for treatment and management.

Sprained ankle is a commonly encountered traumatic lesion in musculoskeletal medicine. Mismanagement can lead to a chronic persistent condition and likely recurrence. Other lesions of the foot and ankle can be attributed to faulty biomechanics, which may also lead to adaptive postures in the lower limb and spine, with consequent problems.

ANATOMY

The foot supports body weight and controls posture by maintaining the centre of gravity. It assists propulsion and lift, as well as restraining gait activities and acting as a shock absorber.

Inert Structures

The foot consists of 26 bones and 57 joints that enable it to act as a rigid structure for weight-bearing (e.g. pointing in ballet) or to be converted into a flexible structure for mobility (e.g. gait activities); (Nordin and Frankel, 2020; Fig. 12.1).

A series of arches, ligaments and muscles provides the foot with both strength and mobility. The main joints and ligaments of clinical concern in musculoskeletal

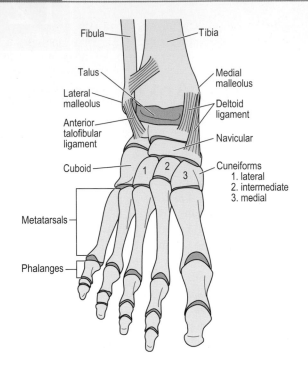

Fig. 12.1 Bones of the ankle and foot, with ankle ligaments.

medicine are described here, followed by a review of the contractile structures.

The *inferior tibiofibular joint* is the articulation between the fibular notch on the lateral aspect of the tibia and the distal end of the fibula. It is considered a syndesmosis because the firm union of the two bones is largely due to the interosseous membrane that extends between the bone shafts. Anterior and posterior ligaments reinforce the joint.

The tibiofibular syndesmosis is established by the *interosseous ligament*, the *posterior inferior tibiofibular ligament* and the *anterior inferior tibiofibular ligament*, which is the weakest of the three. Post-traumatic anterolateral laxity following injury to the anterior talofibular ligament (see below) may lead to anterior extrusion of the talar dome in dorsiflexion, resulting in impingement of the anterior inferior tibiofibular ligament (Bekerom and Raven, 2007).

The deep part of the posterior inferior tibiofibular ligament is the *inferior transverse tibiofibular ligament*, which passes from the tibia into the malleolar fossa of the fibula. It is a thickened band of yellow elastic fibres

forming part of the articulating surface of the ankle joint.

The firm union of the inferior tibiofibular joint is a major factor in the inherent stability of the ankle joint mortise. When the ankle joint is in dorsiflexion, the elastic nature of the inferior tibiofibular joint ligament allows the joint to yield and separate, accommodating the wider anterior aspect of the trochlear surface of the talus. In plantarflexion, the ligament recoils as the narrower posterior aspect of the talus moves into the mortise, approximating the malleoli to maintain a pinch-like grip on the talus.

Dorsiflexion and plantarflexion of the ankle will induce small accessory movements in the inferior tibiofibular joint, affecting the superior tibiofibular joint. Injuries of the syndesmosis usually involve forced dorsiflexion, causing widening or diastasis of the ankle mortise (Edwards and DeLee, 1984; Boytim et al., 1991; Marder, 1994). However, isolated injuries are uncommon, and damage usually occurs associated with other major ligamentous disruption and fracture.

The *ankle joint (talocrural joint)* is a uniaxial, synovial hinge joint between the mortise, formed by the distal ends of the tibia and fibula, including the malleoli and the dome of the talus. Its function is complex, with the talocrural, subtalar and inferior tibiofibular joints working together to allow coordinated movement of the rear foot (Hertel, 2002).

The ankle bears more weight per unit area than any other joint, and any malalignment or instability may lead to degenerative changes (Sartoris, 1994).

The joint surfaces are covered with hyaline cartilage and surrounded by a fibrous capsule that attaches to the margins of the articulating surfaces. The capsule is lined with synovium and reinforced by strong collateral ligaments.

The congruity of the articular surfaces during loading of the joint, the static ligamentous control and the dynamic control of the musculotendinous units all contribute to the stability of the ankle joint (Hertel, 2002).

Movement at the ankle joint occurs about a transverse axis in a sagittal plane, with approximately 20 degrees of dorsiflexion and 35 degrees of plantarflexion, allowing the foot to adjust to different surfaces.

Dorsiflexion achieves the close-packed position of the ankle joint, and no movement of the talus in the mortise should be possible in this position. In full plantarflexion, the loose-packed position, a small amount of side-to-side movement of the talus is usually possible.

The collateral ligaments are roughly triangular in their attachments, radiating downward from the malleoli to a wide base. Each has anterior and posterior components that link with the talus and a central component that links with the calcaneus.

The *medial collateral (deltoid) ligament* forms a strong multiligamentous complex spreading from the apex and anterior and posterior borders of the medial malleolus in a fan shape over the medial aspect of the ankle joint (Fig. 12.2). It has a continuous line of attachment from the navicular in front, along the sustentaculum tali to the talus behind, and has superficial and deep fibres. It is crossed by the tendons of tibialis posterior and flexor digitorum.

As the medial collateral ligament offers such strong support to the medial aspect of the ankle joint, traumatic injuries more commonly cause fracture and disruption of the syndesmosis rather than ligamentous injury. Most strain on the ligament occurs with a dorsiflexion and eversion stress. However, biomechanical problems in the foot can lead to a gradual-onset overuse lesion of the medial collateral ligament, and treatment should be directed to the cause.

The *lateral collateral ligament* consists of three separate bands crossing the lateral aspect of the ankle joint. The contribution of the individual lateral ligaments to ankle joint stability is not constant but depends on the ankle and foot position in space. Forced inversion of the plantarflexed foot commonly affects the lateral collateral ligament (Liu and Jason, 1994; Lee and Maleski, 2002).

The components of the lateral collateral ligament are as follows (Fig. 12.3):
• The *anterior talofibular ligament* is an integral part of the capsule of the ankle joint. It arises from the anterior border and tip of the lateral malleolus and passes deeply and anteromedially across the ankle joint to the neck of the talus in the sinus tarsi. It is a wide, flattened band approximately the width of the patient's index finger.

In the anatomical position, the ligament runs almost parallel to the transverse axis of the foot, while in plantarflexion it runs more parallel to the vertical axis of the leg. In this position of plantarflexion, the ligament is most likely to be sprained, particularly if the foot is inverted (Kannus and Renstrom, 1991; Kumai et al., 2002). It is the most vulnerable of the three components to a forced

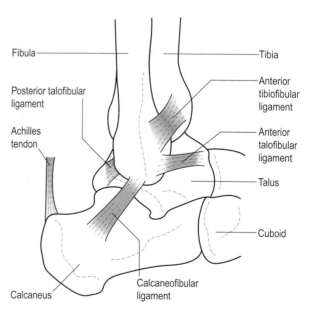

Fig. 12.2 Medial collateral ligament of the ankle joint.

Fig. 12.3 Lateral collateral ligament of the ankle.

plantarflexion and inversion injury (Colville et al., 1990; Hertel, 2002).

- The *calcaneofibular ligament* is a narrow cord separate from the capsule of the ankle joint. It arises from the apex of the lateral malleolus and passes obliquely inferoposteriorly, under the peroneal tendons, to attach to the calcaneus just behind the peroneal tubercle. Here it is closely related to the overlying peroneal sheath containing the tendons of peroneus longus and brevis (Marder, 1994; Miller and Bosco, 2002).

  This component of the ligament crosses both the ankle and subtalar joints and is vulnerable to varus stress; it is taut in dorsiflexion and is most likely to be sprained with forced inversion in dorsiflexion (Colville et al., 1990).

- The *posterior talofibular ligament* is a strong, thick band arising from the posterior border of the lateral malleolus and passing horizontally and posteromedially to the posterior aspect of the talus. Clinically, it is rare to find involvement of this ligament in lateral ligament injuries.

During weight-bearing, stability is maintained by the bony congruency of the mortise. The anterior talofibular ligament has the weakest tensile strength with a load to failure two to three-and-a-half times lower than that of the calcaneofibular ligament, which is rarely injured in isolation (Boruta et al., 1990; Miller and Bosco, 2002).

The *subtalar joint* is a functional unit that includes the talocalcaneal joint posteriorly and part of the talocalcaneonavicular joint anteriorly. Their joint capsules are separated by the sinus tarsi (a narrow tunnel running obliquely forwards and laterally between the talus and the calcaneus).

The subtalar joint works in conjunction with the ankle and midtarsal joints to allow the foot to adapt to the surface of stance and provide shock absorbance. The joints together allow adjustment of the arches of the foot and, in conjunction with muscle activity, provide spring and propulsion to gait. During walking, the subtalar joint adapts to the side-to-side slope of the ground, accompanied by secondary rotation of the tibia (Evans, 1990).

Medial, lateral, cervical and interosseous ligaments stabilise the subtalar joint. The interosseous ligament sits within the sinus tarsi and forms a barrier between the two joint capsules. This division of the subtalar joint has implications for injection of the joint, which is discussed on page 406.

Movements at the subtalar joint are complex due to the shape of the articulating facets, which allow a degree of play to occur simultaneously in three planes. It is quite common to use the terms *supination* and *inversion* interchangeably and *pronation* and *eversion* interchangeably.

Supination is a tri-planar combination of inversion, plantarflexion and adduction, and pronation is a combination of eversion, dorsiflexion and abduction. When the talocalcaneal part of the subtalar joint is considered in combination with the talocalcaneonavicular joint, the movements may be reasonably described as pronation and supination. As a synovial plane joint, the *talocalcaneal joint* in isolation allows only inversion and eversion of the foot (Moore et al., 2017).

The *talocalcaneonavicular joint*, the anterior part of the subtalar joint, is supported by the *spring ligament* (otherwise known as the plantar calcaneonavicular ligament), which spans the gap between the sustentaculum tali on the calcaneus and the navicular below the talar head.

The talocalcaneonavicular joint, can be visualised as a ball-and-socket joint, with the head and lower surface of the neck of the talus as the ball. The osseoligamentous socket supports the head of the talus and is formed by the navicular anteriorly, the sustentaculum tali and calcaneus posteriorly and the spring ligament.

The *midtarsal (transverse tarsal) joints* consist of the talocalcaneonavicular joint medially and the calcaneocuboid joint laterally. These joints together adapt the posture of the foot, keeping the sole in contact with the ground, whatever the slope of the surface or the position of the leg. Together with the ankle and subtalar joints, they act as a shock absorber and provide elasticity and spring to gait.

The *calcaneocuboid joint* is supported by the *dorsal calcaneocuboid ligament*, which is a capsular ligament that runs along the dorsolateral aspect of the joint, and the *plantar calcaneocuboid* (short plantar) and the *long plantar ligaments* (Levangie et al., 2019; Soames and Palastanga, 2018). The dorsal calcaneocuboid ligament can be involved in an inversion sprain of the ankle, as it resists inversion and adduction of the midtarsal joint.

391 Navigation: CHAPTER 12 The Ankle and Foot

Movements at the midtarsal joint (calcaneocuboid and talocalcaneonavicular joint complex) do not occur in isolation (Levangie et al., 2019; Soames and Palastanga, 2018). Accessory movements at the midtarsal joints consist of dorsiflexion and plantarflexion, abduction and adduction and inversion and eversion.

There are medial, lateral and transverse arches that support the foot.

The foot's medial and lateral longitudinal arches are supported posteriorly by the calcaneus and anteriorly by the metatarsal heads. The talus forms the summit of each arch.

- The *medial longitudinal arch* is the larger of the two and has a dynamic role in gait. It consists of the calcaneus, talus, navicular, the cuneiforms and three medial metatarsals. It absorbs and transmits weight backwards through the calcaneus and forwards to the metatarsal heads while providing elasticity for propulsion.
- The *lateral longitudinal arch* has a static role in weight-bearing. It is lower than the medial, making contact with the ground throughout its length to support load in standing. The main supporting mechanism for the longitudinal arches is the plantar fascia (see below). Acting as a cable between the heel and the toes, it locks the joints of the foot and prevents the arches from collapsing during weight-bearing.
- The *transverse arch* is formed by the distal row of tarsal bones and the bases of the metatarsals and acts to support and transmit body weight. As body weight is applied, the metatarsal bones separate and flatten slightly.

The arches of the foot depend on ligamentous and muscular support. The important ligaments are the long and short plantar ligaments, plantar fascia and the spring ligament (plantar calcaneonavicular ligament).

The intrinsic muscles of the foot also maintain the arches, together with some of the long muscles of the leg. Tibialis anterior supports the medial arch, while peroneus longus supports the lateral arch.

The *plantar fascia* (plantar aponeurosis) is a strong structure on the plantar surface of the foot, which, together with the midtarsal ligaments and intrinsic and extrinsic muscles, withstands loading during weight-bearing (Fig.12.4). In addition to its role in supporting the medial longitudinal arch of the foot, it may also have a role in proprioception and peripheral motor coordination (Stecco et al., 2013).

It consists of three variably developed components known as central, medial and lateral cords. The central cord is biomechanically the most important, arising from the medial side of the medial calcaneal tuberosity and consisting of mainly longitudinally arranged fibres of collagen and elastin. The fibres pass distally into the forefoot, widening and thinning before dividing into five distinct bands that extend into the toes (Karr, 1994; Yu, 2000).

The plantar fascia is rich in hyaluronan (Stecco et al., 2013). At its insertion into the calcaneal tuberosity (the enthesis), it has a thickened 'cuff' similar in appearance to the rotator cuff of the shoulder (Yu, 2000). This strong connecting cable passing between the pillars of the longitudinal arch has little ability to lengthen, but under loading 'gives' slightly to act as a shock absorber. The plantar fascia has a close relationship with the paratenon of the Achilles tendon through the periosteum of the heel (Stecco et al., 2013).

The *retrocalcaneal bursa* lies between the distal end of the Achilles tendon, near its insertion, and the superoposterior surface of the calcaneus (Stephens, 1994; Bottger et al., 1998). It is variously described as

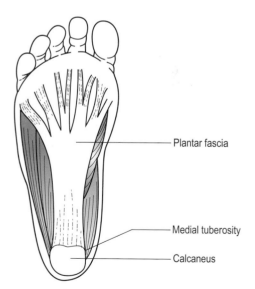

Fig. 12.4 Plantar fascia.

Plantar fascia

Medial tuberosity

Calcaneus

saddle-shaped, horseshoe-shaped or shaped like an inverted boomerang. It rests against the Achilles fat pad superiorly and blends with the Achilles tendon posteriorly (Frey et al., 1992).

Bottger et al. (1998) demonstrated the normal retrocalcaneal bursa to be 1 mm in an anterior–posterior dimension, 6 mm in the transverse dimension and 3 mm in the craniocaudal dimension, but bursal dimensions greater than these were seen in symptomatic subjects.

The nerve supply of the ankle joint is derived from nerve roots L4 -S2 by branches from the deep fibular (peroneal) nerve, as well as from the tibial and sural nerves.

Contractile Structures

The numerous tendons crossing the ankle joint complex contribute to dynamic stability as well as producing movement of the various joints. As tendons cross the ankle joint, they change their direction from running vertically to horizontally. Several retinacula (bands of connective tissue) prevent the tendons from bowstringing under activity, while synovial sheaths protect the tendons as they pass under the retinacula.

The talus provides attachment for ligaments, and many tendons pass over it, although it does not itself give insertion to any contractile unit.

All anterior muscles of the lower leg are supplied by the deep peroneal nerve, and their principal function is dorsiflexion of the ankle and extension of the toes.

Tibialis anterior (L4–L5) takes origin from the upper two-thirds of the lateral tibial shaft and adjacent interosseous membrane. It becomes tendinous in its lower third, passing across the anteromedial aspect of the ankle joint to insert into the medial aspect of the medial cuneiform and the base of the first metatarsal (Fig. 12.5).

Its function is to dorsiflex the ankle during the swing-through phase of gait and to invert the foot. It raises the medial longitudinal arch and works in conjunction with other muscles to counteract gravity and control foot placement.

Tibialis anterior runs a relatively straight course and is not a common cause of pain. However, hill running or irritation from tight-fitting boots, for example, may cause lesions of the muscle or tendon (Frey and Shereff, 1988; Chandnani and Bradley, 1994).

Extensor hallucis longus (L5, S1) takes origin from the middle of the anteromedial border of the fibula and passes downwards and medially to a tendon that inserts into the base of the distal phalanx of the hallux. Functionally it dorsiflexes the ankle and extends the hallux to enable the big toe and foot to clear the ground during the swing-through phase.

Extensor digitorum longus (L5, S1) takes origin from the upper two-thirds of the anterior aspect of the fibula and passes downwards under the extensor retinacula, dividing into four tendons that insert into the dorsal digital expansions of the lateral four toes (Fig. 12.5).

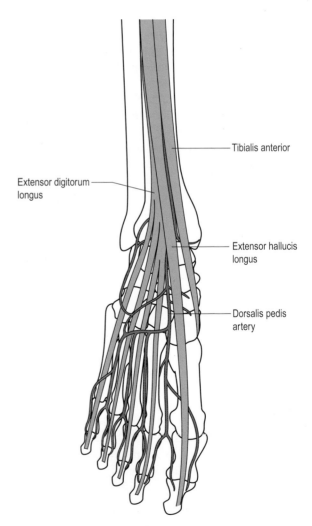

Tibialis anterior

Extensor digitorum longus

Extensor hallucis longus

Dorsalis pedis artery

Fig. 12.5 Anterior aspect of the ankle.

Functionally, it assists dorsiflexion of the ankle and extends the lateral four toes to clear the ground during the swing-through phase.

Peroneus tertius (L5, S1), a divorced part of extensor digitorum longus, arises from the lower anterolateral aspect of the fibula and inserts into the base of the fifth metatarsal. It functions as a weak dorsiflexor of the ankle and an evertor of the foot.

The peroneal tendons pass under two retinacula to reach the lateral side of the foot. The principal function of the lateral muscles is to evert the foot, controlling side-to-side movements in standing and acting as the primary lateral dynamic stabilisers of the ankle (Frey and Shereff, 1988).

Peroneus longus, together with tibialis anterior, forms a stirrup for the foot, maintaining and supporting the arches. Both peroneus longus and brevis are supplied by the superficial peroneal nerve.

Peroneus longus (L5, S1-2) is the main evertor of the foot and causes the foot's medial side to move downwards, as in plantarflexion and eversion. It is the more superficial of the two peroneal tendons and arises from the head and upper lateral two-thirds of the fibula. It becomes tendinous just above the ankle and passes behind the lateral malleolus in a sheath it shares with peroneus brevis (Fig. 12.6).

Continuing, it crosses the lateral surface of the calcaneus, passing below the peroneal tubercle, where it leaves peroneus brevis. It occupies a groove on the lateral and plantar surfaces of the cuboid and crosses the sole obliquely to insert into the lateral side of the base of the first metatarsal and adjacent medial cuneiform.

Peroneus brevis (L5, S1–S2) also produces eversion and plantarflexion (Soames and Palastanga, 2018). It arises from the lower lateral surface of the fibula and lies in front of peroneus longus as the tendons pass behind the lateral malleolus in the common sheath. It crosses the calcaneus above the peroneal tubercle to insert into the base of the fifth metatarsal (Fig. 12.6).

Generally, the more superficial posterior muscles are concerned mainly with plantarflexion of the ankle, while the deep muscles flex the toes. Both groups are supplied by the tibial nerve.

Gastrocnemius (S1–S2) is the most superficial of the posterior muscles and gives the calf its characteristic shape. It has two heads of origin from the appropriate posterior femoral condyle. The medial head is larger, extends more distally and is a common site for muscle belly injuries (Fig. 12.7).

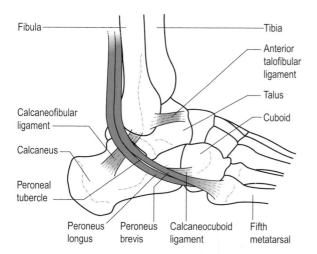

Fig. 12.6 Structures of the lateral aspect of the ankle.

Fibula — Tibia
Anterior talofibular ligament
Talus
Cuboid
Calcaneofibular ligament
Calcaneus
Peroneal tubercle
Peroneus longus — Peroneus brevis — Calcaneocuboid ligament — Fifth metatarsal

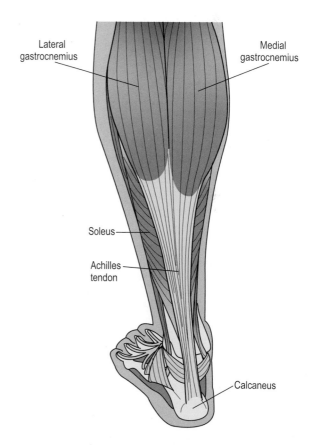

Fig. 12.7 Posterior aspect of the ankle.

Lateral gastrocnemius — Medial gastrocnemius
Soleus
Achilles tendon
Calcaneus

The two muscle heads come together in a broad tendon joined on the anterolateral side by soleus, forming the Achilles tendon. Functionally, gastrocnemius flexes the knee and plantarflexes the ankle.

Soleus (S1–S2) lies deep to gastrocnemius, arising from the upper posterior aspect of the fibula and soleal line of the tibia. The muscle fibres blend into a membranous tendon that lies deep to gastrocnemius, allowing both muscles to function individually. These tendon fibres then merge with the Achilles tendon (Fig. 12.7).

Plantaris (S1–S2) arises from the posterior aspect of the lateral supracondylar ridge of the femur and descends medially to blend with the Achilles tendon. Its function is to assist gastrocnemius.

Gastrocnemius, soleus and plantaris (not shown) form a functional group known as *triceps surae*. Gastrocnemius works with plantaris to flex the knee and plantarflex the foot, providing propulsion to the push-off phase of gait.

Soleus works continuously as a postural muscle through its slow-twitch muscle fibres, maintaining an upright posture (Abrahams, 2019). In standing, the ankle is in a loose-packed position with the centre of gravity falling anterior to the joint. Soleus counteracts the tendency for body weight to move forwards over the stationary foot (Standring, 2015).

The *Achilles tendon* is a long tendon that receives the fibres of gastrocnemius and soleus. It is about 15 cm long (Standring, 2015) is up to 1.5 cm wide and less than 1 cm in anteroposterior thickness (Chandnani and Bradley, 1994; Fig.12.7). It is surrounded by a *paratenon*, a thin gliding membrane, that permits free movement of the tendon within the surrounding tissues. Its insertion into the calcaneus is cushioned by two bursae: the retrocalcaneal bursa on its deep surface and the subcutaneous Achilles bursa on its superficial surface (Smart et al., 1980).

The Achilles tendon has the capacity to withstand high tensional forces, with forces of 12.5 times body weight recorded (Alfredson and Lorentzon, 2000). The tendon consists of approximately 95% type I collagen fibres and elastin embedded in a matrix of proteoglycans and water. The collagen fibres adopt a wavy 'crimp' configuration at rest, and the collagen fibres straighten out as the initial response to tension and activity (Freedman et al., 2014).

The tendon fibres twist as they pass down to their insertion into the middle of the posterior surface of the calcaneus. This twist in the tendon fibres is understood to enhance the tendon's elastic properties, the stored energy providing propulsion to lift the heel during walking, running and jumping activities (Norris, 2004).

The blood supply to the tendon is from the musculotendinous junction, the teno-osseous junction and the surrounding paratenon (Paavola et al., 2002). The tendon has a zone of relatively poor vascularity 2 to 6 cm above its insertion and is prone to overuse, degeneration and rupture, particularly at this site (Chandnani and Bradley, 1994; Pufe et al., 2001; Alfredson et al., 2002).

Tibialis posterior (L4–L5) arises from the upper posterolateral surface of the tibia. It passes behind the medial malleolus in its own sheath, crosses the deltoid ligament and inserts into the tuberosity of the navicular (Fig. 12.8). It sends tendinous slips onto every tarsal bone except the talus. Functionally it is the main invertor of the foot, working with tibialis anterior.

The tibialis posterior muscle is a dynamic stabiliser during the late midstance and push-off phase of walking/running, locking the joints in the mid- and hindfoot (Van de Velde et al., 2017). It gives support to the arches of the foot through its many tendinous insertions

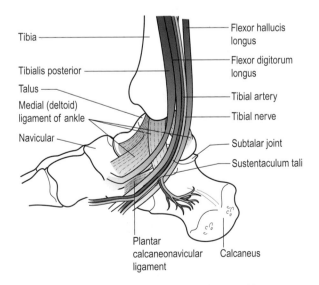

Fig. 12.8 Medial aspect of the ankle.

and decelerates pronation after heel contact (Blake et al., 1994).

Flexor digitorum longus (S2–S3) arises from the middle of the posterior surface of the tibia and passes downwards, becoming tendinous above the ankle joint (Fig. 12.8).

Behind the medial malleolus, it is medial to tibialis posterior and occupies the groove under the sustentaculum tali. Dividing into four tendons, it inserts into the base of the distal phalanx of the lateral four toes.

Functionally, flexor digitorum longus works with the lumbricals to keep the pads of the toes in contact with the ground, increasing the weight-bearing surface. It also assists plantarflexion during the toe-off phase of gait, and repeated push-off activity may cause injury to this tendon (Frey and Shereff, 1988).

The *lumbricals* (S2–S3) arise from flexor digitorum longus tendons and insert into the dorsal digital expansions. They flex the metatarsophalangeal joints and extend the interphalangeal joints; this counteracts the clawing tendency of the flexor digitorum longus. Working together, they maintain the medial arch.

Flexor hallucis longus (S2–S3) arises from the lower posterior surface of the fibula and passes behind the medial malleolus and under the sustentaculum tali to insert into the base of the distal phalanx of the big toe.

It functions to provide the final thrust for toe-off and is important in supporting the medial longitudinal arch. Activities that involve repeatedly pushing off from the forefoot (e.g. ballet, dancing and running) may cause flexor hallucis longus pain and dysfunction (Frey and Shereff, 1988; Newman et al., 2021).

A GUIDE TO SURFACE MARKING AND PALPATION

Medial Aspect

Palpate the short, thick, *medial tibial malleolus*, appreciating that the apex, anterior and posterior borders are all subcutaneous (Fig. 12.8). Compare this with the longer, slender, *lateral fibular malleolus*, which tends to project further distally and lies slightly more posteriorly.

It is difficult to palpate the individual tendons lying behind the medial malleolus, but from medial to lateral, they are **t**ibialis posterior, flexor **d**igitorum longus

and flexor **h**allucis longus (**T**om, **D**ick and **H**arry). The posterior tibial **a**rtery and tibial **n**erve lie between flexor digitorum longus and flexor hallucis longus. The mnemonic can go further to make it **T**om, **D**ick **a**nd **N**aughty **H**arry.

You can palpate the *posterior tibial pulse* by applying light pressure approximately halfway between the medial malleolus and the Achilles tendon.

Consider the triangular *medial collateral (deltoid) ligament*, which fans down from the medial malleolus to attach by a broad base from the navicular in front to the talus behind.

Palpate upwards from the sole to find the *sustentaculum tali* lying approximately one thumb's width directly below the medial malleolus, where it feels like a horizontal, bony shelf.

Move directly forwards from the sustentaculum tali to the next palpable bony bump, the *tuberosity of the navicular*. This gives insertion to *tibialis posterior*. Move directly forwards from the navicular to palpate the *medial cuneiform* and the *base of the first metatarsal*.

Anterior Aspect

Place the ankle joint into plantarflexion and inversion, making the *talus* visible and palpable anterior to the lateral malleolus (Fig. 12.5). Palpate along from the anterior aspect of the lateral malleolus and the lower margin of the tibia to the anterior aspect of the medial malleolus to identify the *ankle joint line*.

Move to the front of the lateral malleolus and feel the depression on the lateral side of the talus; this marks the entrance to the *sinus tarsi* (the narrow tunnel that runs between the talus and calcaneus in front of the subtalar joint).

Palpate the tibialis anterior, extensor hallucis longus, extensor digitorum longus and peroneus tertius tendons (from medial to lateral) as they cross the ankle joint anteriorly.

Palpate the *dorsalis pedis pulse* approximately halfway between the malleoli on the dorsum of the foot, just lateral to the tendon of extensor hallucis longus.

Posterior Aspect

Palpate the *calcaneus*, the largest of the tarsal bones, which forms the bony prominence of the heel (Fig. 12.9).

Palpate the *medial tuberosity of the calcaneus*, which can be located at the posteromedial edge of the plantar surface of the calcaneus; deep palpation may be necessary. This marks the insertion of the central cord of the plantar fascia (Fig. 12.9).

Locate the insertion of the *Achilles tendon* into the middle third of the posterior surface of the calcaneus. Palpate the Achilles tendon, appreciating its thickness, and follow the tendon up to the two fleshy bellies of the gastrocnemius; the medial belly should be felt to extend further distally than the lateral.

Lateral Aspect

Palpate the *lateral malleolus* (Fig. 12.6). Move approximately one finger's width below it and slightly anteriorly to locate the *peroneal tubercle* (Fig. 12.6). This tubercle varies in size and position, so it may not be obvious. It divides the tendons of peroneus longus and brevis.

Consider the individual components of the lateral collateral ligament, which take origin from the lateral malleolus (see Fig. 12.6):

- The *anterior talofibular ligament* is approximately the width of an index finger, and it passes deeply, anteromedially to the talus. Its fibres run roughly parallel to the sole of the foot, and it may be palpated in the region of the sinus tarsi.
- The *calcaneofibular ligament* passes obliquely downwards and backwards, under the peroneal tendons.
- The *posterior talofibular ligament* passes horizontally backwards to attach to the posterior talus; it is difficult to palpate.

Palpate the *base of the fifth metatarsal* and appreciate its prominent tubercle, which gives attachment to peroneus brevis (Fig. 12.6).

To palpate the calcaneocuboid joint line and dorsal calcaneocuboid ligament:
- Place a thumb vertically behind the base of the fifth metatarsal with the interphalangeal joint in line with the sole. A line bisecting the thumbnail will indicate the approximate position of the *calcaneocuboid joint line*.
- Place a finger transversely across the tip of the thumb to form a 'T'. The top cross-bar of the T is now resting over the dorsal aspect of the joint, indicating the approximate position of the *dorsal calcaneocuboid ligament*.

Position your hand to resist eversion of the foot to help palpate the two lateral tendons, *peroneus longus and brevis*, on the lateral aspect of the ankle. Behind the lateral malleolus, peroneus brevis lies in front of longus. They divide at the peroneal tubercle, with brevis running above the tubercle and longus below (Fig. 12.6).

COMMENTARY ON THE EXAMINATION

Observation

Before proceeding with the history, a general observation of the patient's *face, posture and gait* will alert the examiner to abnormalities, particularly the gait pattern.

History

The patient's *age, occupation, sports, hobbies and activities* may indicate the cause of the lesion and alert the

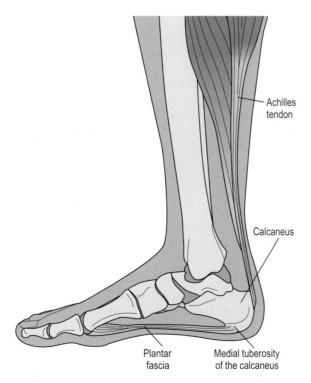

Fig. 12.9 Posterior structures of the ankle.

practitioner to possible biomechanical or postural problems.

The *site and spread* of pain help to localise the lesion, but, as a peripheral joint, pain is usually well localised. The presence of paraesthesia in the foot, or pain in the calf or shin, could suggest a more proximal lesion, radiculopathy or peripheral neuropathy.

The *onset* of the symptoms may be sudden, due to trauma, or gradual, associated with change in use or arthropathy. If the onset is traumatic, the mechanism of injury should be established, particularly to indicate the ligaments involved. A 'snap' or 'popping' sensation at onset may indicate rupture of a tendon or a ligament or fracture.

The *duration* of symptoms indicates the stage of the lesion in the healing process. A history of recurrent episodes indicates possible instability, requiring in-depth biomechanical assessment.

The *symptoms and behaviour* need to be considered. The behaviour of the pain indicates the nature of the lesion: mechanical lesions are eased by rest and aggravated by activity and weight-bearing.

A minor injury is indicated by minimal pain and localised swelling, with the ability to continue weight-bearing activities. More severe injuries will produce diffuse swelling and an inability to weight-bear, suggesting ligamentous rupture or fracture.

Other symptoms described by the patient could include the ankle giving way; this is a symptom of ligamentous instability or possible loose body in the joint. A 'clicking' or 'snapping' sensation on the lateral aspect of the ankle could be due to disruption of the peroneal retinaculum, allowing subluxation of the tendons.

An indication of *medical history, other joint involvement and medications* will aid diagnosis and establish whether contraindications to treatment techniques exist. Rheumatoid arthritis may affect the small joints of the foot.

Practitioners should routinely *screen* for psychosocial factors and consider relevant health co-morbidities and lifestyle factors (see Chapter 1). These factors may contribute to patients' presenting condition or form a barrier to their recovery and normal function, which should be addressed as an integral part of patient management.

In addition to medical history, establish any ongoing conditions and treatment. Explore other previous or current musculoskeletal problems with previous episodes of the current complaint, any treatment given and the outcome of treatment.

Inspection

Inspection should be conducted in both weight-bearing and non-weight-bearing postures.

Bony deformity and functional abnormalities of the medial arch, in particular, will usually be seen in the weight-bearing position.

Check the height of the medial and longitudinal arches. Pes planus is a structural flat foot visible in both weight-bearing and non-weight-bearing positions, while a functional flat foot is only observed on weight-bearing.

The presence of functional flat foot can be estimated by looking for a difference in the height of the medial longitudinal arch in the non-weight-bearing and weight-bearing positions. Estimate the distance between the tuberosity of the navicular and the ground, first in a non-weight-bearing sitting position and second in the standing weight-bearing position (Evans, 1990).

Observe the position of both Achilles tendons from behind for any asymmetry and deviation from the normal straight alignment, which may indicate postural deformity and poor biomechanics. Look for redness, thickening and/or swelling at the Achilles insertion, which may suggest insertional tendinopathy.

Although it is important to note postural abnormalities of the foot, this should be relevant to the patient's presenting signs and symptoms. A detailed biomechanical assessment is unnecessary for uncomplicated lesions, but recurrent symptoms or failure to resolve the patient's symptoms may require referral to a podiatrist or a physiotherapy specialist in lower limb biomechanics.

Abnormal callus formation indicates abnormal weight-bearing. It is worth inspecting the patient's shoes for irregular areas of weight-bearing. This is particularly relevant to athletes and should include their training shoes. In a normal gait pattern, wear is seen on the lateral side of the heel and the medial side of the forefoot (Kannus, 1992).

Camber running or worn out or incorrect training shoes can alter angles of contact between the foot and the ground and be an external cause of overuse (Evans, 1990). Advice will need to be given regarding the type of shoe best suited to the patient's activities (Brukner et al., 2017).

Colour changes such as cyanosis, erythema or pallor may indicate circulatory involvement, and a change in

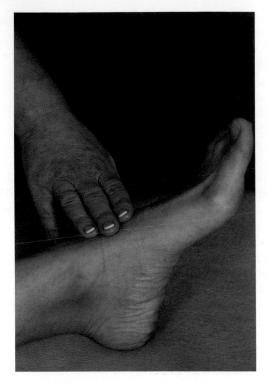

Fig. 12.10 Palpation for dorsalis pedis pulse.

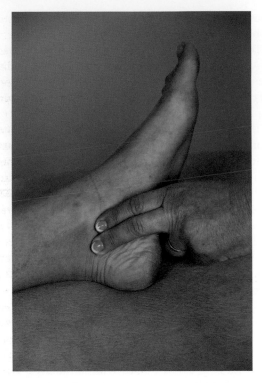

Fig. 12.11 Palpation for posterior tibial artery.

colour in transferring from the weight-bearing to the non-weight-bearing position should be further investigated by palpating for the presence of arterial pulses (Figs 12.10 and 12.11).

Bruising is often associated with a recently sprained ankle or gastrocnemius muscle belly lesion and tracks distally. A severe sprain of the ankle can cause traction injury of the superficial peroneal nerve and vascular structures. Consideration should be given to these possibilities if changes in skin colour persist (Acus and Flanagan, 1991).

Muscle wasting may be seen in the calf or peroneal muscles.

Swelling and any bruising on the lateral aspect of the ankle may be diffuse, indicating a moderate or major ligamentous lesion. Often, a rounded mottled egg-shaped swelling lies in front of the lateral malleolus, known as the *signe de la coquille d'œuf* (Litt, 1992).

Minor swelling may be indicated by loss of the hollows behind the malleoli, and thickening of the Achilles tendon may be observed. Local swellings and ganglia should also be noted.

Palpation

As peripheral joints, the ankle and foot are palpated for signs of activity. The presence of heat is assessed (Fig. 12.12), and synovial thickening is palpated most easily along the anterior joint line (Fig. 12.13).

Swelling can usually be seen on observation, but it is also possible to palpate for swelling, particularly around the malleoli. If the history indicates major ligament sprain, the malleoli and talus can be palpated for any focal areas of tenderness, which may indicate a fracture (Lee and Maleski, 2002).

State at Rest

Before any movements are performed, the state at rest is established to provide a baseline for subsequent comparison.

Examination by Selective Tension

The suggested sequence for the examination is now given, followed by a commentary that includes the reasoning in performing the movements and the significance of the possible findings. Comparison should always be made with the other side.

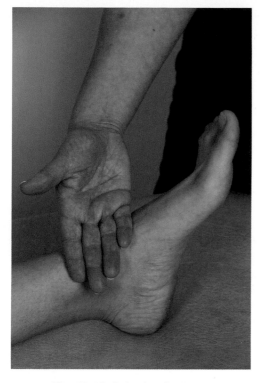

Fig. 12.12 Palpation for heat.

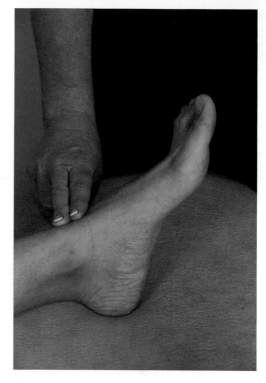

Fig. 12.13 Palpation for synovial thickening.

Ankle Joint
- Passive dorsiflexion (Fig. 12.14)
- Passive plantarflexion (Fig. 12.15)

Subtalar Joint
- Passive inversion (varus stress; Fig. 12.16)
- Passive eversion (valgus stress; Fig. 12.16)

Midtarsal Joints
- Passive dorsiflexion and plantarflexion (Figs 12.17 and 12.18)
- Passive abduction and adduction (Figs 12.19 and 12.20)
- Passive inversion and eversion (Figs 12.21 and 12.22)

Gross Ligament Tests
- Passive inversion in plantarflexion for lateral collateral ligament (Fig. 12.23)
- Passive eversion for medial (deltoid) ligament (Fig. 12.24)

Contractile Structures
- Resisted dorsiflexion (Fig. 12.25)
- Resisted plantarflexion (Fig. 12.26)
- Resisted inversion (Fig. 12.27)
- Resisted eversion (Fig. 12.28)

Accessory Ligament Tests
- Drawer test for the anterior talofibular ligament (Fig. 12.29)
- Talar tilt test for the calcaneofibular ligament and integrity of the mortise (Fig. 12.30)
- Test for the dorsal calcaneocuboid ligament (Fig. 12.31)

Toes
- Passive and resisted testing of the toes is not performed routinely but is included if appropriate

Palpation
- Once a diagnosis has been made, the structure at fault is palpated for the exact site of the lesion

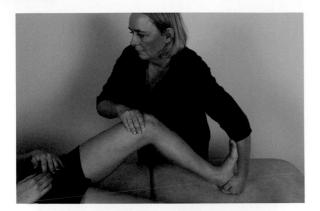

Fig. 12.14 Passive ankle dorsiflexion.

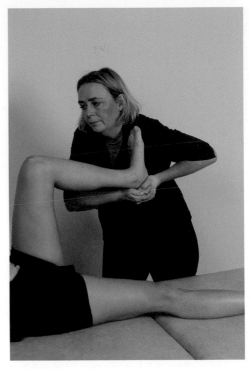

Fig. 12.16 Hand position for varus and valgus stress, subtalar joint: valgus stress shown.

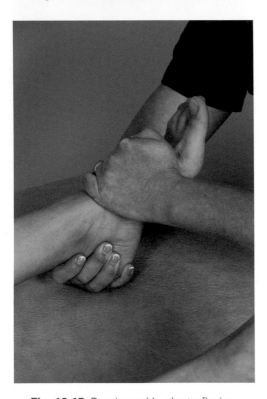

Fig. 12.15 Passive ankle plantarflexion.

The examination is carried out in non-weight-bearing with the patient positioned comfortably in supine lying. The joints are examined first, assessing the range of movement, pain and end-feel.

Passive dorsiflexion normally has a hard end-feel, and to achieve end-range, it must be performed with the knee in flexion to take the tension off the gastrocnemius muscle complex, which spans both the knee and ankle joints.

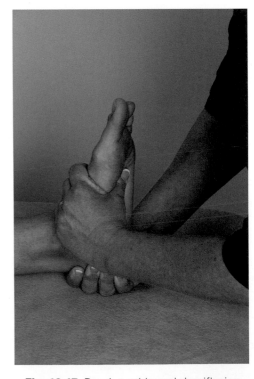

Fig. 12.17 Passive midtarsal dorsiflexion.

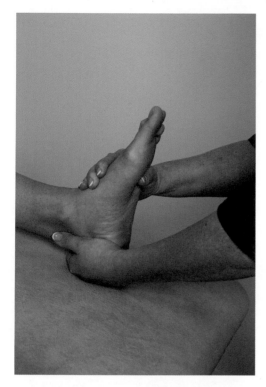

Fig. 12.18 Passive midtarsal plantarflexion.

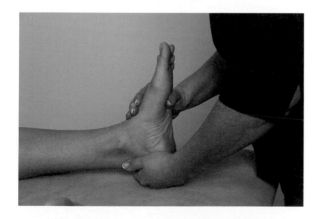

Fig. 12.19 Passive midtarsal abduction.

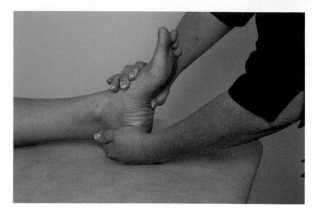

Fig. 12.20 Passive midtarsal adduction.

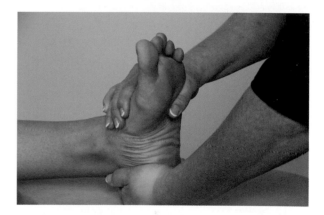

Fig. 12.21 Passive midtarsal inversion.

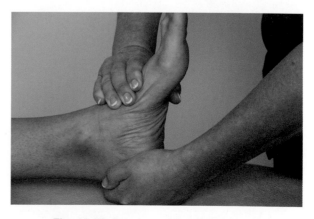

Fig. 12.22 Passive midtarsal eversion.

Passive plantarflexion normally has a firm elastic end-feel due to tension in the tissues on the dorsal aspect of the foot. The presence of the capsular pattern should be noted.

Although individual passive movements can be produced at the ankle joint, it is difficult to produce isolated passive movements at the subtalar and midtarsal joints.

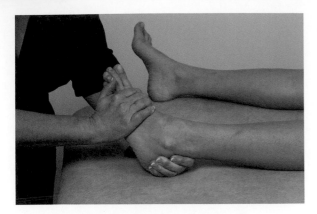

Fig. 12.23 Passive inversion in plantarflexion for lateral collateral ligament.

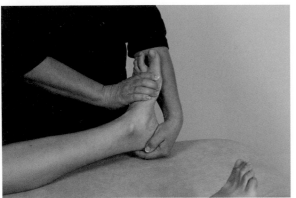

Fig. 12.24 Passive eversion for medial (deltoid) ligament.

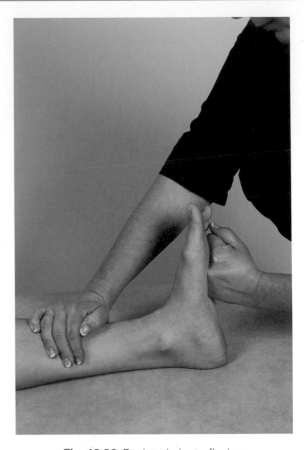

Fig. 12.26 Resisted plantarflexion.

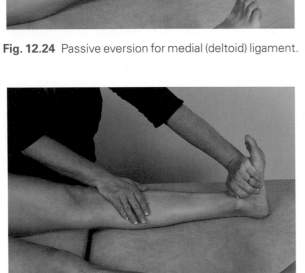

Fig. 12.25 Resisted dorsiflexion.

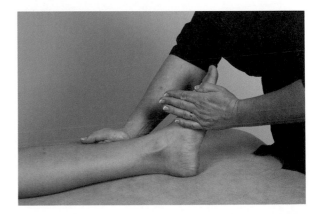

Fig. 12.27 Resisted inversion.

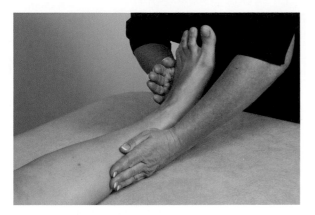

Fig. 12.28 Resisted eversion.

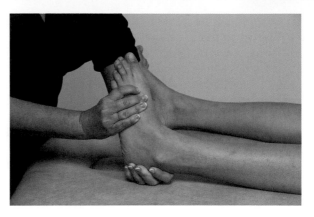

Fig. 12.31 Test for the dorsal calcaneocuboid ligament.

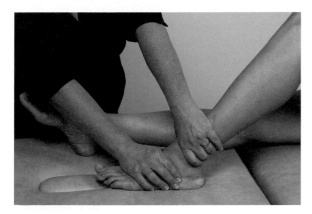

Fig. 12.29 Drawer test for the anterior talofibular ligament.

To assess the small range of movement available at the subtalar joint (Fig. 12.16):
- Grasp the calcaneus with both hands.
- Flex the knee to allow relaxation of the gastrocnemius complex and to push the ankle joint into the close-packed position of dorsiflexion with your shoulder.
- The varus and valgus stresses are then applied to the calcaneus through the heels of both hands, using body weight and rotating your body clockwise and anticlockwise.

The amount of passive movement available at the subtalar joint is limited to a few degrees of inversion and eversion, and the normal end-feel is hard for both.

To assess movements occurring at the midtarsal joints (see Figs 12.17–12.22):
- Pull down on the calcaneus to place the ankle joint into dorsiflexion.
- Place fingers and thumb on either side of the first metatarsal. This can be approached from the medial or lateral aspect of the foot, considering your dominant hand and how you can best perform and observe the movement. Try to have as few changes of hand position as possible as you test the movements.
- Move the midtarsal joint through its range of passive movements, plantarflexion and dorsiflexion, abduction and adduction, inversion and eversion.

These movements are minimal and difficult to produce in isolation.

Assessing passive movements of the toes is not part of the routine ankle examination, but the movements

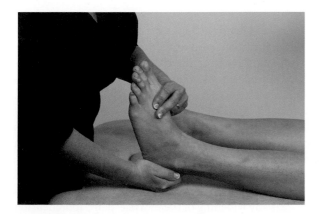

Fig. 12.30 Talar tilt test for the calcaneofibular ligament and integrity of the mortise.

can be applied as necessary to assess for the presence of the capsular pattern.

The main ligaments at the ankle are tested by two gross composite movements: passive inversion in plantarflexion for the lateral collateral ligament and passive eversion in dorsiflexion for the medial collateral ligament. Should it be necessary, the ligaments can be assessed individually, and accessory tests can be applied for joint instability (see below).

The contractile structures are assessed by resisted tests for pain and power. The joints are placed in the mid-position and maximum resistance applied.

Movement	Main Muscles	'Assistors'
Dorsiflexion	Tibialis anterior	Extensor hallucis longus, extensor digitorum longus
Plantarflexion	Gastrocnemius, soleus, plantaris	Flexor hallucis longus, flexor digitorum longus
Inversion	Tibialis anterior, tibialis posterior, extensor hallucis longus	Flexor digitorum longus, flexor hallucis longus
Eversion	Peroneus longus, peroneus brevis, peroneus tertius	Extensor digitorum

Resisted dorsiflexion tests mainly tibialis anterior and resisted plantarflexion tests gastrocnemius. Testing the gastrocnemius group in lying may not produce symptoms, and the test may need to be repeated in standing against the resistance of body weight.

Resisted inversion tests mainly tibialis posterior and resisted eversion tests the peroneal muscles.

Accessory ligament and instability tests are applied if appropriate. The gross ligament test of passive inversion mainly tests the anterior talofibular ligament, which crosses the ankle joint and is taut in plantarflexion. It is the most common ligamentous injury found at the ankle. It is further assessed by the drawer test, which assesses its integrity (Marder, 1994; Hattam and Smeatham, 2020).

DRAWER TEST
- Flex the leg to allow the foot to rest on the couch (Fig. 12.29)
- Position yourself to view movement of the fibula on the lateral side of the ankle
- Place one hand over the talus to fix it and the other just above the ankle joint
- Apply pressure backwards against the fibula and tibia
- Compare the degree of posterior movement of the fibula with the other side

---

Increased posterior movement of the fibula is a positive sign and indicates laxity or rupture of the anterior talofibular ligament. A 'suction sign' or dimple may be observed on the lateral aspect of the ankle if the anterior talofibular ligament is ruptured (Lee and Maleski, 2002; Hattam and Smeatham, 2020).

The calcaneofibular ligament crosses both the ankle joint and the subtalar joint. Injury to this ligament does not often occur in isolation and is usually in conjunction with the anterior talofibular ligament. The calcaneofibular ligament resists varus stresses to the calcaneus in dorsiflexion. Combined rupture of the anterior talofibular and calcaneofibular ligaments results in an increased talar tilt (Boruta et al., 1990; Wilkerson, 1992; Marder, 1994).

TALAR TILT TEST
- With the knee straight, passively dorsiflex the ankle (this allows it to fall just short of the close-packed position) (Fig. 12.30)
- Apply a strong varus stress to the calcaneus
- Compare the range of movement with the other side

This test may also be graded 1 to 3 relative to the contralateral ankle (Lee and Maleski, 2002).

Disruption of the inferior tibiofibular joint may be due to a forced dorsiflexion injury, which can cause widening (diastasis) of the ankle mortise (Marder, 1994). In clinical practice, such an injury would usually only occur in conjunction with other major ligamentous damage and possible fracture, but the talar tilt test can also be applied to test the integrity of the mortise.

Apply the talar tilt test as above (it can only be applied accurately if the lateral collateral ligaments are intact). If there is any widening of the mortise, pain, apprehension and excessive movement will be appreciated. A 'clunk' may be felt as the talus tilts excessively in the enlarged mortise or as the stress is released (Cyriax and Cyriax, 1993; Hattam and Smeatham, 2020).

The dorsal calcaneocuboid ligament crosses the calcaneocuboid joint, part of the midtarsal complex, and may be involved in a lateral collateral ligament sprain or injured in isolation. To assess its involvement, apply stress to the dorsal calcaneocuboid ligament as described below.

> **TEST FOR DORSAL CALCANEOCUBOID LIGAMENT SPRAIN**
> - If testing the left foot, hold the calcaneus with your left hand and apply a small amount of distraction to fix the ankle and subtalar joints (Fig. 12.31)
> - Place your right hand around the lateral border of the foot, with your thumb across the sole, the ulnar border of your hand just distal to the calcaneocuboid joint and your fingers resting over the metatarsals
> - Apply passive adduction and inversion of the midtarsal joints, looking for increased pain at the site of the dorsal calcaneocuboid ligament as it spans the calcaneocuboid ligament on the lateral aspect of the foot
> - Adapt the instructions to test the right foot

Based on the history and clinical examination, the practitioner should be able to establish the most likely diagnosis using clinical reasoning and clinical judgement.

It is important to recognise potential serious pathology, such as infection, malignancy, fracture and inflammatory arthritis, and to make any appropriate onward referral promptly. Should additional information be required to aid diagnosis or to add value to management, further investigations can be considered to inform decision making and planning.

If indicated, the practitioner may consider further investigations such as blood tests, radiological imaging, and other diagnostic procedures (see Chapter 1). Investigations should be guided by the suspected causes and differential diagnosis as an extension to the clinical examination process.

Further investigation should be considered with suspected red flags such as fracture, infection, inflammatory arthritis or suspected malignancy. Blood tests or Doppler ultrasound examinations may be appropriate if a specific underlying cause is suspected, such as vascular claudication, hypothyroidism or diabetes. Blood tests can be considered with suspected peripheral inflammatory arthritis.

Achilles tendinopathy is usually a clinical diagnosis, and imaging (such as ultrasound or MRI) is not routinely recommended in primary care (NICE, 2020a). If a deep vein thrombosis or compartment syndrome is suspected, urgent onward referral for further investigation is required.

CAPSULAR LESIONS

The presence of a capsular pattern at any of the joints in the ankle and foot indicates an arthropathy. The history will have established the cause of the arthropathy, which could be degenerative, inflammatory or traumatic.

Differential diagnosis of ankle arthropathy includes gout, tendinopathy of the ankle and foot, sinus tarsi syndrome, stress fracture, ankle impingement, peripheral neuropathy, instability, malignancy, septic arthritis.

It is not unusual for patients to present with co-morbidities such as lumbar pathology, venous insufficiency, or infection (Demetriades et al., 1998; Simpson and Howard, 2009; Russo et al., 2013).

> **CAPSULAR PATTERN OF THE ANKLE JOINT**
> - More limitation of plantarflexion than dorsiflexion

Degenerative arthropathy is uncommon at the ankle unless predisposed by fracture, poor foot posture or instability caused by recurrent sprain. An alteration in lower limb biomechanics may predispose any of the joints to degenerative arthropathy. Localised degenerative arthropathy of the subtalar joint may follow fracture of the talus or calcaneus (Evans, 1990).

A lateral ligament sprain often produces a traumatic arthritis in the ankle joint and, if unresolved, the joint can be injected with corticosteroid.

A stepped approach to the management of degenerative arthropathy of the ankle and foot is currently recommended. Less invasive treatments are generally offered first, including education/watchful wait, activity and work modification, simple analgesics and non-steroidal anti-inflammatory drugs (NSAIDs) medication, physiotherapy (e.g. exercise, mobilisation), podiatry assessment (e.g. orthotics and biomechanical assessment) and then injection therapy (e.g. corticosteroid, local anaesthetic, hyaluronic acid). If symptoms persist, further investigation and onward referral to a foot and ankle specialist may be required.

The principles of mobilisation for capsular lesions may be applied, and distraction techniques can also be helpful. Corticosteroid injection may be given for symptomatic arthritis. Rheumatoid arthritis is more common in the smaller joints of the foot, and corticosteroid injection is considered.

INJECTION OF THE ANKLE JOINT
Suggested needle size: 23 G × 1 in. (0.6 × 25 mm) blue
   needle or a 21 G × 1½ in. (0.8 × 40 mm) green needle
Dose: 20–40 mg triamcinolone acetonide in a total volume of 3 mL

- Position the patient in supine with the foot resting on the couch. This places the ankle in a degree of plantarflexion and opens the joint.
- Several needle entry points are possible, and it may be necessary to palpate for a suitable opening over either malleolus or between the tibialis anterior and extensor hallucis longus tendons, which avoids the dorsalis pedis artery (Fig. 12.32).
- Having selected a needle entry point, give the injection as a bolus (Fig. 12.33).

The patient should minimise or modify activities for two weeks following injection.

CAPSULAR PATTERN OF THE SUBTALAR JOINT
- Increasing limitation of inversion
- Eventual fixation of the joint in eversion

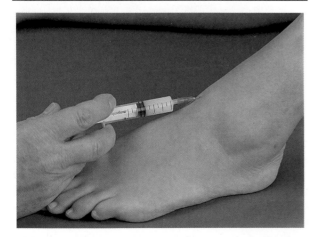

Fig. 12.32 Injection of the ankle joint.

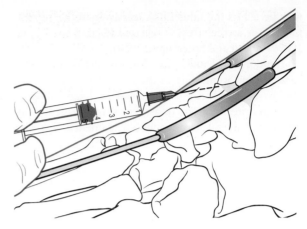

Fig. 12.33 Injection of the ankle joint showing direction of approach and needle position.

Pain from the subtalar joint tends to refer to the sole and heel, and the patient may describe the sensation of walking on a stone. With arthropathy, the capsular pattern will be present with pain and limitation on inversion. It is usually associated with rheumatoid arthritis, but degenerative arthropathy can also affect this joint.

Subtalar impingement syndrome can be a cause of sharp twinges in the joint, and the pain worsens through the day, often with a background ache. The syndrome usually settles without surgical treatment in 2 to 8 weeks.

Fractures of the calcaneus or talus are caused by high impact trauma such as jumping from a height or road traffic accidents. The history and inability to weight-bear would lead to the suspicion of a hindfoot fracture, and X-ray investigation would confirm the diagnosis.

INJECTION OF THE SUBTALAR JOINT (CYRIAX, 1984; CYRIAX AND CYRIAX, 1993)
Suggested needle size: 23 G × 1 in. (0.6 × 25 mm) blue
   needle
Dose: 10–20 mg triamcinolone acetonide in a total volume of 2 mL

The interosseous ligament, which sits within the sinus tarsi, forms a barrier between the two joint capsules, and each compartment must be considered when injecting the joint.
- Locate the joint line immediately above the sustentaculum tali.

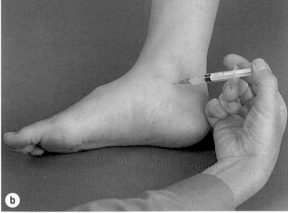

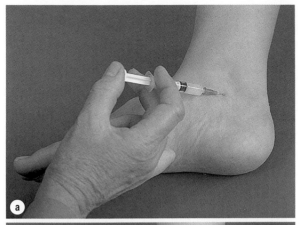

Fig. 12.34 Injection of the subtalar joint.

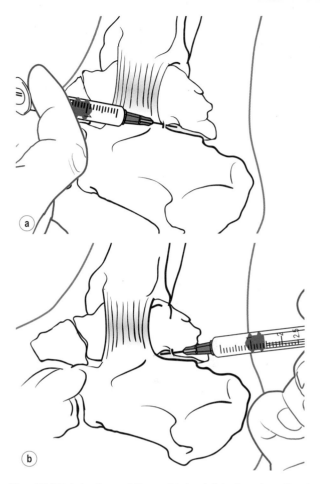

Fig. 12.35 Injection of the subtalar joint showing direction of approach and needle position.

- Insert the needle approximately halfway along the joint line, angling it posteriorly to inject the posterior compartment first (Figs 12.34a and 12.35a).
- Inject half the volume as a bolus.
- Withdraw the needle a little and reinsert it anteriorly to inject the anterior compartment (see Figs 12.34b and 12.35b).
- Give the remainder of the injection as a bolus.

The patient should minimise or modify activities for two weeks following injection.

CAPSULAR PATTERN OF THE MIDTARSAL JOINTS
- Limitation of adduction and inversion
- Forefoot fixes in abduction and eversion

The patient complains of pain in the mid-tarsal region, especially on weight-bearing. The cause is usually poor foot posture, and the pain may come on after unaccustomed activity, such as walking or jogging for a long distance. Footwear may also have a role in the onset. Symptoms may also be associated with rheumatoid arthritis. The capsular pattern will be present with pain and limitation of adduction and inversion.

INJECTION OF THE MIDTARSAL JOINTS (CYRIAX, 1984; CYRIAX AND CYRIAX, 1993)
Suggested needle size: 23 G × 1 in. (0.6 × 25 mm) blue needle
Dose: 10–20 mg triamcinolone acetonide in a total volume of 1.5 mL

The injection site will depend on which joints are affected: the talocalcaneonavicular joint, calcaneocuboid joint or both.

- Locate the appropriate joint line dorsally by palpation, avoiding the tendons and the dorsalis pedis artery if injecting the talocalcaneonavicular joint medially. (Figs 12.36 and 12.37 demonstrate injection of the calcaneocuboid joint.)
- Insert the needle.
- Once intracapsular, give the injection as a bolus.

The patient should minimise or modify activities for two weeks following injection.

> **CAPSULAR PATTERN OF THE FIRST METATARSOPHALANGEAL JOINT**
> - Gross limitation of extension
> - Some limitation of flexion

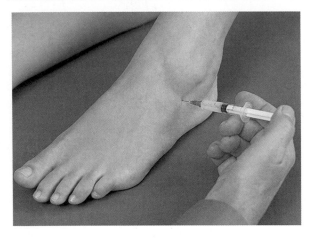

Fig. 12.36 Injection of the midtarsal calcaneocuboid joint.

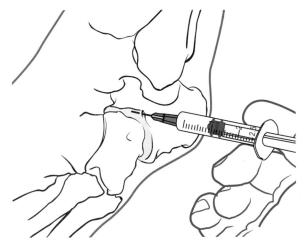

Fig. 12.37 Injection of the midtarsal calcaneocuboid joint showing direction of approach and needle position.

Arthropathy and gout of the first metatarsophalangeal joint cause a loss of the functional range of extension essential to gait activities. Prolonged standing in high heels can also aggravate the condition and can become impossible with inflammatory or degenerative arthropathy. The pain is localised to the joint, and the capsular pattern is present.

Injection is appropriate for arthropathy but never for gout, which is usually far too painful to touch or inject.

> **INJECTION OF THE FIRST METATARSOPHALANGEAL JOINT (CYRIAX, 1984; CYRIAX AND CYRIAX, 1993)**
> Suggested needle size: 25 G × 5/8 in. (0.5 × 16 mm) orange needle
> Dose: 10–20 mg triamcinolone acetonide in a total volume of 0.5 mL

- Identify the joint line dorsally by palpation and distract it to allow easier access
- Choose a point of entry to one side of the extensor tendon (see Fig. 12.38).
- Give the injection as a bolus (see Fig. 12.39).

The patient should minimise or modify activities for two weeks following injection.

The distraction component of this technique can be useful to mobilise this joint in degenerative osteoarthropathy.

The capsular pattern of the other metatarsophalangeal and interphalangeal joints is usually associated with

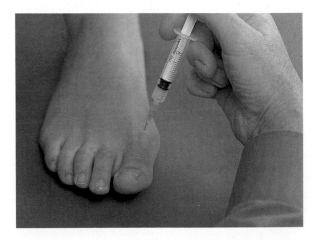

Fig. 12.38 Injection of the first metatarsophalangeal joint.

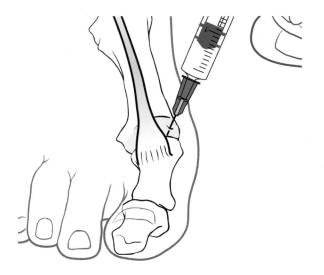

Fig. 12.39 Injection of the first metatarsophalangeal joint showing direction of approach and needle position.

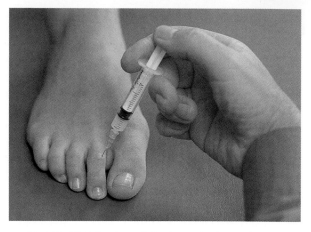

Fig. 12.40 Injection of the interphalangeal joint.

rheumatoid arthritis. As peripheral joints, the patient can indicate the specific joint accurately. The capsular pattern will be evident.

CAPSULAR PATTERN OF THE OTHER METATARSOPHALANGEAL JOINTS (MAY VARY)
- More limitation of flexion than extension
- Joints fix in extension

CAPSULAR PATTERN OF THE INTERPHALANGEAL JOINTS
- Joints fix in flexion

INJECTION OF THE OTHER METATARSOPHALANGEAL AND INTERPHALANGEAL JOINTS
Suggested needle size: 25 G × 5/8 in. (0.5 × 16 mm) orange needle.
Dose: 5–10 mg triamcinolone acetonide in a total volume of 0.5 mL.

- Identify the joint line dorsally by palpation.
- Insert the needle, avoiding the extensor tendons (Figs 12.40 and 12.41)
- Give the injection as a bolus.

The patient should minimise or modify activities for two weeks following injection.

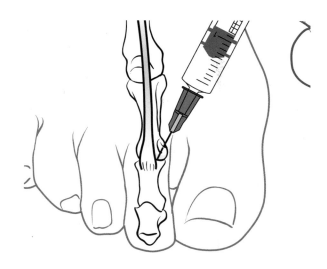

Fig. 12.41 Injection of the interphalangeal joint showing direction of approach and needle position.

NON-CAPSULAR LESIONS

Lateral Collateral Ligament Sprain

Sprain of the lateral collateral ligament is the most common ankle injury, accounting for approximately 85% to 90% of ankle sprains, with approximately 2,000,000 injuries per year (Stanley, 1991; Liu and Jason, 1994; Hur et al., 2020). The injury is more common in those involved in sport or the military, and approximately 85% of all ankle sprains result in injury to the lateral ligament complex (Hur et al., 2020).

The anterior talofibular ligament is the weakest of the ligaments in the lateral ligament complex and is involved in nearly all lateral ligament sprains. When the ankle is plantarflexed, the bony anatomy of the ankle provides less stability and constraint, and the ligament is more vulnerable to injury in this position (Hur et al., 2020).

The calcaneofibular ligament is involved in 50% to 75% of all lateral ligament injuries, and the combination of injury to the anterior talofibular ligament and the calcaneofibular ligament is the second most common injury (Hur et al., 2020).

The posterior talofibular ligament is rarely injured (Ferran and Maffulli, 2006) unless there is gross dislocation of the ankle joint and it is almost always injured in combination with the anterior talofibular ligament and the calcaneofibular ligament (Hur et al., 2020).

The mechanism for lateral ligament sprain is a forced inversion injury (Sartoris, 1994; Kerkhoffs et al., 2002). The injury occurs commonly in activities requiring rapid direction changes, especially on uneven surfaces, or in sports such as basketball, volleyball and netball when a player may land on another player's foot after jumping (Brukner et al., 2017). Apart from sport, the patient may simply have tripped or slipped.

The most common predisposing factor to receiving a lateral ligament injury is a history of at least one previous strain, but an estimated 55% of patients do not seek treatment for a sprained ankle (Hertel, 2002).

Lateral collateral ligament sprains most commonly involve the anterior talofibular ligament, with more severe injuries involving other ligaments and structures on the lateral side of the ankle (Litt, 1992; Liu and Jason, 1994; Hertel, 2002). They are graded according to the severity of the signs and symptoms (Boruta et al., 1990; Stanley, 1991; Litt, 1992; Wilkerson, 1992; Liu and Jason, 1994; Kerkhoffs et al., 2002; Brukner et al., 2017).

Grade I

This is mild stretching of the ligament and surrounding structures. The patient presents with mild swelling and tenderness over the ligament, little or no haemorrhage, some limitation of movement and some difficulty in weight-bearing. On examination, no clinical instability is noted, and the prognosis is good. The injury takes approximately 8 to 10 days to resolve with early mobilisation.

Grade II

This is partial rupture of the anterior talofibular ligament with mild instability of the joint. The patient presents with moderate to severe swelling, bruising, pain, local tenderness, a limited movement range, and great weight-bearing difficulty. There is limitation of movement in the capsular pattern, and a mild degree of ligamentous instability may be detected clinically. Prognosis remains good, the injury taking approximately 15 to 21 days to resolve with early mobilisation.

Grade III

This is complete rupture of the anterior talofibular and calcaneofibular ligaments and lateral capsule with gross instability of the joint. The patient presents with diffuse swelling and marked evidence of haemorrhaging. There is severe pain and tenderness, loss of movement and great difficulty with weight-bearing. It may be difficult to assess for ligamentous laxity clinically as this may be masked by the swelling and the protective reflex muscle spasm produced by the pain.

Diagnosis of sprain can be made mostly on clinical grounds. Ultrasound imaging is used if rupture is suspected, and X-ray investigation is only necessary if there is clear clinical evidence of fracture (e.g. marked bony tenderness to palpation); (Auletta et al., 1991; Litt, 1992). The 'Ottawa ankle rules' have been developed as a guideline to help decide whether an X-ray is necessary and are based on identifying bone tenderness in specific areas (Patel and Subramanian, 2007).

The fibular end of the ligament is more likely to be involved in avulsion fractures than the talar end, which is protected by greater bone density (Kumai et al., 2002). Forced inversion may cause avulsion of lateral structures or undisplaced fracture of the lateral malleolus, while impactive forces may stress medial structures (Sartoris, 1994). Other fractures and dislocations at the ankle should be considered differential diagnosis but are outside the scope of this book.

Injuries to consider within differential diagnosis include lesions of the contractile units; subluxation of the peroneal tendons (through partial or complete rupture of the retinacula); damage to the subtalar and midtarsal joints; and injury to the various neurovascular structures crossing the region (Marder, 1994; Lee and Maleski, 2002). Anterolateral impingement is rare, occurring in only 3% of ankle sprains. It can arise from a meniscoid lesion, synovitis or impingement of the distal fascicle of the anterior inferior tibiofibular ligament (Bekerom and Raven, 2007). Fracture, unstable mortise, ankle instability and complex regional pain syndrome are also possible causes of symptoms (Simpson and Howard, 2009).

A stepped approach to the management of ankle lateral ligament sprain is currently recommended. Less invasive treatments are generally offered first, including education/watchful wait, activity and work modification, simple analgesics medication, physiotherapy (e.g. exercise, mobilisation, strengthening), and podiatry assessment (e.g. orthotics and biomechanical assessment). If symptoms persist, further investigation and referral to a foot and ankle specialist may be required for a surgical opinion.

Recurrent ankle sprains with clinical laxity may need a stress X-ray to measure the laxity before proceeding to eventual surgical repair. In general, surgical intervention for grade III sprains is considered where recurrent injury has failed to respond to conservative management and produces functional disability (Vuurberg et al., 2018).

Persistent symptoms 1 year after the primary injury can lead to chronic lateral ankle instability. Up to 70% of patients who sustain an acute lateral ankle sprain can develop chronic ankle instability, and acute ligament injury must be managed well in the initial stages.

Mechanical impairments may develop due to laxity of the ankle joint, which can lead to recurrent instability, sprains, a gradual weakening of the lateral ligament complex and decreased neuromuscular control. Sensory impairments can develop, leading to persistent pain, perceived instability, and fear of reinjury, leading to a chronic cycle of pain and dysfunction (Hur et al., 2020).

Early mobilisation and exercise are the keys to restoring function in all grades of ligamentous sprain (Kerkhoffs et al., 2002; Vuurberg et al., 2018). Kerkhoffs et al. (2002) present a review of randomised controlled trials in the literature to evaluate the effectiveness of immobilisation as the treatment for acute sprained ankle in adults. Overall, results were better with functional treatment rather than immobilisation, with a higher percentage of patients returning to work and sport, a reduced incidence of persistent swelling, limited movement and instability, and higher patient satisfaction rates.

Functional treatment is, therefore, the treatment of choice for acute sprained ankle. Treatment is directed at all components involved in the sprain and depends on the stage reached in the healing process.

Acute Lateral Collateral Ligament Injury

A complete examination of the ankle and foot is not usually possible following an acute lateral collateral ligament sprain as the swelling and muscle spasm prevent movement. The history will indicate the mechanism of the injury, and the amount of heat and swelling will indicate the severity.

Any movement, active or passive, particularly into inversion, will be painful, and pain is experienced on weight-bearing, leading to an antalgic gait.

Initial treatment follows current guidelines for the management of soft tissue lesions (see Chapter 4). Care should be taken with the use of non-steroidal anti-inflammatory drugs (NSAIDs) to reduce pain and swelling with an acute lateral ligament sprain, as they may suppress the healing process (Vuurberg et al., 2018).

The principles of treatment for acute ligament sprain in the musculoskeletal medicine approach are applied.

Transverse frictions are begun as early as possible, according to the irritability of the lesion, together with Grade A mobilisation, aiming to maintain mobility. Treatment is delivered regularly during the early acute phase, and the patient is encouraged to maintain a normal heel–toe gait, possibly with the aid of crutches. Ankle supports or tape may be applied to provide compression during the early acute phase, especially if there is instability (O'Hara et al., 1992; Vuurberg et al., 2018).

From days 3 to 5 onwards, again dependent upon irritability, there should be sufficient tensile strength in the wound to allow an increasing depth of transverse frictions and a greater range of Grade A mobilisation to be applied. Treatment continues until a full range of pain-free movement is achieved.

Depending on the severity of the injury, the patient should be relatively pain-free and walking normally within 8 to 21 days, if seen within a day or two from onset.

The lateral ligaments require the support of the peroneal tendons to resist inversion stresses; rehabilitation aims to restore muscle strength and re-establish the protective reflexes (Boruta et al., 1990; Brukner et al., 2017).

Functional rehabilitation should involve muscle balance, peroneal strengthening and proprioceptive work to re-establish normal balance and coordination (Cornwall and Murrell, 1991; Karlsson and Lansingeer, 1992; Brukner et al., 2017). Progression to running, sprinting, jumping, figure-of-eight running, twisting and turning follows, depending on the patient's functional requirements.

Specific balance training includes wobble board exercises, closed-chain exercises, core stability and sport-specific manoeuvres (Laskowski et al., 1997; Brukner et al., 2017).

TRANSVERSE FRICTIONS TO THE LATERAL COLLATERAL LIGAMENT COMPONENTS

(Cyriax, 1984; Cyriax and Cyriax, 1993)

The anterior talofibular ligament is usually involved at its fibular end, but palpation will establish the exact site of the lesion, which may also be at the talar insertion or across the joint line.

- Stand on the patient's good side, placing an index finger reinforced by the middle finger onto the anterior edge of the lateral malleolus.
- Direct the transverse frictions back against the malleolus and sweep transversely across the fibres (Fig. 12.42).
- Start gently and maintain the technique for an appropriate time, according to the irritability of the lesion and stage of healing, to achieve analgesia and mobilise the tissues.
- Follow the transverse frictions immediately with Grade A mobilisation together with gait correction.

If the calcaneofibular ligament is involved, the transverse frictions are directed up under the apex of the lateral malleolus and immediately followed by Grade A mobilisation (see Fig. 12.44).

Treatment of any involvement of the peroneal tendons is covered under contractile lesions.

Chronic Lateral Collateral Ligament Injury

There is usually a history of a past sprained ankle that may have resolved without treatment. The patient complains of pain and some swelling on the lateral side of the ankle after exertion.

Symptoms of recurrent giving way may indicate mechanical instability (ankle movement beyond the physiological limit that occurs due to anatomical

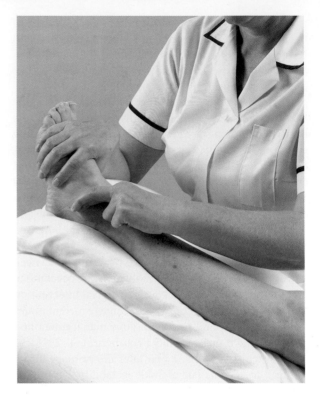

Fig. 12.42 Transverse frictions to the anterior talofibular ligament, acute sprain.

changes such as ligamentous laxity) or functional instability (a subjective feeling of instability that occurs due to neuromuscular and proprioceptive deficits that provide dynamic control); (Tropp, 2002; Hur et al. 2020).

On examination, there is usually pain on full passive inversion, indicating involvement of the anterior talofibular ligament. Pain on passive dorsiflexion with a varus stress to the calcaneus (talar tilt test) indicates involvement of the calcaneofibular ligament. Pain on passive adduction and inversion applied to the midtarsal joints indicates involvement of the dorsal calcaneocuboid ligament.

Provocative tests such as the drawer and talar tilt tests, as described above, can indicate mechanical instability.

The treatment approach for residual chronic ankle instability should be based on mechanical correction and functional rehabilitation, emphasising proprioceptive re-education, muscle balance and postural control, and taping may be appropriate for sporting activities.

As well as chronic lateral ligament sprain and instability, differential diagnosis of continuing lateral ankle pain following inversion injury includes osteochondral fracture, ruptured peroneal tendon, synovitis and ligamentous impingement of the anterior aspect of the ankle, which is uncommon (Bekerom and Raven, 2007).

The importance of continuing rehabilitation for several months after the symptoms of acute ligamentous injury have subsided is paramount in preventing chronic recurrence (Hertel, 2002).

The treatment principle is to increase the range of pain-free movement with one Grade C manipulation at each session once the ligament has been numbed by transverse frictions.

Following the manipulation, the patient is instructed to mobilise vigorously to maintain the movement gained through manipulation.

Functional or structural instability is addressed by proprioceptive exercises and balance work (Lentell et al., 1990). Treatment is usually successful and requires approximately 1 to 3 sessions.

TRANSVERSE FRICTIONS TO THE LATERAL COLLATERAL LIGAMENT COMPONENTS INVOLVED IN A CHRONIC INJURY

(Cyriax, 1984; Cyriax and Cyriax, 1993)

Transverse frictions to the anterior talofibular (Fig. 12.43) and calcaneofibular ligament (if involved; Fig. 12.44) are applied as described above.

If the dorsal calcaneocuboid ligament is involved:
- Apply the transverse frictions from a position on the patient's 'good' side.
- Locate the dorsal calcaneocuboid ligament on the dorsum of the foot, where it crosses the calcaneocuboid joint line.
- Deliver the transverse frictions using an index finger, reinforced by the middle finger (Fig. 12.45).
- Direct the transverse frictions onto the ligament and apply until the analgesic effect is achieved.

The transverse frictions are applied to all involved ligaments to gain the analgesic effect prior to the Grade C manipulation, which follows immediately.

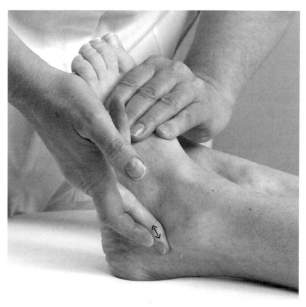

Fig. 12.44 Transverse frictions to the calcaneofibular ligament.

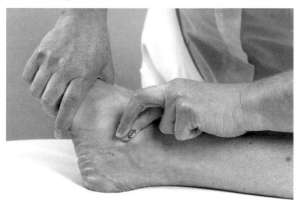

Fig. 12.43 Transverse frictions to the anterior talofibular ligament, chronic sprain.

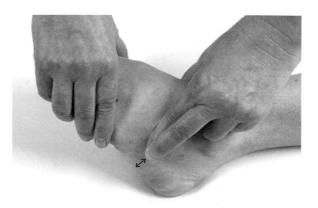

Fig. 12.45 Transverse frictions to the dorsal calcaneocuboid ligament.

CLINICAL TIP

Transverse frictions are only applied before performing a peripheral Grade C manipulation to gain some analgesia, and they should not be continued post numbing. The Grade C manipulation should follow immediately.

GRADE C MANIPULATION FOR CHRONIC LATERAL COLLATERAL LIGAMENT SPRAIN

(Cyriax, 1984; Cyriax and Cyriax, 1993)

The treatment described is for the left ankle:

- With the patient lying supine, stand at the foot of the couch.
- Grasp the patient's left calcaneus with your left hand and apply a varus movement to pull the subtalar joint into inversion (Fig. 12.46). Keep your thumb alongside the palm of your hand to avoid pressing against the lower leg, which will tend to block the movement and is uncomfortable for the patient.
- With a 'flipper' grip, wrap your right hand around the base of the first metatarsal (Fig. 12.47), with the heel of the hand well down alongside the lateral border of the foot, and pull the foot into maximum plantarflexion (Fig. 12.48a). Be careful not to put your thumb round onto the sole, as this is uncomfortable for the patient and makes the technique less efficient.
- Maintain the maximum plantarflexion while you step to the left, turning your body to the left through

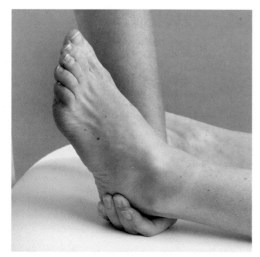

Fig. 12.46 Grade C manipulation: calcaneum grasped and placed into inversion.

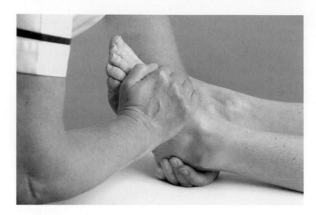

Fig. 12.47 Grade C manipulation: 'flipper' grip handhold.

90 degrees to achieve maximum inversion (Fig. 12.48b and c).

- This step and turn automatically pull the forefoot into maximum adduction and inversion, taking up the slack (Fig. 12.49).
- Apply a minimal amplitude, high-velocity thrust by a sharp adduction movement of your right arm.

The increased range of movement must be maintained by vigorous exercise.

Medial Collateral Ligament Sprain

Eversion sprains of the ankle represent 5% to 15% of all ankle injuries and are not common, as the medial collateral ligaments are 20% to 50% stronger than the lateral ligaments. The mechanism of injury involved is forced eversion with possible damage to the syndesmosis, or fracture of the malleoli, and injury to the medial ligament (Roberts et al., 1995; Lee and Maleski, 2002).

More chronic involvement of the medial collateral ligament is usually associated with biomechanical factors and poor foot posture.

The principles of a stepped approach to management are applied as for the acute and chronic stages of the lateral collateral ligament if the injury is traumatic. The various directions of the ligament fibres need to be borne in mind to apply the frictions transversely. A Grade C manipulation is not applied in the chronic stage due to the multidirectional nature of the fibres.

A secondary medial ligament sprain may develop through poor foot posture. This is especially evident with flattening of the medial arch in the elderly.

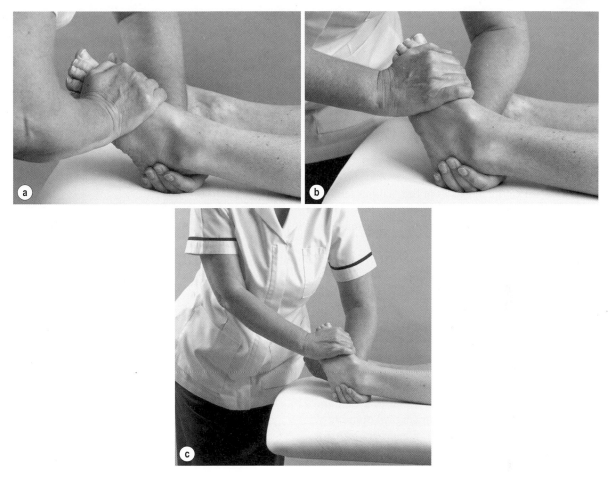

Fig. 12.48 (a) Pulling foot into maximum plantarflexion. (b,c) Pulling foot into inversion and adduction.

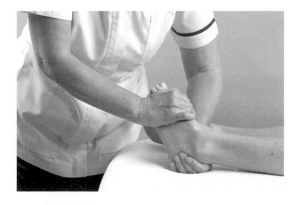

Fig. 12.49 Grade C manipulation: body turned, pulling the forefoot into maximum adduction and inversion before application of the final thrust.

A biomechanical assessment of the foot is indicated, together with orthotic correction to address the cause.

Retrocalcaneal Bursitis

It is difficult to differentially diagnose a retrocalcaneal bursitis clinically, and as it may coexist with an Achilles tendinopathy, ultrasound imaging is usually required.

Ohberg and Alfredson (2003) used ultrasound and colour Doppler to scan patients with chronic heel pain and identified thickened retrocalcaneal bursae, calcifications, bone spurs, and loose fragments in the adjacent tissues.

Frey et al. (1992) demonstrated the existence of the retrocalcaneal bursa on X-ray using an injection of contrast medium. The normal bursa contains approximately 1 mL of fluid. Patients with retrocalcaneal bursitis accepted less of the contrast medium than normal subjects, leading the authors to propose that this was due to inflammatory fluid, thickened oedematous bursal walls, hypertrophic synovial infoldings and pain.

Retrocalcaneal bursitis presents with posterior heel pain and a muddle of signs that may include pain on passive dorsiflexion, which squeezes the inflamed bursa under the stretched Achilles tendon, and/or passive plantarflexion, which may squeeze the bursa between the Achilles tendon and the calcaneus.

Swelling and tenderness to palpation may be present, just anterior to the insertion of the Achilles tendon. Retrocalcaneal bursitis may be a manifestation of rheumatoid arthritis or one of the spondyloarthropathies, such as Reiter's disease (Hutson, 1990; Frey et al., 1992; Baxter, 1994).

A stepped approach to the management of bursitis is currently recommended. Less invasive treatments are generally offered first, including education/watchful wait, activity and work modification, footwear advice, simple analgesics and NSAIDs medication, physiotherapy (e.g. exercise, mobilisation), podiatry (e.g. orthotics and biomechanical assessment), and then injection therapy (e.g. corticosteroid, local anaesthetic). If symptoms persist, further investigation and referral to a foot and ankle specialist may be required for surgical opinion.

Treatment in the musculoskeletal approach consists of a corticosteroid injection. This is normally performed under image guidance, and it is recommended to check local policy before injecting.

The patient should minimise or modify activities for two weeks following injection.

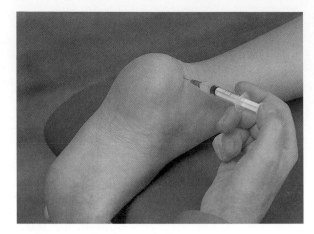

Fig. 12.50 Injection of the retrocalcaneal bursa.

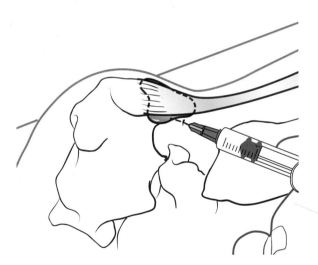

Fig. 12.51 Injection of the retrocalcaneal bursa showing direction of approach and needle position.

INJECTION OF THE RETROCALCANEAL BURSA
Suggested needle size: 23 G × 1 in. (0.6 × 25 mm) blue needle.
Dose: 10 mg triamcinolone acetonide in a total volume of 0.75 mL.

- Position the patient in prone with the foot in a degree of plantarflexion.
- Palpate for the tender area anterior to the distal end of the Achilles tendon and insert the needle from either the medial or lateral aspect, running parallel to the anterior aspect of the Achilles tendon (Figs 12.50 and 12.51).
- Give the injection as a bolus if possible, or pepper the bursa if you feel the resistance of the synovial folds.

Plantar Fasciopathy

Plantar fasciopathy, commonly referred to as plantar fasciitis, usually occurs in middle age, with obesity associated with inactivity as possible predisposing factors (Brukner et al., 2017). It may also be precipitated by an alteration in footwear (e.g. wearing flip-flops or other similar unsupporting shoes) or by prolonged standing on hard surfaces while at work (Trojian and Tucker, 2019). It is a relatively common injury in the running athlete, where it constitutes approximately 10% of running injuries seen (Kibler et al., 1991).

Postural foot deformity such as pes planus and over-pronation lowers the medial longitudinal arch and may overstretch the plantar fascia. Pes cavus may also be associated with the condition (Trojian and Tucker, 2019).

Tightness of the Achilles tendon limits dorsiflexion and may contribute to overpronation (Evans, 1990; Karr, 1994; Trojian and Tucker, 2019). Due to the constant-length phenomenon, extension of the toes increases the height of the longitudinal arch so that activities involving long-term tiptoe standing (e.g. high heels) may excessively stress the plantar fascia. It may also be associated with rheumatoid arthritis or the spondyloarthropathies.

The mechanism of the lesion is thought to be repetitive microtrauma through overloading of the longitudinal arch, which produces focal tears at the insertion of the plantar fascia at the bone–fascia interface (the enthesis; Kibler et al., 1991; Gibbon and Cassar-Pullicino, 1994; Karr, 1994). It may be a traction injury occurring through repeated intrinsic muscle contraction against a stretched plantar fascia during the push-off phase of gait, the plantar fascia acting as an aponeurotic attachment for the first layer of the plantar muscles.

Both mechanisms could possibly lead to the development of calcaneal spurs (Gibbon and Cassar-Pullicino, 1994). Cole et al. (2005) note that calcaneal spurs are present in 50% of patients with plantar fasciopathy and in up to 19% of patients without, but they are not considered to be helpful towards either diagnosis or prognosis (Trojian and Tucker, 2019).

Plantar fasciopathy produces a typical history of a gradual onset of pain felt over the medial plantar aspect of the heel at the enthesis of the central cord into the calcaneal tuberosity (Yu, 2000).

The chronic nature of the condition produces changes in the strength of the plantarflexors, with loss of range of dorsiflexion, and there may be alterations in the length of the stride (Kibler et al., 1991; Chandler and Kibler, 1993).

Its particular characteristic is pain under the heel when the foot is first put to the floor in the morning, easing after taking a few steps (Kibler et al., 1991; Karr, 1994). It is worse after prolonged periods of standing and on initial exercise, easing as the foot warms up but often returning at the end of the day (Trojian and Tucker, 2019).

Passive extension of the toes, with the foot in dorsiflexion, may reproduce the pain by its 'windlass' effect on the plantar fascia arch (Canoso, 1981; Sellman, 1994)

and tenderness to palpation is usually found over the medial calcaneal tuberosity. Diagnosis is made on the typical history and the absence of other findings on examination of the foot and ankle.

Differential diagnosis should exclude fat pad contusion, which tends to occur acutely following a fall onto the heel, or chronically through poor heel cushioning (Brukner et al., 2017). The patient will experience pain on palpation of the heel, and treatment aims to address the cause, advice on footwear and activity modification.

Other conditions to consider are tarsal tunnel syndrome, medial calcaneal nerve entrapment, stress fracture, plantar fibromatosis and enthesopathy (Hossain and Makwana, 2011).

Although unusual, cases of spontaneous rupture of the plantar fascia have been reported, particularly among athletes. It usually occurs during rapid acceleration as the foot forcibly pushes against the ground or may occur over time in association with sustained activity such as walking. The plantar fascia will be tender to palpation, a painful lump may appear, and bruising may be evident; scanning will confirm the lesion. The rupture is usually partial and responds to conservative management. For a complete tear, surgical intervention may be needed (Yu, 2000).

Occasionally infection may occur, but this is usually associated with systemic disease such as diabetes mellitus with heel ulcerations, extension of a surrounding soft tissue infection, or through penetration by a foreign object. The calcaneus is the most commonly infected tarsal bone (Yu, 2000).

A stepped approach to the management of plantar fasciopathy is currently recommended. Less invasive treatments are generally offered first, including education/watchful wait, activity, work and footwear modification, simple analgesics and NSAIDs medication, physiotherapy (e.g. exercise, mobilisation, taping), podiatry (e.g. orthotics and biomechanical assessment) and then injection therapy (e.g. corticosteroid, local anaesthetic, hyaluronic acid and platelet rich plasma (PRP) injections). If symptoms persist, more invasive treatments can be considered, such as night splints, extracorporeal shockwave therapy or fasciectomy.

The National Institute for Health and Care Excellence (NICE) Guidelines (2020b) recommend that patients should be advised that most people will recover in one year, with self-care advice to relieve foot pain, promote healing and prevent future episodes. Simple analgesics and NSAIDs for pain relief as well as other methods, such as applying ice packs or stretches specifically to the plantar fascia, which are more effective than Achilles tendon stretches (DiGiovanni et al., 2006; Trojian and Tucker, 2019).

If a corticosteroid injection is considered for short-term relief of pain, patients should be advised that the injection is painful and there is the risk of fat pad atrophy or rupture. If corticosteroid is still considered to be appropriate, then it should preferably be performed under ultrasound guidance (if this facility is available locally). If it proves to be beneficial, but symptoms return, the NICE Guidelines (2020b) recommend that the treatment may be repeated once only with a minimum of 6 weeks between injections.

The high hyaluronan concentration in the plantar fascia also points to the feasibility of using hyaluronan injections to treat plantar fasciopathy, and platelet-rich plasma (PRP) injections may also be an option (Yang et al., 2017).

If self-care, and following advice and an exercise programme have not been effective after a few months, the advice is to refer to a podiatrist or physiotherapist. Extracorporeal shockwave therapy could be included, and if pain persists, referral to an orthopaedic or podiatric surgeon would be appropriate where surgical division of the plantar fascia could be considered.

Other techniques, including taping and supports, may be applied, and a heel raise or cushion may help to reduce the stretch or pressure on the plantar fascia. All components of dysfunction should be considered when planning a rehabilitation programme and, due to its close relationship with the paratenon of the Achilles tendon, rehabilitation of the triceps surae structures is appropriate (Stecco et al., 2013).

In the musculoskeletal medicine approach, treatment of plantar fasciopathy is by transverse frictions or local corticosteroid injection.

Either treatment is combined with rest from overuse activities and a full rehabilitation programme, which may include intrinsic muscle exercises and foot posture correction, if appropriate.

TRANSVERSE FRICTIONS TO THE PLANTAR FASCIA

- Position the patient in supine lying with the foot held in dorsiflexion, the leg in some lateral rotation.
- Stand on the affected side
- Direct the pressure posteromedially against the origin of the plantar fascia, either with one thumb alone or with one thumb reinforced by the other

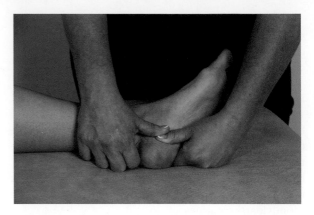

Fig. 12.52 Transverse frictions to the plantar fascia.

- Friction transversely across the fibres (Fig. 12.52).
- Maintain the technique for an appropriate time, according to the irritability of the lesion and stage of healing, to achieve analgesia and mobilise the tissues.

It is important to assess foot posture and to instruct the patient in intrinsic foot exercises. Care should be taken when teaching intrinsic foot exercises to avoid clawing of the toes, which reinforces the activity of the long plantar flexors.

Relative rest is advised where functional movements may continue within the pain-free range.

It is strongly recommended that an ultrasound scan is performed prior to injection to assess the degenerative state of the fascia as a safeguard against possible rupture. It is also important to check local policy before injecting.

INJECTION OF THE PLANTAR FASCIA (CYRIAX, 1984; CYRIAX AND CYRIAX, 1993)
Suggested needle size: 21 G × 1½ in. (0.8 × 40 mm) or 21 G × 2 in. (0.8 × 40 mm) green needle.
Dose: 20 mg triamcinolone acetonide in a total volume of 1.5 mL.

- Position the patient in prone lying with the knee flexed and the lower leg resting on a pillow. Hold the foot in dorsiflexion to apply some tension to the plantar fascia.
- Insert the needle at the heel, anterior to the point of tenderness, and angled posteriorly toward the site of tenderness (Figs 12.53 and 12.54).
- Deliver the injection to the origin of the plantar fascia by a peppering technique, with the needle point in contact with the bone at the anterior edge of the medial tubercle.

The patient should minimise or modify activities for 2 weeks following injection.

Loose Bodies

Although relatively rare, loose bodies can occur in the ankle or subtalar joints. They may be due to degenerative changes in the joint or be associated with fragmented spurs on the tibial or talar side, or by avulsion from the dome of the talus or the malleolus (Scranton et al., 2000).

The patient presents with a history of twinging pain with giving way or a momentary inability to weight-bear; this symptom may also indicate mechanical ankle instability due to ligamentous laxity.

On examination, a non-capsular pattern may be present. The principle of treatment for a loose body is applied: strong traction and Grade A mobilisation. The direction selected for the mobilisation is not important.

Differential diagnosis of loose bodies in the joint includes degenerative, traumatic or inflammatory arthropathy, osteochondritis dissecans or stress fracture.

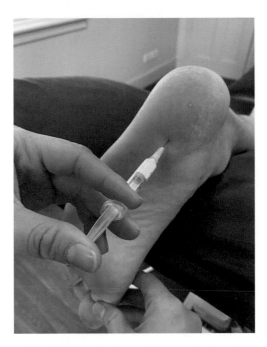

Fig. 12.53 Injection of the plantar fascia.

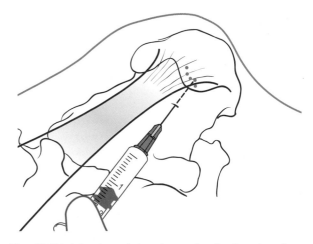

Fig. 12.54 Injection of the plantar fascia showing direction of approach and needle position.

LOOSE-BODY MOBILISATION TECHNIQUE FOR ANKLE JOINT

(Cyriax, 1984; Cyriax and Cyriax, 1993)

- Position the patient in supine with the foot level with the end of the couch.
- Grasp the calcaneus and hold it to act as a fulcrum.
- Grasp the dorsum of the foot with the web of the other hand and lean back to apply strong traction (Fig. 12.55).
- Allow the traction to establish, then apply a circumduction movement with the hand placed around the dorsum of the foot.

The distraction component of the technique can also be useful, especially if the loose bodies are associated with the capsular pattern of pain and limitation of joint movement.

LOOSE-BODY MOBILISATION TECHNIQUE FOR SUBTALAR JOINT

- Position the patient prone with the foot just off the end of the couch.
- Cross your thumbs over the posterosuperior aspect of the calcaneus and wrap your hands around the talus anteriorly.
- Lean back to apply strong traction and apply a varus and valgus stress to the calcaneus with the heels of your hands by rotating your body from side to side (Fig. 12.56).

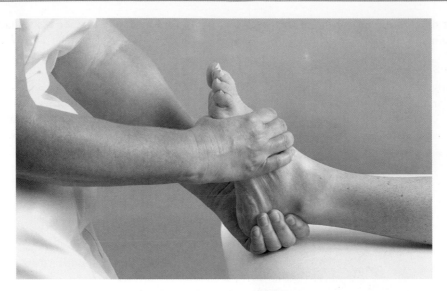

Fig. 12.55 Loose-body mobilisation technique for ankle joint.

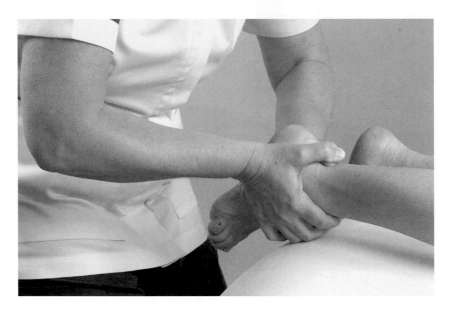

Fig. 12.56 Loose-body mobilisation technique for subtalar joint.

The distraction component can be useful as a mobilising technique in the treatment of arthritis in this joint.

CONTRACTILE LESIONS

The following contractile lesions have been chosen for discussion since they occur relatively commonly in clinical practice. However, the principles of diagnosis and treatment can be applied to any other contractile lesion.

Peroneal Tendinopathy

Peroneal tendinopathy may be a chronic overuse injury (e.g. walking or training on unaccustomed surfaces) predisposed by altered foot biomechanics, or it may have an acute onset as tenosynovitis if the tendons are involved in an inversion sprain of the ankle.

A few cases of rupture of the peroneus longus tendon secondary to repetitive inversion injury or forced eversion injury against resistance have been reported, presenting as chronic lateral ankle instability (Patterson and Cox, 1999).

Pain is felt on the lateral side of the ankle on resisted eversion of the foot. Acute tenosynovitis may also produce pain on passive inversion.

The exact site of the lesion is determined by palpation and it may be at the musculotendinous junction; the tendons above, behind or below the malleolus; or at the insertion of peroneus brevis into the base of the fifth metatarsal.

Disruption of the retinacula may cause 'snapping' of the peroneal tendons due to subluxation or dislocation, which is usually obvious. However, to confirm this, the ankle should be actively dorsiflexed and everted against resistance, which dynamically recreates the subluxation of the tendons (Lee and Maleski, 2002).

Differential diagnosis for peroneal tendinopathy is fracture (talus, fibula, fifth metatarsal), lateral ankle impingement, fibular or sural nerve irritation, and cuboid subluxation (Goode, 2006).

A stepped approach to the management of peroneal tendinopathy is currently recommended. Less invasive treatments are generally offered first, including education/watchful wait, activity and work modification, simple analgesics and NSAID medication, physiotherapy (e.g. exercise, mobilisation, taping), podiatry (e.g. orthotics and biomechanical assessment), and then injection therapy (e.g. corticosteroid, local anaesthetic). If symptoms persist, further investigation and onward referral to a foot and ankle specialist may be required.

Transverse frictions are applied with the tendons on the stretch if the lesion involves the tendons in their common sheath behind or below the malleolus. If the lesion lies in the common sheath below the malleolus, corticosteroid injection is also a treatment option.

TRANSVERSE FRICTIONS TO THE PERONEAL TENDONS

(Cyriax, 1984; Cyriax and Cyriax, 1993)

Stand on the patient's 'good' side and apply treatment to the appropriate site:

Musculotendinous Junction

- Locate the site of the lesion
- Apply the transverse frictions with the index finger, reinforced by the middle finger (Fig. 12.57). Maintain downward pressure as the frictions are applied transversely across the fibres.

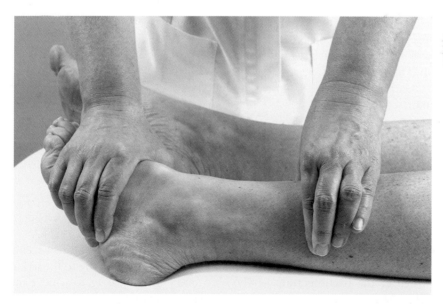

Fig. 12.57 Transverse frictions to the peroneal tendons, musculotendinous junction.

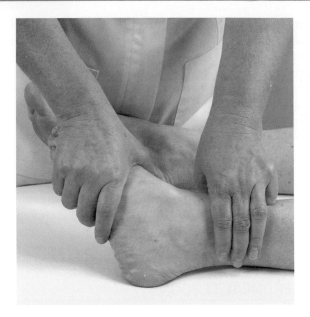

Fig. 12.58 Transverse frictions to the peroneal tendons, above the malleolus.

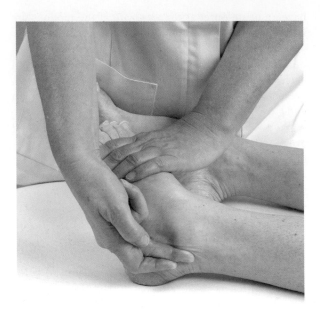

Fig. 12.59 Transverse frictions to the peroneal tendons, behind the malleolus.

Above the Malleolus

- Three fingers are required to cover the extent of the lesion (Fig. 12.58).
- Maintain downward pressure over the tendons as the transverse frictions are applied.

Behind the Malleolus

- Here the tendons run in a common sheath and must be put on a stretch into inversion, as far as discomfort allows.
- Use the middle finger reinforced by the index.
- Apply the transverse frictions by pronating and supinating the forearm (Fig. 12.59).

Below the Malleolus

- Two fingers are required to cover the extent of the lesion (Fig. 12.60).
- The tendons here continue in their common sheath; therefore they are also treated on the stretch. Maintain downward pressure over the tendons as the transverse frictions are applied.

At the Insertion of Peroneus Brevis into the Base of the Fifth Metatarsal

- Apply an index finger, reinforced by the middle, to the insertion and deliver the frictions transversely across the fibres (Fig. 12.61).

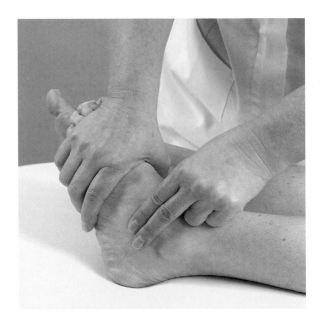

Fig. 12.60 Transverse frictions to the peroneal tendons, below the malleolus.

- Start gently and maintain the technique for an appropriate time, according to the irritability of the lesion and stage of healing, to achieve analgesia and mobilise the tissues.

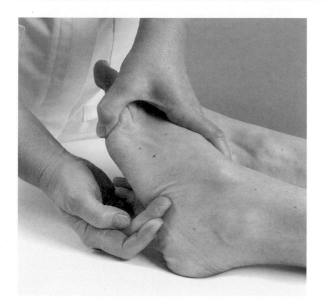

Fig. 12.61 Transverse frictions to the insertion of peroneus brevis into the base of the fifth metatarsal.

Relative rest is advised where functional movements and optimal loading may continue, but no overuse or stretching until the structure is pain-free on resisted testing.

INJECTION TECHNIQUE FOR TENOSYNOVITIS OF THE PERONEAL TENDONS IN THE COMMON SHEATH

Suggested needle size: 23 G × 1 in. (0.6 × 25 mm) blue needle.

Dose: 10 mg triamcinolone acetonide in a total volume of 1 mL.

- Locate the peroneal tubercle, which indicates the distal end of the common sheath.
- Insert the needle into the sheath at the point of diversion of the tendons, aiming the needle toward the malleolus, parallel to the tendons (Fig. 12.62).
- Give the injection as a bolus into the sheath (Fig. 12.63).

The patient should minimise or modify activities for 2 weeks following injection.

INJECTION TECHNIQUE FOR TENDINOPATHY AT THE TENO-OSSEOUS JUNCTION OF PERONEUS BREVIS AT THE BASE OF THE FIFTH METATARSAL

Suggested needle size: 25 G × 5/8 in. (0.5 × 16 mm) orange needle.

Dose: 10 mg triamcinolone acetonide in a total volume of 1 mL.

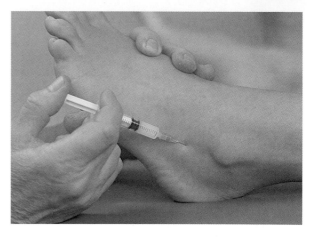

Fig. 12.62 Injection technique for tenosynovitis of the peroneal tendons in the common sheath.

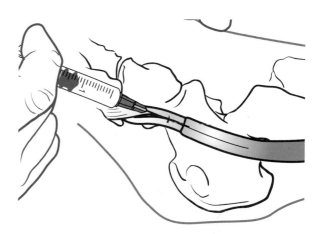

Fig. 12.63 Injection technique for tenosynovitis of the peroneal tendons in the common sheath showing direction of approach and needle position.

- Locate the base of the fifth metatarsal and mark the tender point.
- Deliver the injection by a peppering technique at the teno-osseous junction (Figs 12.64 and 12.65).

The patient should minimise or modify activities for 2 weeks following injection. An appropriate progressive loading rehabilitation programme should be applied.

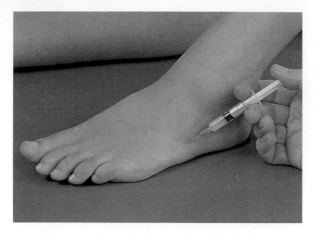

Fig. 12.64 Injection technique at the teno-osseous junction of peroneus brevis: base of the fifth metatarsal.

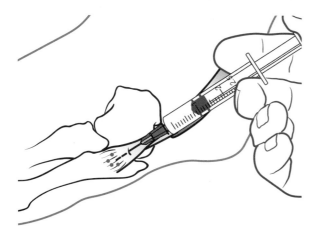

Fig. 12.65 Injection technique at the teno-osseous junction of peroneus brevis: base of the fifth metatarsal showing direction of approach and needle position.

Achilles Tendinopathy

Achilles tendinopathy can involve a range of lesions at different sites in the tendon:

- Approximately 2 to 6 cm proximal to the tendon's insertion, the midportion, which is the zone considered to be of relatively poor vascularity in normal tendons (Chandnani and Bradley, 1994).
- The teno-osseous insertion into the calcaneus.
- The paratenon itself can also be involved.

A lesion at the musculotendinous junction is covered below with the gastrocnemius muscle belly.

Achilles tendinopathy may come on gradually if associated with prolonged over- or underuse or more quickly if associated with sudden trauma or unaccustomed activity. It is diagnosed clinically and can affect the distal insertion or the midportion of the tendon (van der Vlist et al., 2021).

It can affect athletes at all levels, and often a return to activity after a break from training may be involved. Symptoms are common in recreational athletes within the 35 to 50 age group, particularly those who participate in middle- or long-distance running.

However, Achilles tendinopathy can also be caused by less strenuous activities or may even develop without an obvious cause (Alfredson et al., 2002; Ohberg and Alfredson, 2004). Apart from athletes, the condition also occurs in the general population, often in those with a sedentary lifestyle (Alfredson and Lorentzon, 2000; Paavola et al., 2002). There is a higher incidence in older postmenopausal women (J.L. Cook, conference lecture, 2008).

Several aetiological mechanisms have been proposed, including malalignment of the rear foot, leading to functional overpronation Koenig et al. (2004). This supports the value of assessing the biomechanics of the lower limb as part of the examination of the ankle and foot.

Several other proposed mechanisms include incorrect or worn-out footwear, pressure from heel counters, one-off incidents of direct trauma, changes in training surfaces, excessive training, training errors or indirect trauma, muscle weakness and/or imbalance, reduced flexibility, joint stiffness, obesity or leg-length discrepancy.

The plantaris tendon can occasionally cause compression of the Achilles tendon, because it is enlarged and/or ensheathed within the Achilles peritenon, where it may provoke tendinopathy (Brukner et al., 2017).

Wise et al. (2012) observed a strong association between the use of quinolone antibiotics and an increased risk of Achilles tendinopathy and rupture. The association was more pronounced amongst elderly and non-obese persons and where there was concurrent use of oral glucocorticoids. The effect for tendon rupture was stronger in women.

Patients with diabetes mellitus and dyslipidaemia (high level of blood lipids or a low high-density lipoprotein (HDL) cholesterol level) are also more at risk of developing Achilles tendinopathy (NICE, 2020a).

Achilles tendinopathy pain or spontaneous rupture can also be associated with spondyloarthropathies (Jebaraj and Rao, 2006).

Tendinopathy is covered in more detail in Chapter 3.

Patients normally present with a history of a gradual onset of pain felt locally at the back or just above the heel (Ohberg and Alfredson, 2004). They may or may not recall the causative factor. In the early phase of the condition, pain usually follows strenuous activity, whereas, in the more chronic condition, pain occurs during all activities and can be present at rest (Paavola et al., 2002). The tendon is usually sore and thickened, impairing gait (Alfredson et al., 2002; Koenig et al., 2004).

The pain is worse when the foot is first put to the floor in the morning, easing after several steps (the location of the pain distinguishes it from plantar fasciopathy). The thickened tendon is tender to palpation, and crepitus may be present due to movement of the tendon within the paratenon, which may be filled with fibrin exudate (Paavola et al., 2002; Figs 12.66 and 12.67).

On examination, resisted plantarflexion is painful, but it usually needs to be performed against gravity, with body-weight resistance, to reproduce symptoms in minor or chronic lesions. A combination of pain in the Achilles tendon, stiffness, thickening and impaired performance, together with pain on resisted plantarflexion, provides a clinical diagnosis of Achilles tendinopathy (Paavola et al., 2002; NICE, 2020a).

Pain and swelling at the insertion to the posterior calcaneus, with functional impairment, suggests insertional Achilles tendinopathy. Pain 2 to 6 cm proximally

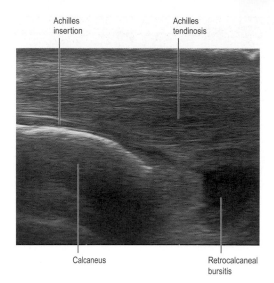

Fig. 12.67 Ultrasound scan demonstrating tendinopathy and retrocalcaneal bursitis. (Provided by Kjetil Nord-Varhaug.)

to the tendon insertion indicates mid-portion Achilles tendinopathy. Some people may have symptoms at both the insertion and mid-portion (NICE, 2020a).

Differential diagnosis for Achilles tendinopathy includes full thickness or partial rupture, retrocalcaneal or superficial bursitis, impingement between the posterior part of the calcaneus and the Achilles tendon, calcification or avulsion fracture, or occasionally mixed pathology (Alfredson and Lorentzon, 2000). Pain associated with pathology in the plantaris tendon itself is usually sited medially with tenderness higher than the usual midportion tendinopathy (Brukner et al., 2017).

Whether partial or complete, rupture may occur through indirect violent trauma (e.g. push-off with knee extension during weight-bearing as in sprinting), unexpected, forced dorsiflexion (e.g. missing a step or stumbling), or forced dorsiflexion of the plantarflexed foot, as in falling from a height. It is accompanied by a sudden onset of pain (Smart et al., 1980; Mahler and Fritschy, 1992). Partial rupture and degenerative tendinopathy may coexist or possibly be regarded and managed as the same condition (Alfredson and Lorentzon, 2000).

Total rupture presents with a history of intense pain at the time of injury, as if being kicked or 'shot' in the tendon, but there is little pain following injury. The tendon's function is disrupted, and the patient is unable to tiptoe stand. A gap may be palpable immediately after injury, and the Thompson's test (also known as Simmond's test) and/or Matles test is positive (Hattam and Smeatham, 2020).

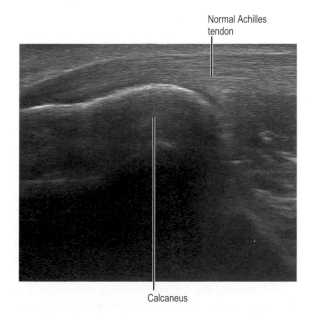

Fig. 12.66 Ultrasound scan of normal Achilles tendon. (Provided by Kjetil Nord-Varhaug.)

THOMPSON'S TEST
- Position the patient in prone lying with the foot hanging off the couch
- Squeeze the bulk of the calf muscle
- If intact, the Achilles tendon plantarflexes the foot

The Matles test is a further aid to diagnosis of rupture, particularly if chronic.

MATLES TEST
- In prone lying, ask the patient to actively flex the knee through 90 degrees
- Observe the foot and ankle
- Normally the foot should remain slightly plantarflexed throughout the movement
- The test is positive if the foot falls into a neutral or a dorsiflexed position (Frey and Shereff, 1988; Lee and Maleski, 2002)

Ultrasound or magnetic resonance imaging MRI are used to confirm diagnosis.

Differential diagnosis of pain in the region of the Achilles tendon includes plantaris tendinopathy, dislocation of the peroneal or other plantar flexor tendons, posterior ankle impingement, Haglund's syndrome, os trigonum syndrome, fascial tears, calcaneal fracture, irritation or neuroma of the sural nerve, fat pad irritation, and systemic inflammatory disease (NICE, 2020a).

There is some debate regarding the optimal treatment for acute, complete ruptures of the Achilles tendon. Both conservative and surgical treatments have their own risks and benefits. The decision on whether conservative or surgical is best for the patient depends on many factors, such as age, and patient factors including functional and activity level, general health, lifestyle and patients' preference. Surgical management usually has a lower re-rupture rate, compared to conservative management.

However, more complications (infections, tendinitis) have been reported after surgical treatment, although they were not statistically significant. Studies have demonstrated that early weight-bearing of an injured tendon does increase collagen production and stimulates the healing process (Manent et al., 2019).

Treatment of Achilles Tendinopathy

At all sites, a stepped approach to the management of Achilles tendinopathy is currently recommended. Less

invasive treatments are generally offered first, including education/watchful wait, activity and work modification, simple analgesics and NSAID medication and physiotherapy (e.g. exercise, progressive loading, mobilisation, acupuncture, extracorporeal shock wave therapy). If symptoms persist, more invasive treatments can be considered, such as PRP injections, sclerosants and surgery.

Despite the general stepped approach outlined above, van der Vlist et al. (2021) found no support for watchful wait for patients with Achilles tendinopathy in their living systematic review, and all treatments appeared to be superior to watchful wait at 3 months.

Treatment objectives are to limit tissue injury and stimulate a healing response (Tasto et al., 2003). For acute injuries, the current regime for the management of soft tissue injuries should be followed (see Chapter 4).

In the reactive stage of Achilles tendinopathy, reducing the load on the tendon will generally allow the tendon to adapt and the matrix to assume a more normal structure; this is also likely to relieve pain (Cook and Purdam, 2009).

The latter stages associated with disrepair and degeneration may be irreversible, but the application of treatment modalities that aim to stimulate cell activity, increase protein synthesis (collagen or ground substance) and restructure the matrix are suitable for Achilles tendinopathy at this stage (Cook and Purdam, 2009). These can include transverse frictions, extracorporeal shock wave therapy and ultrasound, along with progressive loading exercises.

Careful progressive loading through exercise is required to avoid pain aggravation and promote reversal of the tissue changes. Brukner et al. (2017) describe a 4-stage programme for midportion Achilles tendinopathy that passes through pain relief with isometric exercises, isotonic strength endurance (where appropriate), energy storage exercises and energy storage and release exercises. The latter three stages aim to develop tendon capacity.

The final part of rehabilitation, to return to activity or training, must be guided carefully (Scott et al., 2013) and should only be permitted when the energy storage and release exercises (stage 4 above) can be performed repeatedly with no increase in symptoms the following morning (Brukner et al., 2017).

Alfredson and Cook (2007) devised a treatment algorithm for managing Achilles tendinopathy with eccentric training at its heart, but following the modification of the theoretical basis of the management of tendinopathy, eccentric exercises are more appropriate for the latter stage of disrepair and degeneration.

In degenerate tendons, in contrast to the optimal loading progression in reactive tendinopathy, an increased pain level is acceptable while performing eccentric exercise. This appears to be tolerated by the tendon since there is less irritability in this stage of tendinopathy (Cook and Purdam, 2009). It may also be that a combination of both eccentric and concentric exercises are as beneficial as eccentric exercises alone (Brukner et al., 2017).

The analgesic effects of exercise on central pain mechanisms contributing to tendinopathy may have an important role, and Scott et al. (2013) suggest that some pain whilst performing exercise is necessary to maximise these effects.

Apart from exercise, other modalities have been used in the management of Achilles tendinopathy, including extracorporeal shock wave therapy and ice, which can decrease the extravasation of blood and protein from the new capillaries in tendinosis; suspected as a cause of the pain Kader et al. (2005).

Injection therapy for Achilles tendinopathy includes:
- Autologous blood and PRP injections, which aim to stimulate tendon healing via normal physiological pathways (Jo et al., 2012; Pearson et al., 2012; Scott et al., 2013).
- Sclerosant, or prolotherapy, injections that appear to close down new vessels that have become established in degenerative tendinopathy, which (as mentioned above) are proposed as a cause of pain (Ohberg and Alfredson, 2003; Brukner et al., 2017).
- High-volume image-guided injections of normal saline, local anaesthetic and aprotinin (a substance that reverse the vasoactive effect of associated enzymes; Maffulli et al., 2013).

Corticosteroid injections are no longer advocated, due to safety concerns relating to the potential deleterious effect on the tendon tissue and risk of rupture (Coombes et al., 2010), unless all other conservative treatment approaches have failed (van der Vlist et al., 2021), and/or the benefits outweigh the risks.

Surgical treatment requires extensive postsurgical rehabilitation and is reserved for tendons that have failed to respond to conservative treatment. Procedures range from percutaneous tenotomy to open procedures where tendon pathology is removed. A minimally invasive Doppler-guided mini surgical scraping technique has been developed to allow quick rehabilitation and a return to full tendon loading activity after 2 to 6 weeks (Scott et al., 2013).

Within the stepped approach to management, the musculoskeletal medicine technique is to apply transverse frictions to all sites of Achilles tendinopathy, aiming to mobilise the tissue structure, provide pain relief and improve function.

As mentioned in Chapter 4, evidence to support their effectiveness is mainly anecdotal (J. Kerr, unpublished work, 2006), and although clinical experience should not be ignored, further research would be valuable to gain evidence to underpin the extensive use of this technique for this condition. Other mobilisation techniques such as specific soft tissue mobilisations (Hunter, 1998) can also be included in the programme.

Treatment should be accompanied by education in activity modification, particularly addressing the causative factors. A full explanation should be given of the prognosis and expected recovery time, which may well be in excess of 3 months due to the slow progression of tendon healing (Scott et al., 2013; Brukner et al., 2017).

TRANSVERSE FRICTIONS TO THE ACHILLES TENDON

(Cyriax, 1984; Cyriax and Cyriax, 1993)

The sites for Achilles tendinopathy are the anterior aspect and sides of the tendon of the mid-portion of the tendon and the insertion into the calcaneus. The affected site is identified by palpation.

Anterior Aspect of the Tendon

- Position the patient in prone lying with the foot relaxed into plantarflexion on a pillow.
- Push the relaxed Achilles tendon laterally with a finger, placing your middle finger reinforced by the index against the exposed anterolateral surface of the tendon (Fig. 12.68).
- Apply the transverse frictions by a pronation and supination movement of your forearm.
- Maintain the technique for an appropriate time, according to the irritability of the lesion and stage of healing, to achieve analgesia and mobilise the tissues.
- Repeat the same procedure, if required, with the tendon pushed medially to gain access to the anteromedial side (Fig. 12.69).

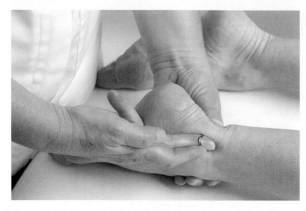

Fig. 12.68 Transverse frictions to the anterolateral aspect of the Achilles tendon.

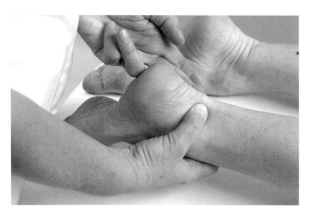

Fig. 12.69 Transverse frictions to the anteromedial aspect of the Achilles tendon.

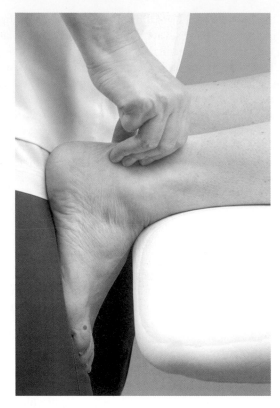

Fig. 12.70 Transverse frictions to the sides of the Achilles tendon.

Sides of the Tendon

- Position the patient in prone lying with the foot resting on a pillow over the edge of the couch. Rest your leg against the patient's foot to place it in a degree of dorsiflexion, applying enough tension to the Achilles tendon to stabilise it for treatment.
- Grasp the tendon between your fingers and thumb, covering the extent of the lesion and friction transversely across the fibres (Fig. 12.70).
- Maintain the technique for an appropriate time, according to the irritability of the lesion and stage of healing, to achieve analgesia and mobilise the tissues.

Insertion of the Achilles Tendon into the Calcaneus

- Position the patient in prone lying, with the head of the couch slightly elevated, preferably with a pillow under the foot to relax it into plantarflexion (Fig. 12.71).

- This puts you into a position of mechanical advantage and allows you to stabilise the calcaneus.
- Make a ring formed by the index fingers, one reinforced by the other, and the thumbs.
- Rest your index fingers on the calcaneus at the tender site and wrap your thumbs around the heel (Fig. 12.71).
- Direct the pressure through your index fingers down onto the insertion.
- Impart the transverse frictions transversely across the fibres by rotating your body side to side.
- Maintain the technique for an appropriate time, according to the irritability of the lesion and stage of healing, to achieve analgesia and mobilise the tissues.

Relative rest is advised for all sites, where functional movements may continue, but no overuse or stretching until the structure is pain-free on resisted testing.

The 'heel drop' eccentric exercise programme is not as effective for lesions at the Achilles insertion into the

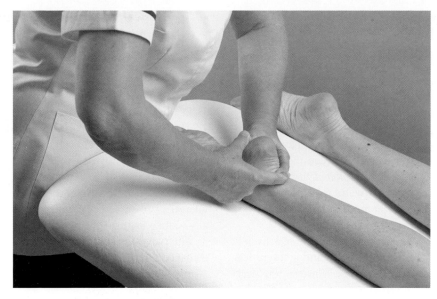

Fig. 12.71 Transverse frictions to the insertion of the Achilles tendon into the calcaneus.

calcaneus as for 'mid-portion' (Thomas et al., 2001; J.L. Cook, conference lecture, 2008; Brukner et al., 2017).

A compression component is proposed in insertional Achilles tendinopathy, which is important and may explain why stretching and full-range eccentric loading are not as effective as in midportion tendon pathology.

Full-range dorsiflexion increases compression on the tendon, and it is advisable to limit dorsiflexion to plantigrade only (i.e. avoiding heel drop over the edge of a stair) when devising eccentric exercise programmes for lesions at this site (Cook and Purdam, 2009). A heel raise can be helpful.

Insertional Achilles tendinopathy and retrocalcaneal bursitis commonly occur together, and both should be addressed within the context of the rehabilitation of the whole musculotendinous unit.

Gastrocnemius Muscle Belly

Strain of the gastrocnemius muscle belly often has an acute onset following a sudden sprinting action such as accelerating from a stationary position with the ankle in dorsiflexion, or lunging forward as in squash or tennis. Sudden eccentric overstretching of the muscle, such as missing a step on the kerb or stairs, is another mechanism (Brukner et al., 2017).

The medial head has a longer attachment to the Achilles and may be more susceptible to injury.

In addition to recent trauma, risk factors may include recent surgery or immobilisation, recent long-haul travel and oestrogen use, as well as family history or previous vascular problems (Taylor, 2002).

A chronic strain of the gastrocnemius muscle belly may result from a past acute lesion or chronic overuse.

In an acute strain, patients feel as though they have been kicked or hit in the calf; the pain is acute, and weight-bearing is difficult. The limb becomes swollen, and bruising develops within 24 to 48 hours.

The diagnosis is conclusive from the history, and palpation often localises the lesion to the medial head of the gastrocnemius muscle belly or to the musculotendinous junction where a dip may be felt. Pain is reproduced by resisted plantarflexion and on passive dorsiflexion.

Differential diagnosis should include deep vein thrombosis, which can be associated with calf injuries and may be difficult to exclude. Taylor (2002) suggests that the force required to damage a muscle or the compressive effects of oedema may be sufficient to cause intravascular damage or microtears leading to roughening of the vessel, and platelet aggregation and thrombus formation.

Risk factors should be considered that may give rise to the combination of factors leading to thrombus formation as described in the so-called Virchow's triad, comprising alterations in blood flow, vascular endothelial injury and changes in normal blood flow or consistency.

Diagnosis of deep vein thrombosis is confirmed in the presence of constant pain, tenderness, heat, swelling and a positive Homan's sign, involving pain on passive overpressure of dorsiflexion with the knee in extension (Brukner et al., 2017). Imaging may also be used to confirm the diagnosis.

A stepped approach to the management of a gastrocnemius muscle belly lesion is currently recommended. Less invasive treatments are generally offered first, including education/watchful wait, activity and work modification, simple analgesics and NSAID medication, physiotherapy (e.g. exercise, mobilisation, acupuncture).

Healing of a mild gastrocnemius muscle tear usually takes about 1 to 3 weeks for recovery, and a severe tear may take 8 to 12 weeks for recovery. However, the healing rate also depends on individual patient factors within medical history and social history, such as occupational and leisure activities. If symptoms persist, alternative causes of symptoms should be considered.

TREATMENT OF ACUTE GASTROCNEMIUS MUSCLE BELLY LESION

Apply the treatment principles for acute soft tissue lesions (see Chapter 4) as soon as possible after the onset and for 2 to 3 days after injury.

- Transverse frictions are applied across the full extent of the lesion with the muscle belly in a relaxed position (Fig. 12.72). This mobilises the muscle tissue, which broadens as the muscle contracts.
- Maintain the technique for an appropriate time, according to the irritability of the lesion and stage of healing, to achieve analgesia and mobilise the tissues.
- Transverse frictions are followed immediately by Grade A mobilisations.

The patient is taught to maintain a normal heel–toe gait with the aid of crutches if necessary. A heel raise takes the pressure off the muscle belly and can be gradually reduced as movement is regained.

The patient is seen regularly. An increasing depth of transverse frictions and progressively greater range of Grade A mobilisation is applied until full painless function is restored.

TREATMENT OF CHRONIC GASTROCNEMIUS MUSCLE BELLY LESION

- Transverse frictions are applied across the full extent of the lesion with the muscle belly in a relaxed position (Fig. 12.72). This mobilises the muscle tissue, which broadens as the muscle contracts.
- Maintain the technique for an appropriate time, according to the irritability of the lesion and stage

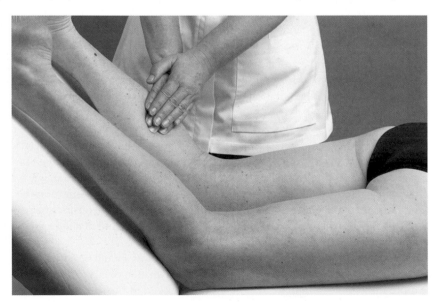

Fig. 12.72 Transverse frictions for acute and chronic gastrocnemius muscle belly lesion.

of healing, to achieve analgesia and to mobilise the tissues.

- Progressive Grade A exercises are performed immediately.

The patient is treated until normal, painless function is restored. Should the muscle need to be stretched, it is applied once the muscle is pain-free on resisted testing, but this should not be necessary if the Grade A exercises have been performed to nudge progressively into the end of pain-free range.

TREATMENT OF GASTROCNEMIUS MUSCULOTENDINOUS JUNCTION

If the lesion is in the musculotendinous junction, it may be treated with transverse frictions.

- Locate the tender site and apply transverse frictions across the full extent of the lesion (Fig. 12.73).
- Maintain the technique for an appropriate time, according to the irritability of the lesion and stage of healing, to achieve analgesia and mobilise the tissues.

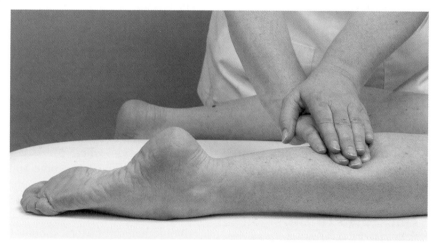

Fig. 12.73 Transverse frictions to the gastrocnemius musculotendinous junction.

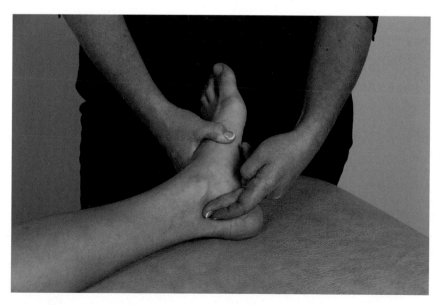

Fig. 12.74 Transverse frictions to the tibialis posterior tendon, behind the malleolus.

Tibialis Posterior

The patient presents with a history of pain felt on the medial aspect of the ankle, and the causative factors may not be known. It is often due to the repetitive microtrauma of overloading associated with overpronated foot postures and flattening of the medial longitudinal arch. It more commonly affects obese, working-aged women who may also be hypertensive. When left untreated, it can develop into an 'adult-acquired flat foot' (Van de Velde et al., 2017).

Activities that involve rapid changes in direction (e.g. soccer, tennis, hockey) place increased stress on tibialis posterior and make it vulnerable to acute injury in these situations (Frey and Shereff, 1988).

On inspection, oedema may be present. There can be obvious thickening of the tendon along its course behind and below the medial malleolus, and heat may be felt on palpation. The positive sign is pain on resisted inversion, and palpation for tenderness localises the lesion. There is usually an inability to perform a single heel raise (Van der Velde et al., 2017).

The lesion may be above, behind or below the medial malleolus or at the tendon insertion.

TRANSVERSE FRICTIONS TO THE TIBIALIS POSTERIOR TENDON

- Transverse frictions are applied with the tendon on the stretch in tenosynovitis, as the tendon is enclosed within a synovial sheath on its course around the malleolus (see Fig. 12.74).
- Apply one finger reinforced with another (usually middle finger reinforced with the index finger) firmly against the tender portion of the tendon.
- Perform the transverse frictions with a rolling movement by pronating and supinating the forearm.
- Maintain the technique for an appropriate time, according to the irritability of the lesion and stage of healing, to achieve analgesia and mobilise the tissues.
- The technique may need to be repeated at a slightly different site if the contact of the fingers cannot cover the full length of the lesion.

Alternatively, corticosteroid injection can be given applying the principles given above for the peroneal tendons.

Tarsal Tunnel Syndrome

Tarsal tunnel syndrome is a compression neuropathy of the posterior tibial nerve. The nerve becomes trapped in the tarsal tunnel as it winds around the medial malleolus. It can be associated with poor foot posture, benign bony projections into the tarsal tunnel, varicose veins and diabetes.

The patient complains of a diffuse burning, tingling, 'electric shock' or numb sensation on the plantar aspect of the foot that may radiate into the toes (Brukner et al., 2017).

Behaviour of the symptoms varies. With some patients, the symptoms are worse in bed at night and relieved by moving (as in carpal tunnel syndrome), and in others, the symptoms are made worse by activity and relieved by rest.

Tinel's test, gently tapping the nerve, may reproduce the patient's symptoms, and electromyography and MRI may also be useful for diagnosis.

Differential diagnosis should include L5 or S1 nerve root compression, where paraesthesia is usually felt in the distal end of the dermatome, within a similar distribution. Occasionally similar symptoms are also experienced with medial plantar nerve entrapment and plantar fasciopathy.

Biomechanical factors should be addressed with orthotics if necessary. Neural mobilising techniques may be appropriate. Surgical decompression is a last resort, and the diagnosis needs to be certain. The surgery outcomes are generally not good, although minimally invasive techniques are being developed that have a lower risk of complications and reduced recovery time (Brukner et al., 2017).

REVIEW QUESTIONS

1. Review the injection procedure for the first metatarsophalangeal joint.
2. How do you test for the integrity of the ankle mortise?
3. Describe the manipulation technique for chronic ankle lateral ligament injuries and consider any contraindications.
4. What are the capsular patterns of the ankle, midtarsal and subtalar joints?
5. What are the possible sites of Achilles tendinopathy, and how would the treatment differ for the various sites?

CASE SCENARIOS

Case 1

History

- Hilary, a 66-year-old housewife, recently took up ballroom dancing inspired by a TV show. She sustained an inversion injury to her left ankle 2 weeks ago whilst doing a tango. Pain was immediate, but she could weight-bear, and swelling occurred a few hours later. Pain is over the lateral malleolus and is worse first thing in the morning and with any inversion movements. She is of good health.

Examination

- She is able to fully weight-bear and has swelling below her left lateral malleolus. Pain at end range of passive ankle plantarflexion and painful limited inversion. Resisted tests are pain-free. Pain end-range midtarsal inversion and adduction. Tender on palpation over two of the lateral ligaments.

Task

- Which two lateral ligaments appear to be injured in this lady? How do we test for ligament instability? Review the anatomy and consider your treatment approach and aftercare.

Case 2

History

- Josh, a 21-year-old Marine, has pain in his left heel following intensive training with a heavy load while wearing newly distributed expedition boots. This has been present for 4 weeks and is affecting his ability to work. Pain is worse with walking, running and first thing in the morning. He has had previous inversion sprains of both ankles and shin splints in the last year.

Examination

- Overpronation and poor balance/proprioception on both feet, left worse than right. Full ankle passive and resisted movements. Some laxity of bilateral anterior talofibular ligaments on testing. He has a tight left gastrocnemius and is tender on palpation of the medial tubercle of the left calcaneus.

Task

- Consider factors contributing to diagnosis. What would your treatment plan and his rehabilitation regime need to consider? Is this young man a candidate for orthotics? Is injection an option? Justify reasoning.

Case 3

History

- Janine, a 49-year-old housewife, is a keen runner and has worn orthotics and the same brand of trainers for years. Two months ago, she bought new trainers with no medial arch support and ran in them for the first time in a 10k race. She has had pain in her right Achilles tendon since the race and cannot run without pain. She is currently taking glucosamine.

Examination

- Overpronated feet bilaterally, with slight thickening around mid-portion of the Achilles tendon. Her pain on the right is reproduced by standing on tiptoe. She is tender on palpation of the medial side of the mid-portion of her Achilles tendon.

Task

- How would you differentiate between Achilles tendinopathy and retrocalcaneal bursitis? What advice would you give this lady regarding footwear and training? Consider the manual treatment and rehabilitation protocol for her.

REFERENCES

Abrahams, P.H., 2019. Abrahams' and McMinn's Clinical Atlas of Human Anatomy, eighth ed. Elsevier, Oxford.

Acus, R.W., Flanagan, J.P., 1991. Perineural fibrosis of superficial peroneal nerve complicating ankle sprain: a case report. Foot Ankle 11, 233–235.

Alfredson, H., Bjur, D., Thorsen, K., et al., 2002. High intratendinous lactate levels in painful chronic Achilles tendinosis. An investigation using microdialysis technique. J. Orthop. Res. 20 (5), 934–938.

Alfredson, H., Cook, J., 2007. A treatment algorithm for managing Achilles tendinopathy: new treatment options. Br. J. Sports Med. 41, 211–216.

Alfredson, H., Lorentzon, R., 2000. Chronic Achilles tendinosis: recommendations for treatment and prevention. Sports Med. 29 (2), 135–146.

Auletta, A.G., Conway, W.F., Hayes, C.W., et al., 1991. Indications for radiography in patients with acute ankle injuries: role of the physical examination. Am. J. Roentgenol. 157, 789–791.

Baxter, D.E., 1994. The heel in sport. Clin. Sports Med. 13, 683–693.

Bekerom, M.P.J., Raven, E.E.J., 2007. The distal fascicle of the anterior inferior tibiofibular ligament (AITFL) as a cause of tibiotalar impingement syndrome: a current concepts review. Knee Surg. Sports Traumatol. Arthrosc. 15 (4), 465–471.

Blake, R.L., Anderson, K., Ferguson, H., 1994. Posterior tibial tendinopathy. J. Am. Podiat. Med. Assoc 84, 141–149.

Boruta, P.M., Bishop, J.O., Braly, W.G., et al., 1990. Acute lateral ankle ligament injuries: a literature review. Foot Ankle 11, 107–113.

Bottger, B.A., Schweitzer, M.E., El-Noueam, K.I., et al., 1998. MR imaging of the normal and abnormal retrocalcaneal bursae. Am. J. Roentgenol. 170, 1239–1241.

Boytim, M.J., Fischer, D.A., Neumann, L., 1991. Syndesmotic ankle sprains. Am. J. Sports Med. 19, 294–298.

Brukner, P., Clarson, B., Cook, J., et al., 2017. Clinical Sports Medicine, fifth ed. McGraw-Hill, Sydney, Volume 1: Injuries

Canoso, J.J., 1981. Bursae, tendons and ligaments. Clin. Rheum. Dis. 7, 189–221.

Chandler, T.J., Kibler, W.B., 1993. A biomechanical approach to the prevention, treatment and rehabilitation of plantar fasciitis. Sports Med. 15, 344–352.

Chandnani, V.P., Bradley, Y.C., 1994. Achilles tendon and miscellaneous lesions. MRI Clin. N. Am. 2, 89–96.

Cole, C., Seto, C., Gazewood, J., 2005. Plantar fasciitis: evidence-based review of diagnosis and therapy. Am. Fam. Phys. 72 (11), 2237–2242.

Colville, M., Marder, R., Boyle, J., et al., 1990. Strain measurements in lateral ankle ligaments. Am. J. Sports Med. 18 (2), 196–200.

Cook, J.L., Purdam, C.R., 2009. Is tendon pathology a continuum? A pathology model to explain the clinical presentation of load-induced tendinopathy. Br. J. Sports Med. 43, 409–416.

Coombes, B.K., Bisset, L., Vicenzino, B., 2010. Efficacy and safety of corticosteroid injections and other injections for management of tendinopathy: a systematic review of randomised controlled trials. Lancet 376 (9754), 1751–1767.

Cornwall, M.W., Murrell, P., 1991. Postural sway following inversion sprain of the ankle. J. Am. Podiat. Med. Assoc. 81, 243–247.

Cyriax, J., 1984. Textbook of Orthopaedic Medicine, eleventh ed. Baillière Tindall, London.

Cyriax, J., Cyriax, P., 1993. Cyriax's Illustrated Manual of Orthopaedic Medicine. Butterworth Heinemann, Oxford.

Demetriades, L., Strauss, E., Gallina, J., 1998. Osteoarthritis of the ankle. Clin. Orthop. Rel. Res. 349, 28–42.

DiGiovanni, B.F., Nawoczenski, D.A., Malay, D.P., et al., 2006. Plantar fascia – specific stretching exercise improves outcomes in patients with chronic plantar fasciitis. J. Bone Joint Surg. 88A, 1775–1781.

Edwards, G.S., DeLee, J.C., 1984. Ankle diastasis without fracture. Foot Ankle 4, 305–312.

Evans, P., 1990. Clinical biomechanics of the subtalar joint. Physiotherapy 76, 47–81.

Ferran, N., Maffulli, N., 2006. Epidemiology of sprains of the lateral ankle complex. Foot Ankle Clin. 11, 659–662.

Freedman, B.R., Gordon, J.A., Soslowsky, L.J., 2014. The Achilles tendon: fundamental properties and mechanisms governing healing. Muscle Ligaments Tendons J. 4 (2), 245–255.

Frey, C., Rosenberg, Z., Shereff, M.J., et al., 1992. The retrocalcaneal bursa: anatomy and bursography. Foot Ankle 13, 203–207.

Frey, C., Shereff, M.J., 1988. Tendon injuries about the ankle in athletes. Clin. Sports Med. 7, 103–118.

Gibbon, W.W., Cassar-Pullicino, V.N., 1994. Heel pain. Ann. Rheum. Dis. 53, 344–348.

Goode, L., 2006. Ankle Differential Diagnosis. Office of Inspector General, Washington DC.

Hattam, P., Smeatham, A., 2020. Handbook of Special Tests in Musculoskeletal Examination, second ed. Elsevier, Oxford.

Hertel, J., 2002. Functional anatomy, pathomechanics, and pathophysiology of lateral ankle ligament instability. J. Athl. Train 37 (4), 364–375.

Hossain, M., Makwana, N., 2011. 'Not Plantar Fasciitis': the differential diagnosis and management of heel pain syndrome. Orthop. Trauma 25 (3), 198–206.

Hunter, G., 1998. Specific soft tissue mobilization in the management of soft tissue dysfunction. Man. Ther. 3 (1), 2–11.

Hur, E.S., Bohl, D.D., Lee, S., 2020. Lateral ligament instability: review of pathology and diagnosis. Curr. Rev. Musculoskelet. Med. 13 (4), 494–500.

Hutson, M.A., 1990. Sports Injuries – Recognition and Management. Oxford Medical Publications, Oxford.

Jebaraj, I., Rao, A., 2006. Achilles tendon enthesopathy in ochronosis. J. Postgrad. Med. 52, 47–48.

Jo, C.H., Kim, J.E., Yoon, K.S., et al., 2012. Platelet-rich plasma stimulates cell proliferation and enhances matrix gene expression and synthesis in tenocytes from human rotator cuff tendons with degenerative tears. Am. J. Sports Med. 40 (5), 1035–1045.

Kader, D., Maffulli, N., Leadbetter, W.B., et al., 2005. Achilles tendinopathy. In: Maffulli, N., Renström, P., Leadbetter, W.B. (Eds.), Tendon Injuries: Basic Science and Clinical Medicine. Springer-Verlag, London, pp. 201–208.

Kannus, V.P., 1992. Evaluation of abnormal biomechanics of the foot and ankle in athletes. Br. J. Sports Med. 26, 83–89.

Kannus, P., Renstrom, P., 1991. Treatment for acute tears of the lateral ligaments of the ankle. J. Bone Joint Surg. 73A, 305–312.

Karlsson, J., Lansingeer, O., 1992. Lateral instability of the ankle joint. Clin. Orthop. Clin. Res. 276, 253–261.

Karr, S.D., 1994. Subcalcaneal heel pain. Orthop. Clin. N. Am. 25, 161–275.

Kerkhoffs, G.M., Rowe, B.H., Assendelft, W.J., et al., 2002. Immobilization and Functional Treatment for Acute Lateral

Ankle Ligament Injuries in Adults (Cochrane Review). Cochrane Library. Update Software, Oxford, Issue 2

Kibler, W.B., Goldberg, C., Chandler, T.J., 1991. Functional biomechanical deficits in running athletes with plantar fasciitis. Am. J. Sports Med. 19, 66–71.

Koenig, M., Torp-Pederson, S., Ovistgaard, E., et al., 2004. Preliminary results of Doppler guided intratendinous glucocorticoid injection for Achilles tendonitis in five patients. Scand. J. Med. Sci. Sports 14 (2), 100–106.

Kumai, T., Takakura, Y., Rufai, A., et al., 2002. The functional anatomy of the human anterior talofibular ligament in relation to ankle sprains. J. Anat. 200 (5), 457–465.

Laskowski, E.R., Newcomer-Aney, K., Smith, J., 1997. Refining rehabilitation with proprioception training: expediting return to play. Phys. Sports Med. 25 (10), 89–102.

Lee, T.K., Maleski, R., 2002. Physical examination of the ankle for ankle pathology. Clin. Podiat. Med. Surg. 19, 251–269.

Lentell, G.L., Latzman, L.L., Walters, M.R., 1990. The relationship between muscle function and ankle stability. J. Orthop. Sports Phys. Ther. 11, 605–611.

Levangie, P., Norkin, C., Lewek, M.D., 2019. Joint Structure and Function: A Comprehensive Analysis, sixth ed. F.A. Davis, Philadelphia.

Litt, J.C.B., 1992. The sprained ankle: diagnosis and management of lateral ligament injuries. Aust. Fam. Phys. 21, 447–457.

Liu, S.H., Jason, W.J., 1994. Lateral ankle sprains and instability problems. Clin. Sports Med. 13, 793–809.

Maffulli, N., Spiezia, F., Longo, U.G., 2013. High volume guided injections for the management of chronic tendinopathy of the main body of the Achilles tendon. Phys. Ther. Sport 14, 163–167.

Mahler, F., Fritschy, D., 1992. Partial and complete ruptures of the Achilles tendon and local corticosteroid injections. Br. J. Sports Med. 26, 7–13.

Manent, A., López, L., Corominas, H., et al., 2019. Acute Achilles tendon ruptures: efficacy of conservative and surgical (percutaneous, open) treatment-a randomized, controlled, clinical trial. J. Foot Ankle Surg. 58 (6), 1229–1234.

Marder, R.A., 1994. Current methods for the evaluation of ankle ligament injuries. J. Bone Joint Surg. 76A, 1103–1111.

Miller, C.A., Bosco, J.A., 2002. Lateral ankle and subtalar instability. Bull. Hosp. Joint Dis. 60 (3), 143–149.

Moore, K.L., Daley, A.F., Agur, A.M.R., 2017. Clinically Oriented Anatomy, eight ed. Lippincott Williams & Wilkins, Philadelphia.

Newman, D.P., Holkup, K.C., Jacobs, A.N., et al., 2021. Recalcitrant flexor hallucis longus dysfunction: a case study demonstrating the successful application of an adaptable rehabilitation program with a two-year follow-up. Cureus. 13 (4), e14326.

National Institute for Health and Care Excellence (NICE), 2020a. How should I assess suspected Achilles tendinopathy? NICE, Washington DC. https://cks.nice.org.uk/topics/achilles-tendinopathy/diagnosis/diagnosis-of-achilles-tendinopathy/. Accessed 5 September 2021.cc

National Institute for Health and Care Excellence (NICE), 2020b. Plantar fasciitis. https://cks.nice.org.uk/topics/plantar-fasciitis/. Accessed 5 September 2021.

Nordin, M., Frankel, V.H., 2020. Basic Biomechanics of the Musculoskeletal System, fifth ed. Wolters Kluwer, Philadelphia.

Norris, C.M., 2004. Sports Injuries: Diagnosis and Management for Physiotherapists, second ed. Butterworth Heinemann, Oxford.

O'Hara, J., Valle-Jones, J.C., Walsh, H., et al., 1992. Controlled trial of an ankle support MalleoTrain in acute ankle injuries. Br. J. Sports Med. 26, 139–142.

Ohberg, I., Alfredson, H., 2003. Sclerosing therapy in chronic Achilles tendon insertional pain – results of a pilot study. Knee Surg. Sports Traumatol. Arthrosc. 11 (5), 339–343.

Ohberg, I., Alfredson, H., 2004. Effects on neovascularisation behind the good results with eccentric training in chronic mid portion Achilles tendinosis? Knee Surg. Sports Traumatol. Arthrosc. 12 (5), 465–470.

Paavola, M., Kannus, P., Järvinen, T.A., et al., 2002. Current concepts review: achilles tendinopathy. J. Bone Joint Surg. 84A (11), 2062–2076.

Patel, V.M., Subramanian, A., 2007. Ottawa ankle rules and the use of radiography in acute ankle injuries. CME Orthop 4 (3), 65–67.

Patterson, M.H., Cox, W.K., 1999. Peroneus longus tendon rupture as a cause of chronic lateral ankle pain. Clin. Orthop. Relat. Res. 365, 163–166.

Pearson, J., Rowlands, D., Highnet, R., 2012. Autologous blood injection to treat Achilles tendinopathy? A randomized controlled trial. J. Sport Rehab. 21, 218–224.

Pufe, T., Peterson, W., Tillmann, B., et al., 2001. The angiogenic peptide vascular endothelial growth factor is expressed in foetal and ruptured tendons. Virchows Arch. 439 (4), 579–585.

Roberts, C.S., DeMaio, M., Larkin, J.J., et al., 1995. Eversion ankle sprains. Orthopaedics 18 (3), 299–304.

Russo, A., Zappia, M., Reginelli, A., et al., 2013. Ankle impingement: a review of multimodality imaging approach. Musculoskelet. Surg. 97 (Suppl. 2), S161–S168.

Sartoris, D.J., 1994. Diagnosis of ankle injuries: the essentials. J. Foot Ankle Surg. 33, 102–107.

Scott, A., Docking, S., Vicenzino, B., et al., 2013. Sports and exercise-related tendinopathies: a review of selected topical issues by participants of the second International Scientific Tendinopathy Symposium (ISTS) Vancouver 2012. Br. J. Sports Med. 47, 536–544.

Scranton, P.E., McDermott, J.E., Rogers, J.V., 2000. The relationship between chronic ankle instability and variations in mortise anatomy and impingement spurs. Foot Ankle Int. 21 (8), 657–664.

Sellman, J.R., 1994. Plantar fascia rupture associated with corticosteroid injection. Foot Ankle Int. 15, 376–381.

Simpson, M.R., Howard, T.M., 2009. Tendinopathies of the foot and ankle. Am. Fam. Physician. 80 (10), 1107–1114.

Smart, G.W., Taunton, J.E., Clement, D.B., 1980. Achilles tendon disorders in runners – a review. Med. Sci. Sports Exerc. 12, 231–243.

Soames, R., Palastanga, N.R., 2018. Anatomy and Human Movement, seventh ed. Elsevier, Oxford.

Standring, S., 2015. Gray's Anatomy: The Anatomical Basis of Clinical Practice, forty-first ed. Churchill Livingstone, Edinburgh.

Stanley, K.L., 1991. Ankle sprains are always more than 'just a sprain'. Postgrad. Med. 89, 251–255.

Stecco, C., Corradin, M., Macchi, V., et al., 2013. Plantar fascia anatomy and its relationship with Achilles tendon and paratenon. J. Anat. 223, 665–676.

Stephens, M.M., 1994. Haglund's deformity and retrocalcaneal bursitis. Orthop. Clin. N. Am. 25, 41–46.

Tasto, J., Cummings, J., Medlock, V., et al., 2003. The tendon treatment centre: new horizons in the treatment of tendinosis. Arthroscopy 19, 213–223.

Taylor, A., 2002. Deep vein thrombosis following calf strain: a case study. Phys. Ther. Sport 3, 110–113.

Thomas, J., Christensen, J.C., Kravitz, S.R., et al., 2001. The diagnosis and treatment of heel pain. J. Foot Ankle Surg. 40 (5), 329–340.

Trojian, T., Tucker, A.K., 2019. Plantar fasciitis. Am. Fam. Physician 99 (12), 744–750.

Tropp, H., 2002. Commentary: functional ankle instability revisited. J. Athl. Train. 37 (4), 512–515.

Van de Velde, M., Matricali, G.A., Wuite, S., et al., 2017. Foot segmental motion and coupling in stage II and III tibialis posterior tendon dysfunction. Clin. Biomech. 45, 38–42.

van der Vlist, A.C., Winters, M., Weir, A., et al., 2021. Which treatment is most effective for patients with Achilles tendinopathy? A living systematic review with network meta-analysis of 29 randomised controlled trials. Br. J. Sports Med. 55, 249–255.

Vuurberg, G., Hoorntje, A., Wink, L.M., et al., 2018. Diagnosis, treatment and prevention of ankle sprains: update of an evidence-based clinical guideline. Br. J. Sports Med. 52 (15), 956.

Wilkerson, L.A., 1992. Ankle injuries in athletes. Prim. Care 19 (3), 377–392.

Wise, B.L., Peloquin, C., Choi, H., et al., 2012. Impact of age, sex, obesity, and steroid use on quinolone-associated tendon disorders. Am. J. Med. 125 (12), 1228. e23–1228.e28

Yang, W.-Y., Han, Y.-H., Cao, X.-W., et al., 2017. Platelet-rich plasma as a treatment for plantar fasciitis. Medicine. 96 (44), e8475.

Yu, J.S., 2000. Pathologic and postoperative conditions of the plantar fascia: review of MR imaging appearances. Skelet. Radiol. 29, 491–501.

The Lumbar Spine

CHAPTER CONTENTS

SUMMARY

This chapter outlines the relevant anatomy of the lumbar spine to support the following discussion of the possible causes of back pain and differential diagnosis. The clinical examination procedure is described, and the models used in musculoskeletal medicine are identified, to act as a guide to management.

Low back pain presents a challenge to the practitioner, with most back pain having no structural cause. Diagnosis is not simple, and the clinical data collected may indicate complicated lesions, with several factors contributing to the signs and symptoms. Psychosocial factors need to be considered along with lifestyle factors, comorbidities and red flags.

Emphasis is placed on the selection of patients suitable for treatment, and contraindications to treatment are discussed. Treatment techniques are described, and guidelines for safety in the application of treatment techniques are recommended.

ANATOMY

The lumbar spine is the lowest region in the series of motion segments that make up the spinal column, each of which consists of an interbody joint and its two adjacent facet joints. It supports the weight of the upper body and is designed to be stable while allowing mobility.

Lumbar Joints

There are five lumbar vertebrae, each with a large vertebral body (Fig. 13.1). Each vertebral body consists of a shell of cortical bone surrounding a cancellous cavity of supporting struts and crossbeams, called trabeculae. This provides a lightweight box with the strength to support longitudinally applied loads.

The spaces between the trabeculae provide channels for the blood supply and venous drainage of the vertebral body, and the presence of blood helps with transmitting load and absorbing force (Bogduk, 2023). The intervening intervertebral discs also provide a mechanism for shock absorption, as well as distribution of forces and movement (Jensen, 1980).

The stabilising function of the lumbar spine is achieved by the bony processes that make up the posterior elements of the lumbar vertebrae (i.e. the pedicles and laminae) and the articular, spinous and transverse processes.

The *pars interarticularis* is the short portion of vertebra that sits between the inferior and superior articular processes of the *facet (zygapophyseal) joint*. The cortical

bone in this region is thicker to help to withstand the forces placed through it, but in some individuals, it is insufficient, leaving the area vulnerable to fatigue and stress fractures (Bogduk, 2023).

The position and direction of the *articular processes* that form the synovial facet joints prevent forward sliding and rotation of the vertebral bodies, while the *spinous and transverse processes* act as leverage and provide attachment for muscles.

The *vertebral foramen* is surrounded by the vertebral body in front and the posterior elements behind. It is triangular in the lumbar spine and is larger than the foramen in the thoracic spine but smaller than in the cervical spine. Together the vertebral foramina form the *vertebral canal*, which contains the spinal cord, terminating opposite the L1 to L2 disc, and the cauda equina. The vertebral canal can vary in shape, and this may be relevant to pathology.

The lumbar lordosis compensates for the inclination of the sacrum and maintains the upright posture. The wedge-shaped lumbosacral disc and vertebral body of L5 contribute to the lordosis, along with the constant antigravity effect of the activity in the erector spinae muscles, which prevents the trunk from falling forwards (Middleditch and Oliver, 2005).

The *facet (zygapophyseal) joints* are synovial joints that provide stability of the spine, control of movement, and protection for the intervertebral discs (Taylor and Twomey, 1994).

The articular facets are covered with articular cartilage (Figs 13.2 and 13.3). The *superior articular facets* face posteromedially to join with the *inferior articular facets* of the vertebra above, which face anterolaterally. The resultant plane of the joint facilitates flexion and extension movements but prevents rotation. It also restricts translation in healthy joints, helping to protect the lumbar disc from the shearing forces responsible for fissuring (Bogduk, 1991; Taylor and Twomey, 1994).

The facet joints are surrounded by a fibrous capsule lined with synovium. The *fibrous capsule* consists of an outer layer of regularly arranged connective tissue and an inner layer of yellow elastic fibres. Anteriorly the capsule is replaced by the *ligamentum flavum*, while some of the deep fibres of *multifidus* give the capsule reinforcement medially (Yamashita et al., 1996).

The superior and inferior aspects of the capsules are loose and contain intra-articular structures consisting of

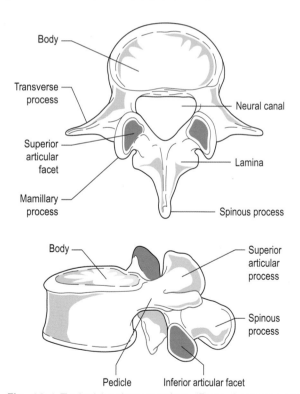

Fig. 13.1 Typical lumbar vertebra. (From Anatomy and Human Movement by Soames and Palastanga, 2018. Reprinted by permission of Elsevier Ltd.)

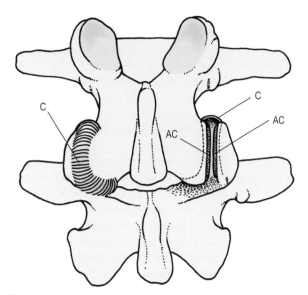

Fig. 13.2 A posterior view of the L3–L4 zygapophyseal joints. On the left, the capsule of the joint (C) is intact. On the right, the posterior capsule has been resected to reveal the joint cavity, the articular cartilages (AC), and the line of the attachment of the capsule (- - -). The upper joint capsule (C) attaches further from the articular margin than the posterior capsule. (From Clinical Anatomy of the Lumbar Spine and Sacrum by Bogduk, 2023. Reprinted by permission of Elsevier.)

fat and meniscoid structures (Bogduk, 2023). Fine nerve fibres, thought to conduct nociceptive and proprioceptive sensations, have also been found within the joints (Yamashita et al., 1996).

As synovial joints, the facet joints may be subjected to trauma or arthropathy and could be a cause of back pain. Degenerative changes usually coexist in the intervertebral joint of the same segment (Urban and Roberts, 2003; Jaumard and Welch, 2011). In 21% to 41% of patients, low back pain is considered to originate from facet joint degenerative arthropathy (Manchikanti et al., 2010).

The *ligaments of the lumbar spine* provide stability but allow mobility. Anterior and posterior longitudinal ligaments are well developed in the lumbar region where both stabilise the vertebral bodies and control movement (Fig. 13.4).

The *anterior longitudinal ligament* is widest in the lumbar spine where it covers most of the anterior and lateral surfaces of the vertebral bodies and intervertebral discs.

The *posterior longitudinal ligament* is relatively weaker and has a denticulate arrangement that permits the passage of vascular structures. Superficial fibres bridge several vertebrae while deeper fibres pass over

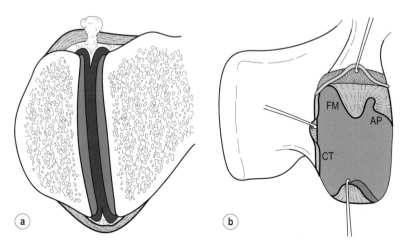

Fig. 13.3 Intra-articular structures of the lumbar zygapophyseal joints. (a) Coronal section of a left zygapophyseal joint showing fibroadipose meniscoids projecting into the joint cavity from the capsule over the superior and inferior poles of the joint. (b) Lateral view of a right zygapophyseal joint, in which the superior articular process has been removed to show intra-articular structures projecting into the joint cavity across the surface of the inferior articular facet. The superior capsule is retracted to reveal the base of a fibroadipose meniscoid (FM) and an adipose tissue pad (AP). Another fibroadipose meniscoid at the lower pole of the joint is lifted from the surface of the articular cartilage. A connective tissue (CT) rim has been retracted along the posterior margin of the joint. (From Clinical Anatomy of the Lumbar Spine and Sacrum by Bogduk, 2023. Reprinted by permission of Elsevier.)

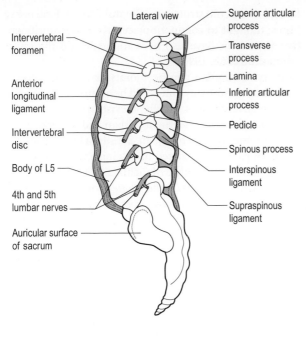

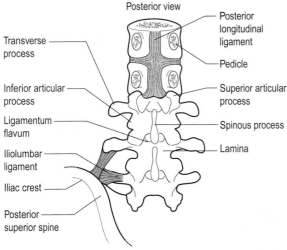

Fig. 13.4 The ligaments of the lumbar spine.

two joints and have lateral extensions intimately related to the intervertebral disc (Parke and Schiff, 1971).

The strong central portion of the posterior longitudinal ligament provides resistance to central disc displacement, deflecting it laterally, where the lateral extensions are deficient and offer a space for potential posterolateral displacement.

The *ligamentum flavum* consists of predominantly yellow elastic fibres and connects adjacent laminae. It controls lumbar flexion by 'braking' the separation of the laminae and assisting the return to the upright posture. The elastic fibres also restore the ligament to its normal length after stretching, to prevent buckling into the spinal canal and compression of the spinal cord or cauda equina. Loss of elasticity in the degenerate ligament can contribute to stenosis.

The *iliolumbar ligament* provides stability for the lumbosacral junction (Yamamoto et al., 1990), attaching the L5 transverse process to the pelvis. Sometimes a band also passes from the transverse process of L4. This anchorage of L5 to the pelvis restricts the amount of movement available to accommodate disc herniation. Disc herniation at the L5 to S1 level can produce severe pain, with the patient fixed in flexion, whereas herniation above this level, usually L4 to L5, may be accommodated more readily by a lateral shift that will reduce pain.

Intervertebral Discs

The intervertebral disc has special biomechanical requirements. It is strong to sustain weight and transmit loads while being able to deform to adjust to movement.

The intervertebral disc has three parts: a central nucleus pulposus surrounded by a peripheral annulus fibrosus, which blends above and below into vertebral endplates. Although the nucleus and annulus are distinct regions within the disc, there is no clear boundary between them (Bogduk, 2023). Both the nucleus and the annulus participate in weight-bearing.

The *nucleus pulposus* accommodates movement and transmits compressive loads from one vertebral body to another. It is composed of irregularly arranged collagen fibres and cartilage cells scattered within ground substance. The collagen fibres are composed of type II collagen, suited to accept pressure and compression (see Chapter 2).

The nucleus has great water-binding capacity through its proteoglycan content. The fluid nature of the nucleus allows it to deform under pressure, but its volume cannot be compressed. Under pressure, the vertebral endplates prevent its superior and inferior deformation but it can deform away from the centre to transmit the applied pressure towards the annulus (Bogduk, 2023), so contributing to the intervertebral disc's ability to support and transmit load.

The *annulus fibrosus* consists of a geometrically organised arrangement of collagen and approximately 10% of elastic fibres (Bogduk, 2023). These are bound together by a proteoglycan gel, allowing it to support weight without buckling.

Types I and II collagen are found in the annulus fibrosus, but the majority of fibres are type I, suited to withstand tensile stress. The fibres are arranged in concentric lamellae around the central nucleus. These tightly packed lamellae are arranged circumferentially at the periphery and can sustain high compressive loads. Adams et al. (2012) suggest an analogy to the stiffness of a telephone directory rolled into a cylinder and stood on its end.

In each lamella, the collagen fibres lie parallel to each other, inclined at an angle of approximately 65 to 70 degrees to the vertical (Fig. 13.5). The direction of fibres alternates in adjacent lamellae (Bogduk, 2023).

The posterior portion of the annulus is thinner than the rest of the annulus, and Marchand and Ahmed (1990) noted a number of irregularities within the laminate structure of the annulus, particularly at the posterolateral corners, where a number of incomplete layers were seen. This is supported by Bogduk (2023), who suggests that up to 40% of the lamellae are incomplete throughout the disc and as many as 50% are incomplete in the posterolateral quadrants, making this area particularly vulnerable to increased stress.

The annulus fibrosus acts like a ligament, restraining excessive movement to stabilise the intervertebral joint while allowing flexibility to permit normal movement. The alternating oblique annular fibres resist horizontal and vertical forces, allowing the annulus to oppose movement in all directions (Bogduk, 1991). The elastic fibres in the annulus also help to reform the nucleus after the stress has been removed.

The *vertebral endplates* are thin layers of cartilage, approximately 1 mm thick, covering the superior and inferior surfaces of the discs. They cover the entire nucleus but not the periphery of the annulus (Bogduk, 2023) and form a permeable barrier for diffusion, mainly between the nucleus and the cancellous bone of the vertebral bodies (Fig. 13.5). The endplates are attached strongly to the disc and weakly to the vertebral bodies where they are vulnerable to being torn away in certain types of spinal trauma (Bogduk, 2023). They also fail relatively easily under excessive compressive loading.

Nerve Supply to the Intervertebral Disc

The outer half of the annulus, at least, is known to have a *nerve supply* (Cavanaugh et al., 1995; Coppes et al., 1997). Adams et al. (2023) specify further that the nerve fibres are abundant in the outer third of the annulus, fewer in the middle third and absent in the inner third and nucleus pulposus.

In the degenerate disc however, nerve fibres have been seen to extend deeper into the inner third of the disc, where they appear to be new growth arising from granulation tissue (Edgar, 2007).

A proliferation of mechanoreceptors is also observed in degenerate discs, along with Golgi tendon organs, which are thought to have a nociceptive function, as well as a mechanoreceptor function, and could be stimulated by increased muscle tone (Edgar, 2007).

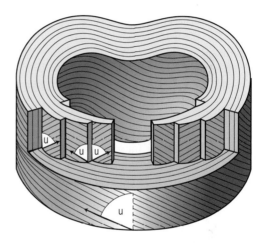

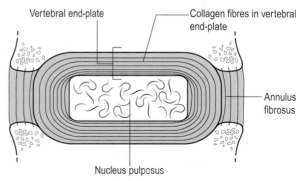

Fig. 13.5 Laminate structure of the disc.(From Clinical Anatomy of the Lumbar Spine and Sacrum by Bogduk, 2023. Reprinted by permission of Elsevier.)

Anteriorly and laterally the annulus is supplied by a plexus of nerves derived from branches of the sympathetic trunks and their grey rami communicantes; the plexus also supplies the anterior longitudinal ligament. The vertebral endplates are supplied in a pattern similar to that of the outer annulus, particularly in the central area adjacent to the nucleus pulposus (Edgar, 2007).

The posterior annulus, posterior longitudinal ligament and anterior dura mater are supplied by branches from a plexus that covers the floor of the vertebral canal and is derived from the sinuvertebral nerves (Adams et al., 2012) (Fig. 13.6). Each sinuvertebral nerve supplies the disc at one level and the disc above (Bogduk, 2023) which could in part explain the poor localisation of low back pain.

Properties of the Intervertebral Disc

The intervertebral disc at rest possesses an intrinsic pressure due to the compressive effect of the elastic ligamentum flavum (Middleditch and Oliver, 2005). This preloaded or prestressed state provides it with an intrinsic stability to resist applied forces such as body weight (Jensen, 1980).

The resting pressure is affected by posture and loading, being lowest in the lying position and highest in the sitting position, with a further increase if external loading is applied (Nachemson, 1966). In the sitting position the spine usually rests in a degree of flexion, and the activity in psoas major contributes a compressive effect on the disc as it stabilises the spine.

Both somatic and radicular pain (see Chapter 1) are affected by movements and posture, and can be increased by straining, coughing or laughing.

Movement of the spine involves simultaneous tension, compression and shear at different locations of the disc. Flexion, extension and side flexion stretch the annulus on one side of the disc and produce compression on the other side, affecting intradiscal pressure and fluid flow (Jensen, 1980).

Flexion includes a component of forward translation that is stabilised by the facet joints, while extension is limited by bony impaction of the inferior articular processes against the lamina of the vertebra below. Axial rotation produces torsion in the intervertebral discs, with tension in half the annular fibres that are inclined towards the direction of the rotation,

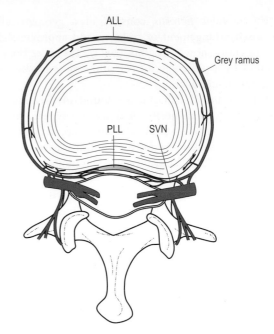

Fig. 13.6 The nerve supply of a lumbar intervertebral disc depicted in a transverse view of the lumbar spine. Branches of the grey rami communicantes and the sinuvertebral nerves (SVN) are shown entering the disc and the anterior and posterior longitudinal ligaments (ALL, PLL). Branches from the sinuvertebral nerves also supply the anterior aspect of the dural sac and dural sleeve. (From Clinical Anatomy of the Lumbar Spine and Sacrum by Bogduk, 2023. Reprinted by permission of Elsevier.)

and impaction of the facet. Side flexion is a composite movement that includes side flexion and rotation and their combined effects on the discal structure (Bogduk, 2023).

As a viscoelastic material, the intervertebral disc is subject to the phenomena of creep, hysteresis and set (Twomey and Taylor, 1982; Oliver and Twomey, 1995; Bogduk, 2023), as discussed in Chapter 2. The creep behaviour of flexion and extension is similar, with the amount of creep increasing with load and progressing with time. Creep also increases with age when the recovery through hysteresis is slower.

Flexion creep, in particular, has implications for occupations that require a constant flexed posture (e.g. manual workers). It may also be responsible for fatigue in the disc, making it vulnerable to a sudden applied force—the 'straw that breaks the camel's back'.

Nutrition of the Intervertebral Disc

The lumbar discs have a relatively poor blood supply as no arteries enter the disc, and it is the largest avascular tissue in the human body (Adams et al., 2012; Paesold et al., 2007). Nutrition of the intervertebral disc occurs through two routes: the blood vessels situated around the peripheral annulus and those in the central portion of the vertebral endplate.

The outer annulus may be supplied with nutrients from blood vessels in the adjacent longitudinal ligaments, but the supply to the nucleus pulposus is almost completely dependent on diffusion via the endplate capillary network (Paesold et al., 2007). The mechanisms involved are diffusion and fluid flow and both are affected by posture and motion (Adams and Hutton, 1986).

The water content of the disc represents a balance between two opposing osmotic and hydrostatic pressures: that is, a swelling pressure (imbibition), which hydrates the disc, and a mechanical pressure (posture, movement, loading and creep), which dehydrates the disc. Diurnal (daily) decrease in the total length of the spine is offset by its recovery in the supine position overnight (Parke and Schiff, 1971; Porter, 1995).

Flexion postures cause a larger fluid outflow from the disc than erect or lordotic postures, with the outflow being reduced further when the spine is unloaded by lying down. Alternating between rest and activity will enhance fluid flow (Adams and Hutton, 1983, 1986).

Factors that influence the nutrition of the disc are increased loading, vibration or spinal deformity. Factors that compromise the vascular supply include smoking, vascular disease and diabetes (Buckwalter, 1995).

The most marked aging or degenerative changes occur in the nucleus of the intervertebral disc. There is a reduction in the water and proteoglycan content and a change in the number and nature of the collagen fibres (Paesold et al., 2007; Bogduk, 2023). Degenerative changes may be well advanced, but they do not necessarily correlate with signs and symptoms (Fig. 13.7).

Lumbar Spinal Nerves

The termination of the *spinal cord* lies approximately level with the L1 to L2 disc, and the lumbar and sacral nerve roots descend vertically in the *cauda equina*, surrounded by the dural sac, to exit via their appropriate lumbar or sacral intervertebral foramina (Fig. 13.8).

Dorsal (sensory) and ventral (mainly motor) nerve roots join to form the relatively short spinal nerve that occupies the intervertebral foramen, together with the dorsal root ganglion (Fig. 13.9). The *dorsal root ganglion* is the collection of the cell bodies of all the sensory nerve fibres related to that segment. The cell bodies of the motor axons are located in the anterior horns of the grey matter in the spinal cord.

The dura of the dural sac extends to envelope the nerve roots in a *dural nerve root sleeve* (Bogduk, 2023). At a point just beyond the dorsal root ganglion, the dural nerve root sleeve blends with the epineurium of the nerve. Immediately after leaving the intervertebral foramen the nerve divides into dorsal and ventral rami.

Spinal nerves do not possess the same protective connective tissue sheaths as peripheral nerves and are said to be vulnerable to direct mechanical injury (Rydevik and Olmarker, 1992).

There are five pairs of lumbar nerves, five pairs of sacral nerves and one pair of coccygeal nerves. Their dorsal and ventral nerve roots pass in the cauda equina in an inferolateral direction to reach their appropriate level, before joining to emerge through the intervertebral foramina as the spinal nerves. Until the coccygeal level is reached there are several nerve roots passing vertically in the cauda equina (Fig. 13.8).

The clinical implications of this should be recognised, as it is possible for a lumbar disc herniation to encroach on more than one nerve root. It also explains how a lumbar disc herniation could compress the S4 nerve root to affect bladder, bowel and sexual function; could produce saddle and/or genital sensory disturbance; and could cause severe or progressive bilateral neurological deficits in the legs (Gardner et al., 2011).

Muscles

The back muscles provide a pool of possible actions that may be recruited to suit the needs of the vertebral column (Bogduk, 2023). In the lumbar spine, isolated 'pulled' muscle strains are rare and muscle lesions are mostly contusions associated with direct trauma.

Myofascial pain can arise from overuse, stretching or diffuse and localised muscle spasm (e.g. trigger points) (Knezevic et al., 2021). When present, it can also be associated with other primary causes of low back pain and is usually included within the classification of non-specific low back pain.

Within the musculoskeletal medicine approach, myofascial pain is not treated specifically and the muscles of the spine are not covered within this chapter. Rehabilitation is also outside the scope of this text. The reader is referred to anatomy texts for further detail that

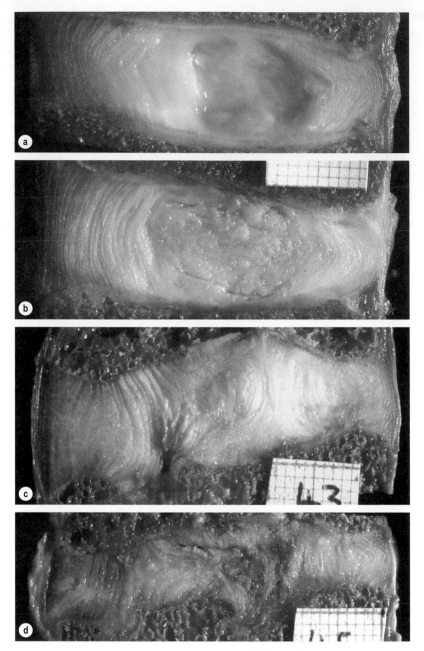

Fig. 13.7 Lumbar intervertebral discs sectioned in the mid-sagittal plane, anterior on left. These discs, which were not subjected to any post-mortem loading, represent the first four stages of disc degeneration. (a) Grade 1 disc, typical of ages 15–40 years (male, 35 years). (b) Grade 2 disc, typical of ages 35–70 years. The nucleus appears fibrous, and there is some pigmentation (brown degeneration) typical of ageing. However, the disc's structure is intact and not 'degenerated' (male, 47 years, L2–L3). (c) Grade 3 disc, showing moderate degenerative changes. Note the annulus bulging into the nucleus, damage to the inferior end-plate, and the lack of pigmentation in some regions of the disc (male, 31 years, L2–L3). (d) Grade 4 disc, showing severe degeneration. Note the pigmentation, the disruption to both end-plates, and internal collapse of the annulus, with corresponding reduction in disc height (male, 31 years, L4–L5). (From Adams et al., 2012. Reprinted by permission of Elsevier Ltd.)

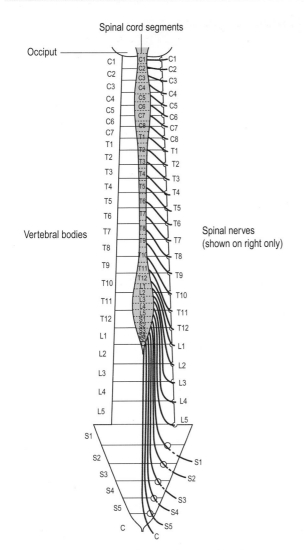

Fig. 13.8 The cauda equina and emerging nerve roots. (From Middleditch and Oliver, 2005. Reprinted by permission of Elsevier.)

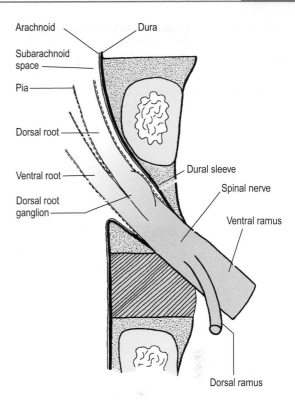

Fig. 13.9 A lumbar spine nerve, its roots and meningeal coverings. The nerve roots are invested by pia mater and covered by arachnoid and dura as far as the spinal nerve. The dura of the dural sac is prolonged around the roots as far as the spinal nerve. The dura of the dural sac is prolonged around the roots as their dural sleeve, which blends with the epineurium of the spinal nerve. (From Bogduk, 2023. Reprinted by permission of Elsevier Ltd.)

may be relevant to other approaches, including those that focus on muscle strengthening and stretching as part of rehabilitation.

CLINICAL DIAGNOSIS AND MANAGEMENT AT THE LUMBAR SPINE

An understanding of the anatomy at the lumbar spine, together with a detailed history and examination of the patient, will help with the selection of patients suitable for manual therapy and will contribute to safe practice.

Assessment of the lumbar spine is covered in detail in the 'Commentary on the Examination' (page 454).

A diagnostic triage approach is used to identify patients who fall into the non-specific back or leg pain classification, and those that fall into a different classification, which could include serious pathology (including malignancy, infection, fracture); neurological deficit (cauda equina syndrome, radiculopathy, stenosis); inflammatory disease (spondyloarthritis) or other visceral or circulatory causes (Almeida et al., 2018).

This clinical diagnosis section is divided into two parts:

- The first part defines non-specific back pain, with or without leg pain, and lists incidence, risk factors, diagnosis, management and prognosis.
- The second part looks at other causes of back pain and associated signs and symptoms, diagnosis and management. Most of these conditions have a more specific or identifiable cause. On the whole, these patients are not appropriate for treatment with manual musculoskeletal medicine treatment techniques and require onward referral.

Non-Specific Low Back Pain

For nearly all patients presenting with non-specific low back pain, a specific nociceptive source cannot be identified.

The experience of non-specific low back pain is a combination of biological, psychological and social factors. Low back pain is a complex condition with multiple contributors to both pain and associated disability, including comorbidities, and pain-processing mechanisms (Hartvigsen et al., 2018). Therefore, all factors should be addressed when deciding on the management package for each patient, through shared decision-making.

In 2015, low back pain was responsible for 60.1 million disability-adjusted life years, which was an increase of 54% from 1990, with the highest increase seen in low-income and middle-income countries. It occurs in all age groups, from children to the older population although it is uncommon in the first decade of life, with prevalence increasing during teenage years. Most adults have an episode of non-specific low back pain at some point in their life and it is more common in women than men (Hartvigsen et al., 2018)

Risk factors for non-specific low back pain include smoking, poor mental health, obesity and lower levels of physical activity, which relate to poorer general health. There is also an increased risk of new episodes of low back pain if there is a history of previous episodes (Parreira, 2018).

Diagnosis of non-specific low back pain is clinical and further investigation is not normally required.

The management of patients with non-specific low back pain can be challenging; however, many published guidelines suggest a similar approach to their assessment and management.

Foster et al. (2018) produced a series of papers on low back pain and advocated a shift in the way non-specific low back pain is managed. They put forward strategies based on greater emphasis on self-management, physical and psychological therapies and some forms of complementary medicine, with less emphasis on pharmacological and surgical interventions.

The National Low Back and Radicular Pain Pathway (2017) supports the implementation of recommendations in the NICE guideline on low back pain and sciatica (NICE, 2020a). The pathway's stepped approach to care and recommendations for non-invasive management are as follows:

- Use of risk stratification (such as STarT back risk assessment) for each new episode of low back pain, with or without sciatica, to inform shared decision making.
- Provide reassurance - non-specific low back pain is a common problem that usually resolves itself within a few weeks.
- Provide education and advice to keep active, to encourage the patient to maintain normal activities and to give guidance on self-management at all steps of the treatment pathway. The person's specific needs, preferences and capabilities should be taken into consideration.
- Offer oral analgesics (e.g. paracetamol, oral non-steroidal anti-inflammatory drugs (NSAIDS) at the lowest effective dose for the shortest period of time. The choice depends on the severity of the pain, personal preference, tolerance and the risk of adverse effects.
- Consider a weak opioid, with or without paracetamol, for acute low back pain, if NSAIDs are contraindicated, ineffective or not tolerated. Opioid medication is not recommended for chronic sciatica.
- Consider muscle relaxants (benzodiazepines are recommended (NICE, 2020a)) for the management of sciatica, if necessary.
- Consider neuropathic medication as the initial treatment for neuropathic pain or for severe neuropathic pain (NICE, 2020d).
- Consider referral to physiotherapy for a multimodal treatment strategy, which may include stretching and strengthening exercise, with or without manual therapy and with or without a combined physical and a psychological programme (CPPP), using a cognitive behavioural therapy (CBT) approach.
- Consider a group exercise programme, such as biomechanical, aerobic, mind–body or a combination of approaches.

- Consider referral to psychological therapy if appropriate.
- Consider referral to occupational health for people with back pain related to their job.

Both documents (NICE, 2020a; NSN, 2017) also provide guidelines and recommendations on invasive treatment for low back pain and sciatica, including referral to pain team/specialists where interventions such as spinal epidural injection, radiofrequency denervation or other surgical procedures can be considered for recalcitrant pain.

A toolkit developed by NHS England and NHS Improvement (The Best MSK Health Collaborative workspace on Future NHS, 2022) offers best practice clinical guidance and evidence-based resources to local services and other musculoskeletal stakeholders, for patients with spinal pain and sciatica across the entire musculoskeletal pathway. This provides a wealth of resources to support musculoskeletal transformation and a collaborative delivery of musculoskeletal services - so that the patient can be seen by the right person, at the right time and in the right place.

Clinical practice guidelines state that recovery from acute low back pain is rapid and complete. Most people with acute back pain experience improvement in pain and disability, and return to work within 1 month (Pengel et al., 2003; Hartvigsen et al., 2018).

However, low levels of pain and disability can persist from 3 to 12 months (Hartvigsen et al., 2018), and recurrence is common (Pengel et al., 2003). It is not always clear whether chronic low levels of pain and disability are due to the persistence of the original episode or to recurrent episodes.

The recommendations within all back pain management programmes are intended to avoid the development of persistent pain, and the aspect of self-management is an important component towards this.

Almost 40% of people presenting to primary care with low back pain are at a high risk of developing chronic disability (Henschke et al., 2008). It is generally accepted that a one-size-fits-all approach cannot be adopted in the management of low back pain and practitioners are encouraged to adopt a personalised and holistic approach for their patients.

There has been extensive research on prognostic factors associated with the transition from acute/subacute (<3 months) to persistent low back pain (>3 months). Prognostic factors include physical factors, such as leg pain and widespread symptoms (Turner et al., 2008); lifestyle factors (e.g. sedentary lifestyle, obesity and smoking) (Knezevic et al., 2021); high pain intensity and a high level of disability (Woby et al., 2007, 2008; Thomas et al., 2010); and traumatic injuries (Knezevic et al., 2021).

Psychological factors include fear-avoidance behaviour (Thomas et al., 2010; Ramond et al, 2011; Knezevic et al., 2021) and distress (Gatchel and Gardea, 1999; Pincus et al., 2002). Personal factors include previous back pain (Shaw et al., 2001), secondary gain, work-related factors (such as job satisfaction and hostile work environment), and the duration of sickness absence (Truchon, 2000; Knezevic et al., 2021). Cognitive and behavioural factors include patient expectations and patients' perception of pain control (Ramond et al., 2011).

Several screening tools have been developed to identify patients who might be at risk of developing persistent pain. The Keele STarT Back Tool (SBT), for example, provides practitioners with a valid and consistent screening tool to guide the management of patients with low back pain, and to facilitate shared decision-making. It is a brief questionnaire for screening prognostic indicators (both physical and psychosocial risk factors) for persistent, disabling back pain, with a stratified care approach (Hill et al., 2011).

Based on the SBT-scores, patients can be categorised into three subgroups: patients with a low, medium or high risk for developing persistent low back pain and limitation of activity (Hill et al., 2008, 2010; Betten et al., 2015).

The management recommendations for each group are that the low-risk group should receive minor attention from health professionals, and education and self-management strategies are recommended. The medium risk group should be offered physiotherapy, such as supervised exercise therapy and manual therapy, and for the high-risk group, a combined physical and psychological treatment programme is recommended (Hill et al., 2008, 2010; Magnussen et al., 2010).

Prevention of recurrence is an important part of the advice to be given to patients and exercise programmes play a vital role in rehabilitation. Patients should be encouraged to return to work and normal activities as soon as possible.

All guidelines recommend exercise for persistent low back pain, but group exercise is now recommended along with the endorsement for various types of exercise, such as Pilates and yoga, swimming and general aerobics (Almeida et al., 2018; NICE, 2020a). Increased, regular activity is an important part of patients' self-management of non-specific low back pain.

Other Causes of Back Pain

The differential diagnosis of back pain includes musculoskeletal lesions (sacroiliac or hip joint pathologies), trauma, arthropathy, lumbar radicular pain/radiculopathy and non-musculoskeletal conditions. Non-musculoskeletal conditions can be classified as inflammatory, vascular, malignant or infectious.

Serious conditions can affect the spine, such as primary or secondary malignancy, infection, acute inflammatory arthritis, fracture or cauda equina syndrome, but these represent a small percentage of the problems compared with non-specific back pain (Swezey, 1993; Finucane et al., 2020b).

Serious spinal pathology is estimated to occur in 1% to 4% of primary care back pain presentations (Henschke et al., 2009). The prevalence at the Emergency Department is often higher, with reported rates of serious pathology as high as 17.9%, being either spinal- (3.3%) or non-spinal- (14.6%) related (Shaw et al., 2020).

The patient may present with signs and symptoms similar to those of a mechanical presentation. A particular feature is an unwell patient with unexplained weight loss, unremitting non-mechanical pain, night pain, possible fever and systemic symptoms.

This part of the chapter considers the other causes of back pain in turn, including serious non-musculoskeletal pathologies that have 'red flags' that should be listened and looked out for in clinical examination.

Sacroiliac and Hip Joint Pathologies

Differential diagnosis at the lumbar spine can be complex, due to the close nerve supply of structures and the overlapping on pain referral patterns. Lumbar spine, sacroiliac joint and hip lesions can all refer pain to buttock and groin, for example, and conditions can co-exist.

Clinical reasoning can be a challenge. It is important to exclude the sacroiliac and hip joints as part of the examination of the lumbar spine, and to conduct a full examination of each if indicated. Sacroiliac and hip joint assessment, diagnosis and treatment are discussed in the relevant chapters.

Traumatic

Spinal fractures make up the largest number of serious pathologies in the spine (Finucane et al., 2020a).

Suspected fractures following major trauma, such as a road traffic accident or a fall from height, will almost always have been dealt with as an emergency.

Spinal fractures associated with osteoporosis (insufficiency fractures) are more commonly encountered within musculoskeletal practice but more so in the thoracic spine where they are discussed in more detail (see Chapter 9).

Lumbar Radicular Pain and Radiculopathy

Radicular leg pain describes pain in one or both legs, often secondary to compression or irritation of nerve roots in the lumbar spine. Typically, the leg pain is worse than the back pain and does not usually follow a specific dermatomal pattern. It is commonly called 'sciatica'.

Lumbar radiculopathy describes a neurological deficit within the lower limb with the presence of motor weakness, loss of reflexes, or loss of sensation, or a combination of all three, with or without radicular pain.

Lumbar radiculopathy stems mainly from disc herniation or spinal stenosis. However, disc herniations are a common finding in asymptomatic people and it is important that the clinical findings match the level of nerve root compression from the disc herniation.

The prevalence of radiculopathy has been estimated to be 3% to 5% of the population, affecting both men and women. Acute lumbar radiculopathy most commonly affects the L5 or S1 root and less commonly the L4 root. It is less common still for the other roots to be affected (Caplan, 1994).

Risk factors include strenuous physical activity, such as heavy lifting, especially while bending and twisting, cigarette smoking and obesity (NICE, 2020a). Other risk factors include prior lumbar radiculopathy and whole-body vibration, for example, driving a vehicle or operating machinery.

In the absence of red flags, plain X-rays of the lumbar spine are unlikely to help and may lead to false-positive findings. MRI is indicated in people with lumbar radiculopathy that has failed to improve after 4 to 6 weeks of conservative management and is significantly affecting quality of life. Earlier MRI can be considered if clinically indicated by severe pain or significant or progressive neurological deficit.

Most people with lumbar radiculopathy will improve regardless of the treatment, and improve spontaneously without surgery (Benoist, 2002; Kesikburun et al., 2019). There is consensus that management of radicular pain should be conservative in the first 6 to 8 weeks and in general pain and related disability resolve within 2 weeks. With conservative management, 80% of the patients are expected to recover within 8 weeks and 95% within 1 year (Legrand et al., 2007).

A relatively rare presentation of referred leg symptoms was described by Cyriax (1982), where symptoms appear in the leg without prior presentation in the back or buttock. It is an uncommon presentation but is encountered in clinical practice from time to time. It usually affects the younger adult patient who complains of relatively minor symptoms, which could be confused with a hamstring or calf injury. However, there is no relevant trauma in the history. A non-capsular pattern of movement is present with lumbar movements provoking the leg symptoms. The condition usually recovers spontaneously over several weeks (Kesikburun et al., 2019) but traction can be a treatment option within the stepped approach.

Surgery for lumbar radiculopathy is usually restricted to people who have persistent or debilitating pain combined with loss of power. Indications for surgery include:
- Signs and symptoms of lumbar radiculopathy, and
- Lumbar radiculopathy with unremitting radicular pain despite 6 to 12 weeks of conservative treatments or progressive motor weakness, and
- MRI that shows nerve root compression.

Some patients may have too many risk factors to consider surgery or may prefer more conservative management for their radiculopathy. In either case, it may be appropriate to refer them to the local multidisciplinary pain management team, where a number of interventions, such as spinal injection, radiofrequency denervation, a combined physical and psychological programme and self-help resources can be offered.

Arthropathy

Arthropathy, in any form, presents with the capsular pattern, which is demonstrated by the lumbar spine as a whole.

CAPSULAR PATTERN OF THE LUMBAR SPINE
- Limitation of extension
- Equal limitation of side flexions
- Usually full flexion

Degenerative arthropathy affects the intervertebral joint and the facet joint. Disruption of the intervertebral joint affects the facet joint, causing the joint surfaces to bear increased weight. In most cases, degeneration of the facet joint is associated with, or preceded by, degeneration of the adjacent disc (Urban and Roberts, 2003; Jaumard and Welch 2011).

Although degenerative changes of the lumbar spine may be obvious on imaging studies, they do not necessarily correlate with symptom severity. For instance, up to 50% to 60% of the healthy population have changes to the intervertebral discs without being symptomatic (Jensen et al., 1994).

The consequences of degeneration and degradation of the intervertebral disc can lead to the increased possibility of disc herniation (Urban and Roberts, 2003) and associated signs and symptoms. Spinal stenosis may be a feature.

Limitation of movement in the capsular pattern will be present but pain may be only mild to moderate. Education and advice on self-management and lifestyle changes, such as weight reduction and postural correction, should be given, along with exercise as the core treatment. Manual therapy and stretching should also be considered (NICE, 2020b).

Spinal Stenosis

Spinal stenosis is a term that has become synonymous with neurogenic or spinal claudication. It is used to define any symptomatic condition in which limited space in the vertebral canal is a significant factor (Porter, 1992).

Lateral stenosis is caused by the narrowing of the lateral recess or neural foramen, which affects the nerve root unilaterally, whereas central stenosis is caused by the narrowing of the central canal, which affects the spinal cord and often results in bilateral symptoms. Cauda equina syndrome may coexist with lateral or central stenosis.

It is important to appreciate that stenosis is part of the aging process, and there is not always an association between spinal stenosis and the presence of symptoms. In the lumbar spine, stenosis is most common at the L4 to L5 level, followed by L5 to S1, and L3 to L4 (Munakomi et al., 2021).

There are several causes of spinal stenosis. Narrowing can have a congenital and developmental cause (Munakomi et al., 2021). It can also occur as a result of degenerative changes through ageing, injury, disease, or as a result of surgery (Lee et al., 1995). Degenerative spinal stenosis can be associated with disc herniation, osteophyte formation at the vertebral body or facet joints, loss of disc height, and ligamentum flavum hypertrophy. These can all lead to narrowing of the central canal and neural foramina (Messiah et al., 2019; Bagley et al., 2019).

The prevalence of spinal stenosis increases with age and is most common in people over the age of 60 (Munakomi et al., 2021). Due to the degenerative nature of the condition, it is rarely seen in people below 50 years of age (Jensen et al., 2020).

It can produce neurogenic or spinal claudication. The patient complains of discomfort, pain, paraesthesia and heaviness in one or both legs on prolonged standing or walking. There may be night cramps and restless legs. A long history of back pain may be present and the patient may have undergone back surgery at some time. The symptoms are usually of several months' duration.

There is usually a threshold distance for walking when the symptoms of claudication develop. There is also a tolerance distance, when the patient has to stop, and the tolerance distance is normally about twice the threshold distance (Porter, 1992).

This pattern of behaviour and symptoms is similar to that of ischaemic pain, associated with intermittent claudication of peripheral vascular disease, and with the age group affected, the two conditions can coexist, making clinical diagnosis difficult.

There are some differences, however. Neurogenic claudication from the spine is usually more proximal to distal, while vascular claudication is more distal and pain is usually around mid-calf. Symptoms from neurogenic claudication often develop more slowly with aggravating activities, take a while to subside, or remain constant, while symptoms from vascular claudication develop more quickly and usually settle quickly when walking stops or with rest.

With neurogenic claudication, there is no colour change and lower limb pulses are expected to be normal. With vascular claudication, there may be changes in skin colour and texture as a result of poor circulation, and lower limb pulses may be weaker.

With neurogenic claudication, stooping or bending forwards relieves the symptoms and allows the patient to continue. Flexion increases the space in the canal and tightens the ligaments, straightening out the buckling that tends to occur with degeneration. The patient can usually walk uphill, which involves a flexed posture,

more easily than walking downhill, which involves a more extended posture. With vascular claudication, forward flexion usually makes little difference.

On examination, the patient often stands with a stooped posture, with flexed hips and knees and a flattened lumbar spine with loss of the lordosis (Knezevic et al., 2021). This posture becomes more evident on walking. The capsular pattern is present with a marked loss of spinal extension.

The rest of the examination may be unremarkable, and back pain itself may not be a feature. Neurological signs are often absent. Bilateral wasting of extensor digitorum brevis, on the lateral dorsum of the foot, has been shown as a reliable clinical bedside marker when assessing underlying lumbar stenosis (Munakomi and Kumar, 2016).

Imaging is not required as part of the initial assessment as there is usually a poor correlation between imaging findings and symptoms (Jensen et al., 2021). Patients may have leg symptoms that are not consistent with the level of stenosis and it can be an incidental finding.

A stepped approach to the management of spinal stenosis is currently recommended. Less invasive treatments are generally offered first, including education, advice on weight loss, watchful wait, activity and work modification, simple analgesics, NSAIDs and neuropathic medication, taking into account the important side effects in older people and the absence of good evidence for efficacy (Jensen et al., 2021).

Physiotherapy (e.g. exercise and manual therapy) may be helpful, with 30% to 50% of patients with mild to moderate symptoms experiencing marked improvement in pain and the ability to walk long distances (Jensen et al., 2021).

Surgery is reserved for those who fail to respond to conservative management. Patients with severe symptoms, progressive neurological deficit, or no improvement after 3 to 6 months of conservative treatment should be referred to a spinal specialist for imaging and further intervention or surgery (Jensen et al., 2021; Munakomi et al., 2021).

Spondylosis

Spondylolysis is a defect or fracture in the pars interarticularis (the neural arch between the lamina and the pedicle). It occurs mostly at the L5 vertebrae (85% to 95%) and also at the L4 vertebrae (5% to 15%). The defect can occur unilaterally or bilaterally. Spondylolysis is one of the most common causes of lower back pain in adolescents, although it remains asymptomatic in the majority of patients (Gagnet et al., 2018).

Lumbar extension generally makes the pain worse. Diagnosis is confirmed by MRI.

Young patients with spondylolysis usually receive conservative management initially. Conservative management generally consists of exercise rehabilitation, activity modification, physiotherapy and pain control (Gagnet et al., 2018). If symptoms persist, onward referral for a surgical opinion is appropriate.

Spondylolisthesis

Spondylolisthesis is an anterior shift of one vertebral body on another, usually involving slippage of L5 on S1. It may be congenital or acquired through degeneration or trauma. It is often associated with bilateral pars articularis defects that usually develop in early childhood and have a family predisposition. Pars articularis defects that develop due to athletic activity (stress fractures) rarely result in spondylolisthesis (Brukner et al., 2017).

If symptomatic, the main symptom is back pain that is usually referred to the buttocks. Spondylolisthesis may also present with symptoms of radiculopathy due to compression of the nerve roots. Symptoms may then also include pain, paraesthesia or weakness in the lower limbs (Gagnet et al., 2018). The pain is normally aggravated by exercise and standing and eased by sitting.

Inspection may reveal excessive skin folds above the defect and a step defect may be felt on palpation (Norris, 2004). On examination, extension is limited, and painful and passive overpressure of the affected vertebra produces the pain.

MRI also assesses the degree or grade of spondylolisthesis, which is measured by the percentage distance the slipped upper vertebra moves forwards on its lower counterpart. There are several classifications of spondylolisthesis and four or five grades may be described.

It is important to consider that a patient's back pain is not necessarily associated with the spondylolisthesis, and it can be an asymptomatic incidental finding (Brukner et al., 2017). However, athletes with more than 50% slippage should be advised to avoid high-speed or contact sports (Brukner et al., 2017).

Spondylolisthesis can be managed conservatively initially, or surgically, depending on the grade of the spondylolisthesis, the symptoms and the impact it is having on the patient's daily activities.

Conservative management of spondylolisthesis consists of activity modification, pain control, bracing (Gagnet et al., 2018) and postural correction. Rehabilitation exercise approaches have also been shown to be effective (Brukner et al., 2017).

Surgical management of spondylolisthesis consists of decompression and fusion (Gagnet et al., 2018). It is usually reserved for slips of over 50% in athletes, where the pain has persisted for over 6 months despite conservative management, or in growing children experiencing progressively worsening neurological signs and radiological evidence of further displacement (Brukner et al., 2017).

Neurological

Cauda equina syndrome (CES) is challenging to diagnose and to manage. It may present in any clinical setting, and practitioners should always consider red flags and indicators for CES to be able to provide judicious and appropriate management. Timely diagnosis is essential to avoid life-changing outcomes such as ongoing bladder, bowel, and sexual dysfunction, along with psychosocial consequences (Finucane et al., 2020a).

The incidence of CES in the United Kingdom has been estimated to be 0.002%. The overall prevalence of CES has been estimated to range from 1 in 33,000 to 1 in 100,000 people. Any space-occupying lesion could cause cauda equina compression but compression of the cauda equina usually arises as a result of disc prolapse. CES is a complication of approximately 2% of all herniated discs (Finucane et al., 2020a).

Relevant symptoms that can be precursors to CES are unilateral or bilateral radicular pain, dermatomal reduced sensation and myotomal weakness. These symptoms can also be associated with disc prolapse, which is why CES is difficult to recognise, but if the symptoms above progress to include any changes in bladder or bowel function, saddle sensory disturbance or sexual dysfunction, then CES should be suspected (Finucane et al., 2020a).

Signs and symptoms of cauda equina syndrome require urgent surgical referral (Dinning and Schaeffer, 1993; Jalloh and Minhas, 2007; Finucane et al., 2020a). Studies have shown that considerable improvements in sensory, motor and sphincter deficits are more likely to be achieved if surgery is performed within 48 hours (Jalloh and Minhas, 2007) but it is common (i.e. 40% to 50%) for these deficits to continue after surgery (Korse et al., 2013).

Patients with suspected CES must be referred in line with local policy and it is important to know local pathways to ensure that people are managed properly. Investigation normally includes emergency MRI and surgical opinion. If there is a suspicion that a person may go on to develop CES, 'safety netting' is essential (i.e. the person must be informed about what to look out for and what to do if symptoms of CES develop) (Finucane et al., 2020a) (see Chapter 1).

Inflammatory

Rheumatoid arthritis can affect the spinal joints. Pain and stiffness in the second half of the night and significant early morning stiffness which lasts over an hour (or a history of prolonged morning stiffness), along with consideration of age, family history and involvement of the small peripheral joints, may lead to the suspicion of the condition (NICE, 2020c).

If suspected, a rheumatological opinion should be sought to confirm diagnosis. Until a rheumatology appointment is available, NSAID medication can be considered at the lowest effective dose and for the shortest possible time (NICE, 2020c).

Spondyloarthropathy refers to a group of inflammatory diseases that include psoriatic arthritis, reactive arthritis, Reiter disease and ankylosing spondylitis (also referred to as axial spondyloarthritis). The predominant feature is joint pain and inflammation, particularly affecting the spine. Ankylosing spondylitis is discussed in Chapter 14.

Axial presentations of spondyloarthritis are often misdiagnosed as mechanical low back pain and there is an average delay of 8.5 years between onset and diagnosis with only around 15% of cases receiving a diagnosis within three months of initial presentation (McAllister et al., 2017).

Vascular Pathology

Aortic aneurysms are commonly abdominal (Feather et al., 2020) and can present with back pain. They can be 'ballooning', caused by a thinning of the arterial wall, or 'dissecting' where a secondary pathway forms within the wall of the aorta. A pulse may be palpable in the abdomen or detected with a stethoscope, and urgent referral is required, where the aneurysm can be confirmed by ultrasound scanning.

Rupture of the aneurysm presents with epigastric pain that radiates through to the back. In addition to a pulsatile mass being palpable, the patient is shocked, and the situation is managed as an emergency.

Malignancy

Malignancy of the lumbar spine, although relatively uncommon, should be considered as a possible cause of low back and leg pain. After fracture, metastatic bone disease is the second most common serious pathology to affect the spine, as a consequence of primary cancer (Finucane, et al., 2020a). The history is especially important here as the primary red flag for the detection of spinal malignancy is a history of previous malignancy (Downie et al., 2013, Finucane et al., 2020a).

The most common cancers to metastasise to the spine are breast (21%), lung (19%), prostate (7.5%), renal (5%), gastrointestinal (4.5%) and thyroid (2.5%) (Ziu et al., 2017). Approximately 30% of all people with one of these primary diagnoses of cancer will develop metastases but it is important not to subject all people with a history of cancer to unnecessary and worrying investigations. In breast cancer, metastatic bone disease can develop at any time, with 50% occurring within the first 5 years after a primary diagnosis of cancer and the other 50% developing 10 years and later (Finucane et al., 2020a).

Malignancy involving the lumbar spine may be clinically silent, may produce pain in isolation, or cause associated neurological deficit (Findlay, 1992). The pain may be due to compression or distortion of pain-sensitive structures and/or to destructive changes in the bone. Neurological deficit is usually of a lower motor neuron type, and it may begin either at the same time as the pain or prior to it.

Metastatic spinal cord compression (MSCC) is usually caused by the collapse or compression of a vertebral body that contains metastatic bone disease. It can also be caused rarely by a direct extension of a tumour into the spine (Robson, 2014). MSCC can lead to irreversible neurological damage. Symptoms can include band-like referral spinal pain, escalating pain and gait disturbance (Finucane, et al., 2020b).

The signs and symptoms of malignancy can mimic a mechanical lumbar lesion, but the pain has characteristic features. It is usually deep-seated, nagging, relatively constant, steadily worsening and often persistent at night. If there is collapse of the vertebral body, the pain will be associated with movement and activity, due to the spinal instability (Findlay, 1992).

Apart from night pain, symptoms of weakness, fatigue and significant weight loss (>10% within 3 months) should be considered to be serious in a patient complaining of back pain. Suspicion of malignancy requires urgent onward referral for further investigation, but MSCC needs emergency referral, in line with local policy.

Infection

Infection may cause *osteomyelitis* or *discitis*, and *spinal abscess* is possible. Spinal infections are uncommon with an incidence of 0.2 to 2.4 cases per 100,000 annually in Western societies. They represent 2% to 7% of all musculoskeletal infections (Finucane et al., 2020a).

Pyogenic (pus-producing) organisms (e.g. *Staphylococcus aureus, Myobacterium tuberculosis* [TB] or, rarely, *Brucella*) may be responsible (Feather et al., 2020). Discitis mostly affects the lumbar spine (58%), followed by the thoracic spine (30%) and cervical spine (11%), whereas TB lesions mainly affect the thoracic spine, and often at more than 2 levels (Finucane et al., 2020a).

The frequency of spinal infections presenting in a clinical setting depends on the demographics of the region or country. Risk factors for spinal infection include immunosuppression due to disease or medications, a primary source of infection, or a personal or family history of tuberculosis (Finucane et al., 2020b).

Spinal infection is rare in high-income countries and the diagnosis is often delayed, since practitioners fail to recognise the relevant red flags and to consider spinal infection as a potential differential diagnosis (Finucane et al., 2020a).

The clinical presentation of spinal infection varies from a complaint of back pain only, to the patient being extremely ill, emaciated and febrile, with a raised erythrocyte sedimentation rate. Clinical features comprise back pain, fever, and worsening neurological dysfunction but many people do not present with all three. Fever is reported in only half of people with spinal infection and the absence of fever does not rule out spinal infection (Finucane et al., 2020a).

On examination, there is tenderness on percussion of the affected vertebra, and widespread muscle spasm may be present. X-ray may show loss of bony contour, cavitation and collapse, and possibly an associated paravertebral abscess (Kemp and Worland, 1974). Albert et al. (2013) proposed that Type 1 Modic changes (bone oedema with some disruption of the endplate and trabeculae) could be due to infection in the adjacent disc.

Suspicion of infection requires emergency onward referral for further investigation, in line with local policy.

The box 'Updated Hierarchical List of Red Flags' presents a weighted list of factors, which, when considered together, in the context of the patient's history, signs and symptoms, helps to raise the practitioner's index of suspicion for serious pathology (see Chapter 1).

UPDATED HIERARCHICAL LIST OF RED FLAGS

- Age > 50 years + history of cancer + unexplained weight loss + failure to improve after 1 month of evidence-based conservative therapy

- Age <10 and >51 years
- Medical history (current or past) of:
  - Cancer
  - Tuberculosis
  - Human immunodeficiency virus (HIV)/acquired immune deficiency syndrome (AIDS) or intravenous drug use
  - Osteoporosis
- Weight loss >10% body weight (3–6 months)
- Severe night pain precluding sleep
- Loss of sphincter tone and altered S4 sensation
- Bladder retention or bowel incontinence
- Positive extensor plantar response

- Age 11 to 19
- loss 5% to 10% body weight (3 to 6 months)
- Constant progressive pain
- Band-like pain
- Abdominal pain and changed bowel habits, but with no change of medication
- Inability to lie supine
- Bizarre neurological deficit
- Spasm
- Disturbed gait

- Loss of mobility, difficulty with stairs, falls, trips
- Legs misbehave, odd feelings in legs, legs feeling heavy
- Weight loss < 5% body weight (3 to 6 months)
- Smoking
- Systemically unwell
- Trauma
- Bilateral pins and needles in hands and/or feet
- Previous failed treatment
- Thoracic pain
- Headache
- Physical appearance
- Marked partial articular restriction of movement

From Greenhalgh and Selfe, 2010. Reprinted by permission of Elsevier Ltd.

COMMENTARY ON THE EXAMINATION

Observation

A general observation of the patient's *face, posture and gait* will alert the examiner to the seriousness of the condition. Patients in acute pain will generally look tired.

They may have adopted an antalgic posture of flexion or lumbar scoliosis. The attachments of the iliolumbar ligament inhibit lateral movement at the lumbosacral junction. Patients with a disc herniation at the L5 to S1 level tend to adopt a flexed posture to reduce pain, whereas at the levels above, the herniation can be accommodated by developing a lateral shift. A lumbar lateral shift is pathognomonic of a disc lesion (Porter, 1995). Patients may not be able to sit during the examination due to discomfort.

The patient's gait may be tense with steps taken cautiously, obviously wary of provoking twinges of pain by sudden movements or pain on weight-bearing. A dropped foot may be evident on walking and will lead you to consider involvement of the L4 and L5 nerve roots affecting the tibialis anterior muscle and interfering with function. A dropped foot of acute onset requires an urgent surgical opinion.

History

A discussion on 'red flags' is included in Chapter 1. The box on page 453 lists the 'red flags' that could indicate the presence of serious pathology and these should be listened for and identified throughout the history and examination.

In isolation, many of the flags may have limited significance, and the contemporary approach is to use a 'cluster' of red flags along with clinical experience to decide whether contraindications to treatment exist and/or whether timely onward referral is indicated (Almeida et al., 2018.)

The history is particularly important at the spinal joints as it informs differential diagnosis and also helps to establish clinical models to guide management.

There is a close relationship between signs and symptoms from the lumbar spine, sacroiliac joint and hip joint. The history will help with the differential diagnosis, but conditions at each of these areas can coexist.

The patient's *age, occupation, sports, hobbies and activities* can give an indication of provoking mechanisms. Often the incident precipitating the episode of back pain is relatively minor, although predisposing factors may have been present for some time.

Patients over age 50 are at increased risk of tumour, abdominal aortic aneurysm and infection. In those over age 65, degenerative spinal stenosis and compression osteoporotic fractures should be ruled out. Prepubescent children can have infection; osteomyelitis and discitis and tumours of the spine or spinal cord are a possibility. Older children up to the age of 18 can have herniated disc or mechanical strain but spondylosis, spondylolisthesis and tumour should be considered.

Many occupations have a sedentary flexion lifestyle, applying postural stress to the lumbar spine joints and it is also helpful to explore the patient's general level of activity as this can also have an influence on the cause and rehabilitation.

The *site* of the pain will give an indication of its origin (see Chapter 1). Lumbar pain can be localised to the back and buttocks or felt in the lower limb. Sacroiliac joint pain is hard to distinguish from pain of lumbar origin. It may also be unilateral, felt in the buttock, or more commonly in the groin, and occasionally referred into the leg.

The hip joint may produce an area of pain in the buttock consistent with the L3 segment, pain in the groin, or pain referred down the anteromedial aspect of the thigh and leg to the medial aspect of the ankle. With such a shared presentation, differential diagnosis between pain of lumbar, sacroiliac joint or hip origin can therefore be difficult based on the site of pain alone.

Dural pain is multisegmental and can be central or bilateral. Pressure on the dural nerve root sleeve refers segmentally into the relevant dermatome. Pressure on the nerve root can refer pain into the leg with accompanying symptoms of paraesthesia at the distal end of the dermatome.

The *spread* of pain will not only give an indication of its origin but also the severity or irritability of the lesion. Generally, the more peripherally the pain is referred, the more irritable the lesion.

A lumbar disc herniation can produce central or unilateral back or buttock pain. If the pain moves into the leg, it can cease or be reduced in the back. Pain of non-mechanical origin does not follow this pattern, and serious lesions usually produce an increasing spreading pain, with pain in the back remaining as severe as that felt peripherally.

The *onset and duration* of the pain can guide the choice of treatment. For example, a sudden and recent onset of pain may respond to manipulation. The whole clinical picture will need to be reasoned through to be able to decide on appropriate management.

The nature and mode of onset are important. The patient may remember the exact time and mode of onset, which could have involved a flexed and rotated posture. If lifting was involved in the precipitating episode, it may only have been a trivial weight. If the patient reports a gradual onset of pain, it is worth questioning further for details of previous activity. A minor traumatic incident some time before the onset may have been the initial cause of symptoms produced later by a prolonged period of sitting.

The gradual onset of degenerative arthropathy is common in the facet joints. Serious pathology tends to develop insidiously but osteoporotic insufficiency fractures can come on suddenly, and with minimal trauma, such as strimming the garden or leaning over a shopping trolley.

If trauma is involved, the exact nature of the trauma should be determined, and any possible fracture eliminated. Direct trauma can produce soft tissue contusions, while fractures may involve the spinous process, transverse process, pars interarticularis, vertebral body or vertebral endplate.

Compression fractures of the vertebral body are common in horse riders, and those falling from a height, and involve the vulnerable cancellous bone of the vertebral body (Hartley, 1995). Hyperflexion injuries may cause ligamentous lesions or involve the capsule of the zygapophyseal joint, while hyperextension injuries compress the zygapophyseal joints. Both forces can injure the intervertebral disc.

The *symptoms and behaviour* need to be considered. Serious pathologies of the spine, including fractures, malignancy or infection, are relatively rare, accounting for less than 1% of all medical cases seen for spinal assessment (Henschke et al., 2008; Friedman et al., 2010). Despite this, the practitioner must remain alert to clinical indicators that need more extensive investigation than the basic clinical examination (Sizer et al., 2007).

Radicular pain is generally a severe lancinating pain, often burning in nature. Typically, the leg pain is worse than the back pain and does not usually follow a specific dermatomal pattern. Radiculopathy is commonly associated with lumbar disc pathology or spinal stenosis and can occur if nerve roots are compressed.

Other symptoms described by the patient can provide evidence for differential diagnosis, contraindications to treatment and the severity or irritability of the lesion. An increase in pressure through coughing, sneezing, laughing or straining can increase the back pain, and this is the main dural symptom.

Paraesthesia is usually felt at the distal end of the dermatome and can be a symptom of nerve root compression. Confirmation of this is made through the signs of nerve root compression (i.e. muscle weakness, altered sensation and reduced or absent reflexes).

Specific questions must be asked concerning numbness or abnormal sensations in the perineum and genital area as well as changes in bladder, bowel and sexual function (i.e. symptoms of cauda equina syndrome). The presence of any of these symptoms indicates compression of the S4 nerve root at the preganglionic extent, which could produce irreversible damage, and indicates emergency referral for surgical opinion.

Manipulation is absolutely contraindicated where S4 root compression symptoms are present. The symptoms of difficulty in passing water, inability to retain urine or lack of sensation when the bowels are opened are important. However, it should also be borne in mind that it is not unusual to find urinary frequency or difficulty in defecating associated with effort in hyperacute lumbar pain, or as a side effect to some medications prescribed to manage pain.

It is also important to differentiate urinary symptoms associated with cauda equina compression from the very common symptoms of stress incontinence and prostate enlargement.

Bilateral sciatica with neurological signs and bilateral limitation of straight leg raise (SLR) suggest a massive central protrusion that may be threatening the cauda equina through the posterior longitudinal ligament, with possible rupture of the ligament (Cyriax, 1982). It is a contraindication to manipulation and needs safety netting advice and further investigation (MRI), since a worsening of the situation could lead to irreversible damage to the cauda equina, as mentioned previously.

The symptoms of cauda equina compression should be distinguished from multisegmental reference of pain into both legs. Notwithstanding, any suspicion of cauda equina compression requires urgent referral, and safety netting advice to patients.

The language used by patients to describe the quality of their pain will indicate the balance between the physical and emotional elements of their pain. Words such as 'throbbing', 'burning', 'twinging' and 'shooting' describe the sensory quality of the pain; emotional characteristics are expressed in such words as 'sickening', 'miserable', 'unbearable' and 'exhausting' or vocal complaints such as moans, groans and gasps (Waddell, 1992, 2004).

The behaviour of the pain will give an indication of the irritability of the patient's condition and provide clues to differential diagnosis.

The pattern of all previous episodes of back pain should be established, as in disc lesions a pattern of gradually worsening and increasing episodes of pain usually emerges.

The patient with a disc herniation and nerve root compression usually complains of pain on movement easing with rest. Changing pressures in the disc affect the pain, and it tends to be worse with sitting and stooping postures than when standing or lying down. In an acute locked back, small movements can create exquisite twinging pain.

The daily pattern of pain is important. Typically, either a disc herniation produces a pattern of pain that is better first thing in the morning after rest, becoming worse as the day goes on, or, since the disc imbibes water overnight, the patient may experience increased pain on weight-bearing first thing in the morning due to increased pressure on sensitive tissues.

It is important to differentiate mechanical back pain from inflammatory arthritis and sacroiliac joint lesions through consideration of other factors, since they also produce early-morning pain, but it is usually associated with significant early morning stiffness that lasts for over an hour.

Patients can usually sleep reasonably well at night, as they are normally able to find a position of ease, but pain can be brought on by movement in bed and disturb sleep. Pain that prevents the patient sleeping and that cannot be eased by changing position could be an indicator of serious pathology.

Questioning the patient about *other joint involvement* will indicate whether inflammatory arthritis exists or if there is a tendency towards degenerative arthropathy. Sacroiliac and hip joint lesions may coexist with pain originating in the lumbar spine.

The *medical history* and the patient's current general health will help to eliminate possible serious pathology, past or present. Visceral lesions can refer pain to the back (e.g. kidney, aortic aneurysm or gynaecological conditions). Infections are usually apparent, with an unwell patient showing a fever. Unexplained recent weight loss may be significant in systemic disease or malignancy.

Malignancy can affect the lumbar and pelvic region, but the pattern of the pain behaviour does not generally fit that of musculoskeletal origin. Past history of primary tumour, especially breast, lung, prostate, renal, gastrointestinal, and thyroid may indicate secondaries as a possible cause of back pain. Serious conditions produce an unrelenting pain; night pain is usually a feature and contributes to the patient looking tired and ill.

In addition to medical history, establish any ongoing conditions and treatment. Explore other previous or current musculoskeletal problems with previous episodes of the current complaint, any treatment given and the outcome of treatment.

Practitioners should *screen* routinely for psychosocial factors and consider relevant health comorbidities and lifestyle factors (see Chapter 1). These factors may contribute to the patient's presenting condition, or form a barrier to recovery and normal function, and should be addressed as an integral part of patient management.

The *medications* taken by the patient will indicate their current medical status as well as alerting the practitioner to possible contraindications to treatment.

Anticoagulant therapy and long-term oral steroids are contraindications to manipulation. It is useful to know what analgesics are being taken and how frequently. This gives an indication of the severity of the condition and can be used as an objective marker for progression of treatment, with the need for less analgesia indicating a positive improvement.

If patients are currently taking antidepressant medication, this may indicate their emotional state and possibly exclude them from manipulation. Care is needed in making this decision, however, since antidepressants can be used in low doses as an adjunct to analgesics in referred leg (radicular) pain.

Assessment of patients with persistent low back pain presents a particular challenge to the clinician. Psychosocial and industrial factors may influence pain perception, while monotony or dissatisfaction at work or home is relevant (Osti and Cullum, 1994). Distinction will need to be made between the true physical symptoms of the presenting condition and those relating to psychosocial factors that influence the way the patient reacts to the pain.

Enquiry should be made about the possibilities of secondary gain factors relating to disability, or the presence of psychological or social stresses that might predispose the patient to persistent pain disorders (Swezey, 1993).

Standard questions on the quality of sleep, tiredness levels, concentration, appetite, etc. may provide information on the patient's mood, which can be assessed further by appropriate questionnaires.

Inspection

The patient should be suitably undressed and in a good light. Difficulty in undressing, especially of socks and shoes, is an indication of the irritability of the lesion.

A general inspection from behind, each side and in front will reveal any *bony deformity*. The general spinal curvatures are assessed (i.e. the cervical and lumbar lordosis and the thoracic kyphosis). The level of the shoulders, inferior angles of the scapulae, buttock and popliteal creases, the position of the umbilicus and the posture of the feet can be assessed for relevance to the patient's present condition.

Any structural or acquired scoliosis is noted. In discal pathology, the patient may be fixed in flexion or have shifted laterally to accommodate the herniation, and this is evident in standing. Small deviations can be noted by assessing the distance between the waist and the elbow in the standing position.

In acute, irritable back pain, the patient may be fixed in a flexed posture and unable to stand upright, and any attempt to do so produces twinges of pain. The level of the iliac crests and the posterior and anterior superior iliac spines gives an overall impression of leg-length discrepancy or pelvic distortion (Fig. 13.10). If these are considered relevant, they can be investigated further.

Postural asymmetry and malalignment are not necessarily indicative of symptoms. It is worth noting them however, since imbalances can be explained to the patient and addressed in the final rehabilitation programme, with the aim of preventing recurrence.

Colour changes and *swelling* are not expected in the lumbar spine unless there has been a history of direct trauma. Any marks on the skin, lipomas, 'faun's beards' (tufts of hair), birthmarks or café-au-lait spots may indicate underlying spinal bony or neurological defects (Hoppenfeld, 1976; Hartley, 1995).

An isolated 'orange-peel' appearance of the skin that is tough and dimpled may indicate spondylolisthesis at that level (Hartley, 1995). Patients with low back pain often apply heat to the area. This can produce an erythematous skin reaction called *erythema ab igne* (redness from the fire), which can be an indicator of the level of pain, through the intensity of heat needed to provide pain relief.

Swelling is not usually a feature, but muscle spasm may give the appearance and feeling of swelling, especially to the patient.

Muscle wasting may not be obvious if the onset of low back pain is recent. Persistent or recurrent episodes of pain may show wasting in the calf muscles or possibly the quadriceps or gluteal muscles.

Palpation is conducted to assess changes in skin temperature and sweating, suggestive of autonomic involvement. Palpation for swelling is not usually necessary at the spinal joints. In standing, the lumbar spine is palpated for a 'shelf' that would indicate spondylolisthesis.

State at Rest

Before any movements are performed, the state at rest is established to provide a baseline for subsequent comparison.

Examination by Selective Tension

The suggested sequence for the examination will now be given, followed by a commentary that includes the reasoning in performing the movements and the significance of the possible findings.

A 'star diagram' assessment tool for recording examination of the lumbar movements is provided in Section 3.

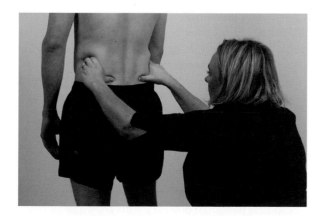

Fig. 13.10 Inspection for pelvic levels.

Articular Signs
- Active lumbar extension (Fig. 13.11)
- Active lumbar right-side flexion (Fig. 13.12a)
- Active lumbar left side flexion (see Fig. 13.12b)
- Active lumbar flexion (Fig. 13.13)
- Resisted plantarflexion, gastrocnemius (Fig. 13.14): S1, S2

Supine Lying
- Passive hip flexion (Fig. 13.15)
- Passive hip medial rotation (Fig. 13.16)
- Passive hip lateral rotation (Fig. 13.17)
- Sacroiliac joint shear tests (Fig. 13.18a–c)
- FABER test (Fig. 13.19)
- Passive straight leg raise (SLR) (Figs 13.20 and 13.21a and b): L4, L5, S1, S2

  Resisted tests for objective neurological signs and alternative causes of leg pain
- Resisted hip flexion, psoas (Fig. 13.22): L2
- Resisted ankle dorsiflexion, tibialis anterior (Fig. 13.23): L4
- Resisted big toe extension, extensor hallucis longus (Fig. 13.24): L5, S1
- Resisted eversion, peroneus longus and brevis (Fig. 13.25): L5, S1, S2

Skin sensation
- Big toe only: L4 (Fig. 13.26)
- First, second and third toes: L5
- Lateral two toes: S1
- Heel: S2

Reflexes
- Knee reflex (Fig. 13.27): L2, L3, L4
- Ankle reflex (Fig. 13.28): S1, S2
- Plantar response (Fig. 13.29)
- Ankle clonus (Fig.13.30)

Prone Lying
- Passive femoral stretch test (FST) (Figs 13.31 and 13.32): L2, L3, L4
- Resisted knee flexion, hamstrings (Fig. 13.33): L5, S1, S2
- Resisted knee extension, quadriceps (Fig. 13.34): L2, L3, L4
- Static contraction of the glutei (Fig. 13.35): L5, S1, S2

Palpation
- Spinous processes for pain, range and end-feel (Fig. 13.36)

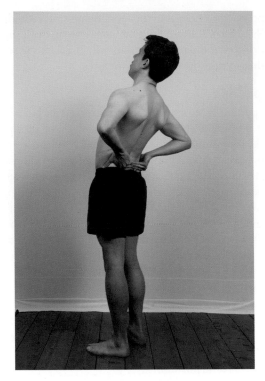

Fig. 13.11 Active extension.

The routine examination of the lumbar spine includes active movements and neurological examination. Since the spinal joints are considered to be a potential focus for 'emotional' symptoms, four active movements are conducted assessing willingness to move, range of movement and pain. The capsular or non-capsular pattern may also emerge from these active movements.

Look for apprehension, guarding or exaggerated movements. An important finding is the non-capsular pattern, usually presenting as an asymmetrical limitation of lumbar movements. The non-capsular pattern is a factor in the clinical models described below that help to guide treatment. The presence of the capsular pattern indicates an arthropathy and it is typically observed with degenerative arthropathy.

Gastrocnemius is assessed for signs of nerve root compression. Testing the muscle group against gravity in standing is convenient at this point, in terms of sequence, before lying the patient down.

In supine lying, other joints are eliminated from the examination to confirm that the site of the lesion is in the lumbar spine. Passive flexion and medial and lateral rotation are conducted at the hip, to assess the hip joint for the capsular pattern or other hip pathology. The sacroiliac joint is assessed within the lumbar examination by three provocative tests and the FABER test (see Chapter 14).

To limit these tests to the hip and sacroiliac joint, it may be necessary to place the patient's forearm under

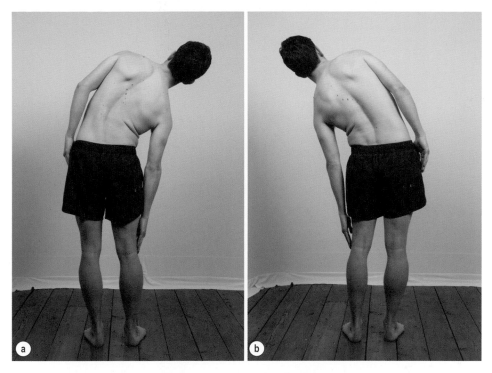

Fig. 13.12 Active side flexions.

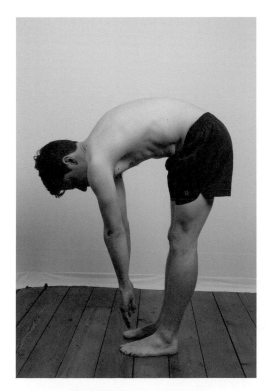

Fig. 13.13 Active flexion.

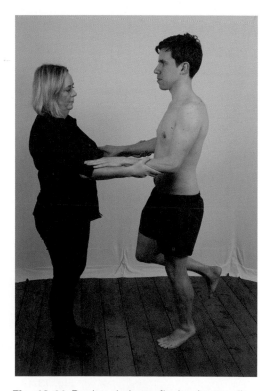

Fig. 13.14 Resisted plantarflexion in standing.

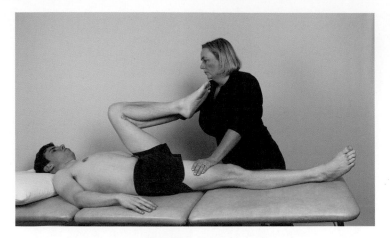

Fig. 13.15 Passive hip flexion.

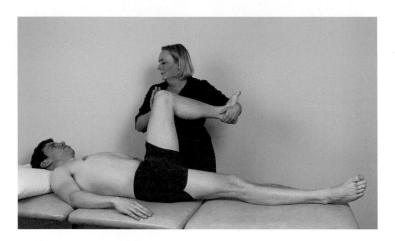

Fig. 13.16 Passive hip medial rotation.

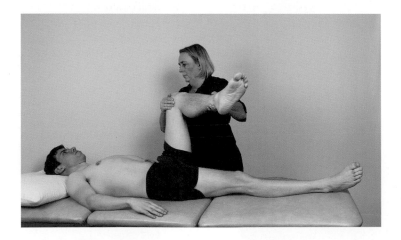

Fig. 13.17 Passive hip lateral rotation.

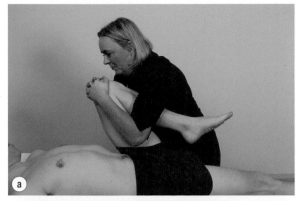

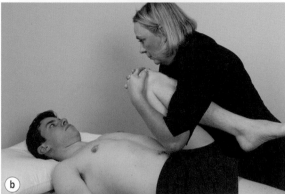

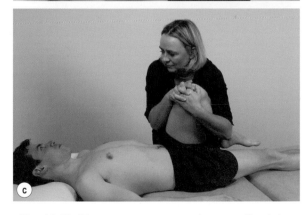

Fig. 13.18 Shear tests to assess the sacroiliac joint.

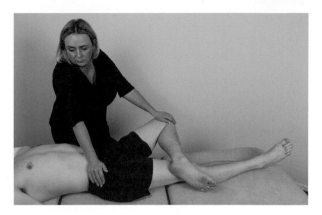

Fig. 13.19 FABER test to assess the sacroiliac joint.

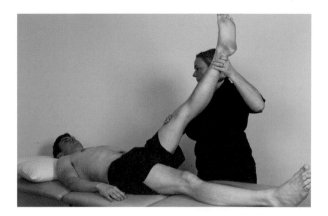

Fig. 13.20 Passive straight leg raise.

the lumbar spine to increase the lordosis and to stabilise the spine. If the lesion in the lumbar spine is very irritable, it may not be possible to conduct these tests adequately. If any of the tests are positive, the full hip or sacroiliac joint examination should be performed.

The SLR is applied passively to each leg in turn, keeping the knee straight. If positive, this can be interpreted as a dural sign, or as an indicator of neural tension affecting the L4, L5, S1, S2 nerve roots.

The normal range of movement for the SLR is between 60 and 120 degrees, with movement being limited by tension in the hamstrings. The range of the SLR should be consistent with the range of lumbar flexion, which is also limited to a certain degree by tension in the hamstrings.

The limited range of the SLR is dependent upon the compression on the dura mater or dural nerve root sleeves and the greater the compression the greater the limitation. A painful arc may be found, which is a useful finding, since it usually implies that manipulation will be beneficial.

The passive SLR is an important clinical test for assessing nerve root tension due to a disc herniation, when back or leg pain is usually produced at 30 and 40 degrees (Supik and Broom, 1994; Jönsson and Strömqvist, 1995). Increased pain on the addition of neck flexion incriminates the dura mater.

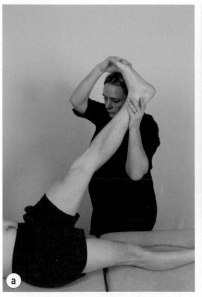
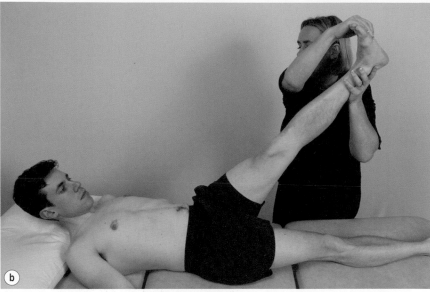

Fig. 13.21 Passive straight leg raise with sensitizing components.

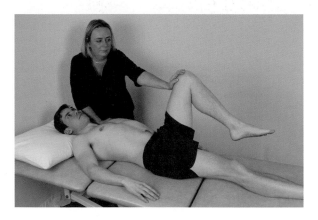

Fig. 13.22 Resisted hip flexion.

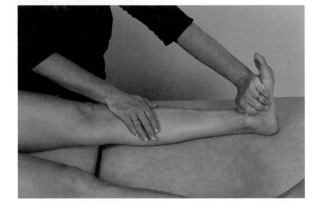

Fig. 13.23 Resisted ankle dorsiflexion.

Further sensitising components such as passive ankle dorsiflexion, passive ankle plantarflexion and inversion, and passive hip medial rotation and adduction can also be added to explore the mobility of the nervous system further as appropriate.

Bilateral sciatica and bilateral limitation of SLR is usually due to a large central disc prolapse compressing the dura mater and can be accompanied by a multi-segmental distribution of pain. If neurological signs are present, it is a contraindication for manipulation and requires urgent onward referral.

A 'crossed' or 'well leg raise' describes the production of the pain in the back or leg on the painful side on SLR of the painless limb. The intensity of the pain induced by the crossed SLR is usually less than that produced on the painful side (Karbowski and Dvorak, 1995). It usually occurs at the L4 level (Cyriax, 1982; Khuffash and Porter, 1989).

Vroomen et al. (1999) identified the crossed SLR test as a strong indicator of nerve root compression, and McCarthy (Evidence Based Management of Back Pain Seminar, July

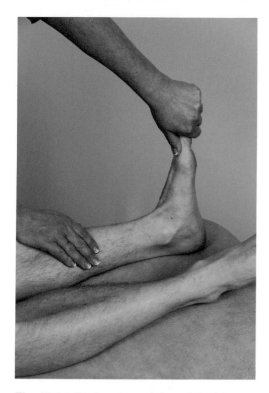

Fig. 13.24 Resisted extension of the big toe.

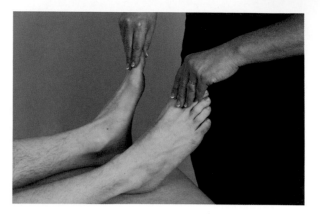

Fig. 13.26 Checking skin sensation.

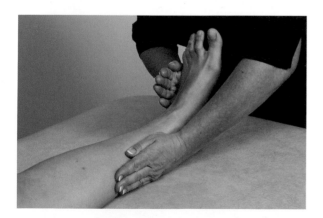

Fig. 13.25 Resisted ankle eversion.

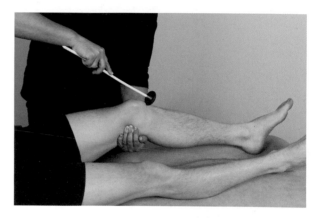

Fig. 13.27 Knee reflex.

2014) endorsed it more strongly still as 'the most useful test in the diagnosis of a lumbar disc herniation'.

The patient is assessed for root signs and alternative causes of pain by the selective application of resisted tests. Signs of muscle weakness, altered skin sensation and brisk, jerky, sluggish or absent reflexes will indicate compression/irritation of a nerve root. Unexplained or abnormal neurology can indicate central compression at higher levels, for example, brain, brain stem or spinal cord, and requires further investigation.

The plantar response is assessed by stroking upwards along the lateral border of the sole of the foot and across the metatarsal heads. The normal response is flexor with flexion of the big toe observed. The Babinski reflex (or Babinski sign) is extension of the big toe. This reflex is a sign of central neuropathology in older children and adults and is indicative of an upper motor neuron lesion, although this is not likely to occur with lumbar lesions since the spinal cord ends at approximately the level of the L1, L2 disc.

The ankle clonus test/reflex is performed by quickly dorsiflexing the foot and holding it in the dorsiflexed position. A positive sign is rapidly repeated oscillations or 'beats' that can be felt and seen by the practitioner and can be indicative of an

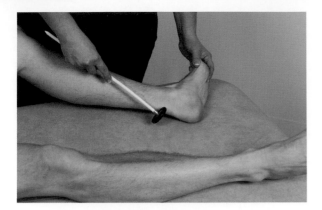

Fig. 13.28 Ankle reflex.

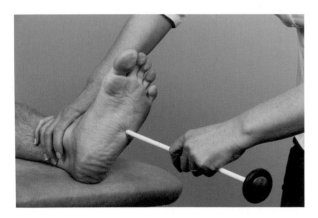

Fig. 13.29 Plantar response.

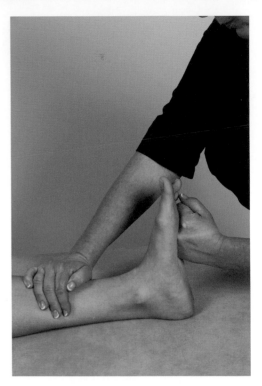

Fig. 13.30 Ankle clonus.

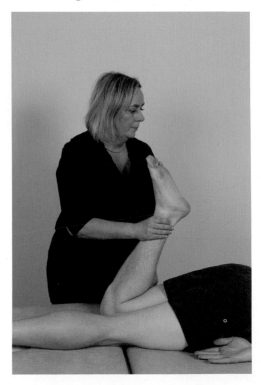

Fig. 13.31 Passive femoral stretch test.

upper motor neuron lesion, in the context of other signs and symptoms.

The femoral stretch test (FST) (prone knee-bending) is applied to assess nerve root tension. The knee is flexed passively and, if positive, pain is usually produced at approximately 90 degrees. A sensitising component of hip extension can be added. Pain is usually felt in the back and the test is limited by tension in the quadriceps. It may be falsely positive due to tight or injured anterior thigh muscles or hip joint pathology (Nadler et al., 2001).

If positive unilaterally, it implicates the nerve roots; if positive bilaterally, central cord compression could be indicated, which requires urgent onward referral to the neurosurgical team. It is theoretically possible to produce a crossed or well-leg FST, but this is not as commonly found in practice (Nadler et al., 2001).

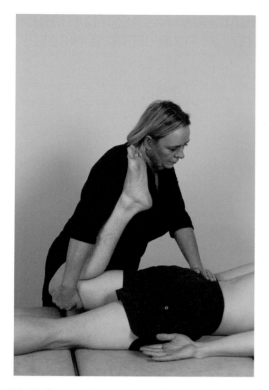

Fig. 13.32 Passive femoral stretch test with sensitizing component.

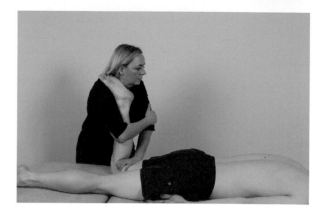

Fig. 13.34 Resisted knee extension.

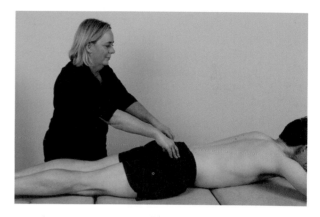

Fig. 13.35 Gluteal contraction, squeezing muscle bulk to assess wasting.

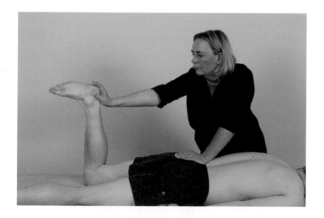

Fig. 13.33 Resisted knee flexion.

The remaining resisted tests for the quadriceps and hamstrings are conducted in prone lying. A static contraction of the gluteal muscles is performed to assess for muscle bulk and palpation is conducted, using the ulnar border of the hand on the spinous processes, for pain, range of movement and end-feel.

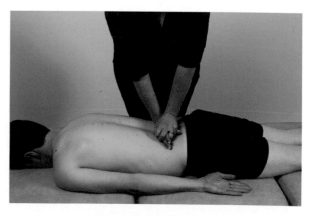

Fig. 13.36 Palpation.

Based on the history and clinical examination, the practitioner should be able to establish the most likely diagnosis, using clinical reasoning and clinical judgement.

If serious pathology is suspected, such as infection, malignancy, fracture and inflammatory arthritis, further tests, including blood tests and radiological imaging, will need to be implemented with appropriate onward referral in a timely manner.

Standard X-ray investigation provides little useful information for mechanical lesions over and above that gleaned from the clinical examination. However, if the patient fails to respond in the expected way, further investigation may be conducted, including MRI, if it would change or add value to management.

It is important to be aware that imaging findings can be misleading, particularly when showing the changes of degenerative arthropathy, which may or may not be symptomatic. Similarly, spondylolysis progressing to spondylolisthesis occurs in approximately 5% of adults but is symptomatic in only half of them (Swezey, 1993). Kalichman et al., (2009) found the prevalence to be slightly higher but observed no significant association between spondylolysis, spondylolisthesis and low back pain.

Any other tests can be added to this basic routine examination of the lumbar spine, including repeated, combined and accessory movements and neural tension testing as appropriate.

TREATMENT OF LOW BACK PAIN

Many patients with diagnosed non-specific low back pain will improve over time, without any treatment, and guidelines now recommend minimal treatment, if any, as a starting point in management (Almeida et al., 2018; Foster et al., 2018; NICE, 2020a; Knezevic et al., 2021).

For most low back pain, with or without leg pain, a stepped approach to management is recommended. Less invasive treatments are generally offered first, including education/advice, watchful wait, activity and work modification, analgesics and NSAIDs medication, physiotherapy (e.g. exercise, mobilisation).

If symptoms persist, further investigation may be required, together with onward referral to a combined physical and psychological rehabilitation programme, or pain team/specialist who may consider pain-relieving injections, radiofrequency or surgery for nerve root compression.

LUMBAR PAIN: A CLASSIFICATION SYSTEM OF FOUR CLINICAL MODELS

Patient selection is the guiding principle in deciding which patients are appropriate for the treatment techniques for low back pain in the musculoskeletal medicine approach. This section presents clinical models to guide treatment within the context of overall management.

It is appropriate to apply treatment based on sets of signs and symptoms, and several classifications to determine treatment programmes and to assist prognosis have been developed (McKenzie, 1981; Riddle, 1998; Laslett and van Wijmen, 1999; McCarthy et al., 2004; Schäfer et al., 2009; Hill et al., 2011, Atkins et al., 2013).

The presentation of signs and symptoms of low back pain, with or without leg pain, has been classified here into clinical models that have been developed from Cyriax's original theories but acknowledge the absence of a clear pathoanatomical diagnosis.

These models are judgement-based and contribute to the clinical decision-making process to rationalise appropriate treatment programmes; they are not intended to be restrictive. Practitioners are encouraged to be inventive, to draw on other experiences, and to implement the approach into their existing clinical practice when putting a package of care together for individual patients.

The treatment techniques described are by no means a cure-all for every case of back pain. However, uncomplicated lesions of recent onset may respond well to the manipulative techniques of musculoskeletal medicine. The key, as in the cervical spine, is the selection of the right treatment for the right patient through sound clinical reasoning.

For the purposes of the following classification of models, a patient may present with the features described in the following.

Clinical Model 1: Acute/Irritable
History
- Central or short bilateral or unilateral severe back pain with high irritability; often with twinges
- No neurological symptoms
- Gradual or sudden onset. Patient may or may not be able to recall the exact mode of onset; may be precipitated by a period of prolonged flexion
- No red flags or significant yellow flags

Examination

- Antalgic posture
- Non-capsular pattern of pain and limitation of movement
- No red flags or significant yellow flags

Treatment

- Education and reassurance
- Pain-relieving modalities
- Postural advice
- 'Pretzel' technique

The focus is on education, reassurance, pain relief, restoration of mobility and appropriate advice. In the musculoskeletal approach, the 'Pretzel' technique as a mobilising technique for acute, or irritable, lumbar pain is suggested.

Once initial irritability and pain subsides, the treatment may be applied as for Clinical Model 2.

Clinical Model 2: Subacute/Non-Irritable
History

- Central or short bilateral or unilateral pain, less severe back or leg (not referred below the knee)
- Sudden, gradual or mixed onset
- Patient may or may not recall the exact mode and time of onset
- No neurological symptoms
- No red flags or significant yellow flags

Examination

- Non-capsular pattern of pain and limitation of movement
- May have increased pain on side flexion away or towards the painful side
- No neurological signs

Treatment

- If no contraindications, mobilisation, manipulation or traction

Manipulation is considered as part of the package of care for these patients, provided there are no contraindications to treatment.

Increased pain on side flexion away from the painful side can often be an indication that manipulation is appropriate and likely to be successful.

Lumbar lesions of gradual onset may demonstrate side flexion towards the painful side as the more painful movement and this feature can help to guide treatment choice. For lumbar presentations of gradual onset, where manipulation has only been partially successful, traction may be applied, provided that there are no contraindications to treatment.

Clinical Model 3: Referred Symptoms
History

- Initial presentation of central or unilateral back or buttock pain, followed by referred leg pain (the central pain usually ceasing or diminishing)
- Sudden or gradual onset
- Often part of a history of increasing, worsening episodes (i.e. may be a progression of the above models)
- Patient may or may not recall the exact time and mode of onset
- Patient may complain of root symptoms (i.e. paraesthesia felt in a segmental distribution, muscle weakness)
- No red flags or significant yellow flags

Examination

- Non-capsular pattern of pain and limitation of movement reproducing back and/or leg symptoms
- Root signs may be present (i.e. sensory changes, muscle weakness, absent or reduced reflexes); consistent with the nerve root(s) involved

Treatment

- If pain above the knee; neurological signs minimal and stable; subacute level of pain and no contraindications, may try mobilisation/manipulation—often unsuccessful
- Traction—mechanical
- Await spontaneous recovery mechanism

The hypothesis of a compressive disc lesion is more readily rationalised here, due to the nerve root involvement. Disc herniation, presence of osteophytes, thickened ligamentum flavum, reduced vertebral body height, reduced disc height, canal or foraminal stenotic changes of the spine, can all contribute to compression or nerve root irritation. Less frequently, tumours or cysts may also lead to compression or irritation.

Pain may be referred into the leg through compression of the dural nerve root sleeve or the nerve root itself. However, the mechanism of injury to the nerve may be more complicated than expressed here and may also involve chemical and ischaemic factors, which could affect the quality of the pain response.

To fall into this model, from the history, the pain should be worse in the leg than in the back (Koes et al., 2007). The pain can radiate to the foot or toes and the paraesthesia will tend to be in the same distribution. Straight leg raising will increase leg pain, usually on the affected side, but the crossover SLR test might be positive, which has high specificity for nerve root irritation, and is usually associated with a herniated disc.

Koes et al. (2007) suggest that, although there is the possibility for more than one nerve root to be affected, due to the obliquity of the nerve roots, it is more usual that local neurology is limited to one nerve root. Acute lumbar radiculopathy most commonly affects the L5 or S1 root and less commonly the L4 root. It is less common still for the other roots to be affected (Caplan, 1994).

Treatment is aimed at relieving pain.

The more peripheral the symptoms, the less likely manipulation is to be successful. Manipulation may be applied in the presence of neurological signs, provided they are minimal and stable (i.e. non-progressive) and that no other contraindications exist. If the neurological deficit is severe and progressing, further investigation and onward referral should be considered.

A caudal epidural of corticosteroid and local anaesthetic may be indicated for acute or persistent severe radicular pain (Cyriax, 1984; Cyriax and Cyriax, 1993; Vroomen et al., 2000; Boswell et al., 2007, NICE, 2020a).

Alternatively, spontaneous recovery is likely (Kesikburun, et al., 2019) and may be awaited with suitable reassurance and/or analgesia being given to the patient.

If patients fail to improve with conservative treatment, and the persistent pain lasts for more than 6 to 8 weeks, without major neurological deficit, then the choice is between prolonged non-surgical and surgical treatment (Valat et al., 2010; Deyo, 2007). However, the patient's treatment preference is influenced by a number of considerations, such as the severity of symptoms, impact on patients' function, patients' willingness to wait for spontaneous recovery, their aversion to surgical risk and whether they have risks that would prevent them from having surgery. It is important to weigh the risks and benefits of available treatment options on a case-by-case basis.

Clinical Model 4: Persistent
History
- Pain for more than 3 months
- Acute/subacute exacerbation of symptoms
- Persistent with no previous input; or non-responder to treatment
- 'Aching' central or unilateral back, buttock and/or leg pain
- Pain worsened by movement
- Often part of a history of increasing, worsening episodes
- Lumbar stiffness
- No red flags or significant yellow flags

Examination
- Capsular or non-capsular pattern of movement producing back and/or leg symptoms

Treatment
- Multifactorial management; education, reassurance, advice on exercise and self-management
- Biological—acute/subacute exacerbation may be treated as the models above, as appropriate, provided there are no contraindications
- Psychosocial—a combined physical exercise and psychological educational programme (such as cognitive-behavioural approach)
- A multidisciplinary pain management programme

The NICE Guideline (2020a) recommends that a combined physical and psychological programme can be considered for people with persistent low back pain or leg pain. This can incorporate a cognitive behavioural approach (preferably in a group context that takes into account a person's specific needs and capabilities), when previous treatments have not been effective or when there are significant psychosocial obstacles to recovery (e.g. avoiding normal activities based on inappropriate beliefs about their condition). Referral to the pain management team may be appropriate.

Manual therapy can be considered for acute exacerbations of pain as part of a package of care, provided there are no contraindications to treatment. Patient selection is important, and tools discussed earlier in this chapter can be helpful towards this.

Musculoskeletal medicine aims to apply techniques of manipulation, mobilisation, traction and injection to treat low back and leg pain as appropriate. The choice of treatment will depend on the nature of the pain, the irritability of the lesion, the reference of pain and the mode of onset.

Musculoskeletal medicine spinal manipulation techniques aim to reduce the signs and symptoms. In terms of expectations of treatment outcomes, the ideal patient for manipulation is Clinical Model 2.

Ebell (2009) proposed a validated simple two-item rule for the 'ideal' patient, including symptom duration of less than 16 days and no symptoms distal to the knee. In the musculoskeletal medicine approach, Clinical Model 2 expands on Ebell's proposal, but these two factors are key features of the model (Atkins et al., 2013).

Manipulation can be attempted for patients within Clinical Model 3 with leg pain, but it is not indicated in patients with the severe radicular pain or severe or progressive neurological deficit. It can also be used for patients with persistent back pain as in Clinical Model 4, provided there are no contraindications.

CONTRAINDICATIONS TO LUMBAR MOBILISATION

It is impossible to be absolutely definitive about all contraindications and nothing can substitute for a rigorous assessment of the presenting signs and symptoms and an accurate diagnosis of a mechanical lumbar lesion.

'Red flags' are signs and symptoms found in the patient's history and examination that may indicate serious pathology and provide contraindications to lumbar manipulation (Sizer et al., 2007; Greenhalgh and Selfe, 2010) (see 'Updated Hierarchical List of Red Flags' box, page 453).

The absolute contraindications are highlighted in the discussion below but there are several cautions that should be considered as well. It may be useful to use the mnemonic *COINS* (a contraction of 'contraindications') as an aide-mémoire to be able to create categories for the absolute contraindications: Circulatory, Osseous, Inflammatory, Neurological and suspicious features indicating Serious pathology. If the first and last two letters are pushed together as *CONS*, the crucial need for *cons*ent is emphasised.

> **COINS**
> - **C**irculatory
> - **O**sseous
> - **I**nflammatory
> - **N**eurological
> - **S**erious

The treatment regime discussed below is contraindicated in the *absence of informed patient consent* (see Chapter 1).

Signs and symptoms of cauda equina syndrome are a contraindication to manipulation. *Bilateral sciatica from the same level* with *bilateral limitation of SLR* and bilateral neurological signs indicate a large, central disc prolapse threatening the cauda equina. Each provides an absolute contraindication to manipulation (Dinning and Schaeffer, 1993). This presentation must not be confused with multisegmental reference of bilateral pain in the absence of neurological signs, as these patients may benefit from the central treatment techniques suggested below.

Severe or progressive neurological deficit associated with Clinical Model 3 is too irritable for the treatment techniques suggested below. It requires further investigation and possible onward referral.

Radiculopathy in the young is rare and full imaging should be conducted on young patients presenting with numbness, weakness and absent reflexes (Sizer et al., 2007). Manipulation is not appropriate. Similarly, *hyperacute pain* in which the patient has twinges and has difficulty even moving or assuming different postures is too irritable to manipulate.

Manipulation is inappropriate for the patient with symptoms of neurogenic (spinal) claudication, associated with spinal stenosis.

The patient taking *anticoagulant therapy*, such as warfarin, is contraindicated due to the risk of intraspinal bleeding. The patient with blood clotting disorders should also be considered as a caution.

Through a thorough assessment it will be possible to screen the patient presenting with his/her first episode of backache under the age of 10 or over the age of 50 and the patient with a history of primary tumour to ensure that the back pain is not serious in origin. Long-term systemic steroid use, inflammatory arthritis, known osteoporosis or HIV are all cautions for manipulation.

The *systemically unwell* patient or the patient experiencing *constant, progressive non-mechanical pain* or other signs of serious spinal pathology is not appropriate for manipulative techniques and fracture will normally need to be excluded in patients suffering recent traumatic incidents such as a motor vehicle accident.

Caution should be taken with the pregnant patient, although there is no evidence to suggest that manipulation is dangerous (Lisi, 2006). Discussion with the patient of the risks and benefits will allow informed consent, should the practitioner judge the manipulation to be appropriate.

'Yellow flags' from the history and examination may highlight degrees of illness behaviour that make the patient inappropriate for manipulation.

Safety recommendations for spinal manipulation techniques are included in Section 3.

TREATMENT TECHNIQUES

It is recommended that a course in musculoskeletal medicine should be attended before the treatment techniques described are applied in clinical practice (see Section 3).

Two types of manipulative technique are used, the first incorporating a short- or long-lever arm according to the effect required:
- Rotation techniques for unilateral pain
- Extension techniques for central pain

The techniques described below are conducted with the couch at a suitable height for the practitioner. For most techniques, this should be as low as possible.

The techniques may be easier to perform if the patient is asked to take in a small breath, with the technique being applied after the patient has breathed out. This encourages patient relaxation and will allow for the effective application of the overpressure with minimal tissue resistance.

The following techniques are described in a suggested order of progression for the novice manipulator, but, once experience is gained in the application of the techniques, any may be chosen as a starting point and the order presented is not an order of efficacy.

The comparable signs are assessed after every technique and the next technique is chosen based on the outcome. As long as a technique is gaining an increase

in range and/or a decrease in pain, it can be repeated. Improvement may reach a plateau or the feedback from the patient may become unclear.

Only professional judgement will reliably dictate when treatment should be stopped in each treatment session. It is better to err towards the side of caution in the early stages of acquiring manipulative skill.

Rotation Techniques

DISTRACTION TECHNIQUE

- Position the patient in side lying with the painful side uppermost.
- Flex the upper hip and knee with the knee just resting over the side of the bed to assist the rotational stress.
- Extend the lower leg.
- Pull the underneath shoulder through firmly such that the uppermost shoulder is positioned backwards and the pelvis positioned forwards.
- Stand behind the patient at waist level and place one hand 'hooked' against the greater trochanter, pointing outwards.
- Put your other hand comfortably on the patient's uppermost shoulder with your fingers pointing away from your other hand.
- Use the hand hooked onto the greater trochanter to push the pelvis just forwards of the midline so that the patient's waist is facing upwards.
- Apply pressure equally through both hands to impart a distraction force; you will see the patient's waist crease stretch out as you lean through your arms (Fig. 13.37).
- Keep your arms straight as you apply a minimal amplitude, high-velocity thrust once all the slack has been taken up.
- Reassess.

SHORT-LEVER ROTATION TECHNIQUE—PELVIS FORWARDS

- Position the patient in supine lying with the hips and knees flexed (crook lying).
- Ask the patient to lift and rotate the hips so that they are lying with the painful side uppermost and the shoulders relatively flat.
- Position the legs as for the distraction technique.

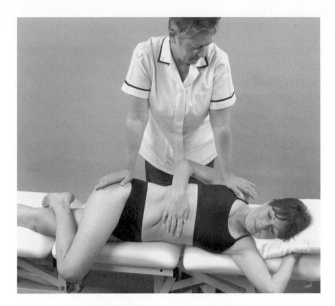

Fig. 13.37 Distraction technique.

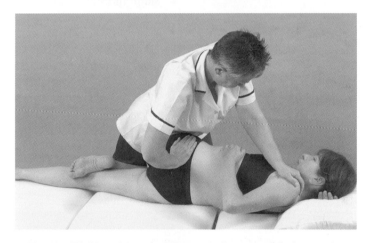

Fig. 13.38 Short-lever rotation technique – pelvis forwards.

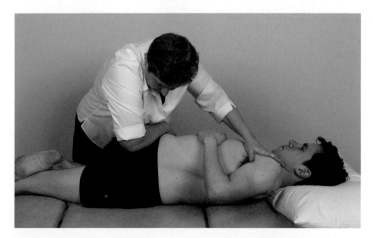

Fig. 13.39 Alternative arm position, short-lever rotation technique – pelvis forwards.

- Stand in front of the patient with one hand fixing the patient's shoulder while the other is placed with the heel of the hand on the blade of the ilium, with the forearm horizontal and your fingers pointing back towards you.
- Apply pressure through the hand on the ilium in a horizontal direction towards you to achieve a rotational strain (Fig. 13.38).
- Apply a minimal amplitude, high-velocity thrust once all the slack has been taken up.
- If you find it difficult to apply the thrust with your hand against the ilium, slide your hand towards you to place your forearm against the bone to give you improved leverage (Fig. 13.39).
- Reassess.

SHORT-LEVER ROTATION TECHNIQUE—PELVIS BACKWARDS

(Cyriax, 1984; Cyriax and Cyriax, 1993)

- Position the patient in side lying with the painful side uppermost.
- Take the lower arm behind the patient and place the upper arm into elevation, resting in front of the patient's face.
- Extend the upper leg and flex the hip and knee of the lower leg. The shoulder will now be positioned forwards and the pelvis backwards.

- Stand behind the patient; place one hand on the scapula to give a little distraction to take up the slack.
- Place the other hand on the front of the pelvis with your forearm horizontal and pointing back towards you (Fig. 13.40).
- Apply a minimal amplitude, high-velocity thrust once all the slack is taken up.
- Reassess.

LONG-LEVER ROTATION TECHNIQUE

(Cyriax, 1984; Cyriax and Cyriax, 1993)

This is a stronger rotational technique and care is recommended in its application to older patients to avoid placing undue strain on the neck of the femur.

- Position the patient as for the short-lever rotation—pelvis forwards technique.
- Stand in front of the patient at waist level, facing the patient's feet to allow the arms to be placed more vertically.
- Fix the shoulder with one hand and place the other hand behind the knee, with your thumb in the knee crease.
- Lean on the knee to produce a rotation strain (Fig. 13.41).
- Apply a minimal amplitude, high-velocity thrust once all the slack is taken up.
- Reassess.

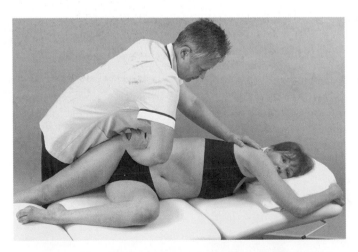

Fig. 13.40 Short-lever rotation technique – pelvis backwards.

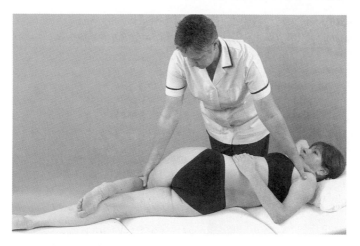

Fig. 13.41 Long-lever rotation technique.

'PRETZEL' TECHNIQUE

This is a strong, long-lever rotation technique when used as a manipulation. It can be broken down into its individual stages and used as a mobilising technique for acute pain when the lesion is too irritable for manipulation. It helps in both instances to be clear on the different stages of the technique. It may be useful for correcting a lateral shift (Cyriax and Cyriax, 1993).

- Stand on the patient's painless side with the patient in supine lying. Flex the knees and cross the good leg over the bad (Fig. 13.42).
- Flex both hips (Fig. 13.43).
- Place your knee that is furthest from the patient's head at the patient's waist to act as a pivot point. Place your hands on the patient's knees and side-flex the lumbar spine to gap the affected side (Fig. 13.44).
- Rotate the pelvis towards you until the patient's knees are resting on your thigh (Fig. 13.45).
- Gently lower your thigh, taking the pelvis further into rotation, ensuring that the other hand fixes the patient's shoulder flat on the couch (Fig. 13.46). Apply a minimal amplitude, high-velocity thrust once all the slack is taken up. Help the patient back to the starting position.
- Reassess.

If the patient is large, an assistant may be required to fix the patient's shoulder.

For *acute pain with high irritability*, each step is conducted individually using gentle mobilisation in the

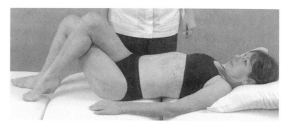

Fig. 13.42 'Pretzel' technique: starting position with knees flexed and 'good' leg placed over the 'bad'.

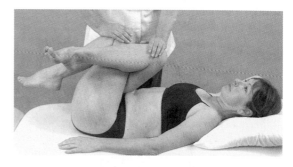

Fig. 13.43 Both hips flexed.

pain free range, constantly monitoring for improvement before progressing to the next step.

Progression through the steps is made cautiously and steadily and may take 5 or 10 minutes to achieve in the very irritable state. The end of range will not necessarily be reached before proceeding to the next step.

The technique should not aggravate the pain and the patient should be firmly and comfortably supported throughout. When applied for acute pain with high

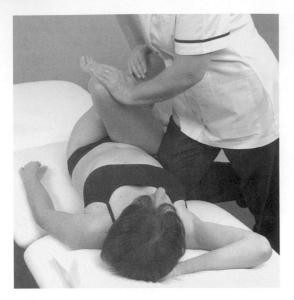

Fig. 13.44 Spine side-flexed around pivot of caudal knee placed in patient's waist.

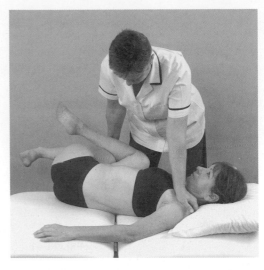

Fig. 13.46 Lowering the patient's knees by removing the thigh, to take the pelvis into rotation, stabilizing the shoulder on the couch. Taking up the slack before applying the Grade C thrust.

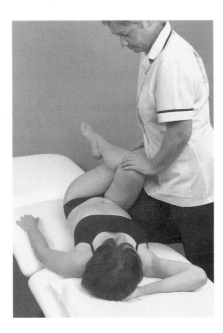

Fig. 13.45 Pelvis rotated forwards to rest patient's knees against thigh.

irritability, this is not a manipulation and any other mobilising technique from other approaches may be applied at each stage.

Extension Techniques

Extension techniques are used for central or short unilateral back pain. They may be used as first-line treatment if a patient presents with central pain or short unilateral back pain, or as a progression of the rotational techniques as the pain centralises.

Extension techniques should be avoided if hypermobility or spondylolisthesis is present.

STRAIGHT EXTENSION THRUST TECHNIQUE

(Cyriax, 1984; Cyriax and Cyriax, 1993)

This technique is indicated for central back pain.

- Position the patient in prone lying and palpate the spinous processes to locate the painful level. Place the ulnar border of your hand over the tender spinous process and reinforce it with the other hand by placing the thumb web over your fingers.
- Apply pressure directly down onto the spinous process through straight arms (Fig. 13.47).

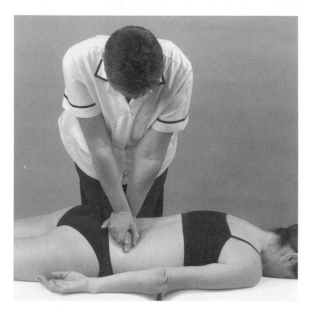

Fig. 13.47 Straight extension thrust technique.

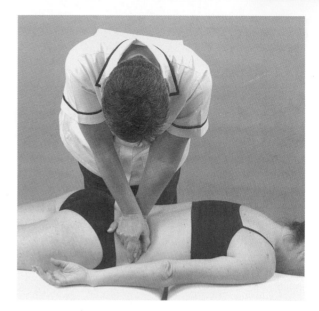

Fig. 13.48 Unilateral extension thrust technique.

- Apply a minimal amplitude, high-velocity thrust once all the slack is taken up by dropping your weight through your straight arms. This can be achieved by lifting and dropping your head down between your shoulders but be careful not to lose the end of range by lifting your hands as you raise your head.
- Reassess.

UNILATERAL EXTENSION THRUST TECHNIQUE

(Cyriax, 1984; Cyriax and Cyriax, 1993)

If the patient presents with a short unilateral back pain, or the pain centralises to a short unilateral pain, this technique may be applied.

- Position the patient in prone lying, stand on the painful side, and palpate the spinous process to locate the painful level.
- Place the ulnar border of the hand over the transverse process at the tender level on the side furthest away from you (i.e. on the painfree or less painful side). The pisiform should be adjacent to the spinous process and the pressure is applied through the paravertebral muscles for patient comfort.
- Stand close to the bed with your knees hooked onto the edge to provide support and to enable you to lean over the patient.

- Direct the pressure back towards your own knees, as you lean down onto the transverse process, through arms as straight as possible (Fig. 13.48).
- Apply a minimal amplitude, high-velocity thrust once all the slack is taken up by lifting and dropping your weight downwards and towards your knees through your straight arms. This can be achieved by lifting and dropping your head down between your shoulders but be careful not to lose the end of range by lifting your hands as you raise your head.
- Reassess.

EXTENSION TECHNIQUE WITH LEVERAGE

(Cyriax, 1984; Cyriax and Cyriax, 1993)

If the above technique fails to clear unilateral pain, this technique is stronger.

- Position the patient in prone lying and stand on the painless side.
- Position one hand flat, just above the painful level and on the painful side, adjacent to the spinous processes.
- Wrap the other hand over and under the leg on the painful side just above the knee.
- Stand close to the couch, lift the leg on the painful side into full extension of the hip and step

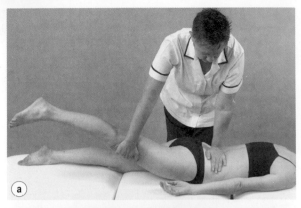

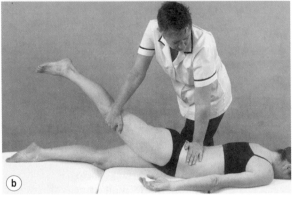

Fig. 13.49 Extension technique with leverage.

backwards to apply side flexion, gapping the painful side (Fig. 13.49a and b).

- Apply a minimal amplitude, high-velocity thrust, continuing the direction of movement, once all of the slack is taken up.
- Reassess.

Lumbar Traction

The major indication for lumbar traction is the presentation of a gradual onset of low back pain, with or without leg pain, as in Clinical Model 2, gradual onset.

The model may be established following thorough assessment of the patient with consideration of the history and the presenting signs and symptoms.

Traction may be applied to any of the presentations within Clinical Models 2 and 3 if other treatments have been unsuccessful or only partially successful, provided that there are no contraindications.

Traction has been documented as a treatment for back pain at least since the time of Hippocrates (Hume

Kendall, 1955). Cyriax himself developed his first traction bed in 1949 and collaborated with his physiotherapists on how it could be used to relieve the symptoms produced by nuclear disc herniation.

Traction's effectiveness has since been questioned by clinical trials (Clarke et al., 2007; Harte et al., 2007; Schimmel et al., 2009). However, it is still a common modality for some practitioners when treating patients with back pain and leg pain (Pellecchia, 1994; Lee et al., 2001), in addition to other treatments.

Several physiological and anatomical effects are claimed for traction therapy. There is evidence for some of these effects, but others remain theoretical and anecdotal. The possible clinical benefits of traction therapy are: to change the position of the nucleus pulposus relative to the posterior annulus fibrosus (Pellecchia, 1994; Cox et al., 1996), to change the disc-nerve interface (Knutsson et al., 2008), to increase intervertebral disc height with lumbar traction (Mathews, 1968; Colachis and Strohm, 1969; Gupta and Ramarao, 1978), to reduce disc herniation/abnormality (BenEliyahu, 1996; Neault, 1992), to reduce intradiscal pressure (Andersson et al., 1983; Sheng et al., 2002), and to stimulate mechanoreceptors (Brumagne et al., 2000; Gay et al., 2005).

Despite the views of the many practitioners who have used traction and 'found it useful' (Swezey, 1983), in these days of evidence-based practice, demands have been made for traction, as an expensive, time-consuming modality, to be stopped as a treatment, until evidence for its use can be found.

The NICE Guideline 'Low back pain and sciatica in over 16 s: assessment and management' (NICE, 2020a) states clearly under 'Manual therapies'—'Do not offer traction for managing low back pain with or without sciatica', which is hard to argue against.

Several trials over many years have failed to demonstrate unequivocal support for applying lumbar traction (Van der Heijden et al., 1995a, b; Beurskens et al., 1997; Van Tulder and Koes, 2002).

A review by Cheng et al. (2020) found that lumbar traction exhibited significantly more pain reduction and functional improvement in the short term but not in the long term. This was also the conclusion of a review and meta-analysis of mechanical traction for lumbar radiculopathy by Vanti et al. (2021), where lumbar traction was added to other physiotherapy modalities. Since many treatments are aiming to provide a window of opportunity for patients to mobilise and return to activities, the short-term effect noted could be helpful towards rehabilitation.

Providing a brief summary of how traction might work, Vanti et al. (2021) suggest that traction hypothetically evokes mechanical consequences through separation of vertebral bodies, distraction and gliding of facet joints, widening of intervertebral foramen, and straightening of spinal curves. 'Modulation of nociceptive inputs in either the ascending or descending pathways, stimulation of proprioceptive receptors, and silencing of ectopic impulse generators' have also been hypothesised.

Cyriax's (1982) hypothesis was that traction would increase the intervertebral space and produce a suction effect within the disc to draw the nuclear material centrally and away from the nerve root. At the same time, a mechanical 'push' would be given to the herniated material by tightening the ligaments spanning the bulge—the posterior longitudinal ligament in particular.

He claimed that to achieve these effects, traction would need to produce separation of the intervertebral and zygapophyseal joints between the vertebrae. To demonstrate this, he compared before and after X-rays of a patient's lumbar spine, which were superimposed upon each other after 50 kg of traction had been applied for 10 minutes, and a widening of the disc space was observed.

The separation effect was supported by Onel et al. (1989) who performed computed tomographic investigation of 30 patients diagnosed as having disc prolapse to observe the effect of traction on lumbar disc herniations. It was apparent that both intervertebral joint and zygapophyseal joint space was increased, with associated stretching of all anatomical structures of the spine.

On observing a second patient, Cyriax (1982) noted that contrast medium appeared to have been drawn into the disc spaces, implying the production of negative pressure, or suction, within the disc. Other authors found the hypothesis of the suction effect to be unfounded, however (Lee and Evans, 2001).

Lee and Evans (2001) examined loads in the lumbar spine during traction therapy and proposed that traction does not simply produce distraction of the spine but also produces a flexion moment, leading to an increase in the posterior height of the discs and a flattening of the lumbar lordosis.

This effect is enhanced using Fowler's position (hips and knees flexed to 90 degrees) and may have clinical significance in tightening the posterior annulus and the overlying posterior longitudinal ligament, theoretically reducing a confined disc prolapse and stimulating mechanoreceptors towards the relief of pain.

Lumbar flexion has been demonstrated to increase the size of the intervertebral foramina (Dolan and Adams, 2001; Punjabi et al. cited in Lee and Evans, 2001) and this would tend to support the use of traction as a treatment tool to enlarge a pathologically narrowed foramen (i.e. with symptoms of spinal stenosis).

A debate of continuous (static) versus intermittent traction developed in the 1960s, with little evidence to support either side. Cyriax proposed that intermittent traction would not be as suitable to produce nuclear movement, since repeated pulls of shorter duration would continually elicit the stretch reflex, producing muscular contraction and preventing joint distraction. His opinion, therefore, was that static traction was more effective at reducing a nuclear protrusion.

Support for sustained, as opposed to intermittent, traction could also lie in the hydrostatic behaviour of the disc (Nachemson, 1980). Sustained traction would be expected to be more effective in producing creep in the viscoelastic tissues and reducing the herniation through the proposed suction effect as well as the 'push' of the ligaments stretched across the intervertebral joints.

Grieve (1981) acknowledged the much wider range of application of traction, irrespective of the disc, suggesting that it could be a useful method of mobilisation of the motion segment, or segments, as a whole.

In the musculoskeletal approach, the selection of appropriate patients for the application of treatment techniques is important. As described at the beginning of this section, if traction is to be used, then it can be considered as an option for patients predominantly falling into Clinical Models 2 and 3 although it could also have a role in treating more persistent back pain (Tanabe et al., 2021).

Since the previous edition of our textbook, intervertebral differential dynamics (IDD) Therapy has become more widespread, alleging to have been developed to decompress intervertebral discs, improve mobility and relieve pain. That sounds uncannily like traction and perhaps we have come full circle.

Contraindications to Lumbar Traction

(See general contraindications page 469.)

- Suspicion of cauda equina symptoms is an absolute contraindication and urgent onward referral is required.
- Absence of consent
- Patients with acute back pain or sciatica, usually associated with twinges and antalgic postures. The application of traction may be quite comfortable but as the traction is released the patient will be far worse and the pain and twinges will be agonising. It may take some hours for the pain to subside sufficiently to allow the patient to get up and the whole experience is awful for both patient and practitioner alike. With patients with less irritable back pain, symptoms are often eased as traction is applied, but be particularly cautious if the history, signs and symptoms reveal an acute situation and the pain is completely relieved by traction.
- Patients with severe cardiac or respiratory problems may not be able to tolerate either the straps or the supine-lying position. A bad cough also contraindicates treatment since the pain could be made much worse.
- Patients with claustrophobia or other psychological disorders may become anxious or experience panic while undergoing traction, although such patients do not usually give consent to its application in the first place.
- Inflammatory conditions affecting the spine are likely to be aggravated by traction.

While not absolute contraindications, there are instances where caution is required, or the technique is unlikely to be successful:

- The pain of disc protrusions with neurological deficit is unlikely to be relieved by traction since the protrusion is too large to be reduced. Manipulation is less likely still to be effective and if the sciatica is acute or severe, a stepped approach is taken with pain management, education and advice, neuropathic medication, injections or surgery, if all other measures have failed.
- Leg pain that has lasted for more than 6 months is unlikely to respond to traction. The patient may be advised to await spontaneous recovery, to try pain management or to seek a surgical opinion, according to the severity of the symptoms and the patient's choice.
- Care is needed with hypermobility.

LUMBAR MECHANICAL TRACTION TECHNIQUE

The selection of patients suitable for mobilisation techniques, including traction, is essential and they should always be part of a package of care derived from shared decision-making and within the context of a stepped approach.

Friction-free electrically operated traction beds have been designed which are usually used in conjunction with electronically operated units that supply options for either rhythmical (intermittent) or static, continuous traction (Fig. 13.50).

Far less sophisticated apparatus may be used that is just as effective, but adjustments may then be needed to calculate the distracting force applied, on the basis of overcoming the frictional forces created between the patient and the couch.

A thoracic and a pelvic harness are attached to either end of a couch and applied to the patient (Fig. 13.51).

Harnesses of modern design are usually comfortable and easy to readjust since they have Velcro® fastenings. A simple device is required for taking up the slack and applying a continuous pull through the pelvic belt, so providing traction to the intervening lumbar spine.

The principle of application is that the pull should be 'as strong as is comfortable'. In the early stages this was the only guideline provided and there was no way of knowing the exact weight being applied. A spring balance was then introduced in series with the pelvic rope, which gave some indication of weight.

Judovitch and Nobel (1957) calculated that a force of $1/2 \times 0.5 = 1/4$ of the patient's body weight is required to overcome the friction between the body and the couch before the distracting force is applied to the spine. This will need to be considered when calculating the weight to apply when using a standard couch. When using a friction-free couch, the weight registering on the accompanying machine is relatively faithful to the actual weight being applied.

Feedback from the patient is important, as mentioned. However, an approximate estimate of the appropriate weight to apply may be made by assessing the size and weight of the patient and, based on clinical experience, the application of one-third of the patient's body weight on a friction-free couch is a suitable starting point.

Before treatment, a thorough explanation should be given to the patient of the reasons for applying the

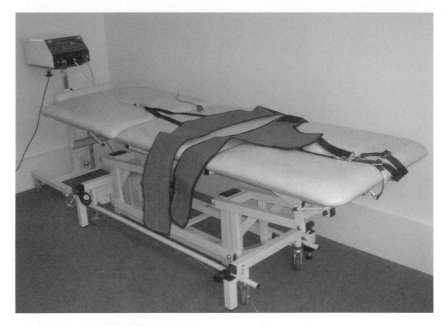

Fig. 13.50 Lumbar traction couch.

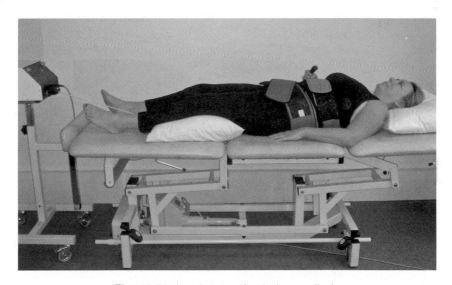

Fig. 13.51 Lumbar traction being applied.

technique and the likely outcome, including any possible adverse effects such as stiffness or increased proximal pain. Consent should then be gained.

A comparable sign should be tested, such as the SLR or lumbar movement(s) in standing, for subsequent comparison.

The patient does not need to be completely undressed for traction. Light clothing may be worn, being careful to remove belts, buckles, car keys, etc., and ensuring that clothing can separate in the middle.

Some practitioners prefer to fix the harnesses to the patient while the patient is standing but many fix the harnesses to the bed and then ask the patient to lie down onto them. The patient is instructed to lie down sideways on the couch before rolling into supine lying.

If using a friction-free couch, ensure that the sliding lumbar section of the table is locked in its fixed position while the harnesses are being applied. The lumbar spine segment being treated should initially be placed over the division in the table.

The usual starting position is in supine lying but the number of pillows under the head and knees may be adjusted for comfort. As the knees are lifted, so the lumbar lordosis will flatten and a stool may be used to achieve Fowler's position (hips and knees flexed to 90 degrees), if the patient is more comfortable with the spine completely flat.

Other positions such as prone lying may be tried if the patient is more comfortable in lumbar extension. Theoretically there are eight combinations of straps varying the patient's position between supine and prone, and choosing to place each of the thoracic and pelvic straps either underneath or on top of the patient.

In practice, however, lying supine or prone, with the straps underneath the patient in both instances, are the two most popular and comfortable positions.

The thoracic belt should be tight enough to grip the chest to prevent it from sliding up towards the axillae, which is very uncomfortable. However, the grip should not be so tight as to restrict breathing, although patients will tend to find that they employ apical breathing more than diaphragmatic breathing while the traction is being applied.

The pelvic harness should sit comfortably above or around the iliac crests where it can pull down on the pelvis, as the traction is applied, but without slipping. The pelvic harness should not be so tight as to compress the abdomen uncomfortably and patients should be warned not to have a large meal before treatment.

The slack is then taken up in the pelvic rope to apply tension to the system.

At the first treatment, 20 minutes of traction is usually sufficient and provides enough time to be effective but not enough to overtreat, causing after-treatment stiffness or soreness. Feedback is encouraged from patients throughout treatment, and it is essential to know if they become uncomfortable or if there is a marked increase in their pain.

Simple adjustments can be made to lessen discomfort from the straps or to reduce the traction as necessary. The patient should always be supplied with a means of summoning help such as a bell or buzzer.

> **CLINICAL TIP**
>
> For lumbar mechanical traction, suggested starting weight is approximately one-third of the patient's body weight on a friction-free couch and for 20–30 min. Start with lower weight and time and progress according to patient response.

In subsequent treatments the time may be increased to 30 minutes. These timings are suggested on an empirical basis and little research has been done on this. Often the time allocated for treatment sessions in the appointment system is the limiting factor.

After treatment, the traction should be released steadily and slowly. The traction belts are then released and patients are encouraged to wriggle for a minute or two. They can bend their knees, and roll onto their side, but should be discouraged from sitting up until the residual stiffness following the application of traction has eased.

When ready, patients should be asked to turn onto their side, and to push themselves up sideways to avoid straining the back. Some patients need to sit for a moment or two until any dizziness or light-headedness arising from postural hypotension has subsided. Patients should be advised to avoid bending while dressing.

The daily treatment originally suggested by Cyriax (1982) has become impractical for most clinical situations and 'as often as possible' would probably be a better aim for current practice.

In the authors' clinical experience, it is still worth applying traction, even if that is once or twice a week. Improvement should become apparent after three or four treatments and if no improvement is evident, modification of the traction position may be made before stopping the modality altogether.

Patients should be given advice on exercise and activity modification, as well as addressing lifestyle factors towards rehabilitation and prevention of recurrence.

Lumbar Injections
Caudal Epidural Injections

In 1901, Sicard introduced local anaesthetic into the epidural space and this technique continued, with the addition of corticosteroid in the 1950s, as a treatment for discogenic sciatica (Dilke et al., 1973; Bush and Hillier, 1991; Bush, 1994). It was reported as a well-tolerated procedure with a high patient satisfaction rate and relatively few side effects.

In 2018 the UK National Health Service proposed to withdraw funding for injections for non-specific low back pain without sciatica due to the lack of supporting evidence (Wang et al., 2021). The NICE Guideline for 'Low back pain and sciatica in over 16 s: assessment and management' (NICE, 2020a) also recommends that spinal injections should not be used for managing low back pain, except for acute or severe sciatic and as part of a stepped approach to management.

Notwithstanding, in light of this being a 'recommendation', we have decided to retain this section, on the basis of possible emerging evidence and changing policy.

Indications for Epidural Injection

- Radicular pain, with or without neurological deficit, which has failed to respond to conservative management during the first 6 to 12 weeks from onset
- As a trial to treat pain before surgical intervention is considered

Several authors have proposed that there is evidence that epidural injection achieves relief for persistent low back pain and radicular pain, at least in the short term (Bush and Hillier, 1991; Boswell, 2007; Dincer et al., 2007; Manchikanti et al., 2008a,b,c,d; Conn et al., 2009). The experience of the clinician performing the injection could be a factor in determining outcome (Dincer et al., 2007).

Cyriax (1984) and Cyriax and Cyriax (1993), advocated the use of local anaesthetic alone and the advantage of adding steroid is not clear. Huntoon and Burgher (2008) supported the use of epidural anaesthesia prior to surgery, as the option with less risk, but they also challenged the addition of steroid, urging a return to an 'earlier time' before the addition of steroid.

Manchikanti et al. (2011) compared the injection of local anaesthetic alone with local anaesthetic and steroid with 120 patients randomised to the two groups. In both groups there was significant improvement at 3-, 6- and 12-month follow-up but the patients who had steroid included showed longer relief and required fewer epidurals overall.

The mechanism by which caudal epidural produces the improvement in pain relief is still debated and several hypotheses exist (Bush and Hillier, 1991; Dincer et al., 2007). Disc material can exert a mechanical effect through compression, a chemical effect through inflammation and an ischaemic effect through oedema.

Introducing corticosteroid into the epidural space may directly affect the chemical and indirectly the ischaemic effects of pain. The introduction of fluid into a fluid-filled space can mechanically affect the relationship between the disc and the nerve root, while the introduction of local anaesthetic may have sufficient short-term effects to break the pain cycle.

Epidural injection via the caudal route can be carried out as an outpatient procedure under image guidance. It is recommended that the procedure should only be conducted by an experienced medical practitioner, after appropriate training.

Once through the sacrococcygeal ligament, the sacral hiatus connects directly to the epidural space (Dincer et al., 2007). The injection involves the introduction of 40 to 80 mg triamcinolone acetonide in 20 to 30 mL of 0.5% procaine hydrochloride via the sacral hiatus using a no-touch technique, with observation of blood or cerebrospinal fluid backflow (Figs 13.52 and 13.53) (Bush, 1994).

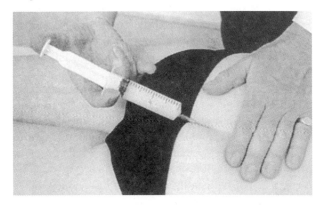

Fig. 13.52 Caudal epidural injection.

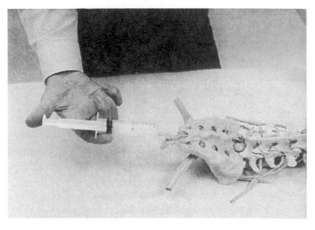

Fig. 13.53 Caudal epidural injection, showing direction of approach and needle position.

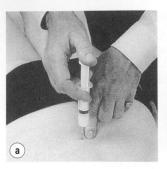 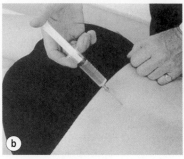 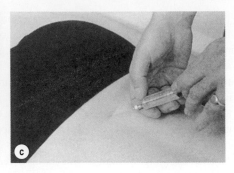

Fig. 13.54 Prolotherapy injection, indicating needle placement to pepper the lumbosacral and sacroiliac ligaments.

The patient is traditionally placed prone to facilitate access to the sacral hiatus, but Makki et al. (2010) concluded that although the reported efficacy of epidural injections via the caudal route remains variable, turning the patient onto the side of their leg pain for at least 15 minutes after the injection enhances pain relief, regardless of the pathology causing the leg pain.

Prolotherapy

Prolotherapy (sclerosant therapy) is used to treat spinal instability and persistent pain (see Chapter 4). It involves the injection of a chemical irritant into the ligaments surrounding an unstable spinal or sacroiliac segment.

The chemical irritant produces an inflammatory response, causing fibroblast hyperplasia and subsequent increase in strength of the supporting ligaments (Ongley et al., 1987).

The patient undergoes manipulation first to ensure that a full range of movement is achievable.

An injection used to be given of a solution called P2G comprising phenol, dextrose and glycerine but these days most practitioners use hypertonic dextrose. Each osseoligamentous junction is infiltrated using a peppering technique (Fig. 13.54a–c).

Injections are given at weekly intervals with a maximum of three or four injections. The patient is instructed to avoid flexion to allow the ligamentous tissue to contract sufficiently to stabilise the joints.

Musculoskeletal medicine courses include the principles of prolotherapy, but a period of supervised clinical practice is recommended.

REVIEW QUESTIONS

1. Which questions in the history are used to rule out suspicion of cauda equina syndrome?
2. What are the differences between Clinical Models 2 and 3?
3. Manipulation is the treatment of choice for Clinical Model 2. However, the presentation needs to be subacute. Explain what subacute means.
4. What is the significance of a crossed SLR?
5. Discuss the contraindications to manipulation and why they are contraindications?

CASE SCENARIOS

Case 1

History

- Alex, a 44-year-old bus driver, had a sudden onset of right-sided low back pain last week whilst digging his bus out of a snow drift. He has no neurological symptoms and describes his pain as intermittent and an ache. His pain is aggravated by sitting, bending and lifting. Pain is slowly resolving and he is currently not working. He has no previous history of low back pain.

Examination

- Hip and sacroiliac (SI) joint tests are all negative. Lumbar flexion and left side flexion are limited by pain, and his right straight leg raise (SLR) limited by 20 degrees. He is tender on palpation to the right of L4–L5.

Task
- Which clinical model is this? What would the appropriate treatment be if the visual analogue scale (VAS) was 3/10 compared to that of VAS 8/10? Review the contraindications to lumbar manipulation.

Case 2
History
- Housewife and mother Louise, age 35, has a gradual onset of central and left-sided low back pain that she associates with lifting her toddler twins. It started 2 months ago and is gradually getting worse. Pain is worse with lifting and bending. Intermittently she feels pain down into her left buttock. There are no neurological symptoms. She has a medical history of gestational diabetes.

Examination
- She has limited and painful lumbar flexion and limited left-side flexion. The left SLR reproduces low back pain but is full range. There are full hip movements and negative findings on stressing the sacroiliac ligaments.

Task
- Which clinical model is this and what are the treatment options?

Case 3
History
- Jemma, 16 years old, has a 2-month history of worsening central low back pain. It started for no particular reason except she had been unwell with the flu and the pain persisted. The pain is fairly constant and is disturbing her sleep and she is unable to sit for longer than 10 min at a time. Pain is worsening over time, and she is now staying home from school.

Examination
- Good lumbar range of movement not affecting pain. Hip and SI joint testing negative. Bilateral SLR limited and brisk lower limb reflexes in general.

Task
- Are there any red or yellow flags for this girl? What would your management be for this patient?

REFERENCES

Adams, M.A., Hutton, W.C., 1983. The effect of posture on the fluid content of lumbar intervertebral discs. Spine 8, 665–671.

Adams, M.A., Hutton, W.C., 1986. The effect of posture on diffusion into lumbar intervertebral discs. J. Anat. 147, 121–134.

Adams, M., Bogduk, N., Burton, K., et al., 2012. The Biomechanics of Back Pain. Churchill Livingstone, Edinburgh.

Albert, H.B., Lambert, P., Rollason, J., et al., 2013. Does nuclear tissue infected with bacteria following disc herniations lead to Modic changes in the adjacent vertebra? Eur. Spine J. 22, 690–696.

Almeida, M., Saragiotto, B., Richards, B., et al., 2018. Primary care management of non-specifc low back pain: key messages from recent clinical guidelines. Med. J. Aust. 208 (6), 272–275.

Andersson, G.B., Schultz, A.B., Nachemson, A.L., 1983. Intervertebral disc pressures during traction. Scand. J. Rehabil. Med. Suppl. 9, 88–91.

Atkins, E., Kerr, J., Goodlad, E., 2013. The Cyriax approach. In: Chevan, J., Clapis, P. (Eds.), Physical Therapy Management of Low Back Pain: A Case-Based Approach. Jones & Bartlett, Burlington.

Bagley, C., MacAllister, M., Dosselman, L., et al., 2019. Current concepts and recent advances in understanding and managing lumbar spine stenosis. F1000Res, 8. F1000, Faculty Rev-137

BenEliyahu, D.J., 1996. Magnetic resonance imaging and clinical follow-up: study of 27 patients receiving chiropractic care for cervical and lumbar disc herniations. J. Manipulative Physiol. Ther. 19, 597–606.

Benoist, M., 2002. The natural history of lumbar disc herniation and radiculopathy. Joint Bone Spine 69 (2), 155–160.

Betten, C., Sandell, C., Hill, J.C., et al., 2015. Cross-cultural adaptation and validation of the Swedish STarT Back Screening Tool. Eur. J. Physiother. 17 (1), 29–36.

Beurskins, S.A.J., de Vet, H.C., Köke, A.J., et al., 1997. Efficacy of traction for nonspecific low back pain: 12-week and 6-month results of a randomized clinical trial. Spine 22 (23), 2756–2762.

Bogduk, N., 1991. The lumbar disc and low back pain. Neurosurg. Clin. N. Am. 2, 791–806.

Bogduk, N., 2023. Clinical and Radiological Anatomy of the Lumbar Spine, sixth ed. Churchill Livingstone, Edinburgh.

Boswell, M., Trescot, A., Datta, S., et al., 2007. Interventional techniques: evidence-based practice guidelines in the management of chronic spinal pain. Pain Physician 10, 7–111.

Brukner, P., Clarson, B., Cook, J., et al., 2017. Clinical Sports Medicine, Volume 1: Injuries, fifth ed. McGraw-Hill, Sydney.

Brumagne, S., Cordo, P., Lysens, R., et al., 2000. The role of paraspinal muscle spindles in lumbosacral position sense in individuals with and without low back pain. Spine 25, 989–994.

Buckwalter, J.A., 1995. Aging and degeneration of the human intervertebral disc. Spine 20, 1307–1314.

Bush, K., 1994. Lower back pain and sciatica—how best to manage them. Br. J. Hosp. Med. 51, 216–222.

Bush, K., Hillier, S., 1991. A controlled study of caudal epidural injections of triamcinolone plus procaine for the management of intractable sciatica. Spine 16, 572–575.

Caplan, L.R., 1994. Management of patients with lumbar disc herniations with radiculopathy. Eur. Neurol. 34, 114–119.

Cavanaugh, J.M., Kallakuri, S., Ozaktay, A.C., 1995. Innervation of the rabbit lumbar intervertebral disc and posterior longitudinal ligament. Spine 20, 2080–2085.

Cheng, Y.H., Hsu, C.Y., Lin, Y.N., 2020. The effect of mechanical traction on low back pain in patients with herniated intervertebral disks: a systemic review and meta-analysis. Clin. Rehabil. 34 (1), 13–22.

Clarke, J.A., van Tulder, M.W., Blomberg, S.E., et al., 2007. Traction for low back pain with or without sciatica. Cochrane Database Systematic Rev. 2007 (2), CD003010.

Colachis, S.C., Strohm, B.R., 1969. Effects of intermittent traction on separation of lumbar vertebrae. Arch. Phys. Med. Rehabil. 50, 251–258.

Conn, A., Buenaventura, R.M., Datta, S., et al., 2009. Systematic review of caudal epidural injections in the management of chronic low back pain. Pain Physician 12, 109–135.

Coppes, M., Enrico, M., Ralph, T., et al., 1997. Innervation of 'painful' lumbar discs. Spine 22 (20), 2342–2349.

Cox, J.M., Feller, J., Cox-Cid, J., 1996. Distraction chiropractic adjusting: clinical application and outcomes of 1,000 cases. Top. Clin. Chiropr. 3, 45–59.

Cyriax, J., 1982. Textbook of Orthopaedic Medicine, eighth ed. Baillière Tindall, London.

Cyriax, J., 1984. Textbook of Orthopaedic Medicine, eleventh ed. Baillière Tindall, London.

Cyriax, J., Cyriax, P., 1993. Cyriax's Illustrated Manual of Orthopaedic Medicine. Butterworth Heinemann, Oxford.

Deyo, R.A., 2007. Back surgery—who needs it. N. Engl. J. Med. 356 (22), 2239–2243.

Dilke, T.W.F., Burry, H.C., Grahame, R., 1973. Extradural corticosteroid injection in management of lumbar nerve root compression. Br. Med. J. 2, 635–637.

Dincer, U., Kirap, M., Caker, E., et al., 2007. Caudal epidural injection versus non-steroidal anti-inflammatory drugs in the treatment of low back pain accompanied by radicular pain. Joint Bone Spine 74, 467–471.

Dinning, T.A.R., Schaeffer, H.R., 1993. Discogenic compression of the cauda equina—a surgical emergency. Aust. N. Z. J. Surg. 63, 927–934.

Dolan, P., Adams, M.A., 2001. Recent advances in lumbar spinal mechanics and their significance for modelling. Clin. Biomech. 16 (Suppl. 1), S8–S16.

Downie, A., Williams, C.M., Henschke, N., et al., 2013. Red flags to screen for malignancy and fractures in patients with low back pain: a systematic review. Br. Med. J. 347, f7095.

Ebell, M., 2009. Predicting benefit of spinal manipulation for low back pain. Am. Fam. Physician 79 (4), 318–319.

Edgar, M.A., 2007. The nerve supply of the lumbar intervertebral disc. J. Bone Joint Surg. 89-B (9), 1135–1139.

Feather, A., Randall, D., Waterhouse, M., 2020. Kumar and Clark's Clinical Medicine, tenth ed. Elsevier, London.

Findlay, G.F.G., 1992. Tumours of the lumbar spine. In: Jayson, M. (Ed.), The Lumbar Spine and Back Pain, fourth ed. Churchill Livingstone, Edinburgh, pp. 355–369.

Finucane, L.M., Downie, A., Mercer, C., et al., 2020a. International Framework for Red Flags for Potential Serious Spinal Pathologies. J. Orthop. Sports Phys. Ther. 50 (7), 350–372.

Finucane, L., Cumming, D., Griffiths, B., et al., 2020b. Guidance to recognise serious pathology as a cause of musculoskeletal symptoms requiring urgent or emergency referral to secondary care. NHS England. https://www.england.nhs.uk/south/wp-content/uploads/sites/6/2020/03/serious-pathology-msk-guidance-v1.5.pdf. Accessed 6 September 2021.

Foster, N.E., Anema, J.R., Cherkin, D., et al., 2018. Prevention and treatment of low back pain: evidence, challenges, and promising directions. Lancet 391 (10137), 2368–2383.

Friedman, B.W., Chilstrom, M., Bijur, P.E., et al., 2010. Diagnostic testing and treatment of low back pain in United States emergency departments: a national perspective. Spine 35 (24), E1406–E1411.

Gagnet, P., Kern, K., Andrews, K., et al., 2018. Spondylolysis and spondylolisthesis: A review of the literature. J. Orthop. 15 (2), 404–407.

Gardner, A., Gardner, E., Morley, T., 2011. Cauda equina syndrome: a review of the current clinical and medico-legal position. Eur. Spine J. 20 (5), 690–697.

Gatchel, R.J., Gardea, M.A., 1999. Psychosocial issues: their importance in predicting disability, response to treatment, and search for compensation. Neurol. Clin. 17 (1), 149–166.

Gay, R.E., Bronfort, G., Evans, R.L., 2005. Distraction manipulation of the lumbar spine: a review of the literature. J. Manipulative Physiol. Ther. 28 (4), 266–273.

Greenhalgh, S., Selfe, J., 2010. Red Flags II: A guide to solving serious pathology of the spine. Elsevier, Edinburgh.

Grieve, G.P., 1981. Common Vertebral Joint Problems. Churchill Livingstone, Edinburgh.

Gupta, R.C., Ramarao, S.V., 1978. Epidurography in reduction of lumbar disc prolapse by traction. Arch. Phys. Med. Rehabil. 59, 322–327.

Harte, A.A., Baxter, G.D., Gracey, J.H., 2007. The effectiveness of motorised lumbar traction in the management of LBP with lumbo sacral nerve root involvement: a feasibility study. BMC Musculoskelet. Dis. 8 (1), 1–12.

Hartley, A., 1995. Practical Joint Assessment: Lower Quadrant, second ed. Mosby, London.1–88.

Hartvigsen, J., Hancock, M.J., Kongsted, A., et al., 2018. What low back pain is and why we need to pay attention. Lancet 391 (10137), 2356–2367.

Henschke, N., Maher, C.G., Refshauge, K.M., et al., 2008. Prognosis in patients with recent onset low back pain in Australian primary care: inception cohort study. Br. Med. J. 337 (7662), a171.

Hill, J.C., Dunn, K.M., Lewis, M., et al., 2008. A primary care back pain screening tool: identifying patient subgroups for initial treatment. Arthritis Rheum. 59 (5), 632–641.

Hill, J.C., Dunn, K.M., Main, C.J., et al., 2010. Subgrouping low back pain: a comparison of the STarT Back Tool with the Orebro Musculoskeletal Pain Screening Questionnaire. Eur J. Pain 14 (1), 83–89.

Hill, J.C., Whitehurst, D.G.T., Lewis, M., et al., 2011. Comparison of stratified primary care management for low back pain with current best practice (STarT Back): a randomised controlled trial. Lancet 378 (9802), 1560–1571.

Hoppenfeld, S., 1976. Physical Examination of the Spine and Extremities. Appleton Century Crofts, Philadelphia, PA.

Hume Kendall, P., 1955. A history of lumbar traction. Physiotherapy 41, 177–179.

Huntoon, M.A., Burgher, A.H., 2008. Back to the future: the end of the steroid century? Pain Physician 11, 713–716.

Jalloh, I., Minhas, P., 2007. Delays in the treatment of cauda equine syndrome due to its variable clinical features in patients presenting to the emergency department. Emerg. Med. J. 24 (1), 33–34.

Jaumard, N.V., Welch, W.C., 2011. Spinal facet joint biomechanics and mechanotransduction in normal, injury and degenerative conditions. J. Biomech. Eng. 133 (7), 071010.

Jensen, G.M., 1980. Biomechanics of the lumbar intervertebral disc: a review. Phys. Ther. 60, 765–773.

Jensen, M.C., Brant-Zawadzki, M.N., Obuchowski, N., et al., 1994. Magnetic resonance imaging of the lumbar spine in people without back pain. N. Eng. J. Med. 331 (2), 69–73.

Jensen, R.K., Jensen, T.S., Koes, B., et al., 2020. Prevalence of lumbar spinal stenosis in general and clinical populations: a systematic review and meta-analysis. Eur. Spine J. 29 (9), 2143–2163.

Jensen, R.K., Harhangi, B.S., Huygen, F., et al., 2021. Lumbar spinal stenosis. Br. Med. J. 373, n1581.

Jönsson, B., Strömqvist, B., 1995. The straight leg raising test and the severity of symptoms in lumbar disc herniation. Spine 20 (1), 27–30.

Judovitch, B., Nobel, G.R., 1957. Traction therapy, a study of resistance forces. Am. J. Surg. 93, 108–114.

Kalichman, L., Kim, D.H., Li, L., Guermazi, A., et al., 2009. Spondylolysis and spondylolisthesis: prevalence and association with low back pain in the adult community-based population. Spine 15, 34 (2), 199–205.

Karbowski, K., Dvorak, J., 1995. Historical perspective: description of variations of the sciatic stretch phenomenon. Spine 20 (13), 1525–1527.

Kemp, H.B.S., Worland, J., 1974. Infections of the spine. Physiotherapy 60, 2–6.

Kesikburun, B., Eksioglu, E., Turan, A., et al., 2019. Spontaneous regression of extruded lumbar disc herniation: Correlation with clinical outcome. Pak. J. Med. Sci. 35 (4), 974–980.

Khuffash, B., Porter, R.W., 1989. Cross leg pain and trunk list. Spine 14, 602–603.

Knezevic, N.N., Candido, K.D., Vlaeyen, J.W.S., et al., 2021. Low back pain. Lancet 398 (10295), 78–92.

Knutsson, E., Skoglund, C.R., Natchev, E., 2008. Changes in voluntary muscle strength, somatosensory transmission and skin temperature R.E. Gay and J.S. Brault. Spine J., 234–242.

Koes, B., van Tulder, M., Peul, W., 2007. Diagnosis and treatment of sciatica. Br. Med. J. 334 (7607), 1313–1317.

Korse, N.S., Jacobs, W.C.H., Elzevier, H.W., et al., 2013. Complaints of micturition, defecation and sexual function in cauda equina syndrome due to lumbar disc herniation: a systematic review. Eur. Spine J. 22 (5), 1019–1029.

Laslett, M., van Wijmen, P., 1999. Low back and referred pain: diagnosis and a proposed new system of classification. N. Z. J. Physiother. 27, 5–14.

Lee, H.-M., Kim, N.-H., Kim, H.-J., et al., 1995. Morphometric study of the lumbar spinal canal in the Korean population. Spine 20 (15), 1679–1684.

Lee, R.Y.W., Evans, J.H., 2001. Loads in the lumbar spine during traction therapy. Aust. J. Physiother. 47, 102–108.

Legrand, E., Bouvard, B., Audran, M., et al., 2007. Sciatica from disk herniation: medical treatment or surgery? Joint Bone Spine 74 (6), 530–535.

Lisi, A., 2006. Chiropractic spinal manipulation for low back pain of pregnancy: a retrospective case series. J. Midwifery Women's Health 51 (910), 7–10.

McAllister, K., Goodson, N., Warburton, L., et al., 2017. Spondyloarthritis: diagnosis and management: summary of NICE guidance. Br. Med. J. 356, j839.

McCarthy, C.J., Arnell, F.A., Strimpakos, N., 2004. The bio-psycho-social classification of non-specific low back pain: a systematic review. Phys. Ther. Rev. 9, 17–30.

McKenzie, R.A., 1981. The Lumbar Spine: Mechanical Diagnosis and Therapy. Spinal Publications, Waikanae, New Zealand.

Magnussen, L.H., Lygren, H., Anderson, B., et al., 2010. Validation of the Norwegian version of Hannover Functional Ability Questionnaire. Spine 35 (14), E646–E653.

Makki, D., Nawabi, D.H., Francis, R., et al., 2010. Is the outcome of caudal epidural injections affected by patient positioning? Spine 35 (15), 687–690.

Manchikanti, L., Cash, K.A., McManus, C.D., et al., 2008a. Preliminary results of a randomized, equivalence trial of fluoroscopic caudal epidural injections in managing chronic low back pain: Part 1—Discogenic pain without disc herniation or radiculitis. Pain Physician 11, 785–800.

Manchikanti, L., Singh, V., Cash, K.A., et al., 2008b. Preliminary results of a randomized, equivalence trial of fluoroscopic caudal epidural injections in managing chronic low back pain: Part 2—Disc herniation and radiculitis. Pain Physician 11 (6), 801–815.

Manchikanti, L., Singh, V., Cash, K.A., et al., 2008c. Preliminary results of a randomized, equivalence trial of fluoroscopic caudal epidural injections in managing chronic low back pain: Part 3—Post surgery syndrome. Pain Physician 11 (6), 817–831.

Manchikanti, L., Cash, K.A., McManus, C.D., et al., 2008d. Preliminary results of a randomized, equivalence trial of fluoroscopic caudal epidural injections in managing chronic low back pain: Part 4—Spinal stenosis. Pain Physician 11 (6), 833–848.

Manchikanti, L., Singh, V., Falco, F.J., et al., 2010. Evaluation of lumbar facet joint nerve blocks in managing chronic low back pain: a randomized, double-blind, controlled trial with a 2-year follow-up. Int. J. Med. Sci. 7, 124e35.

Manchikanti, L., Singh, V., Cash, K.A., et al., 2011. A randomized, controlled, double-blind trial of fluoroscopic caudal epidural injections in the treatment of lumbar disc herniation and radiculitis. Spine 36 (23), 1897–1905.

Marchand, F., Ahmed, A.M., 1990. Investigation of the laminate structure of the lumbar disc annulus fibrosus. Spine 15 (5), 402–410.

Mathews, J.A., 1968. Dynamic discography: a study of lumbar traction. Ann. Phys. Med. 9 (7), 275–279.

Messiah, S., Tharian, A.R., Candido, K.D., et al., 2019. Neurogenic claudication: a review of current understanding and treatment options. Curr. Pain Headache Rep. 23 (5), 32.

Middleditch, A., Oliver, J., 2005. Functional Anatomy of the Spine, second ed. Butterworth Heinemann, Edinburgh.

Munakomi, S., Kumar, B.M., 2016. Wasting of extensor digitorum brevis as a decisive preoperative clinical indicator of lumbar canal stenosis: A single-center prospective cohort study. Ann. Med. Health Sci. Res. 6 (5), 296–300.

Munakomi, S., Foris, L.A., Varacallo, M., 2021. Spinal stenosis and neurogenic claudication. StatPearls Publishing. https://www.statpearls.com/ArticleLibrary/viewarticle/29357. Accessed 6 September 2021.

Nachemson, A., 1966. The load on the lumbar discs in different positions of the body. Clin. Orthop. 45, 107–122.

Nachemson, A., 1980. Lumbar intradiscal pressure. In: Jayson, M.I.V. (Ed.), The Lumbar Spine and Back Pain, second ed. Pitman, London, pp. 341–358.

Nadler, S.F., Malanga, G.A., Stitik, T.P., et al., 2001. The crossed femoral nerve stretch to improve diagnostic sensitivity for the high lumbar radiculopathy: 2 case reports. Arch. Phys. Med. Rehabil. 82 (4), 522–523.

National Institute for Health and Care Excellence (NICE). 2020a. Low back pain and sciatica in over 16s: assessment and management. NICE. https://www.nice.org.uk/guidance/ng59. Accessed 4 September 2021.

National Institute for Health and Care Excellence (NICE). 2020b. Osteoarthritis: care and management. NICE. https://www.nice.org.uk/guidance/cg177. Accessed 4 September 2021.

National Institute for Health and Care Excellence (NICE). 2020c. Rheumatoid arthritis. NICE. https://cks.nice.org.uk/topics/rheumatoid-arthritis/. Accessed 6 September 2021.

National Institute for Health and Care Excellence (NICE). 2020d. Neuropathic pain in adults: pharmacological management in non-specialist settings. https://www.nice.org.uk/guidance/cg173/chapter/Introduction. Accessed 21 April 2022.

National Spine Network (NSN). 2017. National low back and radicular pain pathway. https://nationalspinenetwork.co.uk/National-Back-Pain-and-Radicular-Pain-Pathway. Accessed 21 April 2022.

Neault, C.C., 1992. Conservative management of an L4–L5 left nuclear disk prolapse with a sequestrated segment. J. Manipulative Physiol. Ther. 15 (5), 318–322.

Norris, C.M., 2004. Sports Injuries: Diagnosis and Management for Physiotherapists, third ed. Butterworth Heinemann, Oxford.

Oliver, M.J., Twomey, L.T., 1995. Extension creep in the lumbar spine. Clin. Biomech. 10, 363–368.

Onel, D., Tuzlaci, M., Sari, H., et al., 1989. Computed tomographic investigation of the effect of traction on lumbar disc herniations. Spine 14 (1), 82–90.

Ongley, M.J., Klein, R.G., Dorman, T.A., et al., 1987. A new approach to the treatment of chronic low back pain. Lancet 2 (8551), 143–146.

Osti, O.L., Cullum, D.E., 1994. Occupational low back pain and intervertebral disc degeneration—epidemiology, imaging and pathology. Clin. J. Pain 10 (4), 331–334.

Paesold, G., Nerlich, A., Boos, N., 2007. Biological treatment strategies for disc degeneration: potentials and shortcomings. Eur. Spine J. 16 (4), 447–468.

Parke, W.W., Schiff, D.C.M., 1971. The applied anatomy of the intervertebral disc. Orthop. Clin. N. Am. 2 (2), 309–324.

Parreira, P., Maher, C.G., Steffens, D., et al., 2018. Risk factors for low back pain and sciatica: an umbrella view. Spine J. 18 (9), 1715–1721.

Pengel, L.H., Herbert, R.D., Maher, C.G., et al., 2003. Acute low back pain: systematic review of its prognosis. Br. Med. J. 327 (7410), 323.

Pellecchia, G.L., 1994. Lumbar traction: a review of the literature. J. Orthop. Sports Phys. Ther. 20 (5), 262–267.

Pincus, T., Burton, A.K., Vogel, S., et al., 2002. A systematic review of psychological factors as predictors of chronicity/disability in prospective cohorts of low back pain. Spine 27 (5), E109–E120.

Porter, R.W., 1992. Spinal stenosis of the central and root canal. In: Jayson, M. (Ed.), The Lumbar Spine and Back Pain, fourth ed. Churchill Livingstone, Edinburgh, pp. 313–332.

Porter, R.W., 1995. Pathology of symptomatic lumbar disc protrusion. J. R. Coll. Surg. Edinb. 40 (3), 200–202.

Ramond, A., Bouton, C., Richard, I., et al., 2011. Psychosocial risk factors for chronic low back pain in primary care—a systematic review. Fam. Pract. 28 (1), 12–21.

Riddle, D.L., 1998. Classification and low back pain: a review of the literature and critical analysis of selected systems. Phys. Ther. 78 (7), 708–737.

Robson, P., 2014. Metastatic spinal cord compression. Clin. Med. (Lond.) 14 (5), 542–545.

Rydevik, B., Olmarker, K., 1992. Pathogenesis of nerve root damage. In: Jayson, M. (Ed.), The Lumbar Spine and Back Pain, fourth ed. Churchill Livingstone, Edinburgh, pp. 89–90.

Schäfer, A., Hall, T., Briffa, K., 2009. Classification of low-back related leg pain—a proposed patho-mechanism-based approach. Man. Ther. 14 (2), 222–230.

Shaw, W.S., Pransky, G., Fitzgerald, T.E., 2001. Early prognosis for low back disability: intervention strategies for health care providers. Disabil. Rehabil. 23 (18), 815–828.

Shaw, B., Kinsella, R., Henschke, N., et al., 2020. Back pain "red flags": which are most predictive of serious pathology in the Emergency Department. Eur. Spine J. 29 (8), 1870–1878.

Sheng, B., Yi-Kai, L., Wei-dong, Z., 2002. Effect of simulating lumbar manipulations on lumbar nucleus pulposus pressures. J. Manipulative Physiol. Ther. 25, 333–336.

Schimmel, J.J., De Kleuver, M., Horsting, P.P., et al., 2009. No effect of traction in patients with low back pain: a single centre, single blind, randomized controlled trial of Intervertebral Differential Dynamics Therapy®. Eur. Spine J. 18 (12), 1843–1850.

Sizer, P., Brismée, J., Cook, C., 2007. Medical screening for red flags in the diagnosis and management of musculoskeletal spine pain. Pain Pract. 7 (1), 53–71.

Soames, R., Palastanga, N.R., 2018. Anatomy and Human Movement, seventh ed. Elsevier, Oxford.

Supik, L.F., Broom, M.J., 1994. Sciatic tension signs and lumbar disc herniations. Spine 19 (9), 1066–1068.

Swezey, R.L., 1983. The modern thrust of manipulation and traction therapy. Semin. Arthritis Rheum. 12 (3), 322–331.

Swezey, R., 1993. Pathophysiology and treatment of intervertebral disk disease. Rheum. Dis. Clin. N. Am. 19 (3), 741–757.

Tanabe, H., Akai, M., Doi, T., et al., 2021. Immediate effect of mechanical lumbar traction in patients with chronic low back pain: A crossover, repeated measures, randomized controlled trial. J. Orthop. Sci. 26, 953–961. https://doi.org/10.1016/j.jos.2020.09.018 Epub ahead of print

Taylor, J., Twomey, L., 1994. The lumbar spine from infancy to old age. In: Twomey, L., Taylor, J. (Eds.), Clinics in Physical Therapy: Physical Therapy of the Low Back, second ed. Churchill Livingstone, Edinburgh, pp. 1–56.

The Best MSK Health Collaborative workspace on Future NHS. 2022. MSK guidance toolkit for primary care and community care v3.6 14032022. https://future.nhs.uk (FutureNHS Collaboratation Platform). Accessed 21 April 2022.

Thomas, E.N., Pers, Y.M., Mercier, G., et al., 2010. The importance of fear, beliefs, catastrophizing and kinesiophobia in chronic low back pain rehabilitation. Ann. Phys. Rehabil. Med. 53 (1), 3–14.

Truchon, M.F.L., 2000. Biopsychosocial determinants of chronic disability and low-back pain: a review. J. Occup. Rehabil. 10, 117–142.

Turner, J.A., Franklin, G., Fulton-Kehoe, D., et al., 2008. ISSLS prize winner: early predictors of chronic work disability: a prospective, population-based study of workers with back injuries. Spine 33 (25), 2809–2818.

Twomey, L., Taylor, J., 1982. Flexion creep deformation and hysteresis in the lumbar vertebral column. Spine 7 (2), 116–122.

Urban, J.P.G., Roberts, S., 2003. Degeneration of the intervertebral disc. Arthritis Res. Ther. 5 (3), 120–130.

Valat, J.P., Genevay, S., Marty, M., et al., 2010. Sciatica. Best Prac. Res. Clin. Rheumatol. 24 (2), 241–252.

Van der Heijden, G.J.M.G., Beurskens, A.J.H.M., Dirx, M.J.M., et al., 1995a. Efficacy of lumbar traction. Physiotherapy 81 (1), 29–35.

Van der Heijden, G.J.M.G., Buerskens, A.J.H.M., Koes, B.W., et al., 1995b. The efficacy of traction for back and neck pain: a systematic, blinded review of randomized clinical trial methods. Phys. Ther. 75 (2), 93–104.

Van Tulder, M., Koes, B., 2002. Review – Low back pain and sciatica. Clinical Evidence Concise. BMJ Publishing, London.

Vanti, C., Panizzolo, A., Turone, L., et al., 2021. Effectiveness of mechanical traction for lumbar radiculopathy: a systematic review and meta-analysis. Phys. Ther. 101 (3), pzaa231.

Vroomen, P., de Krom, M., Knotternus, J., 1999. Diagnostic value of history and physical examination in patients suspected of sciatica due to disc herniation: a systematic review. J. Neurol. 246 (10), 899–906.

Vroomen, P., de Krom, M., Slofstra, P., et al., 2000. Conservative treatment of sciatica: a systematic review. J. Spinal Disord. 13 (6), 463–469.

Waddell, G., 1992. Understanding the patient with backache. In: Jayson, M. (Ed.), The Lumbar Spine and Back Pain, fourth ed. Churchill Livingstone, Edinburgh, pp. 469–485.

Waddell, G., 2004. The Back Pain Revolution, second ed. Churchill Livingstone, Edinburgh.

Wang, X., Martin, G., Sadeghirad, B., et al., 2021. Interventional treatments for chronic, axial or radicular, non-cancer, spinal pain: a protocol for a systematic review and network meta-analysis of randomised trials. Br. Med. J. Open 11 (7), e046025.

Woby, S.R., Roach, N.K., Urmston, M., Watson, P.J., 2007. The relation between cognitive factors and levels of pain and disability in chronic low back pain patients presenting for physiotherapy. Eur. J. Pain. 11 (8), 869–877.

Woby, S.R., Roach, N.K., Urmston, M., et al., 2008. Outcome following a physiotherapist-led intervention for chronic low back pain: the important role of cognitive processes. Physiotherapy 94 (2), 115–124.

Yamamoto, I., Panjabi, M.M., Oxland, T.R., et al., 1990. The role of the iliolumbar ligament in the lumbosacral junction. Spine 15 (11), 1138–1141.

Yamashita, T., Minaki, Y., Ozaktay, A.C., et al., 1996. A morphological study of the fibrous capsule of the human lumbar facet joint. Spine 21 (5), 538–543.

Ziu, E., Viswanathan, V.K., Mesfin, F.B., 2017. Spinal metastasis. StatPearls Publishing. https://www.ncbi.nlm.nih.gov/books/NBK441950/. Accessed 6 September 2021.

The Sacroiliac Joint

CHAPTER CONTENTS

SUMMARY

This chapter begins with a presentation of the anatomy of the sacroiliac joint and links it with pathology and differential diagnosis of sacroiliac pain or dysfunction.

Sacroiliac joint problems can be acute or long-lasting and can be difficult to diagnose, often mimicking pain arising from the lumbar spine or hip.

This chapter aims to demonstrate an effective sacroiliac joint assessment procedure and an approach to treating sacroiliac joint pain. In this approach, treatment consists of mobilisation, manipulation and appropriate exercises.

Contraindications to treatment are few, and emphasis is placed on assessment strategies on which to base treatment selection.

ANATOMY

The pelvis is a unique osteoarticular ring consisting of the two innominate bones, which articulate anteriorly at the symphysis pubis and posteriorly at the sacrum (Fig. 14.1). The sacrum is suspended between the innominate bones by its ligaments.

The function of the bony pelvis is to support and transmit body weight between the spine and lower limbs and to dampen the distribution of ground reaction forces occurring during gait activities. It also protects and supports pelvic viscera, provides attachment for ligaments and leverage for muscles.

Because form follows function, small structural differences occur within the pelvis between the sexes, with women exhibiting greater mobility at the sacroiliac joints (Harrison et al., 1997).

Sacroiliac Joints

Each *innominate* bone is made up of the *ilium* above, the *pubis* in front and the *ischium* behind. The *acetabulum* is the cup-shaped hollow on its outer surface at the junction of the three component bones.

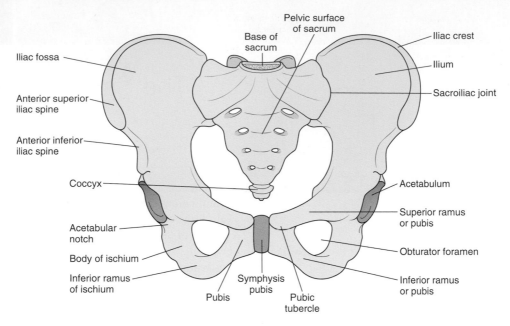

Fig. 14.1 Anterior view of pelvis.

The ilium possesses several palpable bony landmarks. Those relevant here are:

- The iliac crest, which gives an approximate indication of the level of the spinous process of L4
- The anterior superior iliac spine (ASIS), which lies at the anterior end of the iliac crest
- The anterior inferior iliac spine (AIIS), which lies below the superior spine and is not so readily palpable
- The posterior superior iliac spine (PSIS), indicated by a dimple (dimple of Venus) approximately 4 cm lateral to the spinous process of S2
- The posterior inferior iliac spine (PIIS) lying below the superior spine and difficult to palpate

The *iliac fossa* faces medially, and its posterior aspect is thickened, roughened and marked by the iliac tuberosity for the attachment of the posterior and interosseous sacroiliac ligaments. In front of the roughened area lies an articular *auricular surface* corresponding to the articular surface on the sacrum. Laterally the blade of the ilium provides attachment for the gluteal muscles.

The *sacrum* is a large triangular mass of bone formed by the fusion of the five sacral vertebrae (see Fig. 14.2).

The *sacral base* lies superiorly and is angulated upwards and forwards, articulating with the fifth lumbar vertebra to form the lumbosacral angle. Its anterior border is the *sacral promontory*. The apex of the sacrum lies inferiorly and articulates with the *coccyx*, formed by the fusion of approximately four small vertebrae into a small triangular bone (Fig. 14.2).

The pelvic surface of the sacrum is relatively smooth while its dorsal surface is roughened and displays three distinct crests: a *median crest* represents the fused spinous processes of the sacral vertebra, an *intermediate crest* the fused articular processes and a *lateral crest* the fused transverse processes. The lateral crest provides attachment for the posterior sacroiliac ligaments.

The laminae and spinous processes of the fourth and fifth sacral vertebrae are absent, forming an opening referred to as the *sacral hiatus*. Anatomical anomalies are common here, and elements of the other vertebrae may be missing, making this a variably sized opening (Trotter, 1947).

The *sacral cornua* are the remnants of the articular processes of the fourth or fifth sacral vertebra, projecting downwards on either side of the sacral hiatus. They

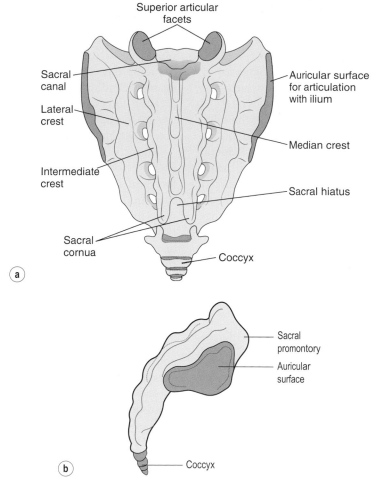

Fig. 14.2 (a, b) Sacrum, showing bony landmarks.

provide palpable bony landmarks for the sacral hiatus, which is clinically relevant for the insertion of a caudal epidural injection.

To palpate the sacral cornua, place the thumb and middle finger of one hand on the PSISs and use the index finger to make an equilateral triangle. The position of the index finger now gives the approximate position of the sacral cornua and hence the sacral hiatus.

The *sacral canal* is triangular in shape and formed by the fused sacral vertebral foramina. The dural sac usually terminates at the level of the lower border of the second sacral vertebra, where it contracts into a filament and continues through the sacral canal to the coccyx to become continuous with the periosteum (Trotter, 1947). Four pairs of sacral foramina provide an exit for the sacral spinal nerves.

The lateral surface of the sacrum is expanded superiorly and provides an articulating surface for the sacroiliac joint. This surface bears an auricular (ear-like) surface anteriorly and a pitted irregular surface posteriorly for the attachment of the posterior and interosseous sacroiliac ligaments.

The sacroiliac joints are highly specialised joints that provide stable but flexible support to the upper body. They are essential for effectively transferring loads between the spine and the legs (Vleeming et al., 2012).

Thawrani et al. (2019) describe the anterior third of the interface between the sacrum and ilium as a true synovial joint, covered by hyaline cartilage, which provides a gliding surface between the bones. The rest of the joint is covered with fibrocartilage and is composed of an intricate set of ligamentous connections, which give inherent stability to the joint.

The hyaline cartilage on the sacral side of the joint is thicker (1.18 mm) than the iliac cartilage (0.8 mm), which appears to be more fibrocartilaginous (Kiapour et al., 2020). The joint is lined with a synovial membrane and surrounded by a fibrous capsule, reinforced by ligaments.

The joint surfaces are relatively planar in the young, allowing gliding in all directions. Following puberty, irregularities develop, more so in the male sacroiliac joint, making it inherently more stable. Vleeming et al. (1990a, 1990b, 2012) describe two types of joint surface irregularities: ridges on one joint surface articulate with complementary depressions on the other, and areas of both coarse and smooth texture exist.

These irregularities also provide the joint surfaces with high coefficients of friction, further contributing to the joint's stability. The irregularities continue to progress with age.

Movement at the sacroiliac joint is restricted to nodding movements along the longitudinal axis of the auricular surface. The range of movement decreases as fibrous ankylosis and osteophyte formation increase with age (Bogduk, 2023), and the joint eventually fuses in the elderly, especially in men (Vleeming et al., 2012).

The restricted movement supports the joint's weight-bearing function and contributes to the stability of the joint. Major subluxation of the joint is not commonly seen clinically, but the interdigitating articular surfaces make minor subluxation a possibility before ankylosis occurs Vleeming et al. (1990b).

The suspension of the wedge-shaped sacrum between the two ilia provides it with a self-locking mechanism. This self-locking mechanism involves both form and force closure (Lee, 2000; Vleeming et al., 2012).

Form closure indicates stability due to the close-fitting joint surfaces, the friction coefficient of the roughened articular cartilage and the integrity of the strong sacroiliac ligaments, so that little or no external forces are required to maintain static stability.

Force closure indicates the dynamic stability of the joint where extra forces are needed to maintain stability. Movements occurring in the sacroiliac joint are small, but as the sacrum moves, activity in the surrounding muscle groups and tensioning of the pelvic ligaments and thoracolumbar fascia enhances the compression forces on the joint. This facilitates the force closure mechanism, making load transfer more efficient (Lee, 2000; Hungerford et al., 2007).

An increase in the weight applied to the sacral base, such as from the effect of gravity or the compression forces of the trunk, will also enhance the force closure mechanism, holding the sacrum more tightly in place through tension in its ligaments (Kapandji, 2019) (Fig. 14.3). This arrangement is similar to the keystone of an arch, where the greater the force applied, the greater the resistance offered, and the more stability is increased (Harrison et al., 1997).

The fibrous capsule is reinforced by strong posterior ligaments and weaker anterior ligaments, while accessory ligaments contribute a stabilising effect on the joint. These strong ligaments prevent translation of the sacrum and separation of the joint and function as a connecting band between the sacrum and the ilium (Cohen, 2005).

The vast *interosseous sacroiliac ligament* forms the main union between the sacrum and ilium, filling the gap between the lateral sacral crest and the iliac tuberosity (Lee, 2000; Vleeming et al., 2012). It is the strongest of the ligaments supporting the sacroiliac joint and provides multidirectional structural stability (Vleeming et al., 2012). It strongly resists separation and translation forces and is a physical barrier to palpation of the sacroiliac joint, which makes intra-articular injection difficult (Harrison et al., 1997; Lee, 2000).

The *posterior sacroiliac ligament* covers the interosseous ligament and has long and short fibres. The ligament imposes the most influence on the mobility of the joint (Vleeming et al., 2012). Short horizontal fibres are placed superiorly where they resist forward movement of the sacral promontory. Longer vertical fibres, continuous with the sacrotuberous ligament, are more superficial and resist a downwards movement of the sacrum relative to the ilium. The long posterior fibres are said to be tense under counternutation, a backward, upwards, nodding movement of the sacrum (Vleeming et al., 1996).

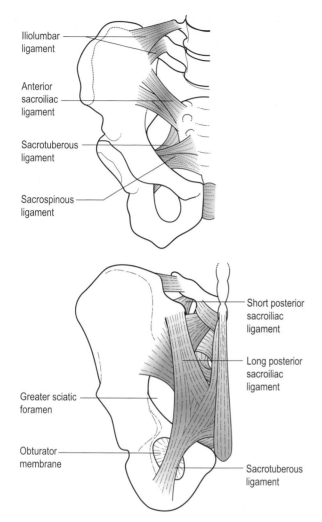

Fig. 14.3 The sacroiliac joint and ligaments. (From Soames and Palastanga, 2018. Reprinted by permission of Elsevier Ltd.)

The *anterior sacroiliac ligament* forms a weak thickening of the anterior joint capsule and has little effect on the mobility of the joint (Vleeming et al., 2012). Accessory ligaments exert a stabilising effect on the joint.

The *sacrotuberous ligament* attaches by a broad base from the PSIS, the side of the sacrum and the coccyx, partially blending with the posterior ligaments. Its fibres converge to pass downwards and laterally, twisting and broadening again at its attachment to the ischial tuberosity, where it blends with the tendon of biceps femoris and the lower fibres of the gluteus maximus.

The *sacrospinous ligament* is thinner and triangular, lying anteriorly to the sacrotuberous ligament. It passes from the lower part of the sacrum and coccyx to the spine of the ischium, and its pelvic surface blends with the coccygeus muscle.

The sacrotuberous and sacrospinous ligaments lie below and lateral to the joint, preventing the tendency for the apex of the sacrum to tilt upwards as body weight is directed down onto the base of the sacrum.

The *iliolumbar ligament* is a large fan-shaped ligament that extends laterally from the transverse processes of the fourth and fifth lumbar vertebrae to the ilium and sacroiliac joint capsule on either side. It stabilises the lumbosacral junction against the tendency of the sacral promontory to move forward under the influence of gravity and body weight, as well as restricting side-flexion (Vleeming et al., 2012).

The *sacrococcygeal joint* is a symphysis between S5 and the first coccygeal segment, but the joint is often obliterated in old age. Flexion and extension movements occur that are largely passive (Lee, 2000; Soames and Palastanga, 2018).

The *symphysis pubis* is the joint between the medial surfaces of the two innominate pubic bones. An interpubic fibrocartilaginous disc is situated within the joint, and the surrounding joint capsule is supported by ligamentous thickenings.

A *superior pubic ligament* is a thick fibrous band joining the pubic crests and tubercles, while an *arcuate pubic ligament* arches between the inferior pubic rami, blending with the intra-articular disc, to support the joint inferiorly (Soames and Palastanga, 2018).

While no muscles act on the sacroiliac joint to produce active movements, it is surrounded by some of the largest and most powerful muscles of the body. These muscles include the erector spinae, psoas, quadratus lumborum, piriformis, abdominal obliques, gluteals, hamstrings, and pelvic floor muscles (levator ani and coccygeus muscles) (Kiapour et al., 2020).

The muscles that cross the joint act on the hip or the lumbar spine and not directly on the sacroiliac joint. Movements of the sacroiliac joint are produced passively by gravity and muscles acting on the trunk and lower limbs rather than by active movements of the sacrum.

Several muscles support the sacroiliac joint. Some of these muscles, including gluteus maximus, piriformis and biceps femoris, are functionally connected to the sacroiliac joint ligaments, and their actions can affect joint mobility (Cohen, 2005).

The ligaments of the sacroiliac joint and lumbar spine fuse with the thoracolumbar fascia and provide attachment for the main trunk-stabilising muscles. Activity in these stabilising muscles provides a 'self-bracing' mechanism, which in turn contributes to stability at the sacroiliac joints (Harrison et al., 1997), and the pelvic floor muscles also act to stabilise the joints (Kiapour et al., 2020).

Movement descriptions applied to the sacroiliac joint refer to the movement of the ilium on the sacrum and include subluxation, upslip, downslip, outflare, inflare, anterior or posterior rotation or torsion (Swezey, 1998; Cibulka, 2002; Middleditch and Oliver, 2005; Standring, 2015). Kapandji (2019) refers to the movements as nutation and counternutation (Latin, *nutare* = to nod) where an anterior (forwards/downwards) and posterior (backwards/upwards) movement of the sacrum on the ilium is described, respectively.

There is general agreement that a small amount of passive movement does occur at the sacroiliac joint, but different methods of measuring the movement give varying results. Normally, movements at the sacroiliac joint are less than 2 degrees (Vleeming et al., 2012) but studies based on changes observed with different positions and movements recorded the lowest change at 0 degrees and the highest change of 9 degrees (Cho and Kwak, 2021).

During symmetrical activities such as sitting or standing, movement normally occurs simultaneously in the two sacroiliac joints with either an anterior or posterior innominate tilt or rotation that brings the two ASISs and PSISs to lie roughly in the same horizontal plane.

During asymmetrical activities such as walking or running, just as one hip flexes and the other extends, one innominate bone tilts posteriorly while the other tilts anteriorly. The movement of one innominate bone leading to reciprocal movement of the other can also be applied to manipulative techniques, which can be reversed and performed on the opposite side if necessary.

Cibulka (2002) suggests that the relationship between the right and left innominate bones should be observed, as patients with sacroiliac dysfunction demonstrate an asymmetrical position even in symmetrical postures such as sitting and standing. This can provide a sign in clinical examination.

The three joints of the pelvic ring, the two sacroiliac joints and the symphysis pubis, are interdependent (Zheng et al., 1997; Vleeming et al., 2012), and functionally, movements at the sacroiliac joint occur in combination with the adjacent joints. Variations between the two joints and between individuals are common, making the examination of these joints difficult.

Nerve Supply to the Sacroiliac Joint

The nerve supply is variable and differs between individuals and often between the two sacroiliac joints in the same person.

A consensus on the nerve supply is hard to establish, but in general terms, the sacroiliac joint and its surrounding ligaments receive a supply derived from L2 to S3 nerve roots anteriorly and L5 to S2 posteriorly (Middleditch and Oliver, 2005). Bogduk (2023) generally agrees with this, stating that the joint is supplied anteriorly by L2–S2 and more widely posteriorly by L4–S3. Both provide 'ballpark' suggestions that would seem to be reasonable in light of current knowledge.

This extensive segmental supply and variation mean that pain patterns can be confusing and may mimic other conditions.

CLINICAL DIAGNOSIS AND MANAGEMENT AT THE SACROILIAC JOINT

This section discusses the differential diagnosis at the sacroiliac joint. Sacroiliac joint pain refers to pain arising from structures associated with the sacroiliac joint, and dysfunction generally refers to an abnormal position or movement of sacroiliac joint structures, which may or may not result in pain.

Pain is the focus in the musculoskeletal medicine approach, and treatment is not applied on the basis of dysfunction alone. However, the dysfunction may also be corrected as an outcome of the treatment techniques applied.

The following section is divided into two parts:

- The first part discusses mechanical sacroiliac joint pain. Assessment of the sacroiliac joint is covered in the next section, 'Commentary on the Examination'.
- The second part looks at other causes of sacroiliac joint pain and associated signs and symptoms, diagnosis and management. Most of these conditions have a more specific or identifiable cause. They are generally not appropriate for treatment with manual musculoskeletal medicine treatment techniques and require suitable referral.

Sacroiliac Joint Pain

Cohen (2005) looked at the prevalence of sacroiliac joint pain by reviewing studies that had used guided anaesthetic injections to confirm a diagnosis. Based on the studies reviewed, he concluded that the prevalence of sacroiliac joint pain in patients presenting with low back pain was in the range of 15% to 20%. Hansen et al. (2007) widened the range to 10% to 27%, and Hungerford et al. (2007) claimed the single figure of 15%.

Although sacroiliac joints are relatively immobile and stable, they are susceptible to mechanical trauma. Joint sprain and minor subluxations can occur, but mechanical lesions are less common in the older age group when ankylosis reduces or prevents movement.

Hypermobility or instability of one sacroiliac joint may be due to a traumatic incident, repetitive microtrauma or hormonal changes in pregnancy (Lee, 2000). The ligaments of the female pelvis relax during pregnancy, increasing the range of movement and making the sacroiliac joint locking mechanism less effective. During this time, the relative hypermobility of the sacroiliac joints makes them susceptible to strain and subluxation.

Typically, patients report a localised buttock pain centred on the PSIS and adjacent sulcus and possibly referring to the groin and into the thigh. It can be difficult to distinguish the pain from lumbar or hip pain, and the different presentations are provided in the discussion below, in the commentary and within the relevant chapters.

Thawrani et al. (2019) acknowledge that there is no reliable specific characteristic pointing to sacroiliac joint pain that can be drawn from the history, clinical examination or imaging studies. However, provocation tests, possibly combined with imaging, could help to identify patients who require treatment or further investigation.

Notwithstanding, diagnosis of sacroiliac joint pain is normally clinical, taking into account the history and the pain provocation tests described below. Palpation for asymmetry in static and dynamic postures can also be helpful but in the context of other signs and symptoms.

The pain provocation tests apply compression, shear and distraction to the joints and can incriminate the joint as a cause of pain. They will be described as part of clinical examination within the 'Commentary on the Examination' section.

Manipulation is appropriate for sacroiliac joint pain, and there is usually a good response. The indications, contraindications and treatment techniques are described later in this chapter.

Applying the manipulative techniques may successfully correct the malalignment of a symptomatic hypermobile sacroiliac joint. Once reduction has been achieved, the joint may need the support of a pelvic belt and correction of any muscle imbalances. The practitioner is referred to other texts focusing on stabilising rehabilitation programmes. Prolotherapy (sclerosant) injections have also been described to stabilise the joint.

Other Causes of Sacroiliac Pain

The sacroiliac joint has an extensive nerve supply, and its close association with the lumbar spine and hip can lead to confusion. Differential diagnosis can include fracture and arthropathy, and other non-musculoskeletal conditions affecting the sacroiliac joint can be classified as inflammatory, malignant or infectious.

Other causes of sacroiliac pain are considered, including serious non-musculoskeletal pathologies that have features and 'red flags' that should alert the practitioner during a clinical examination.

Lumbar and Hip Pathology

Lumbar lesions produce pain felt in one or both buttocks that may refer to the lower limb. Distinguishing features of the history may help to exclude the lumbar spine as a cause of pain, but lesions commonly coexist.

Lumbar lesions are generally aggravated by posture and movement, eased by rest, and often better in the early morning. Radiculopathy may produce objective neurological signs and sensory, neurological symptoms. Degenerative arthropathy of the facet joints and spinal stenosis in the lumbar spine may also produce pain in a similar distribution to sacroiliac joint lesions. Lumbar lesions are discussed in Chapter 13.

Hip joint pathology usually refers pain to the L2–L4 dermatome and may involve unilateral low back and upper buttock pain. Examination of the hip produces positive signs (see Chapter 10).

Greater trochanteric pain syndrome can produce lateral hip and thigh pain (see Chapter 10). Muscle imbalances may need to be addressed, particularly weakness of gluteus medius, within the main hip abductors.

Myofascial pain due to trigger points in the piriformis, gluteus maximus or quadratus lumborum may refer pain to the area of the sacroiliac joint (Chen et al., 2002).

Piriformis syndrome is an entrapment of the sciatic nerve in the gluteal/buttock region that gives rise to a burning or shooting pain or ache down into the back of the leg. It is often aggravated by prolonged sitting. Numbness and tingling may also be described in the sciatic nerve distribution. The cause may be multifactorial, including direct trauma, poor posture or anatomical abnormalities and tumour invasion.

Diagnosis of piriformis syndrome is difficult and is normally made clinically by exclusion. There is usually tenderness on palpation over the sciatic notch and the greater trochanter. Symptoms can normally be reproduced with resisted abduction with the hip in adduction and flexion. Pain may also be reproduced by resisted external rotation with the hip and knee flexed, beginning from a position of internal rotation so that end-range is tested. The straight leg raise is negative (Brukner et al., 2017; Tibor and Sekiya, 2008, Hicks et al., 2020).

A stepped approach to the management of piriformis syndrome is currently recommended, including education/watchful wait, activity and work modification, simple analgesics and non-steroidal anti-inflammatory drugs (NSAIDs) medication and physiotherapy (e.g. soft tissue massage, stretching, exercise). Local anaesthetic injections can have a role in the management of piriformis syndrome, but there does not appear to be any advantage in adding corticosteroid to the injection (Brukner et al., 2017).

Coccydynia is pain in the region of the coccyx, which can arise following direct trauma such as a fall directly onto the bottom. The lumbar spine can also refer pain to the area of the coccyx.

The condition is managed by the use of a cushion or rubber ring, and activity modification, including less sitting and self-mobilisation. An injection can be given if the condition does not settle.

Traumatic

Fracture of the sacrum or pelvic bones is suspected if the patient presents with a history of trauma, severe pain and extensive bruising. The 'sign of the buttock' (see Chapter 10) may be positive, and examination will be difficult due to the level of pain.

Further investigation and onward referral are indicated.

Arthropathy

As synovial joints, the sacroiliac joints are subject to the various forms of *arthropathy*, including *degenerative arthropathy* associated with the ageing process. Reduced mobility appears to occur through a process of fibrous bands or fibrocartilaginous adhesion formation rather than bony ankylosis (Cassidy, 1992; Soames and Palastanga, 2018).

Normally, as described throughout this text, arthropathy will be associated with a capsular pattern. However, at the sacroiliac joint, the small movements of rotation and translation mean that establishing a capsular pattern is difficult. The joint undergoes degenerative changes, reducing the mobility still further and making mechanical lesions less likely in the older age group.

Management is conservative with education, advice and pain medication, i.e. simple analgesics/NSAIDs and physiotherapy (exercise, mobilisation). Some of the manipulation techniques described may be adapted as mobilising techniques in the treatment of degenerative arthropathy.

Inflammatory

Spondyloarthritis describes a group of inflammatory conditions with some shared features. Predominantly peripheral spondyloarthritis includes psoriatic arthritis, reactive arthritis and enteropathic arthritis. Axial spondyloarthritis includes radiographic axial spondyloarthritis (ankylosing spondylitis) and non-radiographic axial spondyloarthritis (McAllister et al., 2017). Each may have some features of the other.

Axial spondyloarthritis primarily affects the joints of the spine, chest and pelvis, but symptoms can be diverse. It may be associated with other comorbidities, for example, uveitis, genitourinary infection, inflammatory bowel disease or psoriasis, but it is also difficult to differentiate from other musculoskeletal conditions, leading to a missed diagnosis or a considerable delay in diagnosis.

There is an average delay of 8.5 years between the onset of symptoms and diagnosis, and only approximately 15% of cases receive a diagnosis within 3 months of initial presentation (McAllister et al., 2017).

Axial spondyloarthritis affects a similar number of women and men and can be present in people who are human leukocyte antigen B27 (HLA-B27) negative and without evidence of sacroiliitis on a plain X-ray; the latter tests being the 'traditional' markers for axial spondyloarthritis (McAllister et al., 2017).

The NICE guideline 'Spondyloarthritis in over 16 s: diagnosis and management' (2017) recommends referral to a rheumatologist for a spondyloarthritis assessment if a person has low back pain that started before the age of 45 years, has lasted for longer than three months and meets four or more of additional criteria that include:

- Low back pain that started before the age of 35
- Buttock pain
- Improvement with movement or within 48 hours after taking NSAIDs
- Waking during the second half of the night due to symptoms
- A first degree relative with spondyloarthritis, and
- Current or past inflammatory conditions.

The later stages involve the whole spine when the X-ray appearance is of a 'bamboo' spine. On examination, there is loss of the lumbar lordosis, increased thoracic kyphosis and decreased chest expansion. Sacroiliitis may be the initial feature, and provocation tests in the clinical examination are likely to be positive.

Pharmacological management begins with the lowest effective dose of an NSAID with ongoing assessment and monitoring and increasing the dose as necessary. If the maximum tolerated dose does not provide sufficient improvement, the NSAID can be changed, or biological disease-modifying anti-rheumatic drugs (DMARDs) may be used.

Patients should also be referred to a specialist physiotherapist to be advised on a stepped and structured exercise programme (which may include hydrotherapy), as well as to other therapists in the allied health professional team as necessary.

Education and advice is an important part of management, and patients should be warned of specific risks, such as any adverse effects from drugs and the risk of osteoporosis and fractures.

Reiter's syndrome is a form of seronegative reactive arthritis that can follow gastrointestinal or genital tract infections (Keat, 1995; Feather et al., 2020). Arthritis affects the lower limb joints, the knees and ankles more readily, but it can also affect the sacroiliac joints. Non-specific urethritis and conjunctivitis may accompany the condition.

Malignancy

Malignant disease can involve the sacroiliac joint directly or indirectly (Silberstein et al., 1992). *Malignancy* involving the sacroiliac joint is uncommon, but metastases may be a cause of pain in the pelvis of older patients. The most common cancers to metastasise to the spine are breast (21%), lung (19%), prostate (7.5%), renal (5%), gastrointestinal (4.5%) and thyroid (2.5%) (Ziu et al., 2017).

Pain can also be referred to the sacroiliac joint region from malignancies in adjacent areas, and Southerst et al. (2012) report a case of multiple myeloma presenting as sacroiliac joint pain.

The history is especially important as the primary red flag for the detection of spinal malignancy is a history of previous malignancy (Downie et al., 2013; Finucane et al., 2020).

The signs and symptoms of malignancy can mimic a mechanical sacroiliac or lumbar lesion, but the pain is usually deep-seated, nagging, relatively constant, steadily worsening and often persistent at night.

Apart from night pain, symptoms of weakness, fatigue and significant weight loss (>10% within 3 months) should be considered to be serious in a patient complaining of sacroiliac pain.

Suspicion of malignancy requires urgent onward referral for further investigation, in line with local policy.

Infection

Infection, as in osteomyelitis in the pelvis or upper femur, produces severe pain felt in the pelvic region, and the patient is unwell, usually with a high fever and marked tenderness over the affected bone.

Septic arthritis, although uncommon in the sacroiliac joint, presents dramatically with pain, heat and swelling. The patient is unwell and febrile.

Suspicion of infection requires emergency onward referral for further investigation, in line with local policy.

The box 'Updated Hierarchical List of Red Flags' presents a weighted list of factors, which, when considered together, in the context of the patient's history, signs and symptoms, helps to raise the practitioner's index of suspicion for serious pathology (see Chapter 1).

UPDATED HIERARCHICAL LIST OF RED FLAGS

🏴 🏴 🏴 🏴

- Age >50 years + history of cancer + unexplained weight loss + failure to improve after 1 month of evidence-based conservative therapy

🏴 🏴 🏴

- Age <10 and >51 years
- Medical history (current or past) of:
  - Cancer
  - Tuberculosis
  - Human immunodeficiency virus (HIV)/acquired immune deficiency syndrome (AIDS) or intravenous drug use
  - Osteoporosis
- Weight loss >10% body weight (3–6 months)
- Severe night pain precluding sleep
- Loss of sphincter tone and altered S4 sensation
- Bladder retention or bowel incontinence
- Positive extensor plantar response

🏴 🏴

- Age 11–19
- Weight loss 5%–10% body weight (3–6 months)
- Constant progressive pain
- Band-like pain
- Abdominal pain and changed bowel habits, but with no change of medication
- Inability to lie supine
- Bizarre neurological deficit
- Spasm
- Disturbed gait

🏴

- Loss of mobility, difficulty with stairs, falls, trips
- Legs misbehave, odd feelings in legs, legs feeling heavy
- Weight loss <5% body weight (3–6 months)
- Smoking
- Systemically unwell
- Trauma
- Bilateral pins and needles in hands and/or feet
- Previous failed treatment
- Thoracic pain
- Headache
- Physical appearance
- Marked partial articular restriction of movement

(From Greenhalgh and Selfe [2010]. Reprinted by permission of Elsevier Ltd.)

COMMENTARY ON THE EXAMINATION

Observation

A general observation is made, including the patient's *face, posture and gait*. Serious conditions of the pelvis may produce severe pain, with night pain as a feature. This may be evident in the patient's face, which looks tired and drawn from lack of sleep.

The posture and gait may show abnormalities, and these need careful assessment to determine if they are relevant to the patient's presenting condition. Sacroiliac joint pain may not alter the gait pattern, but with acute pain, as can be experienced in pregnancy, the patient may not like, or be able, to bear weight on the affected side.

History

See the 'Updated Hierarchical List of Red Flags' box that lists 'red flags' for the possible presence of serious pathology that should be listened for and identified throughout the history and examination. In isolation, many of the flags may have limited significance, but it is for the practitioner to consider the general profile of the patient and to decide whether contraindications to treatment exist and/or whether onward referral is indicated.

A careful history is taken since the differential diagnosis of sacroiliac joint pain is particularly reliant on features of the history.

The patient's *age* is relevant as symptoms arising from all joints in this region tend to present as a condition of the working-aged. Pain associated with the sacroiliac joint in the elderly and in the young should be viewed with suspicion until proven otherwise since mechanical lesions are rare in the sacroiliac joints in these age groups. Younger patients may show postural asymmetry, which may need correction through education and exercise to avoid later problems.

Occupation, sports, hobbies and activities may all have relevance to sacroiliac joint pain. Any occupation or sport that involves increased weight-bearing through one leg may place abnormal stresses on the sacroiliac joint (e.g. driving, ballet, hurdling).

Sacroiliac joint pain affects both sexes but is more common in women. The irregularities in the articular surfaces are more predominant in the male sacroiliac joint, giving it a greater inherent stability.

During pregnancy, the ligaments of the pelvis soften to allow more movement, and the joints are more susceptible to pain and dysfunction. If dysfunction occurs during this time, it could remain once the ligaments tighten in the postpartum phase, and the patient may encounter long-term problems.

The nature of the nerve supply to the sacroiliac joint and its surrounding ligaments makes the *site and spread* of the pain difficult to relate to a specific diagnosis.

Commonly, localised buttock pain is present, often centred on the PSIS and adjacent sulcus and usually below L5. The spread of pain from the sacroiliac joint may be into the groin and front of the thigh, into the buttock and posterior thigh, and possibly into the calf (Fortin et al., 1994a, 1994b; Schwartzer et al., 1995; Dreyfuss et al., 1996; Slipman et al., 2000; Freburger and Riddle, 2001).

The site and spread could be equally indicative of lumbar spine or hip pathology or mimic other conditions. The model of possible pain referral should not be taken in isolation but should be considered within the context of the whole history and examination.

The mode of *onset and duration* of sacroiliac joint pain can be helpful. Sacroiliac joint pain can have a sudden onset when it is usually associated with some form of trauma (e.g. a fall from a height, slipping down the stairs jarring the leg, or a road traffic accident where the foot was placed heavily on the brake). Unidirectional pelvic shear or torsional strain is common, and the mechanism of injury may involve straightening from the stooped position (Leblanc, 1992; Hansen et al., 2007).

Sporting activities that exert repetitive lower intensity forces or a single strong force, such as running, jumping and squatting, may produce excessive movement or stress in the sacroiliac joint and surrounding tissues, leading to overload injuries and soft tissue failure (Chen et al., 2002).

A gradual strain of the sacroiliac joint can also occur through repeated minor trauma, which is often related to occupation (e.g. constant driving over rough ground) or persistent pressure being exerted through one sacroiliac joint. It can also be idiopathic in origin (Hansen et al., 2007).

If female, the patient should be questioned about any significant events during pregnancy that may have provoked symptoms. Obstetric delivery, and gynaecological surgery, can require the use of the lithotomy position: a supine position with the legs separated, flexed, and supported in raised stirrups. This tilts the pelvis posteriorly and may place undue stress on the sacroiliac joints.

The duration is also relevant. Patients may have tolerated the problem for a long time since it produces a dull ache, which can normally be borne more than the pain of acute onset or severe radicular pain associated with lumbar pathology.

The duration of symptoms also gives a prognostic indicator. Adaptive shortening occurs in chronic subluxation, which is unlikely to be corrected by manipulative techniques. However, manipulation may still help the pain, even without correction of the deformity.

The *symptoms and behaviour* need to be considered. Twinges of pain are common, especially after a period of rest, when the patient takes time to 'get going' again. Sit to stand movements may reproduce symptoms, and patients commonly point to the sacral sulcus, which can be tender to palpation (Cibulka, 2002).

Patients may complain of other symptoms that are typical of mechanical sacroiliac pain and distinguish it from other lesions. They cannot sit still or stand for long periods, and the joint likes to be moved and exercised. Sunbathing, for example, is extremely uncomfortable since patients do not like lying flat with legs outstretched and find it hard to lie prone while reading a book. They cannot balance very well on the affected leg. Sleep can be disturbed as the pain wakes the patient when turning at night. The pain may also be worse when lying on the affected side.

The absence of certain symptoms is also relevant in distinguishing sacroiliac joint problems from pain of lumbar origin, particularly arising from nerve root compression. There should be no paraesthesia and no bladder or bowel symptoms.

Symptoms of serious pathology, such as night pain and sweats, fever, generally feeling unwell or unexplained recent weight loss, should be excluded.

The behaviour of the pain indicates the nature of the condition and should distinguish it from lumbar or hip joint pathology. Typically, the patient complains of early-morning stiffness and pain, relieved by movement and made worse with rest, which may be due to the presence of inflammation. As well as being associated with spondyloarthritis, this is also typical behaviour of a ligamentous lesion and consistent with the complex ligamentous structure of the joint.

CLINICAL TIP

Typical findings from the sacroiliac joint history are:
- Female more than male
- Associated with pregnancy, trauma and one-legged activities
- Aching pain around the PSIS
- Aggravated by turning in bed, sitting to stand, extended standing or extended rest periods
- Eased with movement and sitting
- No neurology

Other joint involvement will alert the examiner to possible inflammatory arthritis. However, the initial presentation of axial spondyloarthritis in the sacroiliac joints may occur without other joint signs or symptoms.

Medical history will give information concerning conditions that may be relevant to the patient's current complaint, always with the possible presence of serious illness in mind. An indication of the general health of the patient will indicate any systemic illness, and it may be pertinent to take the patient's temperature.

Recent pregnancy may be relevant to sacroiliac joint problems. Sacroiliac joint pain and dysfunction is a common cause of pain in pregnancy, particularly in the later stages. The increase in weight, change in posture and release of the hormone relaxin all contribute to mechanical instability of the pelvis.

Establish any ongoing conditions and treatment, as well as past medical history. Explore other previous or current musculoskeletal problems with previous episodes of the current complaint, any treatment given and the outcome of treatment.

Practitioners should *screen* routinely for psychosocial factors and consider relevant health co-morbidities and lifestyle factors (see Chapter 1). These factors may contribute to the patient's presenting condition or form a barrier to recovery and normal function and should be addressed as an integral part of patient management.

The *medications* currently being taken by the patient should be listed. This may provide further indication of the patient's medical history or alert the practitioner to possible serious pathology, contraindications to treatment and indications of previous history of malignancy (e.g. tamoxifen) (Ritter et al., 2019).

Anticoagulants and the use of long-term steroids should also be considered. The use of regular analgesia is worth noting as this may provide an objective marker for reassessment.

Inspection

Position the patient in standing, suitably undressed and in a good light. Assessment for *bony deformity* and overall posture is made with particular attention to pelvic asymmetry.

Pelvic asymmetry in the static posture:
- Level of iliac crests (Fig. 14.4)
- Level of ASIS (see Fig. 14.4)
- Level of PSIS (Fig. 14.5)
- Leg length
- General spinal curvatures
- Increased or decreased lordosis

Be aware that these signs cannot be considered in isolation as anomalies and leg-length discrepancies commonly exist. The presence or absence of obvious asymmetry without associated appropriate symptoms is not necessarily relevant to dysfunction of the sacroiliac joint.

The assessment for positional alignment of various landmarks around the pelvis to establish asymmetry in either static or dynamic postures is a popular assessment tool but is not without controversy. It should be recognised that this method lacks reliability and validity and is a subjective interpretation based on the practitioner's eye and experience.

Colour changes, *muscle wasting* and *swelling* are unusual unless there is a history of trauma. In sacroiliac joint strain or subluxation, an area of apparent swelling is sometimes present over the sacrum, usually associated with muscle spasm.

State at Rest

Before any movements are performed, the state at rest is established to provide a baseline for subsequent comparison.

Examination by Selective Tension

The suggested sequence for the examination will now be given, followed by a commentary that includes the reasoning in performing the movements and the significance of the possible findings.

Examination of the sacroiliac joint should include elimination of the lumbar spine and hip joint as possible alternative causes of pain.

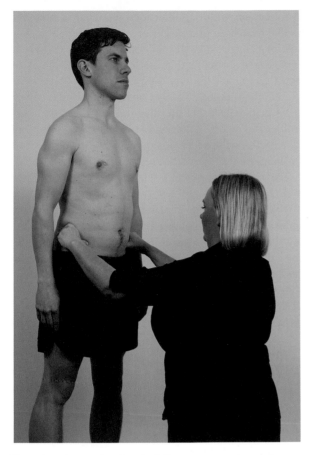

Fig. 14.4 Assessing level of iliac crests and anterior superior iliac spines.

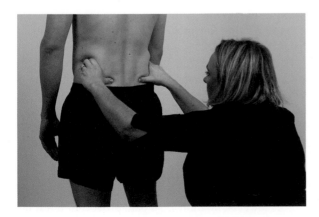

Fig. 14.5 Assessing level of posterior superior iliac spines.

Eliminate the Lumbar Spine
- Active lumbar extension (Fig. 14.6)
- Active right lumbar side flexion (Fig. 14.7a)
- Active left lumbar side flexion (see Fig. 14.7b)
- Active lumbar flexion (Fig. 14.8)
- Passive straight leg raise (Fig. 14.9)
- Check skin sensation in the toes (Fig. 14.10)
- Knee reflex (Fig. 14.11)
- Ankle reflex (Fig. 14.12)
- Plantar response (Fig. 14.13)
- Ankle clonus (Fig. 14.14)

Eliminate the Hip
- Passive hip flexion (Fig. 14.15a)
- Passive hip medial rotation (see Fig. 14.15b)
- Passive hip lateral rotation (see Fig. 14.15c)

Provocative Shear Tests for the Posterior Sacroiliac Ligaments (Saunders, 2000)
- Hip flexion towards the ipsilateral shoulder (Fig. 14.16)
- Hip flexion towards the contralateral shoulder (Fig. 14.17)
- Hip flexion towards the contralateral hip (Fig. 14.18)

Pain Provocation Test for the Anterior Sacroiliac Ligaments
- FABER test (Fig. 14.19)

Further Tests
- Distraction (gapping) test (Fig. 14.20)
- Compression test (Fig. 14.21a and b)
- Sacral thrust test (Fig. 14.22)

Palpation
- For tenderness

Dynamic Asymmetry Palpation Test to Determine Treatment Technique
- The 'walk' test (Fig. 14.23a and b)

The active movements of the lumbar spine and passive hip movements are assessed for range of movement and provocation of pain. If the symptoms are arising from the sacroiliac joint, pain is more commonly felt at the end of the range of these movements, especially lumbar extension and passive hip lateral rotation.

The marked limitation of movement associated with lumbar lesions is not expected. A unilateral reduction of lateral hip rotation has been associated with sacroiliac joint dysfunction (Chen et al., 2002).

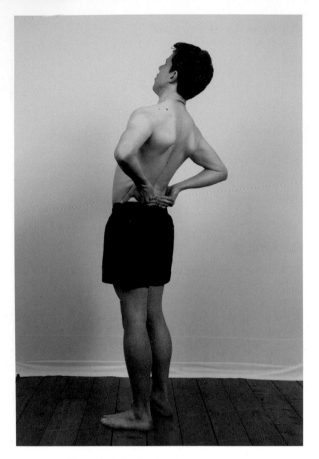

Fig. 14.6 Active lumbar extension.

The patient is assessed for altered skin sensation, and the knee and ankle reflexes are tested. The plantar response is assessed by stroking upwards along the lateral border of the sole of the foot and across the metatarsal heads. The normal response is flexor with flexion of the big toe observed. The Babinski reflex (or Babinski sign) is extension of the big toe. This reflex is a sign of central neuropathology in older children and adults and is indicative of an upper motor neuron lesion.

The ankle clonus test/reflex is performed by quickly dorsiflexing the foot and holding it in the dorsiflexed position. A positive sign is rapidly repeated oscillations or 'beats' that can be felt and seen by the practitioner and can be indicative of an upper motor neuron lesion in the context of other signs and symptoms. Unexplained or abnormal neurology requires further investigation.

In patients with sacroiliac joint pain, palpation of the lumbar vertebrae in a posterior/anterior direction does not normally provoke the patient's pain, but pain may be provoked by springing the sacrum or compression of the sacroiliac joints (Cibulka, 2002).

Radiological and scanning techniques do not appear to be helpful towards the diagnosis of sacroiliac joint problems (Cohen, 2005). Guided anaesthetic injections have traditionally been considered as the 'gold standard' for diagnosis, but the technique is invasive and unwieldy in general clinical practice (Calvillo et al., 2000; Chen et al., 2002).

The use of sacroiliac joint contrast-enhanced injections under fluoroscopic guidance has become more common as a diagnostic and therapeutic option. However, to minimise unnecessary diagnostic injections, several investigators have suggested that only patients with three or more positive provocative clinical tests (or patients with isolated localised sacroiliac pain and positive 'Fortin Finger' tenderness) should receive a diagnostic sacroiliac injection (Thawrani et al., 2019).

The point about the technique being 'invasive and unwieldy' can still be made, however, and the current approach is to use other methods of testing that can be applied more easily in clinical practice.

Pain Provocation Tests

Investigation of intra-articular sources of pain appears to neglect the structures outside the joint capsule and surrounding the sacroiliac joint. Pain provocation tests aim to load the supporting structures surrounding the joint (Robinson et al., 2007), and the ability to make the diagnosis of sacroiliac joint pain through the application of mechanical testing procedures is an important objective (Laslett et al., 2005).

En route to achieving this objective, several studies and reviews have attempted to judge the reliability of various traditional tests for sacroiliac joint pain (Laslett and Williams, 1994; Dreyfuss et al., 1996; Broadhurst and Bond, 1998; Levin et al., 1998, 2001; van der Wurff et al., 2000; Freburger and Riddle, 2001; Kokmeyer et al., 2002).

Most authors agree that pain provocation tests are more reliable than palpation tests for sacroiliac joint dysfunction (Kokmeyer et al., 2002; Robinson et al., 2007). However, no individual pain provocation test has sufficient reliability or validity, leaving this a controversial topic. A battery of tests is used in clinical practice,

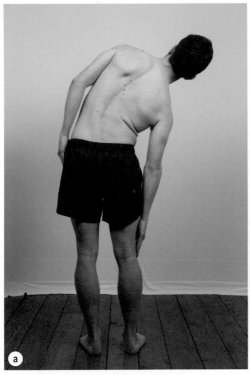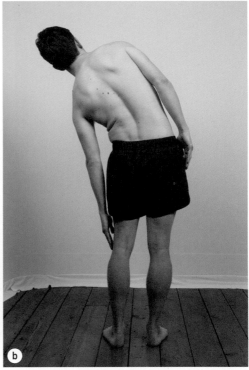

Fig. 14.7 (a, b) Active lumbar side flexions.

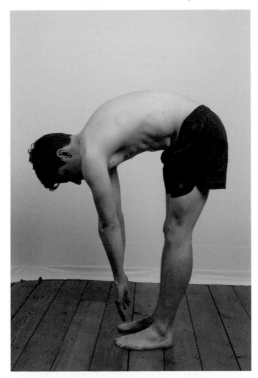

Fig. 14.8 Active lumbar flexion.

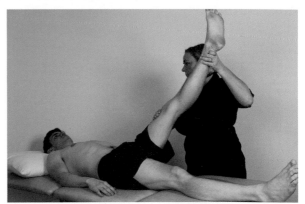

Fig. 14.9 Passive straight leg raise.

and it is commonplace to select three or four individual tests (Broadhurst and Bond, 1998; Chen et al., 2002).

Laslett et al. (2005) selected six provocation tests to explore the ability of the tests, or composites of the tests, to predict the results of fluoroscopically guided, contrast-enhanced sacroiliac anaesthetic block injections. Based on a previous study (Laslett and Williams, 1994), the tests selected were the distraction provocation

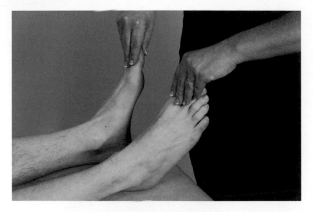

Fig. 14.10 Checking skin sensation.

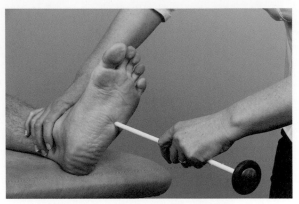

Fig. 14.13 Plantar response.

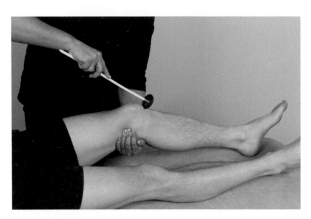

Fig. 14.11 Knee reflex.

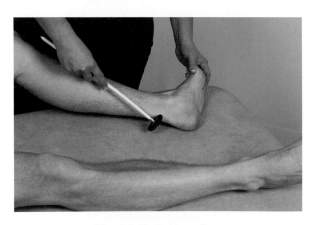

Fig. 14.12 Ankle reflex.

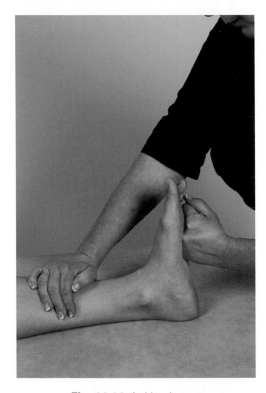

Fig. 14.14 Ankle clonus.

(gapping) test, thigh thrust provocation test, Gaenslen's provocation test, compression provocation test, and sacral thrust provocation test. (The practitioner is referred to the paper itself [Laslett et al., 2005] for a description of the tests as they were applied.)

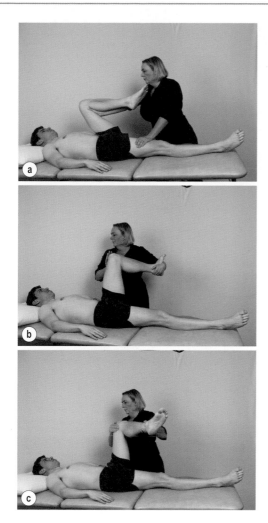

Fig. 14.15 Passive hip movements: (a) flexion; (b) medial; and (c) lateral rotation.

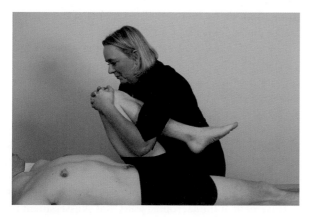

Fig. 14.16 Shear test with the femur pointing towards the ipsilateral shoulder.

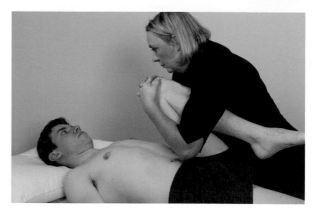

Fig. 14.17 Shear test with the femur pointing towards the contralateral shoulder.

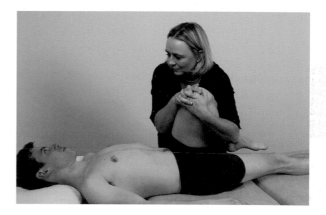

Fig. 14.18 Shear test with the femur pointing towards the contralateral hip.

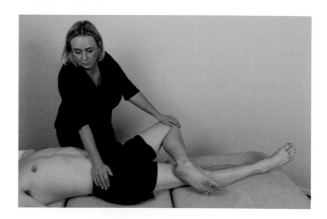

Fig. 14.19 FABER or 4-test.

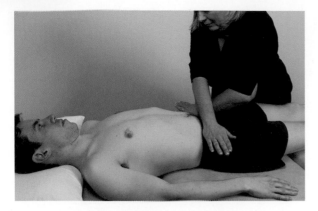

Fig. 14.20 Distraction test.

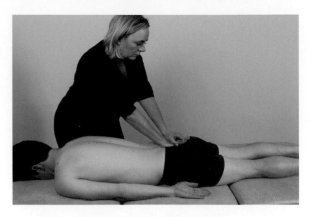

Fig. 14.22 Sacral thrust test.

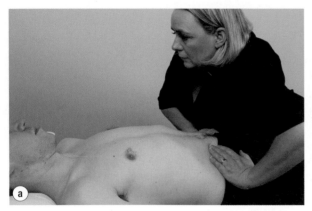

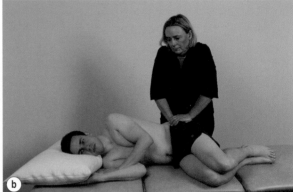

Fig. 14.21 (a, b) Compression test in two positions.

The distraction test was found to have the highest single positive predictive value and was the most specific. The thigh thrust test was the most sensitive and, with the compression and sacral thrust tests, improved the overall diagnostic ability. Gaenslen's test did not contribute positively, and it was suggested that it could be removed from the procedure without affecting the diagnosis.

The key finding of the paper was that the tests should be applied as a composite test, and it was suggested that the distraction, thigh thrust, compression and sacral thrust techniques should be applied, in that order, but to stop when there are two positives. If none of the provocation tests provokes the patient's pain, the sacroiliac joint can be ruled out as the source (Laslett et al., 2005).

Robinson et al. (2007) also looked at an array of one palpation and six provocation tests for sacroiliac joint pain with a focus on interrater reliability. They agreed with Laslett et al. (2005) with regard to the reliability of the thigh thrust test and also supported the value of using a cluster of tests to aid diagnosis.

There is general agreement that the specific tests selected are not as important as the number of the tests that are positive, and two or three positive tests provide good reliability amongst experienced practitioners (Laslett et al., 2005; van der Wurff et al. 2006; Robinson et al., 2007; Arab et al., 2009).

Arab et al. (2009) found that dynamic palpation tests performed well as part of the clusters too, although their use is not as well supported, and they tend to be discounted in studies. In clinical practice, the small amount of movement at the sacroiliac joint makes assessment by palpation difficult and subjective judgements made on sacroiliac static or dynamic alignment alone are not reliable indicators of dysfunction. Correction of alignment is also not necessarily indicative of cure.

O'Sullivan and Beales (2007) suggest active straight leg raising as a means of testing the sacroiliac joint. The test involves the patient lying supine and raising each leg in turn 5 cm off the supporting surface. The test is positive if it brings on the patient's pain and is accompanied by a sensation of profound heaviness in the leg. The pain can usually be relieved by applying compression to the ilia, which may enhance the closure force through the sacroiliac joint and help to confirm a diagnosis.

In the musculoskeletal medicine approach, the sacroiliac joints are tested with the following tests:

- Three thigh thrust provocation tests for the posterior ligaments
- FABER test for the anterior ligaments
- Distraction (gapping) test primarily for the anterior ligaments
- Compression test for posterior ligaments
- Sacral thrust test for posterior ligaments

Reproduction of the patient's pain on the provocation test applied constitutes a positive result for that test. The tests are applied in order of convenience to maintain a flow in the examination sequence described above.

For the posterior ligaments, the aim is to apply a posterior shearing force to the sacroiliac joint via the femur, and the lumbar spine and hip should first be excluded as a cause of pain.

The posterior shear or 'POSH test' applies a shearing force in the combined position of hip flexion with adduction towards the contralateral hip. Saunders (2000) modified the POSH test to include two additional provocative testing positions, and these have been adopted in this approach:

- Hip flexion towards the ipsilateral shoulder
- Hip flexion with adduction towards the contralateral shoulder
- Hip flexion with adduction towards the contralateral hip

With the above tests, care should be taken not to adduct the femur excessively, as this is uncomfortable even in a normal hip joint and may contribute to false-positive results.

The tests are applied as a thrust through the shaft of the femur to assess the posterior ligaments.

PROVOCATIVE SHEAR TESTS FOR THE POSTERIOR SACROILIAC LIGAMENTS (SAUNDERS, 2000)

Perform all three tests on the pain-free side first for subsequent comparison with the painful side.

- Place the patient in supine lying, flex the hip towards the ipsilateral shoulder (Fig. 14.16)
- Grasp the patient's knee with linked hands. Take care to release some pressure from the hip joint flexion before applying the next step of a downward thrust
- Apply a thrust down through the line of the shaft of the femur to stress the posterior sacroiliac joint ligaments. Pain in the buttock on the affected side denotes a positive test
- The test is then repeated twice, but using in turn: (1) hip flexion towards the contralateral shoulder (see Fig. 14.17); and (2) hip flexion and adduction towards the contralateral hip (Fig. 14.18) as the starting positions

---

The FABER test mainly assesses the anterior ligaments and derives its name from the combination of movements applied, being *F*lexion, *Ab*duction and *E*xternal *R*otation of the hip. It is also known as Patrick's test or the '4-test' because of the resultant position of the limb.

The FABER test has not been discounted as strenuously as some of the other tests, and it is commonly used in clinical practice (Cohen, 2005). The test ties in with the limitation of movement and pain that can be provoked in the sacroiliac joint by lateral rotation at the hip, as mentioned previously.

FABER TEST

Perform the test on the pain-free side first for subsequent comparison with the painful side.

- With the patient in supine lying, place the foot of one leg on the knee of the other and allow the leg to rest in lateral rotation and abduction (see Fig. 14.19)
- An assessment is made of the range of movement that is usually limited in sacroiliac joint problems. Pain reported at this stage is more likely to be indicative of hip joint pathology
- Stabilise the opposite side of the pelvis and stress the sacroiliac joint by placing downward pressure gently and steadily on the flexed knee. Pain now reported in the back incriminates the sacroiliac joint as a cause of symptoms (Hoppenfeld, 1976)

DISTRACTION (GAPPING) TEST

- The patient lies supine. Cross your hands over and place the fleshy heel of each hand against the ASISs on the pelvis (see Fig. 14.20)
- This can be an uncomfortable test for the patient as the soft tissues are compressed against the bone as the pressure is applied. Care should be taken to apply the test as comfortably as possible by adjusting your palms, and the patient should be warned before the pressure is applied
- Press downwards and outwards with your hands (posteriorly and laterally)
- The test is positive if the patient's pain is reproduced, which is usually in the gluteal region or posterior thigh

COMPRESSION TEST

- The patient can be placed in a supine position (see Fig. 14.21a), but, as considerable strength can be needed to perform the test on some larger patients, it can also be applied with the patient in a side-lying position, painful side uppermost, which will be described here (see Fig. 14.21b)
- Lower the couch and stand behind the patient, asking the patient to move towards you
- Place your hands on the upper part of the iliac crest
- Press downwards firmly towards the floor with your arms as straight as possible. The test is positive if the patient's pain is reproduced or if there is a sensation of increased discomfort in the region of the sacroiliac joint

SACRAL THRUST TEST

- The patient lies prone
- Place the heel of your hand on the base of the patient's sacrum and reinforce with your other hand on top if necessary (see Fig. 14.22)
- Keep your arm(s) as straight as possible and apply a downwards forward thrust onto the sacrum to cause a shearing force through the sacroiliac joints
- If positive, the test produces pain within the affected joint, and there may be some accompanying referral into the buttock and posterior thigh

It should be acknowledged that the pain provocation tests are non-specific because they stress a number of adjacent structures around the hip, the lower lumbar spine and the sciatic and femoral nerves (Chen et al., 2002). Sacroiliac pain is indicated once two or three of the tests are painful, but if none of the tests reproduces the patient's pain, the sacroiliac joint can be ruled out as the cause (Laslett et al., 2005; van der Wurff et al., 2006).

Palpation may be conducted for tenderness, which is often located over the PSIS, sacral sulcus and surrounding area and is absent on the unaffected side (Dreyfuss et al., 1996; Cibulka, 2002; van der Wurff et al., 2006). However, tenderness is also often present in lumbar and hip pathology and should not be taken by itself as a positive sign of sacroiliac joint involvement.

Based on the history and clinical examination, the practitioner should be able to establish the most likely diagnosis using clinical reasoning and clinical judgement.

It is important to recognise potentially serious pathologies, such as infection, malignancy, fracture and inflammatory arthritis, and to make any appropriate onward referral in a timely manner. Should additional information be required to aid diagnosis or to add value to management, further investigations can be considered to inform decision making and planning.

An investigation should be considered with suspected red flags such as fracture, infection, inflammatory arthritis (including ankylosing spondylitis), suspected malignancy including primary or metastatic tumours and multiple myeloma. Patients with suspected ankylosing spondylitis are typically referred for an X-ray of the sacroiliac joints and blood tests, including testing for the presence of HLA-B27.

In some patients with symptoms of ankylosing spondylitis, inflammation of the sacroiliac joints can be detected on magnetic resonance image (MRI) in the absence of changes on X-ray. The use of MRI enables the detection of non-radiographic axial spondyloarthritis (NICE, 2019, 2020; Royal Australian College of General Practitioners [RACGP], 2013; Royal College of Radiologists, 2017).

TREATMENT OF SACROILIAC JOINT PAIN

A stepped approach to the management of sacroiliac joint pain is currently recommended. Less invasive treatments are generally offered first, including education/watchful wait, activity and work modification, simple analgesics and NSAIDS medication, physiotherapy (e.g. exercise, mobilisation) and then injection therapy (e.g. corticosteroid, local anaesthetic, hyaluronic acid). If symptoms persist, further investigation and onward referral should be considered.

Dynamic Asymmetry Palpation Tests to Determine Treatment Technique

Dynamic palpation tests assess symmetry and movement of the pelvis. Most authors are in agreement that pain provocation tests are more reliable than palpation tests for sacroiliac joint dysfunction (Kokmeyer et al., 2002; Robinson et al., 2007), but they are included here as a guide to treatment technique selection.

The *'walk' test* (Saunders, 2000) may be applied.

'WALK' TEST (SAUNDERS, 2000)

- The patient stands with both hands on a wall or chair for balance (see Fig. 14.23a and b)
- Crouch down so that you are at eye level with the sacrum and the PSISs
- Tuck each thumb up and under the PSIS on either side firmly to locate their position
- Ask the patient to flex alternate hips to 90 degrees without tilting the pelvis, as if taking a marching step, and note the movement of one PSIS in relation to the other
- If normal, the practitioner would expect the PSIS on the non-weight-bearing leg to rotate posteriorly (downwards)
- In order for the test to be significant and to imply hypomobility, a comparison between the two sides is made. If the symptomatic side rotates less posteriorly or more posteriorly than the asymptomatic side, a clue is given to help treatment choice

---

When performing the 'walk' test, it may be difficult for the patient to balance on the standing leg, especially on the symptomatic side, and juddering of the abdominal muscles and/or hip flexors of the non-weight-bearing leg may occur, possibly indicating poor core stability.

The 'walk' test may provide a clue for the application of treatment techniques. If the PSIS on the painful side appears to rotate more posteriorly in relation to the other, then a technique, and appropriate exercises, will be selected to produce anterior rotation. If the PSIS on the painful side appears to rotate less posteriorly in relation to the other, then a technique, and appropriate exercises, will be selected to produce posterior rotation. If no movement abnormality is detected, a more general technique can be applied.

CLINICAL TIP

The 'walk' test is used as a guide to manipulation selection and not for diagnosis.

To recap, diagnosis at the sacroiliac joint relies on the history and positive pain provocation tests. Dynamic asymmetry palpation tests provide clues to treatment.

Treatment for sacroiliac joint pain aims to reduce pain and restore normal function, comprising movement and stability. The assessment and rehabilitation of stability are outside the scope of this text.

With regard to restoring normal movement, having completed the examination, a hypothesis is established relating to the patient's signs and symptoms. If a diagnosis of sacroiliac joint pain is made, and there are no contraindications, manipulation is the treatment of choice.

Due to the mechanical association between the sacrum and low lumbar spine, concomitant lesions are not uncommon, and treatment may need to be directed to both. Most sacroiliac joint treatment techniques will have some effect on the lumbar spine as well as the entire pelvic ring (and vice versa). Notwithstanding, positioning aims to focus forces primarily on the sacroiliac joint.

The progression of treatment is based on the process of constant re-examination. As an examination of the sacroiliac joint is not usually conducted in isolation, the recommended guidelines for the safe practice of manipulation are the same as those covered in the lumbar spine (see Chapter 13). The practitioner must take all due care when applying the treatment techniques.

Indications for Sacroiliac Joint Manipulation

Indications for sacroiliac joint manipulation are as follows:

- Sacroiliac joint pain
- Absence of signs in the lumbar spine and hip
- Two or three positive pain provocation tests
- Tenderness to palpation within 5 cm of PSIS (van der Wurff et al., 2006).

CONTRAINDICATIONS TO SACROILIAC JOINT MANIPULATION

It is impossible to be absolutely definitive about all contraindications, and nothing can substitute for a rigorous assessment of the presenting signs and symptoms and an accurate diagnosis of a mechanical sacroiliac lesion.

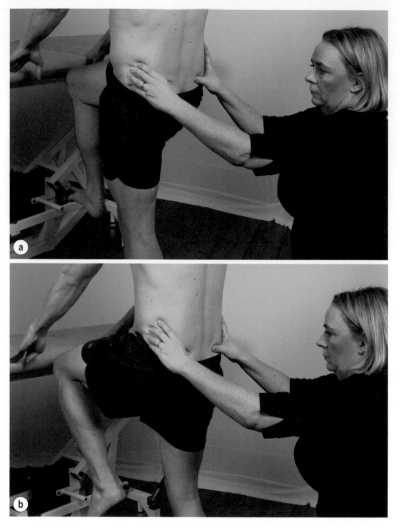

Fig. 14.23 (a, b) The 'walk' test.

'Red flags' are signs and symptoms found in the patient's history and examination that may indicate serious pathology and provide contraindications to sacroiliac joint manipulation (Sizer et al., 2007; Greenhalgh and Selfe, 2010) (see 'Updated Hierarchical List of Red Flags' box on page 498).

In the sacroiliac joint, there are few contraindications, but it may be useful to use the mnemonic *COINS* (a contraction of '*contra*indication*s*') as an *aide-mémoire* to be able to create categories for the contraindications: *C*irculatory, *O*sseous, *I*nflammatory, *N*eurological and suspicious features indicating *S*erious pathology. If the first and last two letters are pushed together as *CONS*, the crucial need for *cons*ent is emphasised.

COINS
- **C**irculatory
- **O**sseous
- **I**nflammatory
- **N**eurological
- **S**erious

The absence of informed patient consent is an absolute contraindication (see Chapter 1). An absence of *dural, cauda equina* and *radicular signs and/or symptoms* would be expected in a sacroiliac joint lesion since they are indicative of lumbar pathology.

The practitioner should be alert to *suspicious features* as indicators of *serious pathology* and any drug history requiring caution. Sacroiliac pain in the elderly is uncommon, and caution is suggested before proceeding with the manipulative techniques described below (Dar et al., 2008).

Occasionally a patient may present with a *highly irritable inflammatory lesion*, and manipulative techniques would be contraindicated.

TREATMENT TECHNIQUES

It is recommended that a course in musculoskeletal medicine should be attended before the treatment techniques described are applied in clinical practice.

For all sacroiliac techniques, the height of the couch is a matter of personal choice. As a suggestion, placing the couch at the level of your mid-thigh gives you the opportunity to facilitate the technique by gapping/distracting the joint. However, the position will ultimately be determined by the relative sizes of the practitioner and the patient – in general, the larger the patient, the lower the bed.

As discussed, the dynamic tests described can provide a guide for technique selection.

SACROILIAC JOINT GAPPING TECHNIQUE

(Saunders, 2000)

The indication for this technique is a diagnosis of sacroiliac joint pain with no observable pelvic asymmetry or difference in the movement of the PSIS during the dynamic palpation tests.

- Position the patient in side-lying, painful side uppermost, pulling the underneath shoulder well through to stabilise the patient.
- Flex the upper leg so that the hip is in a neutral position with the knee over the edge of the bed. Stand in front of and face the patient and place your forearm that is closest to the patient's head comfortably in the patient's waist under the ribs, pushing back against the soft tissues to fix the lumbar spine and allowing the pelvis to fall slightly backwards from the midline.
- Face along the line of the femur and apply gentle downwards pressure with your hand at the patient's knee to gap/distract the sacroiliac joint; maintain this by resting your caudal knee against the patient's flexed knee, then remove your hand.

- Place your forearm on the blade of the ilium to be at right angles with your forearm on the patient's waist (Fig. 14.24a).
- Continue to take up the slack by drawing the forearm on the ilium towards you. Apply a minimal amplitude, high-velocity thrust at the end of the range (see Fig. 14.24b).
- Reassess.

ROTATION OF THE PELVIS DOWN/ POSTERIORLY ON THE PAINFUL SIDE

(Saunders, 2000)

The indication for this technique is a diagnosis of sacroiliac joint pain with either static or dynamic palpation tests, indicating that the PSIS is rotated up or anteriorly on the painful side in relation to the other PSIS.

- Position the patient as above and fix under the rib cage with the forearm as before.
- Place the patient's flexed hip and knee towards more hip flexion to assist rotation of the pelvis posteriorly on the painful side.
- Face along the line of the femur and gap/distract the sacroiliac joint as described above.
- Place the medial epicondyle of your other elbow on the patient's ischial tuberosity.
- Once all the slack has been taken up, by rotating your body and arms to pull the ischial tuberosity towards you, apply a minimal amplitude, high-velocity thrust (Fig. 14.25).
- Reassess.

ROTATION OF THE PELVIS UP/ ANTERIORLY ON THE PAINFUL SIDE

(Saunders, 2000)

The indication for this technique is a diagnosis of sacroiliac joint pain with the palpation tests indicating that the PSIS is rotated down or posteriorly on the painful side in relation to the other PSIS.

- Position the patient as above and fix under the rib cage with one forearm.
- Place the flexed hip and knee towards a hip extension to assist rotation of the pelvis anteriorly on the painful side.
- Face along the line of the femur and gap/distract the sacroiliac joint as described above.

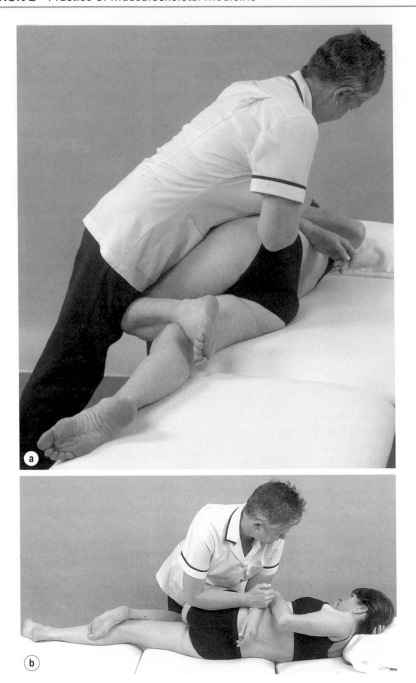

Fig. 14.24 (a, b) Sacroiliac joint-gapping technique.

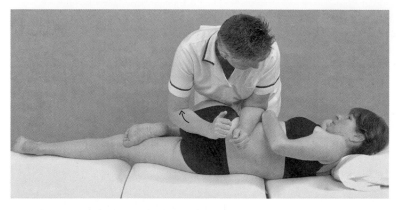

Fig. 14.25 Rotation of the pelvis posteriorly or downwards on the painful side.

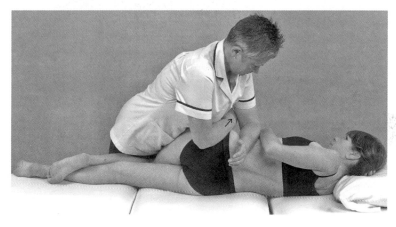

Fig. 14.26 Rotation of the pelvis anteriorly or upwards on the painful side.

- Place the forearm of your other arm to apply pressure just behind the iliac crest, but keep your forearms parallel.
- Pull your arm on the iliac crest towards you and under your other arm and, once all the slack has been taken up, apply a minimal amplitude, high-velocity thrust (Fig. 14.26).
- Reassess.

LEG TUG

The indication for this technique is any diagnosis of sacroiliac joint pain. It is particularly useful during the later stages of pregnancy.
- Position the patient comfortably in supine lying with the couch at about knee height.
- Hold the patient's ankle on the symptomatic side and place your knee against the patient's foot on the

good side to prevent the patient from slipping down the bed.
- Apply a degree of distraction together with a circumduction movement of the hip. Once the patient relaxes, apply a sharp caudal tug (Fig. 14.27).
- Reassess.

The techniques described above can be very successful in treating sacroiliac joint pain. Following treatment, attention should be given to the prevention of recurrence.

Discussion with the patient will allow advice to be given about lifestyle and activity modification that may be contributing to the condition, and any imbalances and postural problems can be addressed. In the later stages of pregnancy, a supportive brace may be helpful after treatment.

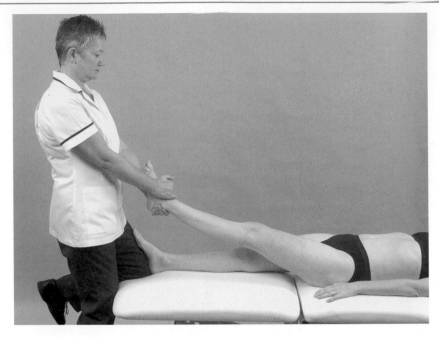

Fig. 14.27 Leg tug.

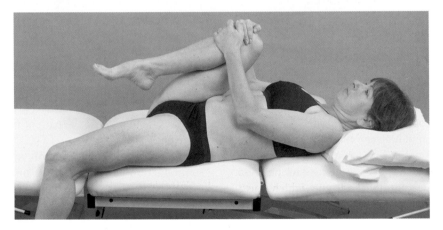

Fig. 14.28 Exercise in supine lying, encouraging movement of the posterior superior iliac spine.

The following exercises may be useful in a maintenance programme and can be adapted to align with the movements applied in the treatment techniques:

- In supine lying, ask the patient to flex one knee to the chest while the other leg hangs over the edge of the couch. Anterior or upwards rotation is encouraged in the extended leg, and posterior or downwards rotation in the flexed leg (Fig. 14.28).
- Standing with one leg on a stool, ask the patient to make a lunging movement forwards, involving flexion at the hip and extension at the lumbar spine. Anterior or upwards rotation of the PSIS is encouraged on the

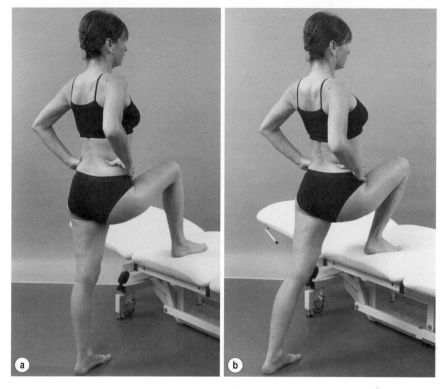

Fig. 14.29 (a, b) Exercise in standing, encouraging movement of the posterior superior iliac spine.

side of the standing, extended leg, and posterior or downwards rotation of the PSIS is encouraged on the side of the flexed leg (Fig. 14.29a and b).

Transverse frictions may be useful to obtain some pain relief, especially after sacroiliac joint manipulation. They may be applied across the tender site, which is usually over the posterior ligaments in the sacral sulcus.

REVIEW QUESTIONS

1. What findings on examination would lead you to a diagnosis of the sacroiliac joint being the source of pain?
2. Consider the main contraindications to sacroiliac joint manipulation.
3. How do you decide which manipulation technique to perform?
4. Would you expect any neurological signs with pain originating from the sacroiliac joint?

CASE SCENARIOS
Case 1
History
- Kirsty, a pregnant 33-year-old nurse, has a 3-week history of left buttock pain. The onset has been gradual, and she is linking it to her increasing baby bump while continuing to work as a nursery nurse. Pain is worse first thing in the morning, after sitting for a long time and on rising from sitting. She has no neurological symptoms

Examination
- Pain end-range lumbar extension, pain on stressing the posterior sacroiliac joint ligaments and a limited FABER test. Equal and full straight leg raise; power, reflexes and sensation normal. Tender on palpation around the left PSIS

Task
- Consider treatment options. Would the number of weeks pregnant have an influence on the treatment selection?

Case 2
History
- Ken, a 45-year-old surveyor, has a 3-month history of left buttock and groin pain following a jump from scaffolding at work. He landed heavily on that side and has felt out of alignment since. His pain is worse with driving and after sitting for long spells at the computer at work; it occasionally wakes him on turning at night. Paracetamol helps. He has a past history of gout

Examination
- Full lumbar movements; pain end-range hip external rotation and positive on testing the sacroiliac joint posterior ligaments and the pelvis distraction test. He is tender around the left PSIS. All neurological testing is negative

Task
- What is the benefit of doing the walk test on this patient, and how will it guide your treatment? How do you differentiate between this and Clinical Model 2 in the lumbar spine?

Case 3
History
- Bobby is a 25-year-old civil servant with a 6-month history of pain in his right buttock. There is no apparent reason for this pain, and it is getting him down, as his back feels really stiff in the mornings. It feels better after he has walked to work. He is awaiting blood test results from his GP. There is no other joint involvement

Examination
- Limited lumbar extension, pain on all sacroiliac joint ligament stress tests on the right and tender around the right PSIS. No obvious asymmetry on the 'walk' test. Neurological testing negative

Task
- Is this a normal sacroiliac joint pain presentation? Discuss differential diagnosis and management of this patient

REFERENCES

Arab, A.M., Abdollahi, I., Joghataei, M.T., et al., 2009. Inter- and intra-examiner reliability of single and composites of selected motion palpation and pain provocation tests for sacroiliac joint. Man. Ther. 14 (2), 213–221.

Bogduk, N., 2023. Clinical and Radiological Anatomy of the Lumbar Spine, sixth ed. Churchill Livingstone, Edinburgh.

Broadhurst, N.A., Bond, M.J., 1998. Pain provocation tests for the assessment of sacroiliac dysfunction. J. Spinal Disord. 11 (4), 341–345.

Brukner, P., Clarson, B., Cook, J., et al., 2017., fifth ed. Clinical Sports Medicine, vol. 1 McGraw-Hill, Sydney.

Calvillo, O., Skaribas, I., Turnipseed, J., 2000. Anatomy and pathophysiology of the sacroiliac joint. Curr. Rev. Pain 4 (5), 356–361.

Cassidy, J.D., 1992. The pathoanatomy and clinical significance of the sacro-iliac joints. J. Manip. Physiol. Ther. 15 (1), 41–42.

Chen, Y.C., Fredericson, M., Smuck, M., 2002. The sacroiliac joint pain syndrome in active patients: a look behind the pain. Phys. Sports Med. 30 (11), 30–37.

Cho, H.-J., Kwak, D.-S., 2021. Movement of the sacroiliac joint: anatomy, systematic review, and biomechanical considerations. Proc. Inst. Mech. Eng. H. 253 (3), 357–364.

Cibulka, M.T., 2002. Understanding sacroiliac joint movement as a guide to the management of a patient with unilateral low back pain. Man. Ther. 7 (4), 215–221.

Cohen, S.P., 2005. Sacroiliac joint pain: a comprehensive review of anatomy, diagnosis and treatment. Anesth. Analg. 101 (5), 1440–1453.

Dar, G., Khamis, S., Peleg, S., et al., 2008. Sacroiliac joint fusion and the implications for manual therapy diagnosis and treatment. Man. Ther. 13 (2), 155–158.

Downie, A., Williams, C.M., Henschke, N., et al., 2013. Red flags to screen for malignancy and fractures in patients with low back pain: a systematic review. Br. Med. J. 347, f7095.

Dreyfuss, P., Michaelsen, M., Pauza, K., et al., 1996. The value of medical history and physical examination in diagnosing sacroiliac joint pain. Spine 21 (22), 2594–2602.

Feather, A., Randall, D., Waterhouse, M., 2020. Kumar and Clark's Clinical Medicine, tenth ed. Elsevier, London.

Finucane, L.M., Downie, A., Mercer, C., et al., 2020. International Framework for Red Flags for Potential Serious Spinal Pathologies. J. Orthop. Sports Phys. Ther. 50 (7), 350–372.

Fortin, J.D., Dwyer, A.P., West, S., et al., 1994a. Sacro-iliac joint – pain referral maps upon applying a new injection/arthrography technique, part I. Asymptomatic volunteers. Spine 19 (13), 1475–1482.

Fortin, J.D., Aprill, C.N., Ponthieux, B., et al., 1994b. Sacroiliac joint – pain referral maps upon applying a new injection/arthrography technique, part II. Clinical evaluation. Spine 19 (13), 1483–1489.

Freburger, J.K., Riddle, D.L., 2001. Using published evidence to guide the examination of the sacroiliac joint. Phys. Ther. 81 (5), 1135–1143.

Greenhalgh, S., Selfe, J., 2010. Red Flags II: A Guide to Solving Serious Pathology of the Spine. Elsevier, Edinburgh.

Hansen, H.C., McKenzie-Brown, A.M., Cohen, S., et al., 2007. Sacroiliac joint interventions: a systematic review. Pain Physician 10, 165–184.

Harrison, D.E., Harrison, D.D., Troyanovich, S.J., 1997. The sacroiliac joint: a review of anatomy and biomechanics with clinical implications. J. Manip. Physiol. Ther. 20 (9), 607–617.

Hicks, B.L., Lam, J.C., Varacallo, M., 2020. Piriformis Syndrome. StatPearls Publishing. https://www.ncbi.nlm.nih.gov/books/NBK448172/. Accessed 5 September 2021.

Hoppenfeld, S., 1976. Physical Examination of the Spine and Extremities. Appleton Century Crofts, Philadelphia.

Hungerford, B.A., Gilleard, W., Moran, M., et al., 2007. Evaluation of the ability of physical therapists to palpate intrapelvic motion with the Stork test on the support side. Phys. Ther. 87 (7), 879–887.

Kapandji, I.A., 2019. The Physiology of the Joints, the Spinal Column, Pelvic Girdle and Head. Handspring Publishing.

Keat, A., 1995. Reiter's syndrome and reactive arthritis. Collected Reports on the Rheumatic Diseases. Arthritis and Rheumatism Council for Research, London, 61–64.

Kiapour, A., Joukar, A., Elgafy, H., et al., 2020. Biomechanics of the sacroiliac joint: Anatomy, function, biomechanics, sexual dimorphism, and causes of pain. Int. J. Spine Surg. 14, S3–S13.

Kokmeyer, D.J., van der Wurff, P., Aufdemkampe, G., et al., 2002. The reliability of multitest regimens with sacroiliac pain provocation tests. J. Manip. Physiol. Ther. 25 (1), 42–48.

Laslett, M., Williams, M., 1994. The reliability of selected pain provocation tests for sacro-iliac joint pathology. Spine 19 (11), 1243–1249.

Laslett, M., Aprill, C.N., McDonald, B., et al., 2005. Diagnosis of sacroiliac joint pain: validity of individual provocation tests and composites of tests. Man. Ther. 10 (3), 207–218.

Leblanc, K., 1992. Sacro-iliac sprain: an overlooked cause of back pain. Am. Fam. Phys. 46 (5), 1459–1463.

Lee, D., 2000. The Pelvic Girdle. Churchill Livingstone, Edinburgh.

Levin, U., Nilsson-Wikmar, L.K., Stendtröm, C.H., 1998. Reproducibility of manual pressure force on provocation of the sacroiliac joint. Physiother. Res. Int. 3 (1), 1–14.

Levin, U., Nilsson-Wikmar, L., Harms-Ringdahl, K., et al., 2001. Variability of forces applied by experienced physiotherapists during provocation of the sacroiliac joint. Clin. Biomech. 16 (4), 300–306.

McAllister, K., Goodson, N., Warburton, L., et al., 2017. Spondyloarthritis: diagnosis and management: summary of NICE guidance. Br. Med. J. 356, j839.

Middleditch, A., Oliver, J., 2005. Functional Anatomy of the Spine, second ed. Butterworth Heinemann, Edinburgh.

National Institute for Health and Care Excellence (NICE), 2017. Spondyloarthritis in over 16s: diagnosis and management. NICE. https://www.nice.org.uk/guidance/ng65. Accessed 6 September 2021.

National Institute for Health and Care Excellence (NICE), 2019. What investigations should I arrange when ankylosing spondylitis is suspected? NICE. https://cks.nice.org.uk/topics/ankylosing-spondylitis/diagnosis/investigations/. Accessed 5 September 2021.

National Institute for Health and Care Excellence (NICE), 2020. Low back pain and sciatica in over 16s: assessment and management. NICE. https://www.nice.org.uk/guidance/ng59. Accessed 4 September 2021.

O'Sullivan, P.B., Beales, D.J., 2007. Changes in pelvic floor and diaphragm kinematics and respiratory patterns in subjects with sacroiliac joint pain following a motor learning intervention: a case series. Man. Ther. 12 (3), 209–218.

Ritter, J.M., Flower, R., Henderson, G., et al., 2019. Rang and Dale's Pharmacology, ninth ed. Elsevier.

Robinson, H.S., Brox, J.I., Robinson, R., et al., 2007. The reliability of selected motion and pain provocation tests for the sacroiliac joint. Man. Ther. 12 (1), 72–79.

Royal Australian College of General Practitioners, 2013. Clinical guidance for MRI referral. https://www.racgp.org.au/getattachment/f8275e83-0489-44a8-893e-461a575ba04a/Clinical-guidance-for-MRI-referral.aspx. Accessed 5 September 2021.

Royal College of Radiologists. 2017. Making the best use of clinical radiology. RCR iRefer Guidelines v. 8. RCR.

Saunders, S., 2000. Orthopaedic Medicine Course Manual. Saunders, London.

Schwartzer, A.C., Aprill, C.N., Bogduk, N., 1995. the sacroiliac joint in chronic low back pain. Spine 20 (1), 31–37.

Silberstein, M., Hennessy, O., Lau, L., 1992. Neoplastic involvement of the sacroiliac joint – MR and CT features. Australas. Radiol. 36 (4), 334–348.

Sizer, P., Brismée, J., Cook, C., 2007. Medical screening for red flags in the diagnosis and management of musculoskeletal spine pain. Pain Pract. 7 (1), 53–71.

Slipman, C.W., Jackson, H.B., Lipetz, J.S., et al., 2000. Sacroiliac joint pain referral zones. Arch. Phys. Med. Rehabil. 81 (3), 334–348.

Soames, R., Palastanga, N., R., 2018. Anatomy and Human Movement, seventh ed. Elsevier, Oxford.

Southerst, D., Dufton, J., Stern, P., 2012. Multiple myeloma presenting a sacroiliac joint pain: a case report. J. Can. Chiropr. Assoc. 56 (2), 94–101.

Standring, S., 2015. Gray's Anatomy: The Anatomical Basis of Clinical Practice, forty-first ed. Churchill Livingstone, Edinburgh.

Swezey, R.L., 1998. The sacroiliac joint. Phys. Med. Rehabil. Clin. N. Am. 9 (2), 515–519.

Thawrani, D.P., Agabegi, S.S., Asghar, F., 2019. Diagnosing sacroiliac joint pain. J. Am. Acad. Orthop. Surg. 27 (8), 85–93.

Tibor, L.M., Sekiya, J.K., 2008. Differential diagnosis of pain around the hip joint. Arthroscopy 24 (12), 1407–1421.

Trotter, M., 1947. Variations of the sacral canal: their significance in the administration of caudal analgesia. Curr. Res. Anesth. Analg. 26 (5), 192–202.

van der Wurff, P., Hagmeijer, R.H.M., Meyne, W., 2000. Clinical test of the sacroiliac joint, part I. Reliability. Man. Ther. 5 (1), 30–36.

van der Wurff, P., Buijs, E.J., Groen, G.J., 2006. A multitest regimen of pain provocation tests as an aid to reduce unnecessary minimally invasive sacroiliac joint procedures. Arch. Phys. Med. Rehabil. 87 (1), 10–14.

Vleeming, A., Stoeckart, R., Volkers, C.W., et al., 1990a. Relation between form and function in the sacro-iliac joint, part I. Clinical anatomical aspects. Spine 15 (2), 130–132.

Vleeming, A., Stoeckart, R., Volkers, C.W., et al., 1990b. Relation between form and function in the sacro-iliac joint, part II. Biomechanical aspects. Spine 15 (2), 133–135.

Vleeming, A., Pool-Goudzwaard, L., Hammudoghlu, D., et al., 1996. The function of the long dorsal sacro-iliac ligament. Spine 21 (5), 556–562.

Vleeming, A., Schuenke, M.D., Masi, A.T., et al., 2012. The sacroiliac joint: an overview of its anatomy, function and potential clinical implications. J. Anat. 221 (6), 537–567.

Zheng, N., Watson, L.G., Yong-Hing, K., 1997. Biomechanical modelling of the human sacroiliac joint. Med. Biol. Eng. Comput. 35 (2), 77–82.

Ziu, E., Viswanathan, V.K., Mesfin, F.B., 2017. Spinal Metastasis. StatPearls Publishing. https://www.ncbi.nlm.nih.gov/books/NBK441950/, Accessed 6 September 2021.

SECTION 3

Practical Resources

INTRODUCTION TO SECTION 3

Section 3 provides resources to support the recording of assessment and to enhance safety, especially whilst learning the musculoskeletal medicine approach.

Information is provided on organisations teaching musculoskeletal/orthopaedic medicine, and the reader is directed to the flexible continuing development pathway provided by the Society of Musculoskeletal Medicine that facilitates ongoing study through advanced courses that culminate in the validated MSc Musculoskeletal Medicine.

A Glossary is provided to define key terms that relate to musculoskeletal medicine practice.

Assessment Tools: Star Diagrams; Pro Forma for Lumbar Spine Assessment; Outcome Measures

STAR DIAGRAMS

Star diagrams can be used as a visual representation of a patient's available range of movement, as well as the amount of pain or other symptoms they are experiencing. The following templates can be used to represent findings for the cervical, thoracic and lumbar spine, and some examples of completed templates are provided below.

Each arm of the star represents a specific spinal movement, with the end of the arm signifying full range of movement.

The available range can be marked along a line, and the amount of pain the patient is experiencing at that point can be noted.

I   Mild pain (1 to 4 on visual analogue scale)
II Moderate pain (5 to 7 on visual analogue scale)
III Severe pain (8 to 10 on visual analogue scale)

In addition to marking pain on the arm of the diagram, it can be helpful to note the site of the pain alongside.

Muscle spasm can be marked with a *z*, a painful arc marked with an *x* and deviation indicated by altering the angle of the line (see below).

The diagram allows for a fast visual recall of the patient's symptoms. It will also highlight whether a patient has a capsular or non-capsular pattern. It is valuable for comparison on retesting, following each spinal mobilisation or manipulation, to be able to visualise improvement.

CERVICAL AND THORACIC SPINE

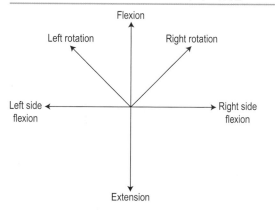

LUMBAR SPINE

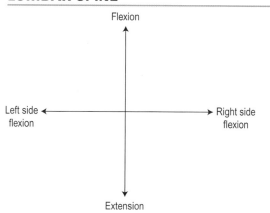

Some examples follow of how the star diagram can be used to represent findings in spinal clinical models.

Please note that for legal purposes you must keep an abbreviations list in your clinic of all symbols or abbreviations used in your clinical notes. This is to enable a non-medical person to translate your patient records if required.

EXAMPLE 1: CLINICAL MODEL 1 IN CERVICAL SPINE

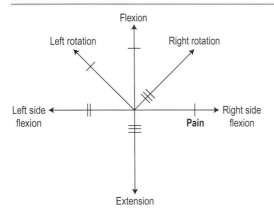

Example 1 demonstrates severe pain and restriction of right rotation and extension, moderate pain but loss of one-half range on left side flexion and some mild pain and limitation of flexion, left rotation and right side flexion.

Movements can be marked on new diagrams at the end of treatment sessions and at ongoing appointments for comparison.

EXAMPLE 2: CLINICAL MODEL 2 IN THE LUMBAR SPINE

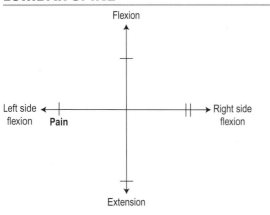

Example 2 demonstrates moderate pain and limitation of right side flexion and mild pain with minimal limitation of left side flexion and extension. There is more loss of range of flexion but only mild pain.

Compared to Example 1, this is a much less severe and irritable clinical finding.

EXAMPLE 3: CLINICAL MODEL 3 IN LUMBAR SPINE

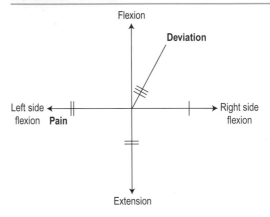

Example 3 represents a deviation on lumbar flexion with severe pain, moderate pain and limitation of left side flexion and extension, and mild pain and limitation of right side flexion.

EXAMPLE 4: LUMBAR SPINE HIGHLIGHTING SPASM AND PAINFUL ARC

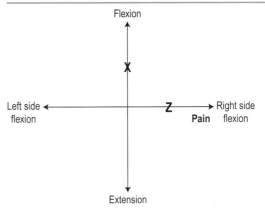

Example 4 demonstrates the highlighting of a painful arc with an *x* and spasm with a *z*.

PRO FORMA FOR LUMBAR SPINE ASSESSMENT

Name (M/F):

OBSERVATION: face, posture and gait (note any abnormalities):

HISTORY:

Age/DOB:

Occupation:

Sports, Hobbies, Activities:

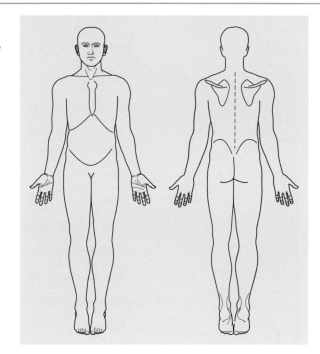

Site & Spread:

Onset: sudden or gradual:

Mechanism of injury:

Duration:

Is it improving/worsening or staying the same?

Any investigation or interventions?

Symptoms:
Description of pain:

NPRS: At best   At worst

Any changes in bladder, bowel or sexual function?

P&Ns or numbness? Draw on body chart:

Edge/ Aspect?

Cough/ Sneeze:

Medical History:

Previous back problems with outcome/treatment and investigations:

Previous malignancy, major operations or illnesses:

Other joint involvement

Medications:

Analgesics:(how much and are they working)
Anti-inflammatories:
Anti-carcinogenics:
Anti-depressants:
Anti-coagulants:

Behaviour:
Constant/intermittent?

Aggravated by:

Eased by:

Night pain:

24 hour pattern:

General Health Checklist:

Diabetes; epilepsy; recent unexplained weight loss; high blood pressure; visceral disease, fever, high cholesterol; infections, viruses, HIV, night sweats; rheumatoid arthritis; osteoarthritis; osteoporosis; smoker; other-including relevant family history.

Muscle relaxants:
Steroids
Others:
Non prescribed drugs:

Clinical impression prior to examination:

INSPECTION:

Bony deformities: **Wasting:**

Colour changes: **Swelling:**

STATE AT REST:

EXAMINATION

Active Lumbar Movements: on star diagram   **Gastrocnemius power (S1/2):**

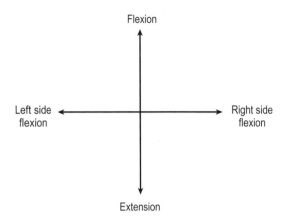

Clear Hips:

                                         Left   **Right**

Passive flexion:

Passive Medial rotation:

Passive Lateral rotation:

Clear Sacroiliac joints:

                                         Left   **Right**

Shear tests

Faber test

Straight leg raise (L & R):

Myotomes in supine: **Femoral nerve stretch:**

Resisted hip flexion (L2/3)   **Myotomes in prone:**

Resisted ankle dorsiflexion (L4/5)   Resisted knee extension (L2/3)

Resisted big toe extension (L5)   Resisted knee flexion (L5/S1)

Resisted ankle eversion (L5/S1)   Gluteal contraction (S1/S2)

Reflexes:

Knee (L2/3)   **Palpation of spinous processes:**

Ankle (L5/S1)

Babinski for plantar response?   **Any additional tests:**

Sensation: Dermatomes, L3, L4, L5, S1, S2

CLINICAL DIAGNOSIS:

TREATMENT PLAN:

OUTCOME MEASURES

An outcome measure is a tool used to assess a patient's current status. Since the mid-2000s, outcome measures have been used increasingly to improve patient care, to improve the health of the population, to compare and contrast interventions and to reduce the cost of healthcare. They reflect the impact of healthcare or an intervention on the health status of the patient.

The two common outcome measures used are 'patient reported outcome measures' (PROMs) and 'patient reported experience measures' (PREMs).

PROMs report patients' perspectives of their health. They are validated, generic and disease specific, allow comparison between specialities and conditions and are typically collected at the start of the treatment and at a subsequent stage after it ends.

Condition-specific PROMs (of which there are some examples below) allow for greater specificity but reduce the ability to compare different pathologies and to extrapolate outcomes from one condition to another.

Generic PROMs measure a variety of aspects of a broad range of medical conditions, allowing for the overall evaluation of care, quality of life and cost effectiveness of interventions.

PREMs report patients' perspectives of their experience of healthcare. They tend to be more functional, for example, asking about waiting times or facilities, and are also personal, asking patients such questions as 'did you feel you were listened to?'

The benefits include that they ensure safety; determine clinical effectiveness; guide treatment decisions; support patient-centred care; evaluate service; identify professional education and training needs; support audit and research; enhance communication with patients/other healthcare professionals; improve care pathways and patient experiences.

The limitations include the choice of the tools (i.e. if the correct tool is chosen for a specific population); the reliability, validity and responsiveness of the tools; data collection, analysing and interpreting data and/or generalising results.

The limitations should not be confused with the barriers to using them which include: they are time consuming; response rates are poor; they have low perceived value; there can be unfamiliarity with the tool; cost (licensing and/or equipment); and training and accessibility.

Notwithstanding the above, practitioners have a responsibility and professional obligation to use them 'wherever practicable', as they play a role in enabling services to demonstrate safety, quality, and clinical and cost effectiveness.

The White paper: Equity and Excellence: Liberating the NHS (2010) (https://assets.publishing.service.gov.uk/government/uploads/system/uploads/attachment_data/file/213823/dh_117794.pdf), and the Chartered Society of Physiotherapy (CSP) page (https://www.csp.org.uk/professional-clinical/research-evaluation/outcome-experience-measures) provide more context and information on outcome measures.

Examples of PROMs

EQ-5D-5L – 'EuroQol – 5 Dimensions – 5 Levels'. This outcome measure comprises five dimensions of health: mobility, ability to self-care, ability to undertake usual activities, pain and discomfort, and anxiety and depression. There are five options (levels) under each dimension.

NPRS – The Numerical Pain Rating Scale (NPRS) is a segmented numeric version of the visual analogue scale (VAS) in which a respondent selects a whole number (0 to 10 integers) that best reflects the intensity of his/her pain.

ODI – The Oswestry Disability Index is the most commonly used outcome-measure questionnaire for low back pain in a hospital setting. It is a self-administered questionnaire divided into 10 sections and is designed to assess limitations of various activities of daily living.

SF36 – The 36-Item Short Form Survey (SF-36) is an often used, well-researched, self-reported measure of health. It comprises 36 questions which cover 8 domains of health.

Examples of PREMs

PREMs tend to be specific to different Trusts, private clinics etc. and standardised tools are generally not available. Topics include time spent waiting; access to services, facilities available, communication with the practitioner (e.g. 'did they give you time to tell your story' and 'did they help you to take control').

Safety Recommendations for Spinal Manipulative Techniques

Following the recommendations given below will help to ensure maximum safety. The practitioner must take all due care while applying the treatment techniques and ensure that they have competence in the techniques to be applied. Shared decision-making and patient consent are crucial before proceeding with treatment.

ENSURE THAT

- A full history and examination have been completed and recorded, sufficient to establish indications and to exclude all contraindications to treatment.
- Specific questions have been asked relating to the following, and the result recorded:

In the Cervical Spine
- dizziness (vertigo), nausea
- past history of trauma
- cardiovascular disease
- blood-clotting disorders
- inflammatory arthritis
- recent trauma
- previous cancer
- unexplained weight loss
- recent infection, fever
- family history of young strokes
- migraine
- high cholesterol
- smoking

The history may steer the clinician to ask further questions relating to:
- visual disturbances
- difficulty in speaking or swallowing
- bilateral paraesthesia in the hands and feet
- unsteadiness in gait or general feelings of weakness in arms or legs
- clumsiness, loss of dexterity

- change in bladder and bowel function, related to symptoms
- medical history
- medications
- general health

In the Thoracic Spine
- unexplained weight loss
- bilateral paraesthesia in the hands and feet
- unsteadiness in gait or general feelings of weakness
- inflammatory arthritis
- past history of trauma
- change in bladder and bowel function related to symptoms
- medical history
- medications
- general health

In the Lumbar Spine
- change in bladder and bowel function related to symptoms
- saddle anaesthesia
- sexual dysfunction
- blood-clotting disorders
- unexplained weight loss
- unsteadiness in gait or general feelings of weakness in legs
- inflammatory arthritis
- past history of trauma
- medical history
- medications
- general health

ENSURE THAT

- From the examination, the following factors are present:
  - A non-capsular pattern of limited movement

- A normal plantar response
- No brisk reflexes
- There is a subacute level of pain.
- There are no contraindications to manipulation. The more peripheral the symptoms, the less likely manipulation is to work, but it may be attempted if minimal neurological signs exist. If neurological deficit is severe and progressing, manipulation should not be attempted but other modalities may be more effective (e.g. traction and mobilisation).
- You have provided sufficient information, including benefits, possible risks, all options for management, including advice, if manipulation is indicated, so that the patient can give informed consent.

- You re-examine the patient after the application of each technique and base decisions to continue on the outcome of the previous technique.
- Any significant adverse response to treatment is reported as appropriate.

Manipulation usually produces immediate results. Therefore, treatment should be progressed following a constant reassessment and clinical reasoning process. If a technique helps, it is repeated; if it is unsuccessful, another technique or alternative modality maybe discussed and applied as part of the shared decision making.

Musculoskeletal Medicine Education

Modules in musculoskeletal medicine are held at a variety of venues both nationally and internationally. The module design usually consists of distance learning packages, modules, intermodular assignments and final practical and theory examinations.

The modules aim to develop practitioners' clinical reasoning in musculoskeletal/orthopaedic medicine and practical skills, with critical analysis of outcomes and skills in reflection and self-evaluation.

The Society of Musculoskeletal Medicine's (SOMM's) foundation module content includes the theory underpinning the approach, applied anatomy, clinical examination and diagnosis, soft tissue treatment techniques – transverse frictions, mobilisation, manipulation and injections. Much of the module is devoted to practical work in small groups with close supervision and feedback. The modules are supported by a comprehensive illustrated manual.

After passing the Society's Membership examinations and completing and passing a summative reflective essay and personal development plan, the SOMM Diploma in Musculoskeletal Medicine is awarded.

The foundation module acts as a pathway to more advanced modules including the 'Theory and Practice of Injection Therapy' and 'Advancing Practice in Musculoskeletal Medicine' modules, and has been accredited as Stage One of the HEE 'Roadmap for First Contact Practitioners' (MSK July21-FILLABLE Final Aug 2021_2.pdf).

The SOMM Diploma in Musculoskeletal Medicine and advanced modules mentioned above form part of a master's pathway towards the achievement of the MSc Musculoskeletal Medicine. The MSc Musculoskeletal Medicine programme has been developed by the SOMM. It was originally validated by Middlesex University in 2000 and moved to Queen Margaret University, Edinburgh, where it was validated in 2018.

Full details of all the Society's courses are available from:

Society of Musculoskeletal Medicine (registered charity no. 802164; www.sommcourses.org)

For details of other courses in musculoskeletal medicine, please contact the following affiliated organisations:

European Teaching Group of Orthopaedic Medicine (www.cyriax.eu)

Irish Society of Orthopaedic and Rheumatological Medicine (www.isorm.ie)

OMI Norden (www.ominorden.com)

Orthopaedic Medicine Seminars (www.stephaniesaunders.co.uk)

Association of Chartered Physiotherapists in Orthopaedic Medicine and Injection Therapy (ACPOMIT) (www.acpomit.co.uk)

GLOSSARY

A

Allodynia Pain produced by a stimulus that is not normally painful (e.g. light touch or a gentle stretch).

Anomalous cross-links An abnormal number of cross-links (adhesions), developing as a result of immobilisation of collagen fibres; responsible for the toughness and resilience of scar tissue.

B

Bursa A closed, fluid-filled synovial sac, which secretes fluid into the bursal space and provides cushioning and a gliding surface to reduce friction between tissues of the body.

Bursitis Inflammation of a bursa.

C

Capsular pattern A limitation of movement in a specific pattern that is peculiar to each joint and indicates the presence of arthritis.

Central sensitisation Increased responsiveness of nociceptive neurons to subthreshold input in the central nervous system.

Close packed position When the joint surfaces fit closely together and are maximally congruent. The position in which a joint is most stable.

Compression A squashing or pushing force, resulting in the structure becoming shortened and broadened.

Corticosteroids Potent anti-inflammatory drugs. In musculoskeletal medicine, injections used to treat chronic soft tissue lesions, acute episodes of degenerative arthropathy and inflammatory arthritis.

Creep A property of viscoelastic structures that consists of a small, almost imperceptible movement, occurring when a constant stress is applied for a prolonged period.

Cross-links Either weak intramolecular hydrogen bonds connecting molecules or stronger covalent intermolecular bonds connecting collagen fibrils and fibres. The links provide connective tissue structures with tensile strength; the greater the number of cross-links, the stronger the structure.

Cyanosis A bluish discoloration of the skin due to poor circulation or inadequate oxygenation of the blood.

D

Deformation A change in length or shape due to the application of a stress, represented as strain on the stress–strain diagram.

Disc herniation/prolapse Discal material passes through a ruptured annulus and/or posterior longitudinal ligament into the vertebral canal or intervertebral canal where it has a secondary effect on pain-sensitive structures: the posterior longitudinal ligament, dura mater, dural nerve root sleeve, nerve root and dorsal root ganglion.

Disc protrusion Degenerate disc material bulges into the weakened laminate structure of the annulus, where it can produce primary disc pain since the outer annulus receives a nerve supply.

Disequilibrium A sensation of being about to fall. It is sometimes described as a feeling that the floor is tilting, or as a sense of floating. The sensation can originate in the inner ear or in the central nervous system and is distinctly different from dizziness/vertigo.

Distraction/traction A force applied in opposite directions across a joint causing the joint surfaces to separate.

Dysaesthesia An unpleasant abnormal sensation; it may be induced or spontaneous.

E

Elastic range Represented on the stress–strain diagram as the range of loading within which a material or structure remains elastic (i.e. it can resume its original form after the deforming force is removed).

Elasticity The property of a material or a structure that allows it to deform when a force is applied. The change is temporary, and the original form is restored when the force is removed.

End-feel A specific sensation imparted through the examiner's hands at the end of passive movement.

Enthesis The point at which a tendon inserts into bone.

Enthesopathy A lesion at the teno-osseous junction (e.g. tennis elbow at the common extensor origin).

F

FABER position A combination of flexion, abduction and external rotation at the hip.

Fatigue A process by which a structure fails when subjected to repetitive low loading cycles.

Force An action that produces movement by pushing or pulling, known as mechanical stress and expressed as the force per unit area.

Force couple The application of equal, but opposite, parallel forces.

G

Glycosaminoglycans (GAGs) Long-chain carbohydrate molecules, the building blocks for proteoglycans.

Grade A mobilisation A passive, active or active/assisted mobilisation performed within the patient's pain-free elastic range in *peripheral* joints. A mid-range movement at *spinal* joints.

Grade B mobilisation A mobilisation applied at the end of available range. A sustained stretching technique into the plastic range aimed to produce permanent lengthening of connective tissue structures in *peripheral* joints. A movement to the end of range in *spinal* joints.

Grade C manipulation A manipulation involving a minimal-amplitude, high-velocity thrust applied at the end of range once all the slack has been taken up. It can be applied to certain *peripheral* or *spinal* lesions.

H

Hyperalgesia An increased response to a stimulus that would be expected to be painful (e.g. a knock or pin prick).

Hysteresis   A property of viscoelastic structures in which the resumption of its original length occurs more slowly than the deformation.

L

Load   A general term describing the application of a force and/or moment (torque) to a structure.

Local anaesthetic   A pain-inhibiting drug. In musculoskeletal medicine injections, it is used for diagnostic and therapeutic effects.

M

Macrofailure   Occurs when there is rupture of a structure, and it is unable to sustain further load. Represented by a rapid fall in the stress–strain curve.

Microfailure   Occurs when a structure reaches its elastic limit with progressive failure of cross-links and fibrils.

Moment   A force that produces bending or torque.

Motion segment   A functional spinal segment consisting of two adjacent vertebral bodies together with their joints and surrounding soft tissues.

N

Neuropathic pain   Caused by damage or disease that affects the somatosensory nervous system that provides information about the body, including the viscera. Can result from disorders of the peripheral or central nervous systems, or both.

Non-capsular pattern   A pattern of limited and/or painful movements that does not fit the capsular pattern of that particular joint.

NSAIDs   Non-steroidal anti-inflammatory drugs.

P

Paraesthesia   An abnormal sensation of the skin (e.g. numbness, tingling, 'pins and needles'). Not necessarily painful.

Peripheral sensitisation   Reduced threshold and increased responsiveness to stimulation of nociceptive neurons in the peripheral nervous system.

Plasticity   The property of a structure that permits it to undergo permanent deformation when the force is large enough to load the structure beyond its elastic range.

Plastic range   Represented on the stress–strain diagram as the range of loading within which a material or structure cannot resume its original form once the deforming force is removed (i.e. the elastic range of the structure is exceeded).

Pressure phenomenon   Pain and paraesthesia occurring on the application of pressure to a nerve root.

Progressive loading   In the rehabilitation of tendinopathy, it is important to increase the load put through the tendon progressively. The activity undertaken should be specific, both to the particular tendon involved, and the normal level of activity of the patient'. Loading may start with isometric exercises and progress towards more challenging concentric/eccentric activities for the tendon. The tendon response to the loading programme is monitored closely by assessing changes to the pain experienced. The exercise programme can then be increased or decreased (regressive loading) accordingly.

Proteoglycans   Protein–carbohydrate complex consisting of glycosaminoglycans (GAGs) covalently bound to protein.

Psychosocial factors   Characteristics that can influence an individual psychologically and/or socially and their perception of pain. Factors can include stress, depression, anxiety, and fear-avoidance behaviour. Often referred to as 'yellow flags'.

R

Radicular pain   Pain evoked from ectopic discharges from a dorsal nerve root or its ganglion. Lancinating, 'electric shock', shooting pain, in narrow bands, rarely follows dermatomal patterns and not clearly defined. May or may not be associated with radiculopathy.

Radiculopathy   Caused by the blocking of conduction along sensory (numbness) and motor (weakness) axons. Objective neurological signs, including numbness, weakness and diminished or absent reflexes. Numbness can be dermatomal and weakness can be myotomal. May or may not be associated with pain.

Red flags   Indicators for possible serious pathology that may be identified from the history and examination.

Release phenomenon   The sensation of deep painful paraesthesia occurring as pressure is released from a nerve trunk.

S

Selective tension   The application of appropriate stress to soft tissue structures in order to test function.

Set   The difference between the original and final length or shape of a structure once the deforming force is removed.

Shear   A force applied parallel to the surface of the structure, causing angular deformation.

Sign of the buttock   Pain on straight leg raise that increases on flexing the knee and hip. It is usually a sign of serious pathology.

Somatic pain   Caused by noxious stimulation of nerve endings within somatic structures. Dull, aching, gnawing. Expanding pressure. Boundary difficult to localise but core of pain clear. Not dermatomal. No neurological signs.

Somatic structures   Skin (superficial) and bones, ligaments, tendons, muscles, fascia and blood vessels (deep).

Stiffness   The resistance of a structure to the deforming force.

Strain   The deformation or change in dimension of a material or structure in response to an externally applied load or force.

Stress   The load or force applied to a structure resulting in strain or deformation.

Stress–strain curve   A diagrammatic representation of the mechanical behaviour of a material or structure, including collagen fibres. Stress is plotted on the y axis and represents the tensile, compressive, shear or torsional force applied. Strain is plotted on the x axis and represents the deformation or elongation of the material.

Synthesis and degradation (lysis)   The production and disintegration of cells or fibres (e.g. collagen) ('turnover').

T

Tendinitis   Inflammation of a tendon.

Tendinopathy   General term for any pathology in a tendon.

Tendinosis   Degenerative tendon changes.

Tenosynovitis   Inflammation of the tendon sheath.

Tensile strength   The maximum stress or load sustained by a material.

Tension A force of equal and opposite loads that results in lengthening and narrowing of the fibres of a material or structure.

Torsion A combination of shear, tensile and compressive force or load applied to a structure causing it to rotate about an axis. The load is called the torque.

Traction/distraction A force applied in opposite directions across a joint causing the joint surfaces to separate.

Translation Parallel movement of two opposing surfaces causing them to slide across one another.

Transverse frictions A specific type of massage applied to connective tissue structures to produce therapeutic movement, traumatic hyperaemia (chronic lesions), pain relief and improved function.

Trendelenburg gait An abnormal gait resulting from weakness of the gluteal musculature, including the gluteus medius and gluteus minimus muscles, which causes the pelvis on the contralateral side to drop while walking.

V

Vertigo An abnormal sensation of motion which can occur in the absence of movement. Spinning vertigo usually originates in the inner ear. Positional vertigo is a sensation of spinning after the patient's head has moved to a new position and may be related to the cervical spine.

Viscoelasticity The property of a material to change when under constant deformation through resistance to shear flow and the ability to reform after stretch.

Viscosity Thickness, or a measure of how resistant a liquid is to flow.

W

Wolff's law A law that states that bone is laid down where it is needed along the lines of stress, and reabsorbed when not needed.

Y

Yellow flags Emotional and behavioural factors that may have an influence on pain. Factors can include stress, depression, anxiety and fear-avoidance behaviour. Also referred to as psychosocial factors.

Yield point The point of the stress–strain curve at which appreciable deformity occurs, without any appreciable increase in load.

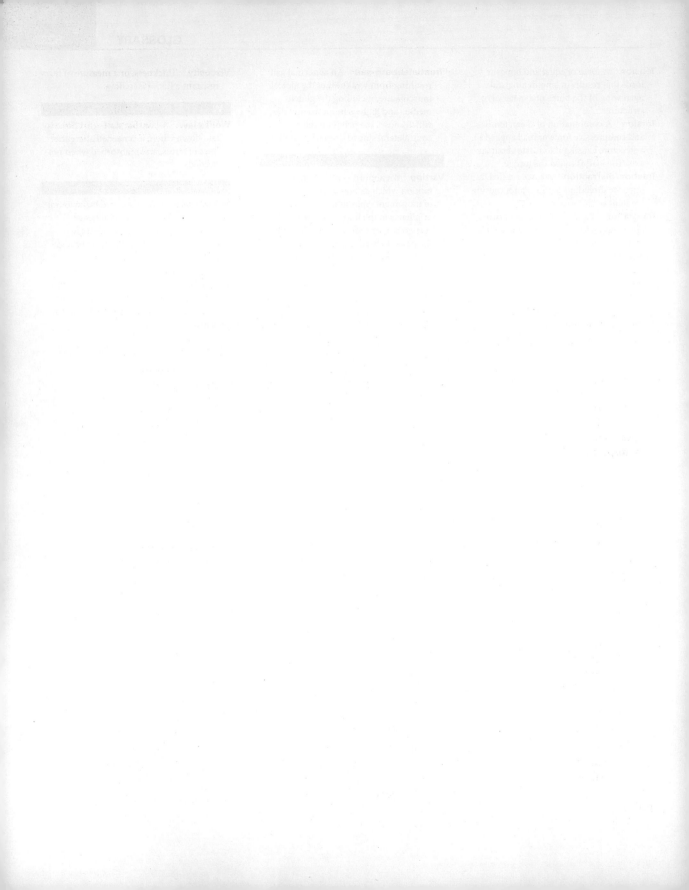

INDEX

Page numbers followed by "*f*" indicate figures, "*t*" indicate tables, and "*b*" indicate boxes.